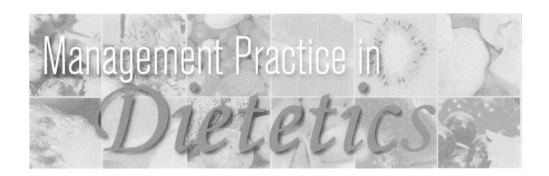

Management Practice in Dietetics

Revised Third Edition

Nancy R. Hudson

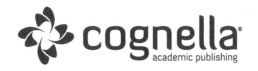

cognella®
academic publishing

Bassim Hamadeh, CEO and Publisher
Michael Simpson, Vice President of Acquisitions
Jamie Giganti, Managing Editor
Jess Busch, Graphic Design Supervisor
Marissa Applegate, Acquisitions Editor
Jessica Knott, Senior Project Editor
Luiz Ferreira, Licensing Associate

First published in the United States of America in 2013 by Cognella, Inc.

Printed in the United States of America

ISBN: 978-1-62661-406-2 (perfect bound) / 978-1-62661-407-9 (binder ready)

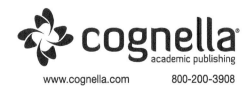

www.cognella.com   800-200-3908

contents

To those of my former students who always met high standards and then went on to exceed expectations. (You know who you are!)

acknowledgments

In preparing the manuscript for the third edition of ***Management Practice in Dietetics***, I drew on the on the expertise of colleagues, friends, and former students. Stacey Dunn-Emke from NutritionJobs assisted me by writing the "In Practice Feature" that follows the Marketing Chapter. Danielle Lee, Linda Adams and Denneal Jamison-McClung from UC Davis contributed their expertise on sustainability, a new chapter in this book. Derek Kerton of The Kerton Group provided information related to technology and information management. Todd Bell and David Zabrowski from the Food Service Technology Center updated me on developments in the foodservice equipment industry. Norma Kobzina from UC Berkeley helped me to hone my Internet and library search skills. And Jessica Knott and her team at Cognella Academic Publishing supported the production of the book. To all of these, I express my sincere thanks.

Special appreciation goes to Francene Steinberg and Joan Frank, academic colleagues at UC Davis who encouraged and supported me throughout the development of this text. I am also indebted to Dustin Burnett from the Western Human Nutrition Research Center who served as my sounding board—giving me the opportunity to "think out loud" without being judged.

And finally, I need to recognize my husband John, whose support through all three editions of this text has been immeasurable. Thank you for the love you have shown over the decades.

part one

overview

The initial three chapters of this text are designed to introduce the reader to management, or—more precisely—management in the dietetics profession. It is likely that dietitians and dietetic technicians will, at some point in their careers, be faced with the need to perform management activities. This is a reasonable expectation for professionals who have been well educated and uniquely prepared as the nutrition experts. Both food and nutrition services are best managed by individuals who have expertise in the field.

It is anticipated that, after studying the materials in Part I, the reader will understand the types of management positions that dietetics professionals hold, the functions that they perform, the roles they play, and the skills that are required to manage successfully. Furthermore, readers will develop a basic understanding of the structure of organizations along with a beginning knowledge of organizational dynamics.

Because it is essential that dietitians and dietetic technicians are both competent managers and strong leaders, leadership is discussed in detail. The reader should learn to appreciate the differences between managing and leading. In addition, recognition of leadership qualities should motivate dietetics managers to develop these characteristics in themselves.

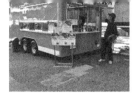

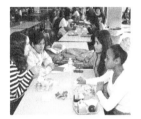

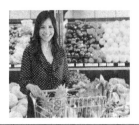

chapter one

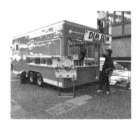

management roles of dietetics professionals

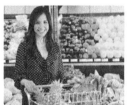

learning objectives

1. Identify the various management roles for dietetics professionals in foodservice.

2. Differentiate between commercial and onsite foodservices.

3. Identify the differences between cook-serve and the cook-chill foodservices.

4. Describe how self-operated foodservices differ from contracted foodservices.

5. Discuss trends that are having an impact on foodservice management.

6. Describe management roles in clinical nutrition.

7. Identify management roles for dietitians in community or public health nutrition.

8. List management roles for dietitians in other areas of practice.

9. Describe the potential areas for upward mobility for dietitian managers.

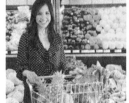

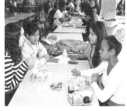

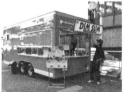

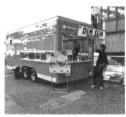

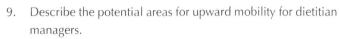

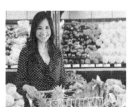

overview

The reasons for becoming a dietitian are many. If you polled a group of **Registered Dietitians (RD)**, you might hear that each entered the field for a different reason. Common reasons include a passion for good food, a love of science, the motivation to be a helping professional, working with sick people to help them get well, and working with healthy people to keep them well. The same is true for **Dietetic Technicians, Registered (DTR)**. Some dietetics professionals enter dietetics with the distinct goal of operating a foodservice, which may be a restaurant, a school lunch program, an employee dining facility, or a hospital nutrition and foodservice department. However, unless the individual has chosen to be a foodservice manager, the motivation that drives individuals to study dietetics seldom stems from a desire to go into management. In fact, many dietitians choose to be dietitians in order to avoid the world of business, of which management is a part.

Those who enter the public health or clinical nutrition areas of the profession do not usually think of their future jobs as ones that will require management skills. Those who choose to develop private practices consider management skills a "future area for development" that they will need as their businesses grow. Even dietitians who work for large, non-service-oriented businesses seldom view themselves as managers. Dietitians are often more comfortable with the designation of *dietitian* than with the title of *manager*. In the practice audit for entry-level practitioners conducted in 2010, the data showed "that entry level RDs overwhelmingly perform activities related to nutrition care delivered to individuals and groups, mostly patients, significantly more than management or research activities."[1] By the fourth and fifth year of practice, however, increases in managing human, financial, and material resources were evident.[2]

At some point in the career of many dietetics professionals, opportunities to enter management arise. Although this may not have been part of their original career plans, there are compelling reasons to take on managerial duties. In 2011, 12% of RDs and 18% of DTRs indicated that their primary area of practice was in "food and nutrition management."[3] A major motivational factor for many is financial. People who take on the additional responsibilities that are required of managers usually receive additional compensation that is commensurate with the increased duties. The highest salaries are associated with positions where managers are responsible for either large numbers of employees or large budgets—or both.[4] However, money is not the only driving force. Some individuals have grown in their jobs to the point where they are no longer challenged; the additional responsibilities of management positions provide an area for growth that keeps the professional stimulated. Others are motivated by the desire to take more control of the work situation (that is, to determine where resources are to be allocated). For many, the transition into a management position is an evolutionary process that occurs without much planning or thought. In short, many dietitians and dietetic technicians who never expected to be managers find themselves changing roles in the course of their careers and taking on managerial responsibilities. Furthermore, it has been noted that RDs in management positions are generally satisfied with their jobs.[5,6]

In this chapter, the various roles of the dietetics managers will be explored. First, the foodservice manager will be considered, because it is this specialty area that, historically, is most closely associated with management practice. Types of foodservice will be discussed, as will the differences between self-operated and contract-managed foodservices. Trends in foodservice that impact today's foodservice manager will be described.

Other management roles for dietitians will be examined. In clinical nutrition, these roles include clinical nutrition manager, chief clinical dietitian, patient services manager, the clinical dietitian, and the DTR. The management roles of public health and community nutritionists, including program management and agency management, will be discussed. Management roles for entrepreneurial dietitians in private practice, the dietitian who owns a business, the dietetics educator, and the dietitian who works in industry will be considered, as will the opportunities for dietetics professionals to develop management skills in voluntary leadership positions. Finally, some of the opportunities available to successful dietetics managers in upper-level management positions and administration will be described. The opportunities for dietetics professionals willing to assume management positions are boundless!

the dietetics professional in foodservice management

Dietitians have been working as foodservice managers since the early days of the profession. The need to provide safe, nutritious food to the military or to hospitalized patients was one of the major factors that contributed to the development of the field of dietetics. Management opportunities outside of the foodservice arena did not become readily available until the latter half of the twentieth century. It is in foodservice where the profession developed its management expertise, and it is there that, historically, dietitians have managed. Though management opportunities now exist in other areas of dietetics, many dietetics professionals still work as foodservice managers.

Foodservice is divided into two major segments—commercial and onsite. **Commercial foodservices** are those with retail outlets that, traditionally, were driven by the profit motive. In the past, the customers of commercial foodservices were viewed as having a choice about whether or not to eat out, and where to eat when they did choose to dine away from home. Restaurants fall into this category, as do independent catering companies and the foodservices associated with lodging and recreation. Other commercial foodservices exist in retail outlets such as department stores,

Commercial Foodservices.
Foodservices that traditionally cater to customers who have choices in where to eat, and which are usually profit driven (for example, supermarkets, food courts, restaurants, and so on).

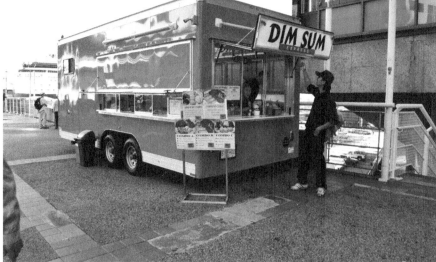

Mobile food vendors are competing with "brick and mortar" restaurants in urban areas.

Mobile Food Vendors. *Food trucks or carts that move from place to place. Originally these were used where restaurants were not located; they have recently expanded their market to other locations.*

Quick Service Restaurants. *Foodservice organizations that provide fast meals, which may be eaten on the premise or carried out. (These are also called fast-food restaurants.)*

Onsite Foodservices. *Foodservices that typically serve people who have little choice in where they eat and that are usually not profit driven (for example, healthcare facilities, schools, prisons, and so on). These are also called noncommercial foodservices.*

supermarkets, and food courts. Though **mobile food vendors** have been around for a long time, their impact used to be limited to areas where "brick and mortar" facilities were not prevalent. The number of these vendors has grown exponentially in recent years, with high-quality (often ethnic) food products being made available in non-traditional and sometimes upscale locations. As more individuals eat more meals away from home, their options continue to increase.

Commercial foodservices are usually divided into market segments that include fine dining restaurants, casual dining restaurants, midscale restaurants (full-service restaurants that do not serve alcohol), fast-casual restaurants (like Chipotle and Panera), and **quick service restaurants** (QSRs). In 2011 it was estimated that Americans eat about 200 meals per year outside the home. About 75% of these are from fast-casual outlets, QSRs, or Convenience Stores.[7]

Onsite foodservices, formerly called noncommercial foodservices, were those that were not designed with the goal of making a profit. In the past, many of these were subsidized by the company or facility in which they were located. It was assumed that their customers had little or no choice about where they ate. Included in this sector are hospitals and other healthcare facilities, schools (ranging from day care for preschoolers through university dining), prisons, the military, businesses with large campuses, and senior citizens' centers. Though it is no longer always feasible to provide subsidies for clients in schools and healthcare organizations, some businesses continue to provide subsidized or even free meals to their employees as a fringe benefit. Historically, dietetics professionals have been most closely associated with onsite foodservices.

Dietetics professionals who work in onsite foodservice find opportunities available to them at many levels. These range from the position of foodservice director in a very

management practice in dietetics

Table 1.1 Foodservice Management Positions

small operation, like a 75-bed nursing home or hospital, to the manager of the school lunch program for a district in a major city where there are 50 or 60 schools and thousands of children to be fed. Larger foodservices will have a variety of positions in foodservice or dietetics management with decidedly different roles and responsibilities. Some of these positions are listed in Table 1.1. In large, onsite foodservices, it is possible to achieve upward mobility while staying at the same facility, or within the same foodservice system.

In today's market, the variables that used to differentiate commercial and onsite foodservices are not as compelling as they once were. Today's onsite foodservices seldom have a "captive" customer base. Commercial restaurants abound on or near educational and business campuses, so that students and employees do not have to eat on campus. Mobile food vendors are not impeded by having a fixed location from which to do business. Customers have ready access to public and private transportation, and can move them from place to place with ease. In fact, the only really captive clients are the very young, the very old, hospitalized patients, those in prisons, and passengers on planes, trains, and ships (and then only for the duration of the trip).

In addition, the profit motive now exists in most onsite foodservices. Hospital cafeteria and catering operations generate enough revenues to subsidize patient foodservices. Lunch programs in public schools may make profits, which can be used to provide books and other teaching materials. University campus dining facilities earn revenues that can be used to offset the cost of building and maintaining facilities such as computer labs in residence halls. Commercial foodservices, including chain-operated restaurants, are moving into traditionally onsite settings and opening retail outlets in schools, hospitals, and universities.

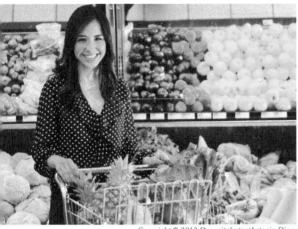

Copyright © 2012 Depositphotos/Antonio Diaz.

Dietitians working in supermarkets may teach classes on grocery shopping, cooking, or menu planning.

As the distinction between commercial and onsite foodservices blurs, there are more opportunities for dietitians to work in the commercial segment of the industry. Commercial foodservices have become concerned about the high fructose corn syrup and the trans fats content of foods that they serve. They also are trying to ensure food safety in their restaurants. Both of these are areas in which dietitians and dietetic technicians have expertise. Individual restaurants are contracting with consultant dietitians to help them with these matters. Larger restaurant and super-market chains are hiring dietetics professionals as staff members to work in product and menu development, nutrient analysis of foods, and food safety.[8]

types of foodservice

In both commercial and onsite operations, four types of foodservice have been characterized.[9] Each of these types is described briefly in Table 1.2. Years ago, it was easy to distinguish among conventional foodservice, commissary foodservice, ready prepared foodservice, and assembly/serve foodservice based on the predominant characteristics described in Table 1.2.

Type	Characteristics
Conventional	Foods are purchased in the unprepared or partially prepared state.
	Production and service take place on the same premises.
	Food is prepared and served in a relatively short time period.
Commissary	Foods are purchased with little pre-preparation.
	Large centralized production facilities are used for food production.
	Prepared foods are transported to remote locations for final preparation and service.
Ready Prepared (also Called Cook-Chill or Cook-Freeze)	Foods are purchased in the unprepared or partially prepared state.
	After food production occurs, the food is chilled or frozen and stored for use at a later time.
	The foods may be stored in bulk or as individual meals or items.
	Foods are rethermalized (heated) just prior to service, which may be on- or offsite.
Assembly/Serve	Food is purchased in a highly processed form and is nearly ready to serve when purchased.
	Food is heated and assembled into meals for service.

Table 1.2 Types of Foodservices—Traditional Definitions

management practice in dietetics

Today, just as the distinguishing features of commercial and onsite foodservices are becoming less distinct, so are the factors that used to differentiate the four traditional types of foodservices.

In contemporary settings, it is probably more useful to differentiate the types of foodservice into two, relatively fluid categories, cook-serve and cook-chill. The **cook-serve foodservice** is one in which hot foods are prepared, brought up to temperature, and served, either at the same or a nearby location. Foods are transported and held at safe temperatures (over 135° Fahrenheit) until service occurs. **Cook-chill foodservices** are those in which hot foods undergo preliminary preparation and then are blast chilled (or frozen). These foods are stored and transported in the chilled mode (at or below 41° Fahrenheit). They are rethermalized to safe serving temperatures just prior to service at the location where the service is to occur. Cook-chill systems can be adapted for use for as individual servings of food, as seen in airline feeding, school lunch programs, and hospital room-service settings. These systems can also be used for bulk foods that are rethermed just prior to service in cafeterias, prisons, and other large-scale feeding operations.

the self-operated foodservice

Many foodservices are independent, one-of-a-kind operations. Within the onsite segment, these are also called **self-operated foodservices**. The designation means that the foodservice is run by the school, healthcare organization, business, or other institution where it is located. In self-operated foodservices, the manager and all of the staff work for the parent organization. The foodservice is run much like any other department in the organization.

There are distinct advantages inherent in the self-operated foodservice. It usually can be very responsive to the needs of the parent organization, because the manager reports directly within that organization. Employees and managers work for the same employer, which gives them a sense of camaraderie and tends to increase loyalty to the organization and to each other. There is freedom for creativity and innovation, and the opportunity to develop a unique foodservice operation.

There are also disadvantages in the self-operated foodservice. These operations are relatively small, which may mean that raw material costs more to buy. This increases the cost of running the business and may cut into the profitability of the foodservice. The foodservice manager, especially one who works in a small operation, often works independently with no built-in opportunity for the cross-fertilization of ideas. A foodservice manager working alone has to work hard at developing networks and keeping up to date on the trends in the foodservice industry. Self-operated foodservices have to develop all of their own menus, recipes, systems, procedures, and other tools. This is labor intensive and time-consuming. Generic tools are available, but seldom can be used without adaptation and individualization.

Cook-Serve Foodservices. *Foodservices in which hot foods are cooked and held at safe (hot) temperatures until they are served.*

Cook-Chill Foodservices. *Foodservices where hot foods are pre-prepared then chilled and held at safe (cool) temperatures then are rethermalized just prior to service.*

Self-Operated Foodservices. *A foodservice in which the organization that receives the service owns and operates the foodservice.*

the contract management company in foodservice management

Several companies offer contract foodservices in the onsite segment. Often these companies specialize in one or more of the following markets: school foodservice, prison foodservice, health care, campus dining, business dining, and so on. The larger of these contract management companies, especially those involved in health care, employ many dietitians.

Contract Management Companies.
Organizations that provide foodservice to other organizations or institutions; contracts vary in the services provided.

When foodservice is contracted out, the **contract management company** provides the contracting organization or institution with varying services, as specified in the contract. At a minimum, the contractor provides the foodservice director and some other services and tools. At the other extreme, all of the employees of the foodservice department, including the clinical dietitians, may work for the management company. The contracts are not standardized; institutions may purchase whatever services they need. The manager of the contracted foodservice may be an RD or a DTR but could also be a person whose background is in business or in the culinary area.

The contract management company is often able to lower the cost of foodservice by providing greater purchasing power and lower food costs. It also provides the tools of the trade such as menus, recipes, manuals, and so on, which may save money because these do not have to be produced for each site. The management company specializes in foodservices and has the expertise of many individuals rather than just one or two. Ideas can be transferred from one client to another through a well-established network. Contract management companies can deliver standardized services to divergent organizations.

There are several disadvantages inherent in operations run by contract management companies. One is that the managers are likely to be loyal to their employer rather than to the contracting institution. Even if this is not true, the manager has two bosses who must be satisfied, and their agendas may not always be in agreement with each other. Frequently, the amount of paperwork increases when a contract management company is in place, because the management and the contracting organization need different types of data. Often, the foodservice workers and the managers work for different employers, creating a potential for interpersonal conflict within the foodservice. In addition, managers need to be concerned with meeting the basic standards of the management company; there is less opportunity to design a truly unique foodservice in contract-managed operations.

Despite the differences between contract-managed foodservices and self-operated foodservices, there is a place for both in today's economy. The appropriateness of either of these options is circumstantial and depends on resources and the short- and long-term goals of the facility or institution where the foodservice is located. In general, the character of a foodservice is set by the operation's manager. There are good and bad managers in self-operated units, just as there are good and bad managers

management practice in dietetics

working for contract management companies. Both situations provide wonderful career opportunities for dietitians who wish to work in foodservice management. An effective manager can succeed in either environment.

trends in foodservice management

The major trends in foodservice management are outlined each year in a variety of publications and Internet sites. (See "To Study Further" section at the end of this chapter.) These and other publications, which deal with both commercial and onsite foodservices, perform market analysis and make projections that are published each year as an industry forecast. This is essential information for managers wishing to remain abreast of new directions and opportunities in foodservice. In addition to overall projected growth for the entire foodservice industry, some current trends include the increase in services for the elderly, changes in campus dining programs, and changes in the offerings of transportation systems, such as specialty dining venues on cruise ships.

School foodservice continues to provide expanding opportunities for dietetics professionals in programs that serve as sites for the National School Lunch Program or the School Breakfast Program. These onsite operations are constantly adapting to changes in governmental regulations and demands from their customers.

National School Lunch Program.
http://www.fns. usda.gov/cnd/ Lunch/

School Meals.
http://www.fns. usda.gov/cnd/

© Bob Nichols (CC BY 2.0) at http://www.flickr.com/photos/usdagov/6282541661/.

Dietitians often manage onsite operations like school foodservices.

Newer requirements for school lunch and breakfast meal patterns, offer-versus-serve options for students, and programs to increase the utilization of whole-grain products and fresh produce, have increased the complexity of these foodservices. RDs and DTRs are uniquely qualified to work in or serve as consultants to this segment of the foodservice industry.

As family dynamics change, fewer meals are prepared and served in the home. The traditional meals that were typical in American homes for generations have been replaced with optional ways to feed families. There has been a growing trend toward dining out, accompanied by rapid growth in QSRs. These and other restaurants are competing with supermarkets in providing food to families. Meals "to go" and home-delivered meals are becoming increasingly popular. In fact, in 2011, 48% of food expenditures in the US were spent on food from restaurants or other foodservices, for a total of $632 billion.[10] Clearly, restaurants and supermarkets are in competition for food dollars. In an attempt to compete, supermarkets are providing more ready-to-eat and convenience foods for home consumption. Lifestyle changes mean that there is limited time for food preparation in the home, even when meals are eaten there. Individuals and families want quality meals that can be put on the table with little effort in the shortest amount of time.

Other opportunities in foodservice management should allow dietetics professionals to become leaders in emerging markets. As more and more food preparation is moved from the home into commercial and onsite foodservice facilities, the opportunities will not only increase but will also become more challenging and require new levels of creativity. Among recent developments are

- emphasis on fresh, sustainable, locally grown ingredients,
- increased use of whole-grain options,
- legislative initiatives to curb the use of sodium, trans fats, and high fructose corn syrup,
- need for effective strategies to deal with the obesity epidemic,
- fusion of ethnic cuisines (like blending Asian and Latin culinary traditions into signature dishes),
- increased use of trained chefs/culinary professionals in onsite operations,
- continuing stress on service management and customer satisfaction,
- innovative meal delivery systems (such as room service) in healthcare foodservices.

clinical nutrition management

In health care, clinical nutrition services are expanding and becoming more technically demanding. In small facilities where there is only one dietitian, that person may be the director of foodservice as well as the clinical dietitian. If the foodservice director in the small facility is not a registered dietitian, it is likely that the clinical dietitian will also be the assistant director of foodservices or the clinical nutrition manager. In larger facilities, several levels of management for clinical dietitians exist. These roles include those of patient services manager, chief clinical dietitian, clinical nutrition manager, clinical dietitian, and dietetic technician. All of these positions have some management responsibilities. In some large facilities, the entire job of the clinical manager is management. The titles for these positions vary from institution to institution, but the general characteristics of these jobs remain the same.

clinical nutrition manager

The **clinical nutrition manager** is the title given to the highest management level in the nutritional care area. Depending on the facility, the clinical nutrition manager may be the head of a clinical nutrition department or, more typically in the United States, an assistant director of the nutrition and food services department of a healthcare facility. (Nutrition services and foodservices are two specialty areas that are usually combined under one umbrella department because of their interdependence.) The department may be under the overall direction of a manager who comes from either a foodservice or a clinical nutrition background. The clinical nutrition manager is responsible for the nutritional care of patients or clients, which includes screening, assessment, diagnosis, intervention, and monitoring.[11] This person usually supervises a group of clinical dietitians, dietetic technicians, and diet clerks and may also take responsibility for patient foodservices, which could be either a direct management responsibility or a coordination function.

chief clinical dietitian

In smaller facilities, the clinical nutrition management function may not be a full-time job. In this case, the dietitian who assumes oversight of clinical services may also be involved in direct patient care. The title often assigned to someone who does both patient care and manages the other dietitians, dietetic technicians, and diet clerks is **chief clinical dietitian**. This position has the responsibility to coordinate patient care with the foodservice side of the department but is not directly responsible for patient foodservice.

patient services manager

In large facilities, there may also be a **patient services manager** who manages foodservices for patients. This position is responsible for the operation of the trayline or other meal delivery system, providing floor stock and between-meal feedings

Clinical Nutrition Manager. *The manager who is responsible for the overall nutritional care of patients who are admitted to a healthcare facility. This person may not do direct patient care on a regular basis.*

Chief Clinical Dietitian. *A managerial title of a dietitian who manages the clinical nutrition area of a healthcare facility and also does direct patient care.*

Patient Services Manager. *A managerial position responsible for managing the foodservice for patients and coordinating the patient foodservice with the clinical nutrition staff.*

as required, measuring patient satisfaction, and coordinating foodservice with the clinical nutrition staff. The reporting relationship for the patient services manager is facility-specific. This person may report to the clinical nutrition manager (if there is one), to the foodservice director, or to both of these positions.

management functions of the clinical dietitian

Clinical dietitians are normally not hired to be managers. However, their educational preparation has provided them with some proficiency in this area, so they are frequently expected to take on some management tasks. The clinical dietitian may be asked to manage a dietetic technician who works in the same clinical area, or may be assigned to manage a project such as the revision of the nutrition screening tool, or the development of a clinical protocol. Some clinicians work on self-managed teams, in which every member of the team assumes some managerial responsibilities, and there is no one person who is identified as the clinical manager. Often, clinical dietitians take on additional management functions in the absence of other management personnel. On weekends and holidays, for example, they may be the only staff member in a facility with authority to make certain types of management decisions.

management functions of the clinical dietetic technician

Dietetic technicians whose jobs are primarily in patient care rather than in foodservice regularly supervise the **trayline**. Though the job may not be classified as a supervisory one, the person who assumes the position of "checker" on a trayline is managing the employees working on that trayline for the duration of the meal service.

management in public health nutrition

Just as there are management roles for clinical dietitians in healthcare facilities, dietitians who work in community or public health nutrition also find themselves in positions that require management expertise. In community nutrition, the community or a group of individuals within a community is identified as the client. Thus, the "client" might be every person who resides in a certain geographic area, or every low-income pregnant woman within the area, or every person with diabetes, and so on. In community nutrition, opportunities exist for dietitians to be program managers or managers in agencies that provide nutritional intervention and care to the community at large or to at-risk groups that have been identified within the community. The agencies involved in community nutrition may be public (governmental) or private (for-profit or nonprofit). Sometimes hospitals provide community nutrition services as part of their outreach efforts.

Management roles in community nutrition are usually assumed by the **public health nutritionist**. This is the title used by an RD who has earned an advanced degree in public health nutrition.[12] The public health nutritionist is focused on populations and systems, rather than on individual clients. **Community dietitian** and **community nutritionist** are terms that are used to describe those dietitians without advanced degrees who work in community nutrition.[13] These dietitians do not usually manage entire programs or agencies, though they may manage a site where community nutrition services are delivered. The major focus of the community nutritionist/dietitian is the individual client or group of clients in the community setting.

agency management

Some public health nutritionists work for agencies whose focus is on nutrition. One example of a public health nutrition program that deals entirely with nutrition issues is the Special Supplemental Nutrition Program for Women, Infants, and Children (WIC). In some states, there may be an agency established to administer WIC funds given to the state by the federal government. A public health nutritionist may manage this type of agency. The agency may be either governmental or private. An example of a private agency that deals exclusively with nutrition issues is the National Dairy Council. (Dairy councils, which are funded by the dairy industry, also exist at the state and regional levels.)

program management

Public health nutritionists frequently manage nutrition programs within an umbrella organization. For example, a senior citizens' agency may serve as a provider of nutrition and other services for the elderly residents of a community. This organization may oversee a variety of services including adult day care, congregate meal sites, social activities, transportation systems, home care services, and the meals-on-wheels program. Within that agency, a public health nutritionist could manage all aspects of that agency that deal with the food and nutritional services for the elderly clients. This would include needs assessment, planning, implementing, and evaluating the services rendered. The job may involve oversight of a food production facility, or contracting with a foodservice management company to provide meals for the congregate feeding sites and for meals-on-wheels clients. Other aspects of a senior nutrition program might include the implementation of the Nutrition Screening Initiative,[14] nutrition education for in-home caregivers, nutrition education for the seniors themselves, monitoring of food safety, menu planning, and so on. In large programs, the public health nutritionist might oversee the activities of several other dietitians, dietetic technicians, or nutrition assistants who provide the direct services to clients.

Public Health Nutritionist.
A dietitian/manager in community nutrition who has an advanced degree in public health nutrition, and whose managerial roles include overseeing community nutrition agencies or programs.

Community Dietitian or Community Nutritionist.
An RD who works in community nutrition by giving direct care to a client or clients.
WIC Home Page
www.fns.usda.gov/wic/

National Dairy Council.
www.nationaldairy-council.org

Nutrition Screening Initiative.
http://www.hospitalmedicine.org/geriresource/toolbox/pdfs/determine.pdf

site management

A large community health agency or program might provide service to clients at multiple sites. For example, a WIC program in a rural county may have five sites where they provide service to geographically dispersed clients. Because of the distances between sites, transportation may be a major issue. A community dietitian might manage one or two individual sites and report to the public health nutritionist who oversees the countywide program. This dietitian manager would be responsible for the operation of the assigned site or sites, and for the supervision of the support staff who work for the WIC program there. Like the chief clinical dietitian, this community dietitian would carry a client caseload, and the managerial duties would be only a part of the overall responsibilities of the position.

managing in other sectors

Though many dietitians work in the types of management positions previously described, these are not the only jobs available. Alternative management positions for dietitians and dietetic technicians include those described in the following section. These are positions that require something "extra" from the practitioner, such as additional resources, education, time to devote to volunteer activities, or a willingness to take risks.

entrepreneurs in private practice

Many dietitians go into private practice at some point in their career. This practice may be limited to individual and group counseling for clients with specific nutrition concerns, or may be a broader type of practice, in which the dietitian becomes an independent contractor. Independent contractors offer a variety of services that range from seeing individual clients to performing nutrition screenings in workplace settings, teaching a food preparation class to a group of elderly men, or writing articles for publication in a wellness letter for a health insurance provider. Some dietitians become consultants in their area of expertise and may have a practice that deals exclusively with marketing, public relations, or recruiting of healthcare professionals. For many dietitians, the private practice is begun on a temporary basis with the intent to return to the regular workforce after a period of time has elapsed (for example, when one's children enter school). Others go into consulting or private practice on a permanent basis because they want the freedom to pick and choose the type of projects they undertake.

Many private practices start as individual efforts with no employees to manage. There is not much thought about management unless the person in private practice happens to be a management consultant. Dietitians tend to think of themselves more as dietitians than as managers. However, just because the personnel management function is minimal, those in private practice are not exempt from utilizing the other management skills that they have acquired. Information management and financial management are crucial to the private practitioner. So are planning and controlling. Self-employed dietitians may need more management skills than those who work as managers for other employers, because the investment is more personal and, therefore, the risk seems greater. If the private practice grows, it eventually becomes necessary to manage human resources, too. Thus private practices, even if they are clinically focused, require that practitioners be managers as well as practitioners.

the business owner/entrepreneur

Some dietitians have taken greater personal risks and, in the true entrepreneurial sense, have opened businesses that are substantially larger than a private practice. Representative ventures include a computer software company, a home nutritional care company, an Internet website, and a commercial food manufacturer. For purposes of this text, these dietitians differ from those in private practice because the initial investment is usually larger and the businesses employ personnel from the outset. The dietitians who establish and run these companies are managers in every sense of the word. They have the overall responsibility for planning, organizing, leading, controlling, and staffing, and for their entire businesses. In order to succeed, these dietetics professionals must be decision makers, negotiators, mentors, delegators, and financial analysts. Owning and nurturing an owner-operated business may be the ultimate management opportunity for a dietitian.

industry

A growing number of dietitians are working in management positions in industry. Initially, positions for dietitians were available in sales and marketing of food, food-service, and nutrition-related products. Some positions in product development also required the skills of dietetics professionals. As individuals in these positions gained experience and expertise within their respective industries, they began to move into management positions. It seems to be a natural transition for many dietitians because of the management skills that they developed during their educational experience. Potential employers in industry include food manufacturers, food distributors, large restaurant chains, equipment wholesalers, and pharmaceutical companies.

education

Dietitians who teach in colleges and universities have management opportunities open to them as well. These positions require that the dietitian hold an advanced degree. Included are the management of didactic or supervised practice programs as well as the management of a department or a college within a university. In addition to their teaching responsibilities, these dietetics educators/managers are responsible for human resources management, strategic planning, financial management, maintaining standards for accreditation, and implementing and evaluating educational programs.

volunteerism

Dietetics professionals find themselves with abundant opportunities to develop and utilize their management skills in voluntary positions. Volunteers can offer their services

Organization	Short Form	Address
Academy of Nutrition and Dietetics www.eatright.org/	The Academy	120 South Riverside Plaza, Suite 2000 Chicago, IL 60606-6995
Dietitians of Canada www.dietitians.ca/	DC	480 University Avenue, Suite 604 Toronto, Ontario M5G 1V2
American Public Health Association www.apha.org/	APHA	800 I Street, NW Washington, DC 20001-3710
American Society for Parenteral and Enteral Nutrition www.nutritioncare.org/	A.S.P.E.N.	8630 Fenton Street Suite 412 Silver Spring, MD 20910
School Nutrition Association www.schoolnutrition.org/	SNA	120 Waterfront Street Suite 300 National Harbor, MD 20745
National Association of College and University Food Services www.nacufs.org/	NACUFS	2525 Jolly Road Suite 280 Okemos, MI 48864-3680
Association for Healthcare Foodservice www.healthcare foodservice.org/	AHF	455 S. 4th Street Suite 650 Louisville, KY 40202
National Restaurant Association www.restaurant.org	NRA	2055 L Street, NW Washington, DC 20036
Society for Nutrition Education and Behavior www.sne.org	SNE	9100 Purdue Road Suite 200 Indianapolis, IN 46268
State, Provincial, and Local Dietetic Associations		

Table 1.3 National Professional Organizations

to a wide variety of professional organizations, like those listed in Table 1.3. Volunteers are welcome at the local, state, and national levels. The positions range from being the voluntary chair of a project, a program, or a committee, to becoming an elected officer of a district, state, or national association. Some dietitians begin to develop management skills in volunteer jobs with such organizations before they have the opportunity to assume a managerial role at work. Demonstration of leadership in volunteer positions enhances one's resume and may increase the chance for promotion at work.

There are voluntary leadership positions available in other agencies such as health departments, hospitals, educational programs, and industry, where dietetics professionals often sit on boards or advisory committees. Whenever dietitians volunteer for groups related to, but not solely concerned with, food and nutrition, they increase the credibility of the profession. In addition, the **pro bono** work that dietetics professionals do helps them to develop their leadership skills while sharing the knowledge and skills that contribute to the nutritional health of the community.

Pro Bono.
Professional services provided free of charge.

upward mobility

In recent years, dietetics professionals have been given opportunities to expand their roles beyond the traditional ones. These opportunities, often called a **career ladder**, are pathways that allow one to progress from an entry-level position to successively higher positions within a profession. For example, a DTR may start as a food service supervisor, progress to catering manager, then on to becoming a food service director, followed by taking the position of director of support services in a healthcare organization. A clinical dietitian may move from that position to that of clinical manager, to food service director, to hospital administrator. Good managers learn to apply the practice of management so that it is not limited to dietetics. They use these principles to manage other areas as well. No longer are dietitians and dietetic technicians limited to managing nutrition or food services or nutrition programs. Some new roles that dietetics managers have taken are described in the following section.

Career Ladder.
A series of progressively more responsible positions that allows one to move from entry level to upper level management over time.

managing multiple departments

The trend toward consolidating various departments in hospitals and other organizations under one manager has been evolving over the past few decades. An assumption was made that management is discipline in itself, and that a manager who can manage effectively in one department is probably able to manage another department. This is not universally true, because there is a degree of technical expertise required to manage certain departments that precludes all managers from being interchangeable. For example, it is unlikely that a dietitian would become the director of the hospital pharmacy. However, some departments, such as environmental services and laundry, are service departments where the technical knowledge requirement is minimal and a good manager can master the information needed in a relatively short period of time. Thus, dietitian managers of foodservice operations are expanding their jobs to include the management of multiple departments in hospitals, schools, and businesses.

upper management

Dietitians are also likely to continue to move upward into positions of increasing authority and responsibility. The positions at the upper-management level are fewer and require a great degree of management experience before they become available. Most of the opportunities in this section are open to both dietitians and non-dietitians. Because these positions are more management than dietetics, the RD credential is not usually required for this type of position. They may also be filled by physicians, pharmacists, nurses, or those with a background in business or healthcare administration.

hospital administration. Within a healthcare organization, some dietitians have been promoted to administrative positions. In this type of position, the administrator coordinates the activities of several departments but does not do direct management within these departments. An administrator may run several of the ancillary services of a hospital, such as pharmacy, laboratory, medical records, foodservice, security, environmental services, and facilities operations.

public health. In state and local health departments and other public health agencies, public health nutritionists can move up the ranks and assume administrative duties for umbrella agencies and for statewide programs. Examples include the manager who coordinates nutrition and nutrition education programs for the state department of education or an administrator in the local health department.

contract management companies. Foodservice managers who work for contract management companies may be promoted into the position of district manager, where they oversee the operations of several foodservices. A district manager may be responsible for administering the contracts in five to ten facilities in a geographic region. District managers report to regional managers, who are responsible for an area covering several states or provinces. Dietitians may also hold regional manager positions within contract management companies. The larger companies that provide contract foodservice to healthcare facilities across the nation usually have dietitians in upper management at the corporate level.

sales and marketing. Dietitians who have demonstrated their management prowess have moved up the ranks in food distribution companies. Some are regional managers, and others hold managerial positions at the national level. Others have become marketing managers for pharmaceutical companies at the regional or national level.

management practice in dietetics

education. When education-based dietitian managers are successful, they can be and are promoted to administrative positions in institutions of higher learning. Dietitians have held the positions of department chair, dean, and provost. Other academic administrative positions that dietitian educators might aspire to are university president or chancellor.

nutrition policy. There are other management positions for dietitians that, technically, fall under the broad heading of public health. These positions deal more with research, policy, resource allocation, and funding issues rather than with the direct provision of service. Some positions exist at the state and national levels; in governmental departments such as education, agriculture, health and human services, and disaster relief; and in the military. Others exist in international agencies such as UNICEF, the Red Cross, the U.S. Agency for International Development, the World Bank, and other private foundations. Management positions in the area of nutrition policy are available to dietitians and other professionals with the appropriate education, credentials, and experience.

conclusion

This chapter has described a variety of positions in which dietetics professionals use management skills. Most of the opportunities described here are those that are routinely available to RDs; many are also available to DTRs. It is likely that individual dietetics professionals have additional management opportunities open to them that are beyond the general scope of this chapter.

1. A variety of foodservice management positions are open to dietitians, especially in onsite operations.
2. More opportunities are becoming available to dietitians in commercial foodservices because of increased interest in the nutrient content of foods and food safety.
3. Clinical nutrition management may be a part-time or a full-time responsibility.
4. Though clinical dietitian and dietetic technician positions are not usually designated as management jobs, they require the use of management skills.
5. Public health nutritionists manage programs or agencies that offer nutrition services in the community.
6. Community dietitians may function as site managers within community agencies.
7. Dietitians have demonstrated managerial skills while self-employed, in industry, in education, and in voluntary positions.
8. Excellent managers can be promoted into a wide variety of upper-level management or administrative positions.

activities

activity 1

Interview a dietitian with management responsibilities.

(You may do this as an individual project, or your instructor may invite a guest speaker to class.) Try to determine:

1. What the motivation was behind assuming a management role.
2. What this dietitian's management responsibilities are.
3. What non-management responsibilities this dietitian performs.
4. If the dietitian perceives herself or himself to be primarily a manager or primarily a dietitian, or views both roles as equally important.
5. The most rewarding part of being involved in management.
6. The most frustrating part of having management responsibilities.

activity 2

Access the National Restaurant Association's website at http://restaurant.org/research/forecast/. Listen to the information provided at that site related to the industry forecast for this year.

1. Describe the trends that are projected to have an impact on each type of commercial and onsite foodservice during the current year.
2. Identify one foodservice in your community for each foodservice type mentioned.
3. Determine which of the foodservices you have identified employs a dietitian or uses one as a consultant.

to study further

Additional information on foodservice management and other management roles for dietitians can be found in a wide variety of places. Notable among these are

- Payne-Palacio, June and Deborah D. Canter. *The Profession of Dietetics: A Team Approach.* 4th ed. Sudbury, MA: Jones and Bartlett Learning, LLC, 2011.
- Winterfeldt, Esther A., Margaret L. Bogles, and Lea Ebro, eds. *Dietetics: Practice and Future Trends.* 3rd ed. Sudbury, MA: Jones and Bartlett Publishers, LLC, 2011.

scholarly journals

- *The Journal of the Academy of Nutrition and Dietetics* (formerly *Journal of the American Dietetic Association*) http://www.elsevier.com/wps/find/journal description.cws_home/727057/description#description
- *Canadian Journal Dietetic Practice and Research* http://dcjournal.metapress.com/home/main.mpx

other relevant periodicals

- *Food Management* www.food-management.com/
- *Foodservice Director* www.foodservicedirector.com/
- *Foodservice Equipment Reports* www.fermag.com/
- *Nation's Restaurant News* www.nrn.com/
- *Today's Dietitian* www.todaysdietitian.com/
- Publications of the management-focused practice groups of the Academy of Nutrition and Dietetics:
  - *Clinical Nutrition Management*
  - *Dietetics in Health Care Communities*
  - *Dietitians in Business and Communications*
  - *School Nutrition Service*
  - *Dietetic Technicians in Practice*
  - *Management in Food and Nutrition Systems*
  - *Nutrition Entrepreneurs*
  - *Public Health/Community Nutrition*
  - *Healthy Aging*

in practice

preamble[15]

The American Dietetic Association (ADA) and its credentialing agency, the Commission on Dietetic Registration (CDR), believe it is in the best interest of the profession and the public it serves to have a Code of Ethics in place that provides guidance to dietetics practitioners in their professional practice and conduct. Dietetics practitioners have voluntarily adopted this Code of Ethics to reflect the values (Figure) and ethical principles guiding the dietetics profession and to set forth commitments and obligations of the dietetics practitioner to the *public, clients, the profession, colleagues, and other professionals*. The current Code of Ethics was approved on June 2, 2009, by the ADA Board of Directors, House of Delegates, and the Commission on Dietetic Registration.

application

The Code of Ethics applies to the following practitioners:

(a) In its entirety to members of ADA who are Registered Dietitians (RDs) or Dietetic Technicians, Registered (DTRs);
(b) Except for sections dealing solely with the credential, to all members of ADA who are not RDs or DTRs; and
(c) Except for aspects dealing solely with membership, to all RDs and DTRs who are not members of ADA.

All individuals to whom the Code applies are referred to as "dietetics practitioners," and all such individuals who are RDs and DTRs shall be known as "credentialed practitioners." By accepting membership in ADA and/or accepting and maintaining CDR credentials, all members of ADA and credentialed dietetics practitioners agree to abide by the Code.

principles
fundamental principles

1. The dietetics practitioner conducts himself/herself with honesty, integrity, and fairness.
2. The dietetics practitioner supports and promotes high standards of professional practice. The dietetics practitioner accepts the obligation to protect clients, the public, and the profession by upholding the Code of Ethics for the Profession of

management practice in dietetics

Dietetics and by reporting perceived violations of the Code through the processes established by ADA and its credentialing agency, CDR.

responsibilities to the public

3. The dietetics practitioner considers the health, safety, and welfare of the public at all times.

    The dietetics practitioner will report inappropriate behavior or treatment of a client by another dietetics practitioner or other professionals.

4. The dietetics practitioner complies with all laws and regulations applicable or related to the profession or to the practitioner's ethical obligations as described in this Code.

    a. The dietetics practitioner must not be convicted of a crime under the laws of the United States, whether a felony or a misdemeanor, an essential element of which is dishonesty.

    b. The dietetics practitioner must not be disciplined by a state for conduct that would violate one or more of these principles.

    c. The dietetics practitioner must not commit an act of misfeasance or malfeasance that is directly related to the practice of the profession as determined by a court of competent jurisdiction, a licensing board, or an agency of a governmental body.

5. The dietetics practitioner provides professional services with objectivity and with respect for the unique needs and values of individuals.

    a. The dietetics practitioner does not, in professional practice, discriminate against others on the basis of race, ethnicity, creed, religion, disability, gender, age, gender identity, sexual orientation, national origin, economic status, or any other legally protected category.

    b. The dietetics practitioner provides services in a manner that is sensitive to cultural differences.

    c. The dietetics practitioner does not engage in sexual harassment in connection with professional practice.

6. The dietetics practitioner does not engage in false or misleading practices or communications.

    a. The dietetics practitioner does not engage in false or deceptive advertising of his or her services.

    b. The dietetics practitioner promotes or endorses specific goods or products only in a manner that is not false and misleading.

    c. The dietetics practitioner provides accurate and truthful information in communicating with the public.

7. The dietetics practitioner withdraws from professional practice when unable to fulfill his or her professional duties and responsibilities to clients and others.

    a. The dietetics practitioner withdraws from practice when he/she has engaged in abuse of a substance such that it could affect his or her practice.

ADA Values	Principles
Customer Focus: Meets the needs and exceeds expectations of internal and external customers	#5, #9
Integrity: Acts ethically with accountability for life-long learning and commitment to excellence	#1, #2, #4, #5, #6, #7, #10, #11, #12, #13, #17, #18
Innovation: Embraces change with creativity and strategic thinking	
Social Responsibility: Makes decisions with consideration for inclusivity as well as environmental, economic, and social implications	#3, #8, #9, #11, #13, #14, #15, #16, #17, #18, #19

Figure. Alignment of American Dietetic Association (ADA) Values to the Principles of the Code of Ethics for the Profession of Dietetics.

    b.   The dietetics practitioner ceases practice when he or she has been adjudged by a court to be mentally incompetent.

    c.   The dietetics practitioner will not engage in practice when he or she has a condition that substantially impairs his or her ability to provide effective service to others.

responsibilities to clients

8.   The dietetics practitioner recognizes and exercises professional judgment within the limits of his or her qualifications and collaborates with others, seeks counsel, or makes referrals as appropriate.

9.   The dietetics practitioner treats clients and patients with respect and consideration.

    a.   The dietetics practitioner provides sufficient information to enable clients and others to make their own informed decisions.

    b.   The dietetics practitioner respects the client's right to make decisions regarding the recommended plan of care, including consent, modification, or refusal.

10. The dietetics practitioner protects confidential information and makes full disclosure about any limitations on his or her ability to guarantee full confidentiality.

11. The dietetics practitioner, in dealing with and providing services to clients and others, complies with the same principles set forth above in "Responsibilities to the Public" (Principles #3–7).

responsibilities to the profession

12. The dietetics practitioner practices dietetics based on evidence-based principles and current information.

management practice in dietetics

13. The dietetics practitioner presents reliable and substantiated information and interprets controversial information without personal bias, recognizing that legitimate differences of opinion exist.

14. The dietetics practitioner assumes a life-long responsibility and accountability for personal competence in practice, consistent with accepted professional standards, continually striving to increase professional knowledge and skills and to apply them in practice.

15. The dietetics practitioner is alert to the occurrence of a real or potential conflict of interest and takes appropriate action whenever a conflict arises.

    a. The dietetics practitioner makes full disclosure of any real or perceived conflict of interest.

    b. When a conflict of interest cannot be resolved by disclosure, the dietetics practitioner takes such other action as may be necessary to eliminate the conflict, including recusal from an office, position, or practice situation.

16. The dietetics practitioner permits the use of his or her name for the purpose of certifying that dietetics services have been rendered only if he or she has provided or supervised the provision of those services.

17. The dietetics practitioner accurately presents professional qualifications and credentials.

    a. The dietetics practitioner, in seeking, maintaining, and using credentials provided by CDR, provides accurate information and complies with all requirements imposed by CDR. The dietetics practitioner uses CDR-awarded credentials ("RD" or "Registered Dietitian"; "DTR" or "Dietetic Technician, Registered"; "CS" or "Certified Specialist"; and "FADA" or "Fellow of the American Dietetic Association") only when the credential is current and authorized by CDR.

    b. The dietetics practitioner does not aid any other person in violating any CDR requirements, or in representing himself or herself as CDR-credentialed when he or she is not.

18. The dietetics practitioner does not invite, accept, or offer gifts, monetary incentives, or other considerations that affect or reasonably give an appearance of affecting his/her professional judgment.

clarification of principle:

    a. Whether a gift, incentive, or other item of consideration shall be viewed to affect, or give the appearance of affecting, a dietetics practitioner's professional judgment is dependent on all factors relating to the transaction, including the amount or value of the consideration, the likelihood that the practitioner's judgment will or is intended to be affected, the position held by the practitioner, and whether the consideration is offered or generally available to persons other than the practitioner.

    b. It shall not be a violation of this principle for a dietetics practitioner to accept compensation as a consultant or employee or as part of a research grant or corporate sponsorship program, provided the relationship is openly disclosed and the practitioner acts with integrity in performing the services or responsibilities.

c. This principle shall not preclude a dietetics practitioner from accepting gifts of nominal value, attendance at educational programs, meals in connection with educational exchanges of information, free samples of products, or similar items, as long as such items are not offered in exchange for or with the expectation of, and do not result in, conduct or services that are contrary to the practitioner's professional judgment.

d. The test for appearance of impropriety is whether the conduct would create in reasonable minds a perception that the dietetics practitioner's ability to carry out professional responsibilities with integrity, impartiality, and competence is impaired.

responsibilities to colleagues and other professionals

19. The dietetics practitioner demonstrates respect for the values, rights, knowledge, and skills of colleagues and other professionals.

a. The dietetics practitioner does not engage in dishonest, misleading, or inappropriate business practices that demonstrate a disregard for the rights or interests of others.

b. The dietetics practitioner provides objective evaluations of performance for employees and coworkers, candidates for employment, students, professional association memberships, awards, or scholarships, making all reasonable efforts to avoid bias in the professional evaluation of others.

references

1. Ward, B., D. Rogers, C. Mueller, R. Touger-Decker, and K. Sauer. "Entry-Level Dietetics Practice Today: Results from the 2010 Commission on Dietetic Registration Entry-Level Practice Audit." *Journal of the American Dietetic Association*, 111:914–941, 2011.

2. Ibid.

3. American Dietetic Association. *Compensation & Benefits Survey of the Dietetics Profession 2011.* Chicago: American Dietetic Association, 2011.

4. Ibid.

5. Sauer, K., D. Canter, and C. Shanklin. "Job Satisfaction of Dietitians with Management Responsibilities: An Exploratory Study Supporting ADA's Research Priorities." *Journal of the American Dietetic Association.* 110 1432–1440, 2010.

6. Sauer, K., D. Canter, and C. Shanklin. "Describing Career Satisfaction of Registered Dietitians with Management Responsibilities." *Journal of the Academy of Nutrition and Dietetics.* 112:1129–1133, 2012.

7. Ashton, Robin. "*Foodservice Equipment Reports* 2012 E&S Market Forecast Update." Presentation on 24 January, 2012.

8. Shanklin, C.W. and R. Dowling. "Opportunities in Commercial Foodservice—The Members' Perspective." *Journal of the American Dietetic Association,* 95:236–238, 1995.

9. Unklesbay, N. "Monitoring for Quality Control in Alternate Foodservice Systems." *Journal of the American Dietetic Association,* 71:423–428, 1977.

10. National Restaurant Association. http://restaurant.org/research/facts/ accessed June 10, 2012.

11. Lacey, K. and E. Pritchett. "Nutrition Care Process and Model: ADA Adopts Road Map to Quality Care and Outcomes Management." *Journal of the American Dietetic Association.* 103:1061–1072, 2003.

12. Mixon, H., J. Dodd, B. Haughton, Public Health/Community Nutrition Practice Group, American Dietetic Association. *Guidelines for Community Nutrition Supervised Experience.* 2nd ed. 2003.

13. Ibid.

14. Moseley, M.J. "Nutrition and Electrolytes in the Elderly." In *Handbook of Nutrition in the Aged.* 3rd. ed. Ed. R.R. Watson. Boca Raton, FL: CRC Press LLC, 2001, p. 6.

15. "American Dietetic Association/Commission on Dietetic Registration Code of Ethics for the Profession of Dietetics and Process for Consideration of Ethics Issues," *Journal of the American Dietetic Association, vol. 109,* issue 8, pp. 1461–1463. Copyright © 2009 by Elsevier Press. Reprinted with permission.

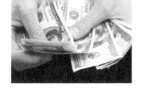

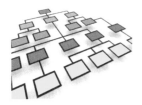

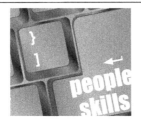

chapter two

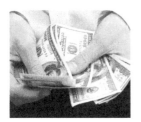

managing within an organization

learning objectives

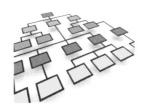

1. Describe what the term *organization* means.
2. Define *worker*, *manager*, and *span of control*.
3. Differentiate between frontline, middle, and top-level managers.
4. Differentiate among the various types of organizational structures.
5. Discuss how an organization's mission and philosophy relate to its structure.
6. List the characteristics of organizational culture.
7. Discuss why internal congruity is important to an organization.
8. Outline the systems approach to viewing an organization.
9. Describe the skills needed by managers at different levels.
10. Identify the functions that managers perform.
11. Describe what is included in the planning function.
12. Describe how managers organize the activities for which they are responsible.
13. State how planning and organizing interrelate with the other managerial functions.
14. Describe each of the four outcome criteria for management.
15. Cite examples of each of the three management roles—interpersonal, informational, and decisional.

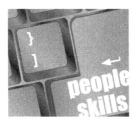

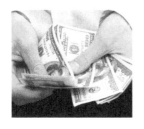

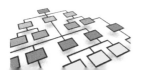

overview

It is safe to say that, when dietetics professionals assume a management position, they usually work in an organization of some sort. The organization may be public or private, commercial or noncommercial, for-profit or not for profit. It may be as small as a local health club or as large as the federal government. Though these organizations are very different, with varying goals, philosophies, missions, and cultures, there are some factors that are common to all organizations. This chapter will describe different kinds of organizations and outline the theory that is common to them all. The process of how an entity evolves from a small operation to become one that is defined in bureaucratic terms will be discussed, as will the different ways that organizations define their missions and their culture. Variations in organizational structure will be considered, as will the concept of internal congruity. Finally, the organization will be examined from the systems perspective, which describes the ways in which the organization interacts with its internal and external environments.

In this chapter, it is also appropriate to spend some time discussing who managers are and what they do. These factors are universal to all management positions, not just management in dietetics and nutrition. Dietetics managers may be found in any of the positions shown in the previous chapter, from a frontline supervisor to the CEO of a large corporation. All managers need technical, human, and conceptual skills, but the relative importance of each is dependent on the level of the management position. The various functions that managers perform will also be discussed. These include planning, organizing, leading, and controlling. This will be followed by a description of the roles that managers play, including interpersonal, informational, and decisional.

the organization

Organization.
A systematic arrangement of people to accomplish a specific purpose.

Because managers work in **organizations**, it is necessary to know something about what an organization is and how organizations are structured. In the simplest terms, an organization is "a deliberate arrangement of people to accomplish some specific purpose."[1] Those three components—people, structure, and purpose—are universally necessary for an organization to exist, be it a family, a church, a sports team, a hospital, a restaurant chain, or a government. The people include both managers and workers, though those are not always the words we use to describe the members of an organization. The structure is the framework within which the people work to accomplish the organizational goals. The purpose is the driving mission, philosophy, or goals of the organization.

organizational structure

An organization usually has some sort of structure. Even the smallest organization, with just a few individuals working together, has to have some sort of division of responsibility in order to function smoothly. In small businesses there is usually a manager (or owner/operator), who makes the decisions and holds the power, and the workers. As more people join an organization, the manager's job becomes more than one person can handle. That is the point at which some sort of structure evolves. It usually starts as a simple structure that is easily altered to meet the challenges faced by the organization, in which the **lines of authority** are obvious. However, as the organization continues to grow, the structure becomes more complex and more formalized. A bureaucracy is born.

The structural framework that is in place in an organization, large or small, is based on five elements, and the interrelationships among them. These elements are hierarchy, span of control, line/staff relationships, centralization/decentralization, and departmentalization. A description of each of these elements follows.

hierarchy

Hierarchy refers to the vertical relationships within an organization—that is, the reporting relationships between **line managers**. As shown in Figure 2.1, the foodservice workers report to the supervisor, who reports to the production manager, who reports to the assistant director of foodservices, and so on. Traditionally, hierarchy assumed that each individual reported to only one superior, and that authority was delegated downward through the organization.

Within the organization, different levels of staff are evident. The individuals at the

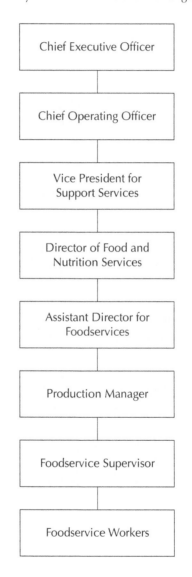

Figure 2.1 Organizational Hierarchy

Lines of Authority. *The vertical relationships within an organization; chain of command.*

Hierarchy. *A description of the vertical relationships in an organization, which dictates the reporting relationship among workers and the various levels of management.*

Line Managers. *Managers whose reporting relationships, both upward and downward, are vertical.*

Worker. *A person who does the work of the organization or produces the product.*

Managers. *People who oversee and direct the work of others.*

Management. *Planning, organizing, leading, and controlling the use of resources to achieve objectives.*

Frontline Managers. *Managers who oversee employees responsible for production; need a high level of technical skills, good human relations skills, and some conceptual skills.*

Top-Level Managers. *Managers who direct the activities of large segments of an organization rather than the actual production; need a high level of conceptual skills, good human relations skills, and some technical skills.*

bottom of the hierarchy actually do the work of the organization; they do not have to direct or monitor the work of others. Each of these people is called a worker or, sometimes, a frontline worker. **Managers** are people who oversee the work of others at some level. They may be frontline managers who do some of the work themselves as well as overseeing the work of others, they may be middle managers, or they may be top-level managers, whose primary role is **management**. Middle and top-level managers do little of the actual production work, if any.

For the most part, the type of position that a manager holds is closely correlated to where that position is located in the organizational hierarchy. When reporting relationships are vertical, with several individuals reporting to a manager, and with that manager reporting to another, higher-level manager, the relationship is said to be linear. The managers in this type of relationship with each other are called line managers. Because there are usually three or more levels in this type of structure, management levels are also defined. The managers who work closest to the customer are called **frontline managers**. They oversee the employees who make the product or deliver the service that the organization produces. On the other end of the spectrum are the **top-level managers**. There are fewer of this kind of manager, and they oversee the work of other (middle) managers rather than the production of goods and services. Indirectly, the top managers have responsibility for all that goes on under them, but with layers of managers between them and the workers to see to the day-to-day operations of the organization. This frees top-level management to attend to more global issues. Between the frontline manager and top-level managers, there may be one or more levels of **middle managers**. The number of middle managers, and the number of levels at which they function, is dependent on a number of factors. These include the size of the organization, the work units that have been identified, the geographic divisions that exist, and the span of control for each manager.

One thing that characterizes line managers is that there is a distinct **chain of command**, both upward and downward. Each person has one boss. Everything (ideas, information, plans, and so on) that moves upward through the organization moves from subordinate to boss, to the next level manager and the next level. When ideas and changes move downward, the reverse pattern is used. When management relationships are vertical and linear, it is often considered taboo to circumvent any managerial level. No one is supposed to deal directly with the boss's boss, or worse yet, to make direct contact with the president of the company on matters related to the organization or its business.

As organizations continue to evolve, however, these assumptions are no longer universally true. Today, teams may function without a manager at all. In other cases, managers may report to more than one superior. An example of this would be the clinical nutrition manager who reports to a physician (or a medical staff committee) concerning medical nutrition therapy and to a foodservice director for matters related to operations and finance.

A second area in which the traditional hierarchy is being questioned is the view that authority is delegated from the top down. Today, authority is sometimes viewed as coming from below—that is, from subordinates who are willing to accept direction from managers. Though the hierarchy still exists, it is no longer characterized by the premise of simple top-down delegation of authority from one individual to another through vertical relationships.

span of control

The second element of organizational structure is **span of control**, which is a way to measure the influence that a manager has in an organization. It is usually reported in terms of the number of people who report directly to that manager. The frontline manager in a cafeteria might supervise eight employees who work in the cafeteria on the morning shift on weekdays. Thus, this supervisor's span of control is eight. The supervisor could report to a middle manager, who is responsible for both the cafeteria and catering functions of a foodservice. If the morning cafeteria supervisor, the afternoon cafeteria supervisor, the cafeteria's relief supervisor (who covers days off for the other supervisors), a catering supervisor (who handles special events), and a clerk all report to this person, the span of control for the cafeteria and catering manager is five. Indirectly, though, all of the workers who report to the supervisors (assume eight each for purposes of this example) are also under the cafeteria and catering manager. Ultimately, this middle management position takes the responsibility for the work of 37 people.

Further up the management ladder is the foodservice director (FSD). Suppose that the following managers report to the FSD: the cafeteria and catering manager, the executive chef/food production manager, the patient services manager, and the clinical nutrition manager. The FSD's span of control is four. However, if these managers have 37, 24, 25, and 18 people reporting to them, respectively, then the FSD's authority would cover 108 people even though the span of control is the four who report directly to the FSD. It would be impossible for the FSD to manage every one of the 108 employees, individually; thus there is a real need for middle managers.

Even though top-level managers do the work of managing through others, it is necessary for them to keep in touch with what is happening at the various levels below them. Though the chain of command described earlier prevents workers from circumventing their immediate supervisor, it does not prevent the top-level managers from keeping in touch with employees at any level. This can be achieved by having councils or advisory groups made up of workers and managers at all levels of the organization. Another method for top-level managers to keep in touch with those

Middle Managers. *Managers whose level is above that of frontline managers, but who are subordinate to top-level managers; need technical and conceptual skills in equal amounts and good human relations skills.*

Chain of Command. *The vertical relationships between members of an organization that are based on authority and power.*

Span of Control. *A measure of the influence a manager has on an organization; usually measured by the number of people who report to the manager.*

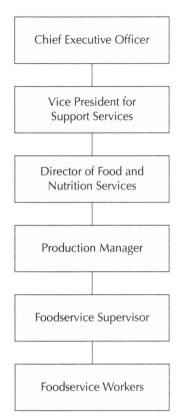

Figure 2.2 A Flattened Organizational Hierarchy

Chief Executive Officer

Vice President for Support Services

Director of Food and Nutrition Services

Production Manager

Foodservice Supervisor

Foodservice Workers

Staff Managers.
Managers who oversee supportive departments or groups; they report laterally, not vertically.

below them is by using the technique known as management by walking around (MBWA). It is amazing what an observant manager can learn when making unscheduled walking rounds through the facility.

In years past, the typical span of control was limited to four or five people reporting to each manager. This limited span resulted in an organization with multiple levels of managers and a great number of layers between the top-level manager and the workers. The current trend is toward training staff more intensely so that individuals are more independent and require less supervision. In general, the more skilled the workforce, the larger the span of control can be; that is, a manager can provide direct supervision to a greater number of subordinates. Depending on the manager's other responsibilities and the skill level of employees, the span of control may range from as few as 4 to as many as 30, or even more, direct subordinates. Increasing a manager's span of control allows for the flattening of the organization, which is the elimination of layers of middle management. When an organization deliberately increases the span of control of its managers in order to flatten the organization, the process is called *downsizing* (or, more positively, *rightsizing*). The newly evolved organization is more efficient because of this flattening. This is illustrated in Figure 2.2, which shows that two levels of management have been eliminated from the hierarchy shown in Figure 2.1, which results in a "flatter" organization. Flatter organizations are often more responsive to customer needs.

line/staff relationships

Not all managers have linear reporting relationships. Consider, for example, the public relations or the human resources departments in an organization. Their services are essential to the entire organization, but they do not do the actual work of producing goods or services, either directly or indirectly. They act in more of an advisory capacity. Both of these departments are fairly close to the top of the organizational structure but are often small departments with no need for multiple managerial levels. Similar departments, like education and training, may exist at lower levels in the organization. The commonality is that all of these departments support the entire organization, rather than one segment of it. The people who manage this type of department are known as **staff managers**, because their functions transcend departments and have an impact on the whole, rather than on any specific part of the organization. Usually, the reporting relationship for staff managers is horizontal rather than vertical.

Despite the non-linear reporting relationship, it is necessary to keep in mind that staff positions represent functions that are critical to the organization. Figure 2.3 illustrates how staff managers fit into an organizational structure. Table 2.1 reviews various types of management positions that might exist in an organization.

management practice in dietetics

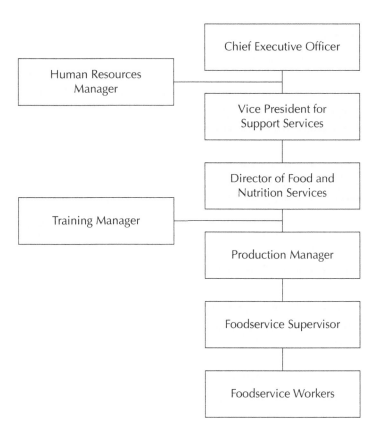

Figure 2.3 Line and Staff Managers

Position Type	Level	Responsibility/Skills Needed
	Frontline Manager	Managers who oversee production tasks; need a high level of technical skills, good human skills, and some conceptual skills
	Middle Manager	Managers who oversee several groups of workers and their supervisors; need some technical and conceptual skills and good human skills
	Top-Level Manager	Managers who direct the activities of large segments of an organization; need a high level of conceptual skills, good human skills, and some technical skills
Line Manager	Various	Managers whose reporting relationships are vertical; skills needed are dependent on the managerial level
Staff Manager	Various	Managers who direct supportive departments or groups and report laterally; skills needed are dependent on the managerial level

Table 2.1 Types of Managers

centralization

Centralization.
The concentration of decision making and power at the upper levels of an organization.

Centralization is the fourth element of organizational structure. It refers to the concentration of power at the upper levels of an organization. In a centralized structure, information flows upward through the various layers of the linear organization. Substantive decisions are made at the upper levels. The decisions are then transmitted down through the organization to be implemented by lower-level managers. The communication, both upward and downward through multiple levels of the organization, can lead to problems because the information may be distorted as it moves through the organization. Also, the information moves very slowly because of the number of layers it must traverse.

Decentralization.
The ability for individuals at lower levels of an organization to make decisions appropriate to their own areas of responsibility.

In this area, too, organizations are changing how they operate. The current trend is toward **decentralization**. As organizations are flattened, and staff is better trained, decisions are being made at lower levels, where the information related to those decisions is most available and where the time between making and implementing the decision is shortest. In some circumstances, the frontline worker is empowered to make the decision without consulting a manager. For example, a member of the waitstaff in a restaurant might have the authority to replace a customer's meal if the customer is unhappy. Decentralization allows the organization to be more responsive to customer needs. It should be noted, however, that not all decisions can or should be made by frontline employees. The waitstaff should not be given the authority to decide whether or not the restaurant should expand to double its current size. The decision related to expansion needs planning, market research, and knowledge of the restaurant's financial status that is probably not available to the waitstaff. More and more organizations are decentralizing the decision-making process by forcing decisions to be made at the lowest *appropriate* organizational level.

departmentalization

Departmentalization.
The specialization of groups in an organization, which may be based on product, function, clients, location, or work processes.

The final element of organizational structure is that of **departmentalization**. Many organizations specialize their functions and group like activities together. Departmentalization might be based on what the products are, or it might be based on the function of the work group, what customers are served, the geographic location, or the work processes.

Within hospital foodservice departments, the typical division would be between patient services and revenue-producing operations (cafeteria and catering). This is a division based on the customers. The patient services might be further departmentalized into meal service, enteral and parenteral feedings, and clinical services such as nutritional screening, assessment, counseling, and other services. These divisions are based on product line. Cash operations might be subdivided into an employee cafeteria, a visitor's café, a convenience store, on-premise catering, and off-premise catering; these are geographic divisions. Back-of-the-house operations might be further segmented into procurement, production, and sanitation, based on work processes. If accounting or quality management were handled as separate entities, the separation from the rest of the operation would be based on function.

There are some problems inherent to departmentalization that need to be considered. One is the lack of coordination between the various work groups. Each group or department works as an independent entity without consideration for what other departments are doing, or for the organization as a whole. Another problem is the competition that arises among work groups. Though competition can be good, in excess it could lead to turf issues, laying blame, and outright sabotage. Classically, both of these problems occur in the division between clinical services and patient foodservice within hospital nutrition and foodservice departments. The two groups do not communicate well with each other. Then, when problems about patient trays arise, the clinical staff blames the kitchen for incompetence, while the kitchen staff maintains that the clinical staff is elitist and makes unreasonable requests that increase their workload, which leads to unnecessary errors.

Such problems need to be identified and addressed by making sure individuals in the different departments or work groups talk with each other, not just through their managers. This type of lateral interdepartmental communication is not a part of the traditional organizational structure. One model that is being used to enhance lateral communication is the interdepartmental team that joins together for problem solving under the accountability process known as total quality management (TQM). (See Chapter 13.) A more complex model, in which all employees have two managers, is also used. In foodservice, the dual-reporting model is widely used for individuals who work for contract foodservice management companies but also report to an administrator in the contracting facility. This two-way reporting relationship is sometimes called matrix management (see Figure 2.4). The remedy for the problems of departmentalization seems to be rooted in communicating horizontally across departmental lines, rather than relying exclusively on vertical lines of communication.

the organization chart

The structure or framework of an organization may be graphically represented in an **organization chart**. This is especially true for large companies with multiple levels of management. (See Figure 2.5.) Organization charts depict horizontal and vertical relationships within an organization and define operating units or departments. Organization charts help the various members of the organization to see how they fit into the overall picture. It is like a map that allows one to visualize working relationships, reporting relationships, the number of levels in an organization, the way the work is divided, and the span of control for various managers.

Organization Chart. *A graphic representation of an organization's structure.*

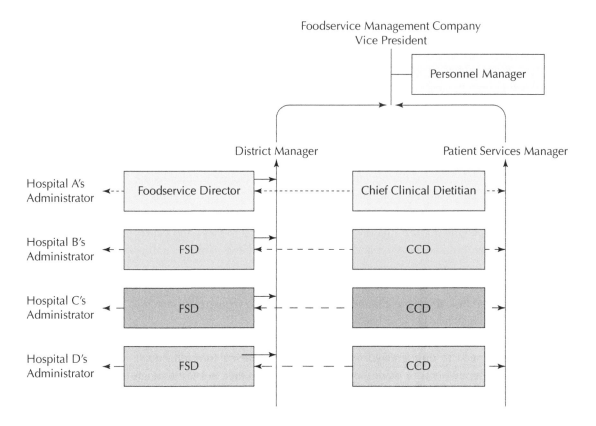

Figure 2.4 A Simplified Matrix Management Model

Organization charts are sometimes limited by the amount of space that it would take to illustrate all the intricacies possible in an organization. Thus, a large establishment might have a series of organization charts. The primary chart could give an overview of the entire organization, listing only the top-level positions like executive officers, vice presidents, and department heads. This could be augmented by other, more detailed charts for specific departments. The detailed charts have the same function as insets on a map or the zoom on a computer screen. They allow for magnification and addition of detail.

There are some things that cannot be illustrated in the organization chart. One such item is the additional, non-vertical work that the manager does. Committee memberships, special projects, and networking outside of the organization are all management functions that are not evident on the organization chart. When a manager appears to have a disproportionately small span of control, it may be that there are other responsibilities that preclude increasing the span of control part of the workload of this manager. Also, it should be noted that the organization chart

management practice in dietetics

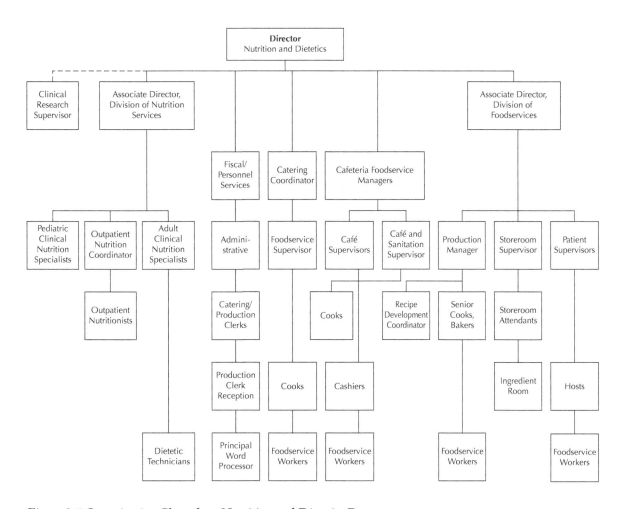

Figure 2.5 Organization Chart for a Nutrition and Dietetics Department

does not usually provide any information about centralization (or decentralization) of power. Therefore, one cannot make assumptions about the level at which decisions can be made by looking at the chart.

Another factor that may not be apparent from the organization chart is the **division of labor** among individuals. This is characterized by the assignment of specialized tasks to individuals. It has been shown that efficiency is gained by giving each worker a few discrete tasks to perform. In a large organization, only a few tasks are assigned to each worker. For example, in a large hotel kitchen, one of the six chefs might be assigned to prepare only soups and sauces. In a small organization, though, each worker may be called on to perform multiple tasks. This can be seen in a small restaurant, where the (only) chef would be responsible for the preparation of appetizers, salads, soups, entrées, side dishes, sauces, and desserts.

Division of Labor.
The practice of assigning each worker a few specialized tasks to perform, rather than a large number of more general tasks.

The contradictions to specialization are that boredom from doing the same task repeatedly can lead to errors. In addition, repetitive stress injury is a real risk for the employees when tasks that involve the same physical movements are repeated over and over again. Included in this category are assembly work, keyboarding, repeated bending and lifting, and other repetitive tasks.

Despite some shortcomings, the organization chart is a useful tool. Organization charts are used for providing data in a concise form to accrediting agencies. They can be used by management to report how the organization "looks" to stockholders or to outside agencies. Moreover, they have a myriad of internal uses, such as orienting new staff to the structure of the organization, "selling" the organization to candidates for employment, and teaching new managers about the way information flows. Candidates for employment would do well to study a business's organization chart before accepting a position in that business. It provides the astute individual with a great deal of insight into the organization.

One last thing should be noted about organization charts. The chart is one of many tools that are used by managers in performing the management function. As with other tools, the organization chart should not be viewed as static. As changes are made in the business, the organization chart should be revised and updated to accurately reflect the existing situation. Much of the usefulness of the organization chart is lost if it is not current.

organizational mission

Earlier it was mentioned that there are three components to an organization—people, structure, and purpose. The people and the structure have been described. The final part of the triad is the organizational purpose, frequently expressed as a **mission statement**. The difference in how the mission is expressed in small and large organizations is noteworthy. Small businesses, with only a few employees, may have a mission that is known by the manager or owner/operator and is communicated to the employees in an informal way. The mission may be to produce a delicious and healthy cookie, to provide congregate meals to the elderly population, or to educate the public about the benefits of increasing their physical activity. Because there are only a few employees, and communication with the manager is direct, there is little chance for the mission to be distorted. As organizations grow, managerial levels increase, and departmentalization occurs, the mission may be less clear to the larger number of individuals in the organization. The finance/accounting department may want to concentrate on making a profit (or breaking even, if the organization is nonprofit). The human resources department may be interested in reducing staff turnover. The material management department may be preoccupied with reducing inventory levels. The overriding purpose of the

management practice in dietetics

organization (producing the delicious and healthy cookie, feeding the elderly, or educating the public) gets lost in the bureaucracy. Thus, it is useful to develop some sort of written statement that embodies the purpose of the organization and reminds everyone what the focus really is.

The written statement should be concise, so that it is useful to employees and understandable to customers and clients. For example, "The mission of Children's Hospital Oakland is to ensure:

- The highest quality pediatric care for all children through regional primary and subspecialty networks
- Strong medical education and teaching programs
- A diverse workforce
- State-of-the-art research programs and facilities
- Nationally recognized child advocacy efforts."[2]

Cal Dining's mission is "… to provide the highest quality services and programs that ease a student's transition through the University and in the greater community, and to provide all our customers—students, faculty, staff and guests—with a quality customer experience."[3] In addition, the Cal Dining website also presents a vision for the program that details how the mission is to be fulfilled.

This declaration may be called a mission, a philosophy, a statement of purpose, a list of values, or a vision statement. Though technically there are some differences between these different formats, what it is called is less important than the function it serves. The most important reason for stating the organization's mission in writing is to make it accessible, familiar, and useful to all members of an organization. To emphasize this point, some organizations use it in their advertising, on business cards, or as wall and desk ornaments.

organizational culture

The mission of the organization is one of the driving forces behind what is known as **organizational culture**. It is "a pattern of shared basic assumptions learned by a group as it solved its problems of external adaptation and internal integration, which has worked well enough to be considered valid and, therefore, to be taught to new members as the correct way to perceive, think, and feel in relation to those problems."[4] Just as families, ethnic groups, and religions have their own cultural norms, so do businesses and workplaces.

Organizational Culture. *The "personality" of an organization.*

Organizational culture helps determines how employees view their jobs, and how they act, both toward their colleagues and toward outsiders. Other factors that play a part in the development of the organizational culture are the leadership styles of the managers, the size and complexity of the organization, its product or service, and the environmental forces that come to bear on the organization.

Organizational culture determines how things are done within the organization. For example, one organization may encourage managers to make decisions related to their area of responsibility and inform their supervisors only when problems arise. Another organization might require that all decisions be cleared with a supervisor before being implemented. The degree to which risk-taking is encouraged, the emphasis on teamwork or rugged individualism, and the accessibility of staff are all a part of what is known as organizational culture. Even something as simple as working out differences in person or through written memos (which leaves a paper trail) is influenced by the culture that exists.

internal congruity

Internal Congruity. *Consistency within the organization, related to managers, employees, processes, communications, philosophy, culture, and so on. It is the thread that unifies the whole.*

Another important factor in the smooth operation of an organization is internal congruity. Essentially, this is the degree to which things work together for the achievement of the overall purpose of the organization. Things go more smoothly when the organization's structure and culture are integrated with each other and supported by the people in the organization. Individual managers must have managerial styles that are consistent with the structure and culture, and employees must know what roles they are expected to play in the organization.

An autocratic manager could be successful in an organization that is multilayered, centralized, and operated in a way that relies heavily on rules and regulations. In such an organization, however, it is unrealistic to expect employees to take risks or express creative ideas; the employees must be willing to do what they are told to do without asking too many questions. On the other hand, a flat organization with a history of decentralized decision making would probably not be a comfortable place for the autocratic manager. This type of organization would encourage employees to take responsibility for their own actions and empower them to make decisions and take risks without fear of reprimand.

When organizations promote from within, there is a distinct advantage in that the new managers know how things are done within the culture that exists. Their role models have been integrated into the structure and culture. New managers learn, from these role models, how to operate in the organization. Outsiders, no matter how successful they have been in previous positions, will have a steeper learning curve when hired into a new organization. Successful integration is not always predictable. It may not be easy for a newcomer to gain acceptance in an organization with a strong culture.

Sometimes, it is necessary for an organization to change either its structure or its mission—or both. Change might have its origin in changing markets, technology, or

management practice in dietetics

result from other external factors. When this occurs, it should be noted that there will be a period of chaos, during which the organization will appear to be dysfunctional. Change takes time; it is not something that can be accomplished overnight. Though it is not always possible to control the rate of change in an organization, the process will be less traumatic if it evolves rather than happens abruptly. Change theory will be discussed in Chapter 18. For the moment, it should be noted that major organizational change is not usually welcomed.

the organization as a system

Thus far, the organization has been identified as having structure, purpose, and people. But organizations also *do* something. The "doing" can be best described using the systems theory of management where inputs are transformed into outputs. (See Figure 2.6.) Nearly any organization can be viewed in this way. Because most organizations interact with environmental forces, the systems that result are open systems. In the rare case that a system does not interact with the external environment, it is called a closed system.

Inputs are whatever is brought into the system. People provide time, energy, skills, and ideas to the organization. All of these are inputs from human resources. Without people, it is unlikely that much work will occur. Another input is in the form of material. It is not necessary that the material be "raw material." For example, a foodservice does not have to buy wheat, grind it into flour, and make bread. The foodservice may purchase sliced bread and "transform" it into sandwiches or French toast. Information is another input. It can come from a variety of sources, including data from market

Inputs. *Resources brought into a system; for example, money, people, technology, and materials.*

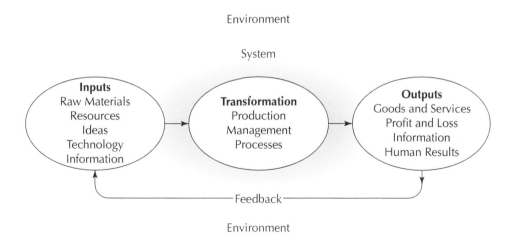

Figure 2.6 *The Organizational System*

research that identify customer wants and needs, data related to customer satisfaction, and historical facts that have been gathered. Other inputs include money, technology, equipment, and so on.

Transformation.
The production or work of an organization that changes inputs into outputs.

Within the system, the inputs are changed into something else. That change, which is the work of the organization, is known as **transformation**. Transformation includes all of the things that happen to the inputs within the organization. Work processes are involved in transformation, as are management functions and the various tasks that workers do. Some processes are relatively simple, like typing a letter. Other processes are more complex, like those involved in performing open-heart surgery. In large organizations, different types of transformations take place in different settings. For example, a hospital would have a system for nursing, one for pharmacy, one for environmental services, one for finances, one for human resources, and so forth.

In dietetics practice, the systems approach was adopted in the foodservice area in the late 1960s. Spears identified four subsystems in foodservice organizations: procurement; production; safety, sanitation and maintenance; and distribution and service.[5] Later, Sullivan and Atlas expanded the number of subsystems to seven[6] (menu, food purchasing, food production, foodservice, finances, personnel, and equipment). This innovative approach, which revolutionized the field of foodservice management, resulted in the dietetics profession equating management with foodservice. In healthcare facilities, nutrition became aligned with clinical systems.[7] For quite a while clinical and community nutrition seemed to lag behind foodservice in the development of management theory and practice. However, it is equally important to apply the systems approach to these areas of dietetics practice. In clinical nutrition, transformation occurs through the first three steps in the nutrition care process that include nutrition assessment, nutrition diagnosis, and nutrition intervention.[8] In community nutrition, the transformation is based upon the subsystems of community assessment, problem identification, program planning, and intervention.[9]

Outputs. *The results that occur when inputs are transformed in a system.*

Outcomes. *The term used for outputs in clinical or community nutrition.*

Outputs are the outcomes that occur after the inputs have undergone transformation. Some outputs are tangible goods, like the sandwiches or the French toast, but outputs do not have to be tangible. Other outputs for foodservices would include number of meals served, revenue generated, and customer satisfaction. In clinical and community nutrition, the word **outcomes** is substituted for outputs. Clinical outcomes are measured as the fourth step of the nutrition care process, nutrition monitoring and evaluation. Examples include the knowledge gained by clients, behavior changes in response to the intervention, and improvement in health, specifically as it relates to the nutritional diagnosis. Such outcomes as a reduction in body weight, lowering of serum cholesterol level, or improved blood glucose levels are clinical outputs. Outcome measurements are also a part of community nutrition systems and include such things as changes in the awareness and behavior of the target population, as well as data on its morbidity and mortality. Schematics of the systems theory as it relates to foodservice, clinical, and community nutrition practice can be seen in Figure 2.7.

Environment

Food Service System

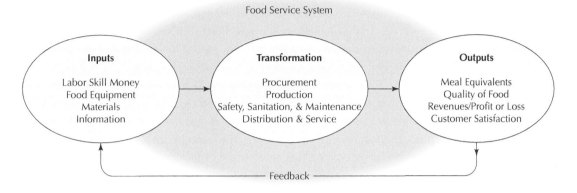

Environment

Clinical Nutrition System

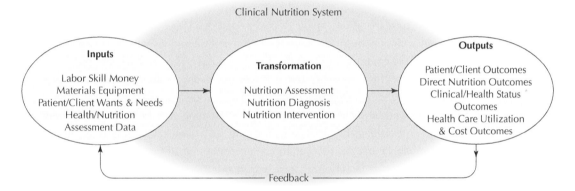

Environment

Community Nutrition System

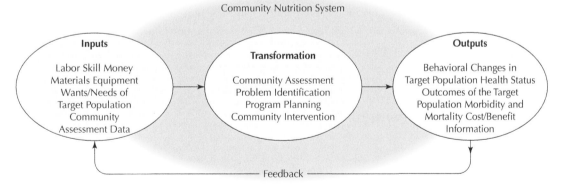

Environment

Figure 2.7 Organizational Systems in Dietetics

It is important to note that outputs are not always positive, nor should they be. Consider that operating profit is good and indicates that the operation is running smoothly. This positive piece of information means that things are going well. Conversely, if there are a large number of worker-related injuries, this information provides evidence that something is not working well and that it needs to be fixed. Both positive and negative outputs become part of the **feedback** that the system then uses as additional input to improve and refine the transformation process. For example, if a foodservice made too many sandwiches, which became stale and had to be discarded, the information gained through that experience should lead the manager to reassess the production of sandwiches. Options include decreasing the production of sandwiches, making the sandwiches to order as customers request them, or packaging the sandwiches so that they do not get stale. Using the informational output data that the system generates as inputs for the system is called feedback. This is an integral part of how a system works. Feedback is like organizational memory; it helps the organization avoid repeated errors and maximize what is positive.

Feedback. *Outputs from a system that are recycled as inputs to prevent errors or to improve the system in the future.*

The entire organization can be viewed as part of a larger system, too. For a foodservice or a clinical nutrition service, the larger system is usually the hospital, which is part of the community, the state, and the country. The external environment has a major impact on how the system behaves. For example, foodservices must provide safe food. Food handling practices are mandated by federal or state regulations and are evaluated by local and state health departments and by voluntary accrediting agencies. If there is an outbreak of illness traced to a hospital foodservice, the media will probably carry the news to the larger community. Physicians and patients may lose faith in the facility and stop patronizing the hospital, which could lead to financial losses.

Every organizational system must be mindful of the environment in which it exists. It must comply with the regulations imposed on it from the outside, as well as with its own internal policies and procedures. It must be responsive to the needs of the greater community from which it draws support. Organizations should be good citizens and good neighbors.

management

In the previous sections of this chapter, the terms "management" and "managers" were used and defined. Different levels of managers were identified, and their responsibilities and the skills that they must have were listed in Table 2.1. Still, it is necessary to look more closely at managers and management, so that their roles and functions within the organization are apparent.

management practice in dietetics

skills needed by managers

Managers need three types of skills. These are technical, human, and conceptual.[10] Although the skills are universal requirements for managers, different managerial positions require the skills in varying degrees. Generally, as a manager moves up through management ranks, proficiency is gained in one skill area (conceptual) and lost in another (technical). The gain or loss is directly related to the degree to which each skill is used. Skills, like muscles, get stronger when used and deteriorate from lack of use.

Technical skills are those that are needed to do the actual production work of the organization. Technical skills are generally acquired through either experience or education, and sometimes through both. For example, a cook would have technical skills in food preparation, a DTR would have technical skills in screening clients for risk, and a clinical dietitian would have technical skills in performing nutritional assessments. Frontline managers who supervise the day-to-day activities of production need to have a high degree of technical skill. They need to know how the various people who report to them go about getting the work done. A good frontline manager will be able to do most or all of the tasks that are performed by subordinates. Proficiency at doing the tasks is not required, only the ability to perform them at some level. The clinical nutrition manager who supervises the work of RDs and DTRs should know how to do nutritional assessments and how to screen clients for nutritional risk. All managers need some technical skills related to the work of the organization, but frontline managers need these to a larger extent than do middle or top-level managers.

The second type of skill set needed by managers is **human skills**. These skills are a universal requirement for managers at all levels, because people are the most valuable resource in any organization. Human skills are a combination of personal attributes, knowledge, and learned behavior. This skill set requires knowing the rules and regulations relative to working with employees, and it requires the ability to communicate with subordinates and with those in authority. Because human relations make up a large part of the job of middle managers, it can be argued that they need this type of skill more than do top-level managers or frontline managers, but these skills are very important for all management personnel. No matter the level, a manager who is poor at human relations has a limited chance of long-term success. Even staff managers, with few people reporting to them, need human skills to communicate with other managers and with their superiors.

The third type of skill that is needed by managers is conceptual. This skill set allows one to see beyond the reality of the immediate situation, and look at the global picture to visualize what is possible. It involves work that is abstract, like developing mission and value statements, strategic planning, working out budgets, evaluating

Technical Skills.
Managerial skills related to the production work of the organization.

Human Skills.
A managerial skill set composed of personal attributes, knowledge, and learned behavior that enables managers to work effectively and communicate with others.

markets, determining growth potential, and bringing projects to successful conclusions. **Conceptual skills** are needed most by top-level managers, who work more with ideas than with things. These managers do very little that relates to the actual production of goods and services.

To reiterate, all managers need each of the three skills described above, with the most important being human skills. Of the other skill sets, the frontline manager relies heavily on technical skills, and the top-level manager needs more conceptual skills. In addition to human skills, the middle manager needs balanced amounts of technical and conceptual skills.

management functions

Managers perform a number of different functions. These include planning, organizing, leading, and controlling.[11] All managers participate in these functions as routine parts of their jobs. These functions, and how dietetics managers go about performing them, are the basis for this entire book. Each function will be covered in detail as the text unfolds. For the moment, a brief description of each function should be sufficient to introduce the concepts.

planning

One of the management functions is **planning**, which involves determining the mission of the organization or work group, setting goals, and outlining a blueprint for action that will enable the goals to be met. The first step in planning is developing a mission statement, a philosophy, or a statement of purpose or values. This is essential to the organization because it provides an overall direction for it, and gives everyone working for the organization a sense of purpose. The mission guides the decision-making process; it is the thread that holds the organization together.

Unfortunately, some managers see the development of a mission statement or a philosophy as an academic exercise and prefer to operate without one. They are much more comfortable "doing" rather than "philosophizing." This attitude is misguided. If a manager proceeds to move forward with the development and implementation of plans without clearly defining the goal of the organization or work unit, then the plans become ends in themselves. This can lead to costly errors, such as growth for the sole purpose of growth, without regard to need or function.

Some managers feel that the mission is intuitive. They "know" what the direction of the organization should be despite the fact that there is no written mission statement. The problem with this is that an unwritten mission is subject to personal interpretations,

management practice in dietetics

which are probably not going to be consistent among management personnel. If there are 15 departments in an organization, there may be 15 interpretations of what the organization's mission is. These inconsistencies lead to internal chaos and turf wars. Eventually, the organization will need to pull back, reorganize, and establish an organizational philosophy if it is to work efficiently and effectively. Once an organizational philosophy has been established, plans can be developed that are consistent with the philosophy, enabling the organization to move forward in a systematic manner.

Under the umbrella of a mission or philosophy, plans for the organization and for its individual units can be developed. In general, three types of plans are made. **Short-term plans** are those goals and objectives that an organization intends to achieve in a twelve-month period of time. The budget (which is the financial plan for an organization) is generally prepared for a 12-month period and is considered to be a short-term plan. **Long-term plans** incorporate goals and objectives that cover a period of three to five years. (In the past, long-term plans often projected five to ten years into the future, but with the rapid expansion of technology, it is difficult to plan that far in advance. The future is less predictable than it used to be.) **Strategic plans** are those that are closely aligned with the organization's mission that set the direction for the organization within the context of its internal and external environments[12]; they tend to be more global in nature than short- and long-term plans.

A long-term plan for a dietitian starting up in private practice might be to have 75 physicians referring patients to the practice within three years. There might also be a goal of seeing the average diabetic client for a total of six visits, another goal of spending 30 hours in individual counseling sessions per week, and another goal of overseeing three group counseling sessions each week. The plan might even include moving from a shared office to a private one and hiring a part-time administrative assistant and another dietitian by the end of the three-year period. The long-term plans are often stated in terms of outcomes, or outcome goals—that is, what one hopes to have accomplished at the end of the time period.

Short-term plans are the interim plans that allow one to move toward the long-term goals. Short-term plans might be measured in months, weeks, or even days. The dietitian starting a private practice might have some short-range plans that include: make three visits to potential referring physicians each week, schedule all referrals to be seen within one week, and send follow-up notes to the referring physicians before the end of the week. Short-term plans are subject to change as circumstances change. For example, if the dietitian reaches the long-term goal of 75 referring physicians and 30 hours of individual counseling per week after 15 months, it might no longer be necessary to continue making three physician visits each week. The goals that are set in short-term plans are sometimes referred to as process goals.

For a foodservice manager, the long-term plan might be to move into a new, cook-chill, commissary-type kitchen in three years. Short-term plans would be the various

Short-Term Plans.
The interim plans of an organization geared toward fulfilling long-term goals; usually projected in days, weeks, or months. These are sometimes called process goals.

Long-Term Plans.
The projected outcomes or strategic plans of an organization based on its mission or philosophy; usually covering a period of from three to five years. These are sometimes called outcome goals.

Strategic Plans.
Global plans that set the direction for the organization within the context of its internal and external environments.

steps along the way, including designing the facility, overseeing the construction, purchasing the equipment, having it installed, training the staff, and so on. With this type of long-term plan, it can be expected that there will be some changes in schedules and dates along the way. This is where the mission statement is useful. For example, assume that the construction project is driven by an organizational statement of purpose such as "To provide safe and high-quality food to the students on the campus of XYZ University in an efficient and cost-effective manner." Then, if a piece of equipment for the new facility is unavailable, the decision about substituting another piece of equipment can be based on safety and cost-effectiveness, not on convenience, pressure to meet a deadline, or a salesperson's persuasive manner. The mission/philosophy should be the driving force behind the establishment and revision of plans.

organizing

Organizing is the establishment of an orderly, systematic method of dealing with work. It entails looking at the work that needs to be done, and figuring out who will do the work and what methods will be used to do it. Organizing usually results in the establishment of an organizational structure, with identified reporting relationships. It also leads to standardized ways of dealing with the process of work as it moves through time and space. Workstations are organized to make them comfortable, efficient, and safe for the worker. Work processes are organized to prevent redundancy and unnecessary backtracking. Production schedules deal with timelines for the work that needs to be done. Policies and procedures are established in order to give guidance to individuals who are performing tasks that are new to them so that they do not have to learn solely from the "trial and error" method. Job specifications, job descriptions, performance appraisals, and personnel action forms are all designed to organize the tasks related to human resources and staffing. Purchase orders, receiving documents, and payment authorizations are all used to organize the acquisition of goods. Nearly everything that managers do repeatedly is, or eventually becomes, organized to facilitate the completion of the work.

Once work has been organized, it becomes easier to do. Part of the reason is that organizing often produces step-by-step directions about how the task is to be done (for example, the standardized recipe used in foodservice). Another reason is that, as an individual does a job repeatedly, it becomes familiar enough so that less thought is given to each step of the process. The activities become routine. Furthermore, organizing produces tools that can be used by many individuals, rather than by just one person; duplication of effort is avoided. It should be noted, though, that the tools should not be used just because they exist. To be useful, tools must facilitate the accomplishment of work. If a tool does not accomplish its purpose, it should be updated so that it works in the current environment.

Organizing work is more structured than organizing one's personal life, because many people are involved in how things happen at work. In a setting where several people do the same or similar jobs, guidelines must be in effect to allow workers to achieve similar results despite their individuality. Indeed, as the number of people doing a job increases, there is more need for standardized processes and less room for creativity. Cooks in quick-service restaurants with thousands of outlets must produce a safe, uniform product, in exactly the same way each time, whereas the chef at a five-star gourmet restaurant is allowed more artistic license with the foods that are produced.

One of the problems encountered when organizing work processes has to do with the tendency of people to resist change. Once work is organized, a system is put into place, and individuals are trained in the process, they become entrenched in that way of doing things. When someone new comes into the system and asks why something is done in a certain way, the answer is likely to be, "Because we've always done it that way." Unfortunately, "that way," which may have been efficient, effective, appropriate, and adequate when it was introduced, may no longer be the best way to do the task. Therefore, the organizing of work should not be viewed as a task that gets completed, but rather as an ongoing process that requires remodeling and updating over time.

leading

Leading is that part of management involving the direction and coordination of the activities of workers. Leaders work with people to achieve a shared organizational vision. Leading is motivating others, managing their activities, communicating, and resolving conflicts. It is the function of management that relies most heavily on the human skills described earlier. An entire chapter of this text is devoted to leadership, because it is often the most crucial management function. It is less tangible than planning, organizing, or controlling, and somewhat more difficult to describe.

Leading. *A management function that deals with the direction, motivation, and coordination of staff and their activities.*

In general, an organization is as good as its leadership. This can be illustrated by looking at several operations run by the same management company—for example, a contract foodservice management company that runs foodservices in healthcare institutions, at business dining sites, on college campuses, in prisons, and for public school systems. All of these foodservices have similar operating systems. Some of the foodservices run smoothly, are profitable, and have a productive and satisfied workforce. Other operations, managed and operated by the same corporation using the same systems, are in upheaval. When this occurs, the operation may be less profitable and there may be dissatisfaction among the staff. The differences are due largely to the individual site managers. The critical factors are generally the leadership style and the human skills of each individual manager. This does not imply that one leadership style is innately better than another, but that the manager's leadership style has to be consistent with the mission of the facility in which the foodservice is located. The success of a foodservice operation is probably more dependent on the individual manager than it is on which, if any, contract management company is operating the foodservice.

controlling

Controlling is following up on the work that is being done to make sure that it is being done as planned and that organizational standards are being met. Essentially, controlling can be summed up in the phrase "inspect what you expect." If quality is expected, then ways must be found to measure quality. If financial goals are a priority, there must be a measure of financial performance. If there is a goal to complete a community assessment by the end of the year, then the progress toward meeting this goal needs to be monitored. All of this monitoring, measuring, and comparison with standards is called controlling.

Control can also be measured by how well procedures are being followed. Most managers understand that the outcomes are as important as, if not more important than, following the procedure. It may be possible to allow some flexibility in the procedures if doing so does not have a negative impact on the safety or health of workers or the quality of the product. For example, consider the procedure that calls for a diet clerk to tally items on the menus on a line-by-line basis by putting hatch marks for each item ordered on a "tally sheet." If one clerk is able to count the items accurately without using the hatch marks, and the individual's procedure results in the same degree of accuracy as the prescribed procedure, there is no justification for insisting that the individual write the hatch marks just because it follows a written procedure. In fact, the elimination of the writing step may save time for that person and lead to better efficiency. Like other management functions, control must be tempered with flexibility and open mindedness.

other management functions

Some management theorists use terminology that differs from that used in this section. Motivating, actuating, directing, or a combination of these terms might be used instead of leading. Sometimes, staffing is added as an additional function of management. However, staffing can be viewed in light of the other four functions rather than as a separate one. For example, a manager must plan for the number and types of employees that are needed to carry out the work. The organizing function includes outlining the job qualifications, as well as recruiting, hiring, and training the appropriate workers. Leading is the motivating and directing of the employees in order to accomplish the actual work. Controlling is the measurement and appraisal of the staff's performance. Whether staffing is identified as a separate function or a part of the other functions is less important than the manager's ability to carry out all of the functions in an effective, efficient, appropriate, and adequate manner.

management practice in dietetics

outcome criteria

Ultimately, the process of management is oriented toward getting the work of the organization done in a manner that is efficient, effective, appropriate, and adequate. **Efficient** is defined as getting the most out of the resources that are used. **Effective** means meeting the goals that have been established. **Appropriate** means that what is being done is correct for the specific situation and **adequate** means that the amount is sufficient. Outcomes of management functions and the decisions that managers make can be measured against these four criteria to determine how well management is performing its tasks to meet the goals of the organization. (See Table 2.2.)

As an illustration, consider the management of a WIC clinic, whose purpose is to provide nutrition education and electronic benefit transfer (EBT) funds for qualified food products to eligible women, infants, and children at nutritional risk. The clinic is effective if it is providing nutrition education and EBT funds to clients who actually use the services to maintain or improve nutritional status. Efficiency is measured by weighing the resources needed to provide the service against the number of clients served. Obviously, if a clinic serves 1,000 clients with a staff of eight, it is more efficient than one that serves 200 clients with the same staffing levels. The service is appropriate if it is able to individualize service to meet client needs, for example by differentiating between families with a lactating mother (EBT funds will be for more foodstuffs) and families with bottle-fed infants (EBT funds will include infant formula). Finally, the program is adequate if all clients who need the service are getting it.

These four criteria can also be used to evaluate the effectiveness of a decision that has been made. For instance, if a manager chose a deep-fat fryer to make French fries for a quick-service restaurant (QSR), the fryer would be effective if it actually fried potatoes. But that is not enough. It also needs to be efficient, which in a fryer means it does not waste fuel, costs little to operate, and conserves cooking oil. Appropriate is a matter of suitability to the facility and its menu. If the QSR touted "healthy, low-fat foods," then a hot-air fryer would be more appropriate than a deep-fat fryer. Finally, the fryer is adequate if it has the production capacity to meet peak customer demand.

Effective. *A criteria for management focused on meeting defined goals and objectives.*

Efficient. *A criteria for management defined as doing things in the best way relative to resource utilization.*

Appropriate. *A criteria for management based on the ability to adapt to the specific environment.*

Adequate. *A criterion for management that considers if what was done was done in the correct amount.*

Effective	Doing the right thing
Efficient	Doing things in the right way
Appropriate	Adapted for the circumstances
Adequate	In the correct amount

Table 2.2 Outcome Criteria

In relation to each of the management functions cited earlier, it is necessary for managers to evaluate their own performance and decisions based on these four outcome criteria.

roles of managers

Managers typically move from activity to activity in rapid succession, performing a variety of roles during the course of a day. The roles can be grouped into three categories—interpersonal, informational, and decisional.[13]

interpersonal

Interpersonal Roles. *A managerial role in which a manager acts as a figurehead, a leader, or a liaison.*

Interpersonal roles are those in which the manager acts as a figurehead, a leader, or a liaison. Figurehead roles are ceremonial and include such things as attending to legal matters or social responsibilities. Signing official documents and attending company picnics, parties, and other rituals are among the duties that fall under this heading. Any activity that involves working with, relating to, or motivating employees falls under the leader role. Networking, both internal and external, is considered to be part

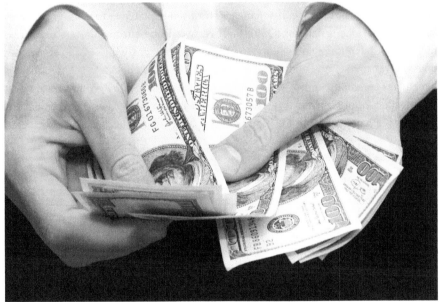

One of the decisional roles of managers is that of resource allocation.

of the liaison role of a manager. This includes activities such as serving on committees and working with local and national professional associations.

informational

Informational roles involve the monitoring or dissemination of information and acting as the spokesperson for the unit that is being managed. The monitor role includes keeping current on professional issues through reading, listserves, and the like. Managers should have their finger on the pulse of the organization and know what internal and external factors are likely to influence it. Managers also pass on information as necessary within the organization; in these instances they act as information disseminators. The final informational role of the manager is to be the spokesperson for the organization or the operational unit, transmitting information to those outside the organization.

Informational Roles. *A managerial role in which the manager monitors and disseminates information or acts as a spokesperson for the organization.*

decisional

Managers have four decisional roles. These are those of entrepreneur, disturbance handler, resource allocator, and negotiator. The entrepreneurial role is one in which the manager determines when to take risks, make changes, or develop new programs. The disturbance handler deals with problems and potential problems in an effort to mediate disturbances before they get out of hand. The resource allocator decides how resources will be used. Finally, the negotiator acts as an intermediary for the organization when making deals and arranging contracts.

Decisional Roles. *A managerial role based on being an entrepreneur, disturbance handler, resource allocator, and negotiator; these roles allow a manager to take charge, make changes, handle conflicts, determine how resources are used, and arrange deals.*

In summary, managers play a variety of roles in carrying out the four functions of management. Different skills are needed as the manager tries to meet organizational goals in an effective, efficient, appropriate, and adequate manner. Furthermore, the manager's personal style should be compatible with the organizational structure and its culture, which were discussed earlier in this chapter.

conclusion

This chapter has included an overview of organizations and how managers and management fit into an organizational structure. The key concepts that can be found in this chapter include:

1. The elements that characterize an organization's structure are hierarchy, span of control, line/staff relationships, centralization, and departmentalization.
2. The organization's purpose is reflected in both its mission and in its culture.

3. The organization can be viewed as a system, in which inputs are transformed into outputs.
4. The skills needed by all managers are technical, human, and conceptual, though different levels of managers need these in differing amounts.
5. Functions of managers are planning, organizing, leading, and controlling.
6. The criteria for measuring management outcomes are efficiency, effectiveness, appropriateness, and adequacy.
7. Roles of managers are interpersonal, informational, and decisional.

activities

activity 1

The school that you attend is an organization with a structure that can be represented in an organization chart. The dietetics program is located within that college or university. For this activity, draw an organization chart that depicts how you view the relationships within the dietetics program, and the relationship of the program to the larger organization.

activity 2

Using the organization chart in Figure 2.5, please respond to the following:

1. Describe what you are able to infer about the organizational hierarchy.
2. What is the span of control of the various managers depicted on the chart?
3. Is the organization a tall one, or does it appear to be flat?
4. Which positions are vertical, line positions?
5. Which positions, if any, are staff positions?
6. Are you able to determine if the organization is centralized or decentralized?
7. What types of departmentalization exist?

to study further

The following resources provide additional information on systems theory, organizations, and organizational structure.

- Alvesson, Mats. *Understanding Organizational Culture*. Thousand Oaks, CA: SAGE, 2004.
- Drejer, Anders. *Strategic Management and Core Competencies: Theory and Applications*. Westport, CT: Quorum Books, 2002.
- Flamholtz, Eric G. *Effective Management Control: Theory and Practice*. Boston: Kluwer Academic Publishers, 1996.
- Hill, Charles W.L. *Strategic Management Theory: An Integrated Approach*. Boston: Houghton Mifflin, 2004.
- Heracleous, Loizos. *Strategy and Organization, Realizing Strategic Management*. Cambridge, UK: University Press, 2003.
- Morris, Langdon. *Managing the Evolving Corporation*. New York: Van Nostrand Reinhold, 1995.
- O'Donovan, Giselle. *The Corporate Culture Handbook*. Dublin: Liffy Press, 2006.
- Sackmann, Sonja A. and Bertelsmann Stiftung. *Success Factor: Corporate Culture: Developing a Corporate Culture for High Performance and Long-Term Competitiveness, Six Best Practices*. Gütersloh: Verlag Bertelsmann Stiftung, 2006.
- Sloane, Robert M., Beverly LeBov Sloane, and Richard K. Harder. *Introduction to Healthcare Delivery Organizations: Functions and Management*. Chicago: Health Administration Press, 1999.
- Tosi, Henry L., John R. Rizzo, and Stephen J. Carroll. *Managing Organizational Behavior*. 3rd ed. Cambridge, MA: Blackwell Publishing, 1994.
- Links to business journals and management magazines http://www.brint.com/magazine.htm#ISJbus

scholarly journals

- *Academy of Management Review*
- *Harvard Business Review*
- *Journal of Healthcare Management*
- *MIT Sloan Management Review*
- *Organization Science*
- *Strategic Management Journal*

other relevant periodicals

- *Healthcare Executive*

in practice

in healthcare facilities, where do nutrition services belong?

In most healthcare facilities, food and nutrition services are rolled together into one department, the name of which usually reflects the mission of the department. For example, "Food and Nutrition Services Department" implies that the department provides both food and nutrition services, and that foodservice is the main focus. "Nutrition and Food Services Department," by its name, tells the observer that nutrition is the centerpiece of the department. In the past, the department that prepared and served foods was known as the "Dietary Department." That name has largely become outdated, in large part because the word "diet" is associated with denial or deprivation of food and thus has many negative connotations.

Some practitioners question the rationale that keeps foodservices and nutrition services in the same department, arguing that the relationship is obsolete and has no basis in today's reality. Let's look back into history to see why food and nutrition services were originally located in the same department, and if this rationale still holds in the twenty-first century.

In the early part of the last century, the profession of dietetics did not exist, and many hospitals relied on the families of patients to bring food in from home. As hospitals evolved, they began to provide foods to their patients; often these foods were grown in gardens and farms on the hospital grounds. When the American Dietetic Association was founded in 1917, the early dietitians were responsible for the preparation and service of food to their patients as well as whatever nutritional care was provided. The only way to nourish people in those days was with food. Intravenous solutions of any type were considered an "extraordinary measure" in the 1920s and the concept of total parenteral nutrition was non-existent. Tube feedings, first used in the 1950s, were made from foods ground in the hospital kitchen; commercial enteral feedings did not become available until the 1960s.

Given these circumstances, it is only reasonable that food and nutrition services went hand in hand. Patients were not billed for food and nutrition services and the cost of the food and nutrition services was included in the room charges. (In many situations, this is still the case.) Hospital dietetics was based on using foods as part of the treatment for diseases.

Foodservice to the non-patient customer used to be incidental to patient services. Dietary departments fed staff so that they could do their work and not have to leave the building to eat. External customers were not encouraged to eat in staff cafeterias. Sometimes, the food for staff was heavily subsidized and external customers were banned.

management practice in dietetics

Fast-forward to the twenty-first century … There are a myriad of ways to feed patients: total parenteral nutrition, peripheral parenteral nutrition, disease-specific tube feedings that can be delivered directly into the stomach or the jejunum, enteral oral supplements, standard and special-use infant formulae, and a wide variety of vitamin and mineral supplements. Food is still used, and indeed it is the preferred method of feeding patients, but it is not the sole means available to the clinical dietitian. Clinical nutrition services (assessment, diagnosis, and intervention), enteral supplements, and alternative feeding solutions and equipment are expensive and in many cases cannot be absorbed as part of the room rate. Some hospitals find it necessary to bill separately for these products and services.

The foodservice has changed, too. It is no longer a matter of walking out to the garden and picking some vegetables. Food is purchased from large wholesale vendors and is delivered to the foodservice in various states of preparedness. Some places have installed elaborate, high-tech cook-chill foodservice systems and operate more like a factory than a kitchen. Foodservices serve patient meals, but that may no longer be their primary focus. The paying customer, who now includes hospital staff, outpatients, patients' families, and visitors, expects high-quality, restaurant-style food. In addition, meals for staff are not generally subsidized and the foodservice is either profit-driven or expected to break even. Healthcare foodservices are focusing more and more on the non-patient customer; the operation must run like any other business.

Given these changes, the foodservices and nutrition services are drawing further and further apart. Nutrition services are patient-driven but foodservices may not be. Nutrition services require the expertise of a dietetic professional, though this is not necessarily true for foodservices, which are often ably managed by foodservice directors who are neither RDs nor DTRs.

From an organizational perspective, too, the services are divergent. Nutrition fits under the umbrella of clinical services. Comparable services include pharmacy, nursing, physical therapy, radiology, and the like. Foodservices are often considered a support service, which is a service that does not provide patient care. Other support services include environmental services, security, parking and transportation, engineering, and so forth.

So, with all of these changes, it is reasonable to think that the two services should be separate and should not remain in a single department. Foodservices should deal with the preparation and service of food and nutrition services should deal with clinical nutrition services and patient nutritional care issues. Theoretically, the departments do not need to interact except for those patients who are eating. It is reasonable to assume that the clinical dietitians can order food for the patients in the same way that physicians order drugs from the pharmacy.

In reality, the separation of the departments may work or it may not. A number of variables will determine if there is adequate reason for separating the two service areas in a given institution. These include at least the following:

- The size of the facility
- Whether the facility is a community hospital or a tertiary care facility
- The acuity of the patient population
- The percentage of patients who are able to eat
- Whether or not the facility is a teaching institution
- The fiscal position of the hospital
- The revenue potential for nutrition services
- Nutrition knowledge of the foodservice department staff
- Communication between the clinical nutrition and foodservice

Generally, large tertiary hospitals with an academic component and high-acuity patients can benefit from an independent nutrition services department. This is especially true in pediatric facilities where fewer than half of the patients may actually be served meals. In addition, the clinical component must be specialized enough to generate revenues of its own, and not merely be a cost center. (Clinical nutrition departments usually do not make a profit.) Typically in the US, if clinical nutrition cannot produce revenue, it stays under the umbrella of foodservices, which subsidizes clinical activities.

When an independent clinical nutrition department is established, a major issue is to determine where it fits in the organization. If clinical nutrition communicates well with the foodservices department, then the two may report to different administrators, the former to clinical services and the latter to support services. However, if the departments do not envision a common goal, then it may be necessary to have both report to the same administrator who will ensure cooperation between the two. It is obvious that, even if the departments are independent of each other, there still needs to be a good working relationship in order to ensure that patients who are eating get the appropriate foods and beverages.

Another area of concern is the ability of the clinical manager to manage an independent department. Traditionally, clinical managers have little financial experience and have been more involved with medical nutrition therapy issues than with management issues. A manager who runs a clinical department must have skills related to clinical issues, procedures, and protocols as well as skills related to management functions. This individual needs to have the ability to plan, organize, lead, and control, just like any other manager. Unfortunately, clinical nutritionists are sometimes ill-prepared in the management area because they concentrated more on their clinical coursework during their education. The biggest knowledge gap for clinical managers seems to be in the area of financial management, since more than half of clinical managers have no budget authority at all.[1] When clinical practitioners have insufficient management skills, it is often easier for the organization to keep the clinical services tied to foodservices, where experienced managers are readily available.

Finally, there is a cost issue of maintaining two separate management structures in an era of consolidation. Many managers are broadening their scope of practice to manage multiple departments. This is being done to flatten organizations and achieve cost efficiencies. Independent clinical nutrition departments may not work in small organizations because the manager's span of control is too limited to work for the organization.

Unfortunately, there is no "best" way to organize these complementary food and nutrition services. No master solution is available that will work in every instance. Each organization must evaluate its own situation and determine what works best for it. Several different models have worked and are working (including one innovative model where clinical nutrition service reports through the Pharmacy Department). The decision should be based on the options that are available, choosing the one that works best in a specific situation. Remember, too, that flexibility is crucial in this time of constant change. Periodic reevaluation of organizational structure in light of changes in the facility, the marketplace, and available management personnel is warranted to determine if and when a change in structure is appropriate.

---

[1]Sauer, K., D. Canter, and C. Shanklin. "Job Satisfaction of Dietitians with Management Responsibilities: An Exploratory Study Supporting ADA's Research Priorities." *Journal of the American Dietetic Association*. 110 1432–1440, 2010.

references

1. Robbins, S. P. and M. Coulter. *Management*. 11th ed. Upper Saddle River, NJ: Pearson Education, Inc., 2012, p. 6.
2. Children's Hospital Oakland. http://www.childrenshospitaloakland.org/about/about_mission.asp accessed June 17, 2012.
3. Cal Dining, University of California at Berkeley. http://caldining.berkeley.edu/vision.html accessed June 17, 2012.
4. Schein, E. H. *Organizational Culture and Leadership*. 4th ed. San Francisco: Jossey-Bass, 2010, p.18.
5. Spears, M. C. and M. B. Gregoire. *Foodservice Systems: A Managerial and Systems Approach*. Englewood Cliffs, NJ: Pearson Prentice Hall, 2004.
6. Sullivan, C. F. and C. Atlas. *Health Care Foodservice Systems Management*. Gaithersburg, MD: Aspen Publishers, 1998.
7. Halling, J. F. and M. A. Hess. "Vision vs Reality: ADA Members as Food/Food Management Experts." *Journal of the American Dietetic Association,* 95:169–170, 1995.
8. Lacey, K. and E. Pritchett. "Nutrition Care Process and Model: ADA Adopts Road Map to Quality Care and Outcomes Management." *Journal of the American Dietetic Association,* 103:1061–1072, 2003.
9. Boyle, M. A. and D. H. Morris. *Community Nutrition in Action: An Entrepreneurial Approach*. 3rd ed. Belmont, CA: Wadsworth Publishing Company, 2003.
10. Katz, Robert L. "Skills of an Effective Administrator." *Harvard Business Review,* 52:90–102, 1974.
11. Robbins, S. P. and M. Coulter. *Management*. 11th ed. Upper Saddle River, NJ: Pearson Education, Inc., 2012, p. 6.
12. Drejer, A. *Strategic Management and Core Competencies: Theory and Application*. Westport, CT: Quorum Books, 2002.
13. Mintzberg, Henry. *The Nature of Managerial Work*. New York: Addison Wesley Longman, 1973.

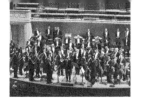

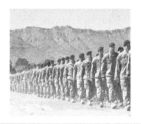

chapter three

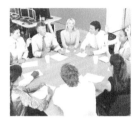

leadership

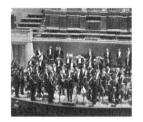

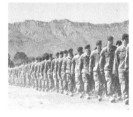

learning objectives

1. Differentiate between the terms *manager* and *leader*.

2. Differentiate between formal and informal leaders.

3. List some of the characteristics of effective leaders.

4. Describe the continuum of leadership styles.

5. Describe the various leadership styles and the advantages and disadvantages of each.

6. Define *transformational* and *transforming leadership*.

7. Discuss the concept of self-managed teams.

8. Describe the five types of power.

9. Differentiate between the ethical use and the abuse of power.

10. Identify the relationship between leadership and trust.

11. Discuss the social responsibility associated with leadership.

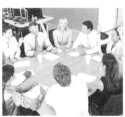

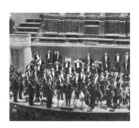

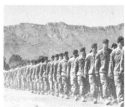

overview

The literature on leadership theory abounds with definitions of leadership. Most of the early studies focused on the characteristics of effective leaders. It was assumed that leadership was a characteristic inherent in certain individuals and was not something that could be learned or cultivated. Today, leadership traits have been identified, and many are behavioral characteristics that can be acquired. However, the level of comfort that the individual leader feels, and the degree to which these traits are compatible with the leader's personality, also contribute to success in leadership.

For the purpose of this chapter, leadership will be defined as that part of management that involves interpersonal relationships. It is the ability of an individual to work with people to achieve a shared organizational vision, as opposed to the management of tasks. Leadership is an essential part of management, but not all managers are effective leaders.

In this chapter, the discussion of leadership will be centered on the manager, and how managers may develop leadership behaviors. Characteristics of leaders will be described as will leadership styles, ranging from autocratic to consensus. This will be followed by a discussion of transformational and transforming leadership and of self-managed teams. There will be a description of the types of power exerted by leaders and the potential for the use and abuse of that power. The chapter will close with a discussion of leadership and social responsibility.

managers and leaders

Within the management structure of organizations, leaders can be found in the ranks of effective managers. But there is nothing inherent in the title of *manager* that guarantees that the person who holds the title will be a good leader. **Managers** who are not effective leaders are often found within organizations. These are the individuals who can effectively manage (plan, organize, and control) finances, production, purchasing, and the like, but have less success when working with staff.

Leaders, in addition to being good managers, are people-oriented. They work well with staff and demonstrate respect, concern, and empathy for others in the work setting. Leaders share with their employees. They share information, decision making, authority, rewards, trust, and vision. Leaders know how to relate to individuals as individuals, finding ways to honor differences while being fair to all employees. And leaders take risks when it will be of benefit to the work group. A more in-depth look at the qualities of effective leaders is found later in this chapter.

Managers.
Individuals found within organizations who can effectively manage (plan, organize, and control) finances, production, and purchasing, but may not be considered effective leaders.

Leaders. *Individuals who are considered good managers, work well with staff, and demonstrate respect, concern, and empathy for employees.*

formal and informal leaders

Within every organization (or other social system), two types of leaders exist. The first is the **formal leader**, who is usually a manager and is endowed by the organization with a position and a title that reflect the individual's status. Such leaders are recognized by the organization and are expected to assume the mantle of leadership, which includes setting the direction for subordinates and facilitating the ability of the staff to fulfill the organizational vision. The other type of leader is the **informal leader**. This is an individual who exhibits many of the characteristics of the formal leader, but is not recognized as a leader by the organization. The informal leaders do not perform the other management functions of planning, organizing, and controlling. Often, they do not have the skills necessary to be managers. These informal leaders have no titles and no authority, but exert a significant influence on colleagues, nevertheless. Examples of informal leaders might include a senior employee, an employee with the greatest degree of technical expertise, or an individual who has a formal leadership post (for example, an elected member of the local school board) outside of the organization.

Because both types of leaders exert an influence in the workplace, both must be considered. In fact, one of the attributes of an effective leader is the ability to recognize leadership traits in others, to nurture those characteristics, and to enlist the support of those individuals in achieving organizational goals. The formal leader should identify informal leaders; earning their respect and support should be a high priority.

Though this chapter will center on the formal leader—that is, the manager who is also a leader—many of the characteristics described in this section and in the section on power can be applied to both the formal and the informal leader. For the remainder of this chapter, the word *leader* means formal leader, unless otherwise noted.

characteristics of effective leaders

There have been decades of study regarding the characteristics of effective leaders. Evidence shows that there are six major traits that characterize leaders—drive, motivation, integrity, self-confidence, intelligence, and expertise. Other traits include charisma, creativity, and flexibility.[1] Additional characteristics have been noted but are not as widely accepted. Though not all leaders are alike, and they do not all exhibit the traits listed above in the same relative proportions, these are the underlying characteristics that differentiate leaders from non-leaders.

Formal Leader.
A type of leader who is usually a manager and is recognized as one with a position and title that reflect the individual's status.

Informal Leader.
A type of leader who exhibits many characteristics of the formal leader but is not recognized as a leader by an organization and holds no title or authority.

intelligence

Intelligence. *A major leadership characteristic that includes the ability to acquire and retain knowledge, and to respond quickly and successfully to a given situation.*

One leadership characteristic that is universally accepted is **intelligence**. A good leader is usually endowed with a great deal of native intelligence. This is not necessarily correlated with educational level, though it is often assumed that people with a high level of education are intelligent. But not all leaders are highly educated, nor should they be. It is the intelligence, the ability to acquire and retain knowledge and to respond quickly and successfully to a new situation, that is the common trait.

The other factor to note regarding intelligence is that leadership is not directly related to measures of intelligence. Smarter individuals do not always make better leaders. In fact, some very intelligent individuals demonstrate none of the other traits of leadership. Intelligence in a leader must be complemented with other leadership traits.

drive

Drive. *A major trait of effective leaders that describes their ambition, efforts, and risks they take in order to succeed.*

Drive is another characteristic of effective leaders. Leaders are achievers, and they need to achieve in order to feel successful. They want to move ahead, take on difficult tasks, and implement new ideas. These people are ambitious and want to "fast track" their own careers. Often, they pull others along with them. To support the need for achievement and ambition, leaders are willing to put a lot of effort into their work, they are willing to take risks, and they are willing to stick with a task until there are successful outcomes.

Leaders expend a high level of energy. They set high standards of performance for themselves and others. But the standards set for employees are usually not as demanding as the standards the leaders set for themselves. Leaders would not expect their employees to do things that they are unwilling to do. For instance, if employees are expected to work overtime to meet a project deadline, the leader would consider it necessary to work overtime, too.

Take, for example, the dietitian who opens a small business, like a nutrition consulting service. This dietitian usually works longer and harder than any of the staff that she employs. There is the routine work and consultations that have to be done, but in addition, this owner/leader has to deal with finances, planning, quality improvement, contracts, growth, information systems, and so on. Furthermore, the risks are very personal in a small business, so she must deal with the added stress of potential personal losses. The success of the business depends not only on how well the leader performs but also how well her employees perform. This dietitian/leader must be driven in order to achieve success in the small business arena. Many individuals try, but fail to achieve success in small business, and often this is related to insufficient drive.

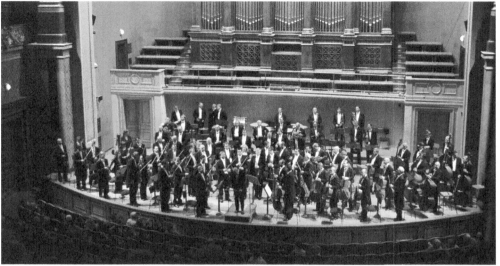

Source: http://commons.wikimedia.org/wiki/File:%C4%8CESK%C3%81_FILHARMONIE,_Rudolfinum_-_Dvo%C5%99%C3%A1kova_s%C3%AD%C5%88_2011.jpg. Copyright in the Public Domain.

One way leaders achieve their vision is by coordinating a well-orchestrated team.

motivation

Leaders want to be leaders. They have **motivation** toward a vision and want others to be able to see and follow that vision. It has been said that leaders actively seek power, and sometimes this is true. But the power that effective leaders seek is social power—that is, power that can be used for the good of all those in the work setting. Though some persons seek power for personal gain, the effective leader will choose to use power for the good of the group. Leaders know that indiscriminate or selfish use of power can, and often does, alienate followers and undermines the leadership role.

Not everyone wants to be a leader. Some think that leadership is a logical step in the career ladder of dietetics. That is, a clinical dietitian works her way from staff dietitian to a dietitian with a clinical specialty (for example, Certified Nutrition Support Dietitian or Certified Diabetes Educator) and then on to Clinical Nutrition Manager. This is a mistake. Some dietitians really want to be primary caregivers and do not want the responsibility of management or leadership. Dietitians who do not want a leadership position should not be coerced into accepting such a position. Without the motivation to lead, success as a leader is unlikely.

On the other hand, an entry-level dietitian may be dissatisfied with the status quo in a local hospital, where dietitians are still performing significant numbers of technical-level tasks each day. This "fresh-out-of-school" dietitian may want to change things and to "protect" the other professional staff from having to perform the less-professional parts of the job. This person has the motivation of a leader and is more likely to achieve leadership success than is a more experienced, but less enthusiastic, colleague.

Motivation. *A common trait in leaders essential to their realization of a vision or goal and part of their need to be a leader.*

integrity

Integrity is also an essential characteristic of a leader. In order to be effective in the leadership role, the leader must exhibit credibility, reliability, and fairness while being as open and honest as possible. Trust must be earned. One way to do this is to demonstrate consistency between what is said and what is done. Consider the clinic manager who states that the patient is the highest priority but then refuses to stay past closing time to see a client who was late for an appointment. The words and the action are not congruent, and such inconsistencies will not support a trusting relationship.

Another way that leaders demonstrate integrity and earn the trust of staff is by exhibiting fairness to all staff members and not "playing favorites." Even though individual employees are different and are motivated and rewarded in different ways, it is essential that good and bad performance be recognized with impartiality. For example, a good leader will not tolerate one employee's chewing gum while serving food to customers because the employee is a "good worker" and then penalize another worker for the same behavior. The performance expectations in a given job must be the same for all individuals doing that job. Other expectations, such as dress code, continuing education requirements, productivity, and so on, must also be consistent and be universally enforced.

self-confidence

Self-confidence is another trait of the effective leader. The leader must have enough of a sense of security to make decisions, to take risks, and to admit mistakes or to say, "I don't know." Those who follow must believe in the leader's self-confidence, too. Individuals who are self-confident and assertive move with ease in the leadership role. It is important that leaders maintain self-assurance in the face of negative comments and criticism, because it is unlikely that even the best leader will be liked by everyone, all of the time. The effective leader will have the poise to demonstrate "grace under pressure." The leader who wants to be everybody's friend will have difficulty making effective business decisions if it appears that a degree of personal stature might be lost, even if the loss is temporary.

expertise

The last trait that is usually considered to be necessary for an effective leader to have is **expertise** in the specific area being managed or in doing the tasks that are required. The type of expertise will vary, however, with the leader's management position. At lower management levels, the expertise required is more technical in nature, whereas at upper-management levels, conceptual expertise is more applicable. It is inevitable,

management practice in dietetics

then, as managers progress upward in an organization that their technical skills will lessen and their management skills will increase. Leadership skills should increase, too (though, unfortunately this does not always happen).

Consider, for example, the nutrition services component of a county health department. Assume that the health department has 15 clinic sites and employs 20 registered dietitians and 30 nutrition assistants. Each clinic site might have a dietitian manager who oversees the nutrition services at that site, including the nutrition assistants, the clerical help, and other dietitians who are assigned to that site. It is usual in this type of setting that the dietitian manager will also have a caseload to follow and must maintain the technical expertise to see clients with a variety of food, nutrition, and medical nutrition therapy needs. These might include issues of food acquisition, nutrition screenings, nutrition assessments, and counseling. This dietitian must be able to teach classes on maternal and child nutrition, give individual diet instructions, and make appropriate referrals for clients, while also fulfilling management functions.

At the county level, however, there is likely to be a chief or executive dietitian who oversees the nutrition services at all 15 clinic sites and to whom the 15 dietitian managers report. This executive dietitian will probably not do direct service and will not need to be as proficient at counseling and group education. However, additional expertise will be needed in the areas of strategic planning, fiscal management, staffing and human resources management, and so on. Once a manager reaches a certain level, the management skills become transferable from one management position to another, even without the accompanying technical skills. The management skills actually become the technical skills for some jobs.

other characteristics of leaders

charisma. Another characteristic that is widely accepted to be found in leaders is a degree of personal magnetism, or **charisma**. Some individuals have an ability to attract others to them and to be followed, sometimes without question. Historical examples of charismatic leaders include both heroes and villains—for example, Martin Luther King, Jr. and Adolf Hitler. The attraction toward a charismatic leader is not usually a physical one, though some persons with charisma may be physically attractive. The attraction is more likely to be based on the leader's ability to describe a vision for the future that is appealing to the follower. In addition, the charismatic leader energizes and enables followers to bring about the changes that are envisioned.[2] It can be a truly awesome trait to have. However, it is probably not essential to have charisma in order to be an effective leader.

It is also true that charisma alone is not enough. Without expertise and intelligence, a charismatic person might not be able to perform the more technical tasks of

Charisma. *A characteristic in leaders that reflects their degree of personal magnetism and their ability to attract others and to be followed.*

management. Without integrity and the ethical use of power, the charismatic leader may lead unquestioning followers into disaster. Charisma is a quality that supplements and enhances the major leadership traits described earlier.

creativity. Leaders must also possess enough **creativity** to look beyond existing paradigms for new ways to get things done. Some leaders actually possess the ability to create solutions on their own, and though this is an enviable trait, it is not absolutely necessary. What is necessary is that the leader be able to find such ideas, wherever they exist, and apply them in the context of current needs.

Consider the clinical nutrition manager who needed to update patient education materials for clients with celiac disease. The update was necessary because of changes in food labeling laws, and because of the growing number of new products in the marketplace that were designed for individuals with gluten intolerance. All previous materials that this hospital had related to nutrition education were printed booklets that could be given to the patient to take home. Since additional gluten-free products were being introduced every day, it was necessary to consider other approaches to presenting this material. It was no longer cost effective to reprint the materials each time a change occurred. In this case, the manager looked at the problem creatively and decided that the materials could be made available online. This allowed for changes to be made to the materials as necessary, but also allowed the dietitians to print the materials for those clients who did not have access to a computer at home. Once the limit of "we've always done it that way" is discarded, lots of options open to the innovative leader.

flexibility. The final characteristic of a leader to be discussed here is **flexibility**. This is a trait that is becoming more essential as information becomes more readily available to organizations. Managers and leaders must be able to react to the new information and are expected to make judgments and adjustments more quickly than ever. A leader who prefers to set a course and then watch events unfold will soon be lost. The nature of business today does not allow for such rigidity. Midcourse adjustments are now a part of management on an everyday basis.

This concept has always been a part of foodservice management, where production requirements change on a daily basis in relationship to customer numbers, weather conditions, market fluctuations, customer income level, and many other external forces. In other areas of dietetics, the need for midcourse adjustments has been less apparent. Patients used to stay in the hospital for much longer periods of time than they do today, and most of the dietitian's interventions took place in that setting. Since patients are going home sooner, it is necessary to move some of the dietitian's patient care activities from the inpatient to the outpatient setting. As cost containment becomes more of an issue under managed care, it is likely that frequent staffing adjustments will have to be made to accommodate this changing caseload. It is inevitable that the effective leader in dietetics must be able to obtain and interpret new information as it becomes available and make adjustments in a timely manner.

management practice in dietetics

Manager/Leader	Manager/Nonleader
Innovates	Administers
Develops	Maintains
Focuses on people	Focuses on systems
Inspires trust	Relies on control
Has a long-term view	Has a short-term view
Asks what and why	Asks why and how
Looks at the horizon	Looks at the bottom line
Is an original	Is a copy

Warren G. Bennis and Robert Townsend, *Reinventing Leadership: Strategies to Empower the Organization*, pp. 6–7. HarperCollins Publishers, 1997.

Table 3.1 Differences Between Managers with and Without Leadership Traits

One must also be cautious not to make the midcourse adjustments prematurely. If one reacts to incomplete information or inaccurate projections, it is possible to suffer irrevocable losses. The effective leader not only will make good decisions but will also know when those decisions must be made. Chapter 4 deals extensively with the decision-making process.

The leadership traits described here differentiate managers who are leaders from managers who are not leaders. See Table 3.1 for a list of how these differences are reflected in how these two groups perform. It is also important to consider these traits as they relate to dietitians and to dietetics as a profession.

Some of the characteristics of leaders listed on the previous pages are inherently found in dietetics professionals. For instance, dietitians usually have the intelligence and the expertise to become leaders if they wish to do so. Otherwise, they would not have been able to obtain their professional credentials. Integrity may also be assumed because the profession is self-regulated and has a published code of ethics under which individuals practice. (See the "In Practice" feature at the end of Chapter 1.) If there is noncompliance with this set of standards, the Registered Dietitian or Dietetic Technician, Registered is subject to disciplinary action that may result in the suspension of the credential.

Other leadership traits are very individual and may or may not exist in dietetics professionals. Drive, motivation, charisma, and creativity are attributes that are highly variable among dietetics professionals. That's to be expected. Not all of these are needed for effective leadership, and not every dietitian needs to assume a formal leadership role. If a dietitian lacks any of these traits and wants to become a leader, it would be appropriate to complete a self-assessment to determine areas for growth and how to strengthen those areas that need improvement.

At one time, it was not considered appropriate for dietitians (or, indeed, for women) to be assertive. Thus, seasoned practitioners may lack this particular trait. This is especially evident in those areas in which they have had little formal education, such as in management (other than foodservice) or in negotiation techniques. Many experienced dietetics professionals would benefit from personal development programs to improve their self-confidence. For some, the acquisition of knowledge in the content area where information is lacking might be needed. For others, assertiveness training would provide support for the practitioners' existing knowledge base. Fortunately, the Professional Development Portfolio established by the Commission on Dietetics Registration allows professionals to set a continuing education program for themselves that meets their learning needs.[3]

Dietitians are sometimes thought to be more rigid than other professionals. This may be a result of working with exact numbers and the degree of precision needed to do diet calculations and nutrient analyses or a function of the type of person who becomes a dietetics professional. Still, this trait is in direct conflict with the need for leaders to be creative and flexible. Dietitians, in general, need to identify ways in which they can develop flexibility and creativity.

Rigidity and lack of assertiveness will actually interfere with the individual dietitian's ability to lead and the profession's ability to produce effective leaders. Dietitians, individually and collectively, need to continue to find ways to nurture self-confidence and flexibility within the profession.

leadership styles

Leadership is partly a learned behavior, and partly a function of the personality of the leader. Most leaders use a variety of leadership styles, which vary with the situation. This variation can best be viewed on a continuum that ranges from autocratic to consensus management. Each leader, however, has a predominant leadership style, which is developed over time and is consistent with that individual's personality. This does not mean that the predominant leadership style is unchangeable, but it takes education, time, experience, discipline, and motivation to effect such a change. In most cases, the leader will be most effective when using the style that is most "comfortable."

Leaders are free to move along the continuum and adjust their own style to the circumstances. For example, a physician leader might have an autocratic style when giving orders regarding the care of patients and having those orders followed without question. However, if that physician is asked to chair the fundraising efforts of a building committee for his favorite hospital, he may use a participative leadership style to enhance fundraising efforts of the committee. Leaders who learn to switch among leadership styles can produce powerful results.[4] The remainder of this section will describe the different leadership styles and some of the pros and cons inherent in each style.

autocratic leadership

The **autocratic leadership** style, also called directive or command-and-control leadership, is illustrated by the leader who takes total control. That leader assumes full authority and takes full responsibility for the area being managed. The autocratic manager makes decisions, tells others of the decision, and expects them to carry out the decision without question. The physician described above is an autocratic manager in terms of patient care, and depends on the subordinates (nurses, dietitians, therapists, pharmacists, and so on) to follow the orders precisely. Thus, the patient's care is entirely the responsibility of the physician, who has assumed responsibility for both the quality of care and the patient outcomes.

Autocratic management is best exemplified by the military model, where the orders are carried out when and as issued; any questions are asked (if questions are asked at all) after the fact. This management style is often described as a traditional male management model, though male gender is not requisite to using this method. Men seem to have more success when using this model than do women.[5,6] It is important to note that this leadership style, though associated with the military, is not the only type of leadership used in the military. Other leadership models are used in noncombat situations, though autocratic leadership is frequently used in combat situations.[7] Outside of the military, autocratic leadership is most effective when used in either a crisis or in situations where there is a limited window of opportunity. It works best when used by a proven leader who has earned the trust and support of subordinates prior to having the need to be autocratic.

Just as the autocratic style of leadership is the dominant leadership style of some managers, it is also preferred by some of the employees who are being managed. Frequently, unskilled workers may feel that it is the responsibility of the manager to tell the worker what to do and how to do it, and that it is the responsibility of the worker to carry out the manager's wishes. These workers want only to do what they are told to do, and to receive fair compensation for their time and effort. This preference may also be held by some individuals who come from places where autocratic leadership is the norm. Such people may find that the leadership style that they are most comfortable with is the one to which they are accustomed. In addition, people who work in an environment where they cannot use their native tongue may fear being misunderstood when asked to contribute ideas to the management process; they often prefer to be told to do tasks that they know and understand and where there is minimal chance for miscommunication. In short, some workers are selling their time and do not feel obligated or inclined to contribute their ideas. For this type of person, a leader with an

Autocratic Leadership. *A leadership style illustrated by a leader who takes total control, assumes full authority, and takes full responsibility for the area managed.*

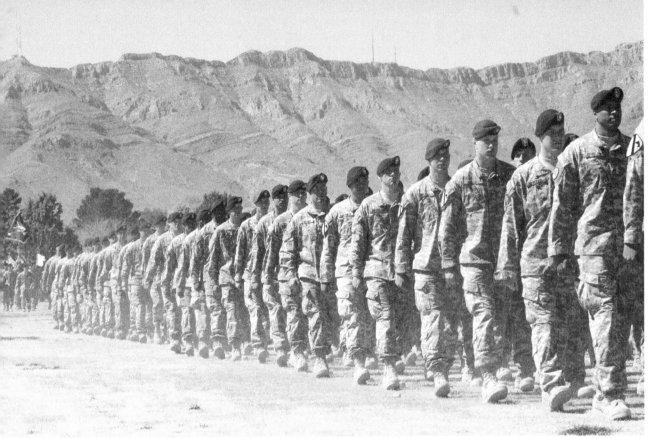

Autocratic leadership is used in military training.

autocratic style is a good fit. Leaders and managers who work with subordinates who prefer an autocratic leadership style would do well to adopt this style in the specific situation, even though this is not their usual method of operating.

There are some distinct advantages to this leadership style. The major benefit is that it saves time. One person gathers the necessary data and moves forward without the necessity of calling meetings and seeking the input of others. It is necessary for all leaders to be autocratic when timeliness is a factor. If, for example, an accident happens in the workplace, the leader must take immediate action to minimize the risk to staff and to the organization. When a decision must be made rapidly, the leader usually assumes an autocratic stance, whether or not it is the preferred style of that leader. It would constitute unjustifiable risk to use participative leadership methods in an emergency situation. For example, it would be very dangerous to seek the input of 12 different middle managers before calling an ambulance to transport an injured employee to an emergency room.

The major disadvantage of the autocratic leadership style is that the leader makes many decisions in a vacuum, not taking advantage of the experience and insights of others on the management team. It is possible to have all the information needed

management practice in dietetics

to make a good decision and still make a poor one because of inexperience or the inability to look at a problem from varying perspectives. Also, the other members of the management team are likely to become alienated and disgruntled if their ideas are not considered by the autocratic manager. Given sufficient time, better decisions come from participative management than from autocratic management.

The autocratic style is also used for making "programmed" decisions. A programmed decision is one that is made routinely and can be made by one individual with information that is on hand. An example might be the decision to call in a replacement worker for one who has failed to report to work. This type of decision making is automatic; it is guided by precedent or by a written procedure for making the decision so that consultation with others is unnecessary.

Individuals whose primary leadership style is autocratic are often labeled as "controlling" or as "micro-managers" because they are reluctant to delegate authority. In general, their subordinates feel disenfranchised and unable to make meaningful contributions to the organization. Many are unhappy with the work situation. In most cases, the predominant use of the autocratic leadership style in today's workplace is counterproductive and should be avoided.

The autocratic leadership style is being used with less frequency than in the past, though under some circumstances it is necessary for a leader to be autocratic. More and more, it is being recognized that a participative management style is usually more effective than an autocratic one.

participative leadership

One of the most widely used leadership styles is **participative leadership**. In this type of leadership, the manager gathers information necessary to take action and then seeks the opinions of colleagues and/or subordinates before doing anything. With the participative management style, the manager still "sets the agenda" and makes the decisions, but this is done only after there has been input from others. In addition to seeking input, the participative manager may share information with subordinates so that the subordinates have enough data to provide the best possible input. Sometimes the subordinates actually generate the data for the manager and deliver it with an analysis that will help the manager to do the best thing.

An advantage of using participative leadership is that one has a variety of ideas from which to work and is less likely to make errors relative to insufficient evidence or narrow perspectives. In addition, subordinates feel that what they have to say is important and has been heard. This allows them to feel some ownership within the organization. The majority of employees in today's workforce, especially those who are middle managers or professionals, want to feel that they "have a say" in how their

Participative Leadership. *A commonly used leadership style in which the leader gathers information and seeks the opinions of colleagues and/or subordinates before taking action.*

organization runs. The participative manager is likely to be rewarded with increased loyalty and support from staff.

It should be noted, too, that managers who elicit information and opinions from their subordinates are expected to use the information and ideas that are generated. Participative management is not just hearing what the subordinate has to offer but also involves using those ideas or, at the very least, informing the staff why the ideas were not used. If employees' ideas are solicited but never used, staff will learn to distrust the manager and will eventually stop participating in the process. This can be related to the earlier discussion of the leader's integrity. There must be congruity between the seeking of information and ideas from subordinates and the use of that material in the management process.

It is also a good idea for a leader who uses the participative methodology to be willing to share the credit for success. A manager who takes full credit for the success of an idea, project, or decision that was accomplished using staff participation may be viewed by subordinates as self-serving or power-hungry. In the long term, this may undermine the manager's credibility. A leader who credits subordinates with the successes in which they participated will gain support from staff. In addition, superiors usually view the success of the group as an indication of the effectiveness of the manager, so that the leader does not lose stature with superiors by sharing credit with staff.

There are disadvantages to this leadership style, too. Participative leadership takes time and energy. Many individuals must be brought up to speed on an issue. In the sharing of information, the leader will lose some sense of "control." There will be a need to incorporate the ideas and information from a variety of sources into a workable whole. In short, the process of management loses a degree of efficiency.

There is also a problem because the manager is not free to share all pertinent information with subordinates. What is shared may be incomplete because of confidentiality issues. For example, a manager cannot share information about the salary of specific people when a group is working on a plan to downsize an organizational unit. This and other information may be subject to "leaks" and should not be shared.

No matter how much the manager prefers to use participative leadership techniques, when time constraints or confidentiality issues are present, staff participation in the management process may have to be limited or eliminated. However, for the leader whose usual leadership style is participative, the situations when autocracy is used will likely be viewed as a demonstration of the leader's strength, rather than as a demonstration of the need for power or control.

With participative management, the manager still takes responsibility for making the final decision, but the decision is based on a more complete data set than if the decision were made autocratically. Communication of the decision, and the materials that supported it, should flow back down to the contributing staff members. This will enhance the leader's credibility. Though participative management is more time-consuming than autocratic management, it is worth the investment because it helps to develop the trust, loyalty, and goodwill that are needed in a productive work setting, and it helps to keep the lines of communication open in both directions.

Sometimes leaders feel that decision making is actually a group function. Thus, they carry participative management a step further and adopt a democratic management style.

democratic leadership

The **democratic leadership** style is one in which decisions are made by the group, rather than by the manager alone. Once again, it should be stated that this technique will not be used for all decisions. Routine decisions will not be taken to the group, nor will those that require immediate attention or those that involve confidential matters. The types of decisions that are typically made by groups are decisions related to policies and procedures, the hiring of new staff, the development of marketing and strategic plans, and so on. The theory behind using the democratic leadership technique is that if people agree with a decision, there is an increased likelihood that these individuals will actively work to make the outcome successful. This technique guarantees that the majority of staff goes on record as agreeing with the decision, and therefore each of them takes partial ownership of the outcome.

When used effectively, this method enhances the probability of reaching a good decision and improves the success rate relative to outcomes. However, those involved in the process must have access to the most relevant information in order to achieve consistently positive outcomes. In the following situation, staff members have access to much but not all of the information needed to complete a task.

The scenario is one in which a search committee has been appointed to make recommendations for hiring a staff dietitian. The process starts with a preliminary screening of the employment applications of several candidates to eliminate those whose qualifications do not meet minimum standards. Depending on the number of qualified applicants, a phone interview may be conducted by a member of the search committee to determine which candidates should actually be brought in for a personal interview. Those candidates selected for an interview will then be interviewed by members of the search committee. At the completion of the interviews, search committee members must meet and arrive at a decision about which candidates are acceptable to the group, and they must rank acceptable candidates. (Because the employment agreement is a two-way contract, it cannot be assumed that the candidate who is the first choice of the committee will accept the position.) The search committee does not make the job offer, because the issue of compensation is the part of the transaction that requires confidentiality. The manager's role is to make

Democratic Leadership. *A leadership style based on "majority rules," in which decisions are made by the group rather than by the manager alone.*

employment (and compensation) offers in the order set by the search committee until a dietitian accepts the position.

Democratic leadership is even more time-consuming than participative leadership. If a majority of staff cannot agree on a course of action, no action can be taken at all. This delays progress and can cause an organization to miss opportunities until a majority of individuals come to agreement. Another disadvantage of the democratic style is the fact that the "majority rules." If the majority of the group reaches agreement, but one member of the group is really opposed to the decision that has been made, that member may (consciously or unconsciously) work against the implementation of the decision to justify his or her position.

A manager who uses the democratic leadership style increases the chances of reaching good decisions and attaining positive outcomes. But the possibility of sabotage always exists for the democratic leader. The management style that avoids the "majority rules" pitfall is known as consensus management.

consensus management

Consensus management is the type of management most often associated with women managers. It is a style that has been evolving over the past decade at the same time as more and more women take on the responsibilities of leadership. Therefore, the apparent association between women and the consensus style may be nothing more than a matter of coincidence. It can be and is used by individuals of either gender. Like the other leadership styles described here, it is one point on a continuum. Probably there are as few purely consensus leaders as there are purely autocratic leaders. Most leaders move along the continuum as the situation dictates.

Consensus leadership requires that decisions or plans be made by a group. Consensus requires that every member of the group must agree with the action that will be taken. The group must work together until all members reach agreement. This is easier said than done. It involves many people making compromises so that each member of the group can be accommodated, because everyone must live with the decision.

In the case of the search committee described earlier, consider that the five members of this group had interviewed all of the candidates and were now meeting to rank the four finalists for the position. (The finalists were Jennifer, Latoya, Glenn, and Mercedita.) Four members of the search committee ranked Mercedita as their first choice, based on her experience and her skill in answering the clinical questions that were part of the structured interview for each candidate. The fifth member of the committee ranked Mercedita last because she was older than the rest of the candidates and "might not have enough energy to carry the workload." Under the democratic model discussed earlier, Mercedita would have been offered the position

Consensus Leadership. *A leadership style that requires that decisions or plans be made by a group and is based on all members working together until agreement is reached.*

management practice in dietetics

Leadership Style	Major Characteristics
Autocratic Leadership	Leader gathers necessary data to make decisions or take action on his/her own, without consulting others; expects others to follow without question. Process is efficient, from the perspective of time. Decisions may be flawed because of limited data.
Participative Leadership	Leader seeks input from others before making management decisions. May or may not use the information gathered to make decisions or take action. May communicate the decision to participants in the process; shares credit with others.
Democratic Leadership	Leader defers to the group for decision-making, with the majority position being the one that is taken. Process is relatively time-consuming. Others may readily support the decision because they actively participated in the process.
Consensus Leadership	Leader requires the entire group reach agreement on a decision before action is taken. Process is extremely time-consuming and may never reach a conclusion. Generally all members of the group support the action, because of the negotiation and compromise involved in the process.

Table 3.2 Leadership Styles

first. Under the consensus model, she cannot yet be offered the position, because all members of the search committee are not in agreement. The committee will have to have further discussions on the relative merits of each candidate until agreement is negotiated. The dissenting member might be convinced that her opinion represents age discrimination and drop her objection, but it is more likely that the group will reach consensus on ranking another candidate first and Mercedita will drop to second or third place.

From this illustration, it becomes obvious that the consensus model is the most time-consuming of all those discussed. It can take months, or even years, to reach consensus. Sometimes the group never reaches consensus. Sometimes it becomes necessary for the manager to revert to the participative model and make the decision.

Another negative aspect of consensus leadership is that, while the process is ongoing, the manager may appear to outsiders to be unable to make a decision. An effective leader will know when it is appropriate to seek consensus and when it would be counterproductive to do so.

The major advantage of this leadership style is that staff members feel that they are an integral and valued part of the team. There is the feeling that each voice is heard in a safe environment and that what is said is important. This is often accompanied by improvement in group cohesiveness and teamwork and fierce loyalty to the manager.

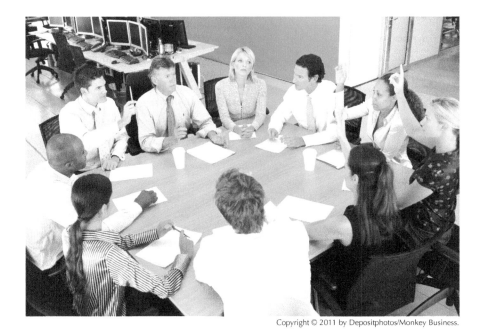

Leaders often encourage their employees to participate in the management process.

Transformational Leadership. *A leadership style that transforms employees who merely carry out their duties to employees who feel comfortable in contributing their input to the management process.*

Transforming Leadership. *A leadership style that prepares the subordinate to take over management functions and, in some cases, to become the successor to the manager.*

transformational and transforming leadership

Within the writings on leadership, there are two additional terms that require some explanation. The first of these is **transformational leadership**, which came into vogue in the late 1970s. It can be defined as the type of leadership that transforms staff from rugged individuals into team players. Transformational leadership provides individuals with the support they need to develop into workers who are willing and able to contribute their input to the management process. All but the autocratic leadership style, described earlier, represent transformational leadership, which deals with two-way interaction between the manager and the staff.

Transforming leadership goes a step further and actually prepares the subordinate to take over management functions, perhaps even to become the successor to the manager. This is less attractive to managers than transformational leadership, because few managers want to work themselves out of a job. Still, good leaders do "succession planning" by developing leadership skills in staff members. Both the democratic and the consensus leadership styles can be a part of transforming leadership. In addition, the staff members who are learning to become leaders must learn to make autocratic and programmed decisions as well.

management practice in dietetics

self-managed teams

The idea for self-managed teams (teams without a designated manager)[8] developed in the 1980s in a scenario that could have been something like this. Some professional work groups that were led by democratic or consensus-style managers lost their leaders through attrition—for example, by retirement or promotion of the manager. While looking for managers to fill the vacant positions, personnel departments were unsuccessful in finding replacement managers who were willing to take on new positions using these leadership models. The work groups were unable to accept other leadership styles. In many cases, the now-absent manager had been a "transforming" leader who was grooming the staff for independence. The parent organizations introduced self-managed teams using the rationale that if the democratic or consensus models worked in the presence of a manager, it could work without an identified leader. As an added benefit to the organization, there are significant cost benefits associated with the self-managed team because there is no need to hire a manager.

The unanswered question is, "Do self-managed teams really work?" Some do, under defined circumstances and in specific situations. However, the long-term effectiveness of this model is unknown. Some of the issues involved in the self-managed team approach follow.

project work

Self-managed teams work well on projects in which the team is established to address a problem or perform a task and knows that it will be disbanded when the project is complete. **Project teams** may be from within a departmental staff (a group of clinical dietitians working to revise patient education materials) or may cross departmental lines (a team that includes a clinical dietitian, a foodservice manager, a foodservice worker, a nursing unit clerk, and a nurse manager to develop a policy for late tray delivery to patients). Project teams have only one item on the agenda and do not deal with day-to-day operational issues. Such groups establish their own processes and timelines. They are frequently used to address issues of quality management.

Self-managed teams also work well during transitional periods, such as the time between when a manager vacates a position and a replacement is hired. Again, there is some definition to the task—in this case, a limited period of time. However, the task is not as well defined because day-to-day operations are subject to a lot of variability, much of which is not predictable.

Self-Managed Teams. *Work groups that function without a designated manager and involve the team members in decision making and in working together to manage themselves.*

Project Teams. *A type of self-managed team whose duties do not include day-to-day operational issues but, instead, a specific issue for which they are free to set deadlines and processes.*

day-to-day operations

It is more difficult for self-managed teams to function in day-to-day operations. This relates to the fact that all members of the group are equal and no one member has authority over other members, nor does one member have the sole responsibility for decision making. Sometimes self-managed teams implement a rotation schedule for making routine decisions, in which each member of the team assumes this responsibility for a week, a month, or a quarter. In other situations, a member of the team who is particularly good at day-to-day operations becomes the team leader and assumes the responsibility for routine decision making, such as scheduling and processing payroll documents. This can create problems because the team leader is performing additional tasks without being compensated. To avoid this dilemma, the team leader may be relieved of some of the routine duties, or may earn additional compensation. If the latter occurs, the team leader becomes the "acting" manager, and the concept of the self-managed team disappears.

why democratic/consensus managers are not hired

There are several reasons it is difficult to hire a democratic or consensus manager. The basic reason is that these leadership styles require that a degree of trust be established between the leader and the staff before implementation. A prospective manager would be ill-advised to create expectations of a certain type of leadership before initially getting to know the staff in a working situation and determining what style would be most appropriate to use. Because managers are free to move along the leadership style continuum, it is common for a new manager to start by using less-participative management models and then to move toward the consensus model.

Another reason that newly hired managers are not inclined to use the consensus model from the outset is that there are many decisions that must be made in the first days and weeks of employment. (This is particularly true if the position is one that has been vacant for a period of time, or if the previous manager did not perform well.) With so many changes to be addressed in a short period of time, there is not enough time to utilize the consensus model.

Finally, the democratic and consensus models are dependent on a functional work group. When a new individual enters such a group, there is a transition period during which the new member is assimilated into the group. During this time, the dynamics of the group change. If the new member happens to be the new manager, the adjustments will be major and the group may need a substantial period of time to adjust to and to accept the new leader. This process takes more time than the new manager has available for decision making in the initial period of employment. Actions cannot be deferred until the group has adjusted to the new member.

It is possible to hire from within the group, especially if the previous manager had done succession planning and had mentored an individual to assume the management role. In such situations, the new manager is familiar with the group processes and protocols and can move more quickly toward the consensus model, if that is desired. But even in this optimal situation, there still must be transition because a replacement for the manager is entering the group and the new manager is adjusting to a change in role. A change in group dynamics is inevitable and will probably necessitate some autocratic behavior on the part of the new manager, who is trying to demonstrate integrity and credibility as well as develop the trust of staff members, and to establish who now has final authority.

The long-term success of self-managed teams is unknown. Many such teams have had difficulty with coordination and with productivity. They are frequently disbanded before their effectiveness can be measured. The frustration is often due to a lack of leadership. It may evolve that the successful self-managed team will actually be a team that is managed with the consensus leadership model.

power

When discussing leadership, it is necessary to consider **power** and the use of power by both managers and leaders. It was stated earlier that an effective (and moral) leader uses power for the social good, rather than for personal gain, but the line between the two is not always clear. Before discussing the use and abuse of power, it is appropriate to look at power itself, and the types of power that a manager or a leader might have.

types of power

It is generally accepted that there are five types of power.[9] These are expert power, referent power, legitimate power, reward power, and coercive power. A brief description of each follows. See Table 3.2 for a synopsis of these types of power.

expert power. **Expert power** is found within the individual and is sometimes referred to as the power of knowledge, experience, or information. Most likely, it is some combination of the three. This type of power is found in both the formal and the informal leader as well as in managers. Individuals who are educated or experienced in a certain field may exert influence on others because of their knowledge in that field.

Earlier in this chapter, a situation related to the development of online patient education materials for celiac disease was used to illustrate the trait of creativity in a clinical nutrition manager. It might even be that the manager or a staff dietitian uploaded these

Power. *The source of a leader's influence over subordinates. It may originate from the leader, from the subordinate, from the position, or from the leader's ability to dispense rewards or punishment.*

Expert Power. *A type of power—also known as the power of knowledge, experience, and information—in which an individual can exert influence on others due to their knowledge in a certain field.*

Expert Power	Power based on knowledge, experience, or information
Referent Power	Power based on the followers' view of the leader as a leader
Legitimate Power	Power derived from the position or title that is held
Reward Power	Power based on the control of resources to compensate individuals for good performance
Coercive Power	Power to punish those who perform poorly

Table 3.3 Types of Power

materials into a user-friendly website. If, however, the clients subsequently had need of a corresponding SmartPhone application (app) for this material, it is unlikely that the clinical nutrition manager could develop such an app. A more probable scenario is that a computer engineer on the project (self-managed) team will be consulted to assist with the development of the app. In this situation, it is the computer engineer who has the "expert" power because it this person knows how to go about meeting the particular technical needs of the project. Conversely, the dietitian is the expert when it comes to developing content that meets the Celiac Disease Evidence-based Nutrition Practice Guidelines from the Academy of Nutrition and Dietetics.[10] It is not necessary for a manager or a leader to have expert power in all situations.

Expert power may be shared with colleagues and subordinates. To do so, however, one must either not seek power in the first place, or be self-confident enough to know that the knowledge is not the only source of one's power. If an individual seeks knowledge and information and is not willing to share it freely with colleagues and subordinates, it might be assumed that the individual is insecure or that the accompanying power is intended for personal, rather than social, gain. Competitive individuals are often unwilling to share their knowledge with others; this is counter to effective leadership, which seeks to build teams to achieve the organizational vision.

Referent Power.
A type of power that comes from the relationship between a leader and his or her followers and is not related to the leader's position but to the ability to create and share a vision.

referent power. **Referent power** comes from the relationship that exists between a leader and the followers. It characterizes both formal and informal leaders, though it may not be present in managers who are not leaders. The leader is viewed as a role model or as a mentor and, as such, possesses power. Referent power is not related to the position one holds, but rather is dependent on one's ability to create and share a vision. It is related to the respect that is shared between the leader and the follower, between teacher and student. Referent power is usually established over a period of time. Charismatic leaders exert a great deal of referent power.

When trying to conceptualize referent power, dietitians and dietetic students would do well to reflect upon those individuals who most influenced their careers. It may have been a practicing dietitian who directed volunteer work for high school students in the local hospital. It may have been a nutrition counselor who helped grandpa to lose weight after his first heart attack. It might have been a teacher who introduced nutrition in a high school health class. All of these individuals have referent power.

legitimate power. **Legitimate power** is bestowed on an individual because of the position held. It is the type of power that usually differentiates the formal from the informal leader. However, informal leaders may have some degree of legitimate power because of positions they hold outside of the workplace, such as captain of the bowling team or school board member, even if it is not recognized in the work setting.

Both managers and leaders hold legitimate power, and both may use that power effectively. In school foodservice, the dietitian who directs the operations for an entire school district would hold legitimate power in the eyes of the managers of an individual school's foodservice.

reward power. **Reward power** gives one the resources to reward staff members. As such, it is a powerful tool. It includes the ability to increase pay, give bonuses, and distribute resources (such as equipment, office space, parking privileges, funding to attend meetings, and so on) to favored individuals. It can also be embodied in other forms of recognition, such as a pat on the back, a private "thank you," or public acknowledgment for a job well done. It should be noted that the reward must be tailored to meet the recipient's needs, not the needs of the manager.

A clinical nutrition manager might feel that four of the six staff dietitians in the department are deserving of some sort of reward for a job well done, but there is a salary freeze and staff members will universally be given a 2 percent pay hike at the end of the calendar year. In order to reward the staff members for good performance, the dietitian should know the needs of individual staff members and find a suitable way to recognize each. For the dietitian who is planning to publish an article in the *Journal of the Academy of Nutrition and Dietetics*, paid time to do a literature search in the hospital's library might be appropriate. Another, who recently passed the registration exam, may benefit from financial support to attend the state dietetic association meeting. The third, who has expressed the desire to move into management, could be rewarded by being given some formal management training within the organization, accompanied by the opportunity to actually perform some management tasks during the manager's vacation. The fourth, a Certified Diabetes Educator who loves teaching, might be encouraged to develop a series of classes for clients with newly diagnosed diabetes mellitus.

Reward power can be a double-edged sword, too. It can build support within an organization if it is administered in an evenhanded way, or it can foster divisiveness if favoritism is suspected. Rewards may buy loyalty and commitment, or may only produce compliance, depending on how they are administered and on how the manager is perceived by subordinates. An effective leader will find ways to use rewards adequately, appropriately, efficiently, and effectively.

Legitimate Power.
A type of power that usually differentiates the formal from the informal leader and is related to the position held by the individual who exerts the power.

Reward Power.
A type of power that is based on the ability to reward employees in terms of material goods (for example, pay raise or privileged parking) or praise (for example, public acknowledgment).

*A type of power
managers have to
punish, which can
be seen in disci-
plining, suspending,
or terminating
employees for
cause, or in laying
off staff when
needed.*

coercive power. Coercive power is the power to punish. Management has the right to discipline, suspend, or terminate employees for cause, or to lay off staff when there is no work for them. In nonunion settings, individuals who are poor performers are the ones who are laid off whenever there is a reduction-in-force (RIF); this illustrates another use of coercive power. This type of power is a very real part of the power that a manager holds, and must be exercised with great care.

In theory, this type of power has been curtailed significantly in the United States, as state and local governments have made it illegal to take arbitrary action or to discriminate on the basis of age, race, or gender. Unions also play a role in protecting individuals from the coercive power of managers. But even with legal protection, workers often feel threatened by managers because of the importance that the job has in the employee's life. People who need to earn money to feed the family, provide medical care, pay the rent, and so on, often feel that they have to put up with abuse from the management in order to keep the job. Even professionals make compromises if they need the job badly enough.

In one very sad situation, a group of clinical dietitians were faced with an RIF in their hospital department. In order to secure their own jobs, which they needed for a variety of personal reasons, they convinced management to lay off the dietetic technicians and the diet clerks. The rationale was that the dietitians were able to do all three jobs (which was true, though dietitians usually do not do clerical work). Over time, the dietitians found themselves so busy with tasks such as answering the phone, processing computer orders, writing diets, tallying menus, and checking trayline that there was little time for the screening, assessment, and care of patients. They compromised their professional standards in order to keep their jobs. After several years, their clinical skills diminished and they no longer functioned as clinical dietitians. Though this is an extreme situation, it illustrates what can happen when individuals feel the need to keep their jobs, no matter the cost.

In addition, more subtle forms of coercion exist in the workplace such as withholding pay increases, increasing workloads, assigning undesirable tasks, scheduling someone to work irregular shifts, and generally making the job so unpleasant that the employee will seek alternatives. These less direct forms of coercion may be implemented consciously or unconsciously by the manager. Effective leaders will avoid the use of subtle coercion because of the negative effect it has on credibility.

Sometimes, subtle coercion encourages the individual to find another job, but more often the resulting stress of working in an unpleasant environment leads to illness. The latter is costly, in terms of insurance, loss of productivity, ill will, and numerous other factors. A manager who is tempted to exercise indirect coercion on a staff member would do well to look at the potential costs. It is often a no-win situation.

A leader will be prudent in the use of coercion for a number of reasons. First, the management position, in and of itself, represents coercive power. The leader doesn't have to flex muscles to demonstrate this power. Second, integrity requires that the leader be evenhanded and fair, and it is unfair to target specific individuals with subtle forms of punishment. And finally, coercion is not consistent with team-building, which is the goal of an effective leader. It is much more effective (and less costly) to work with poor performers to improve their performance, just as the leader works with good performers to enhance their accomplishments.

use and abuse of power

That managers and leaders have power is inevitable. It is how the power is used that is important. Power may be used for the common good or for personal gain. The use of power for the common good is considered to be positive and moral. It is a good thing for a leader to do. Using power for the common good includes such things as providing equal opportunity for all employees, giving bonuses to the staff when a company has had a profitable year, making sure that the working environment is as safe as possible to minimize physical injuries, and protecting staff from having to make compromises, such as the ones described on the previous page (in which the dietitians were faced with an RIF).

Using power for personal gain includes such things as using the company's copier and paper for a personal business or social club activities, shopping for oneself on an office computer during business hours, or selecting a vendor who charges a premium price for a generic product because the vendor is one's cousin. Such abuse of power can be blatant or subtle, but can exist at all levels of management. It is impossible for a leader/manager to be insulated from opportunities to abuse power, so integrity becomes a critical factor.

Unfortunately, the question of abuse of power is not always clear. One common practice is that the executives in a company, a hospital, or a school are given preferred parking. It might be said that this custom prevails because the people who have the authority to confer this privilege are the people who use it, and it constitutes an abuse of power for personal gain. On the other hand, executives justify this privilege with the fact that they work longer hours than others, come in and out at odd hours, and would waste company time if they had to park at the far end of the lot. In fact, they feel that it benefits the organization to provide them with this "perk." This may, indeed, be true. (As an aside, note that many executives could benefit from the additional exercise of having to walk a little more.)

The use of an office computer during business hours for personal correspondence with friends is definitely abuse of power. However, it is probably OK to send a congratulatory e-mail to a colleague who was quoted in an article in *Today's Dietitian* or has just won an election to be an officer in a professional organization. Thus, the same activity carried out under one set of circumstances is appropriate and under a different set of circumstances is inappropriate. It is easy to visualize examples related to phones, copiers, and the like in which the same activity may be abusive or justifiable, depending on the circumstances.

Note, too, that using power for personal gain is not always bad, immoral, or abusive. If an entrepreneur dietitian volunteers time to do committee work for the Canadian Dietetic Association, and by doing so accumulates enough frequent flyer miles to take a free trip to Europe, there should be no cause for question. The free trip was a consequence of the volunteer activities, not the reason for doing them.

Once again, the question of abuse or misuse of power is situational. It is hard to judge from the outside, because outsiders seldom have access to the information that was used to justify the action taken. Because this is true, managers are free to rationalize whatever they do and justify it as being for the common good. They will not usually be questioned by staff, who don't want to disturb the "powers that be." Therefore, it is prudent for the leaders to avoid the appearance of impropriety so that their integrity does not come under discussion.

leadership and social responsibility

Leaders are people-oriented. They recognize that it is people who are ultimately the beneficiaries (or the victims) of what they do. They also know that it is individuals, working in concert as a dedicated team, which will allow them to achieve their vision. Ultimately, the leaders understand their dependence on people and the need to nurture this valuable resource. They need to trust and to be trusted.

trust

Throughout this chapter, the issue of trust has been raised several times. Trust is important in all areas of practice.[11] If clients do not trust dietetic practitioners to give them reliable and valid information, then the credibility of the profession is in jeopardy. Likewise, employers must trust that professional staff will perform their duties in an ethical manner. Even more importantly, staff at all levels must believe that the manager and the management team are trustworthy. In fact, trust is one of the major factors why employees continue to work for an organization. The other factors are fair treatment, care, and concern.[12]

An erosion of trust occurs whenever there is bad management. This could include inconsistent application of standards, tolerating incompetence or bad behavior, problem avoidance, favoritism, and so forth.[13] If a degree of trust is lost, the leader must be forthright in admitting mistakes and taking steps to correct them as soon as possible. Failure to do so will cause trust to be further eroded, possibly to the point where it cannot be rebuilt.

It is imperative that leaders establish and maintain trust if they are to succeed. One trustworthy person will not be able to build trust in an organization or within a work-group. Organizational trust is built on good communication, consistency, support, fairness, recognition of the accomplishments of others, and flexibility at all levels. In order to be trusted, the leader also needs to trust others, be they subordinates, colleagues, or higher-level managers. Problems must be faced with candor rather than disregarded or swept under the rug.

social responsibility

Leaders accept responsibility for safety within the work environment. For example, the workplace should be a safe place for people to come on a daily basis. Physically, this means it should be as free as possible from work-related hazards. Hospital staff who have direct contact with patients should have all the appropriate immunizations, and there should be a policy and procedure in place to guide what is done in case an employee is accidentally pricked by a needle. In a business environment, workstations for clerical staff should be designed to minimize the risk of repetitive stress injury. Employees who work late into the night should have safe access to their cars after dark, such as a well-lit parking area nearby, use of surveillance cameras in the parking lot, or an escort service. The list of other safety concerns is too long to cite here. Though lower-level leaders may not be able to initiate activities to bring about a safe workplace, it is still that leader's obligation to lobby for the safety of the staff.

Safety also includes freedom from undue stress at work. Leaders will not tolerate harassment in any form (ethnic, racial, and gender-related are the most prevalent) in the work setting. If certain work stations are more stressful than others, the leader will find a way to distribute that work evenly among staff so that no one individual is subject to disproportionate amounts of stress. And the leader will act as a buffer to protect staff from external stress when possible. As an example, if a physician is angry with a clinical dietitian over an error on a patient tray, the chief clinical dietitian should intervene to deal with the problem. Leaving the clinical dietitian alone to respond to the physician could have a negative effect on her ability to work with that physician in the future and could impact patient care.

In addition, leaders must deal with all groups of subordinates in an evenhanded way. As an illustration, consider the natural divisions that occur between clinical staff and foodservice staff in a hospital foodservice department. Typically, foodservice takes precedence over clinical because of its relative size. It employs a larger staff, uses a bigger share of the budget, and has a greater profit potential. If a clinical dietitian is promoted to the position of foodservice director, the clinical staff will expect to have their position enhanced because of the dietitian's background in clinical practice. In reality, one of three things can happen. First, the new foodservice director can favor the clinical component of the job (where there is a high comfort level) and ignore the foodservice aspect (which is a major part of the new job responsibility). Second, the new director can ignore clinical while learning the bigger part of the job that is unfamiliar. In either case, this new manager is being unfair to one group of constituents by accommodating the other group while settling into the new job. A leader will choose the third option, which is to deal evenhandedly with both constituencies. Though this strategy may, in the short run, decrease the new manager's popularity with both groups, it will increase the manager's overall chance of long-term success.

Leaders must be willing to make compromises. It is not always possible to satisfy all constituencies at the same time. Leaders seek options with the likelihood of having the most positive consequences for the largest segment of the staff while minimizing the negative impact on others.

And finally, the leader will recognize social responsibility beyond the workplace. This will range from allowing staff dietitians time off to volunteer in professional associations to implementing recycling programs to lessen the organization's negative impact on the environment. Even at the lowest management levels, leaders demonstrate their social commitment by the example they give to staff, colleagues, and even their neighbors.

conclusion

Throughout this chapter, the issue of leadership has been discussed. This includes the traits that differentiate leaders from other managers, the various leadership styles that are employed, and how leaders use power. All of these concepts can be summarized as follows.

1. Leadership skills are not inherent in all managers. People-centered skills are the factors that differentiate leaders from managers.
2. The characteristics of effective leaders include drive, motivation, integrity, self-confidence, intelligence, and expertise and may include charisma, creativity, and flexibility.
3. The continuum of leadership styles ranges from autocratic through participative and democratic to consensus leadership. The autocratic style is the least

people-oriented but the most time-sparing model; the consensus model is time-consuming and person-centered.

4. The five types of power exerted by leaders are expert, referent, legitimate, reward, and coercive. Leaders are expected to use power in an ethical manner.

5. Trust is an essential part of leadership.

6. Leaders demonstrate social responsibility toward their employees and the community at large.

activities

activity 1

Describe a situation from your work experience in which your manager acted more like a manager and less like a leader. What could have been done differently to make you feel better about the situation?

activity 2

Case Study. A foodservice management company provided the following staff to a community hospital: the foodservice director (FSD), an assistant director for patient services (ADPS), an assistant director for nonpatient services (ADNS), a production manager (PM), 3.4 clinical dietitians, and 3.0 foodservice supervisors.

Weekdays, the staff included the FSD, ADPS, ADNS, PM, three clinical dietitians, two dietetic technicians, and two foodservice supervisors. Weekend staffing consisted of one clinical dietitian, one dietetic technician, and two foodservice supervisors. The contract management company was new to the account.

The clinical dietitians felt that they had very little clinical work to do on Sundays and that, therefore, they should not have to work on Sundays. Their manager, the ADPS, was a consensus manager. She agreed with the clinical dietitians that the workload on Sundays was light, and that many of the tasks that the dietitians performed on the weekends were either technician tasks (such as calorie counts and screenings) or foodservice tasks (like food substitutions and production issues). When the subject was introduced in a staff meeting, the group decided that the issue should not be addressed at this time because the contract was new and any proposed change might be interpreted as a cut in service. There was agreement that to move forward with such a proposal, hard data were needed to substantiate the anecdotal information that the clinical dietitians had gathered to describe their weekend workload. Thus, the clinical staff agreed to keep productivity records on Saturdays and Sundays to determine what they actually did on the weekends. They designed a form to record all of the tasks that the clinical dietitians performed on weekends.

Ten months later, when the management company was secure with its position within the facility, the issue again appeared on the agenda. Data indicated that clinical dietitians performed, on average, 0.3 nutritional assessments, 2.1 kcal counts, and 3 screenings on Sundays. The rest of their day was spent catching up on office work, resolving foodservice issues (4.2 each Sunday), or reading journals. Interestingly,

management practice in dietetics

Saturday activities were similar. Average tasks performed included 1.2 discharge instructions, 2.4 kcal counts, and 1.8 screenings, plus 3.8 foodservice-related tasks. On most Saturdays, no nutritional assessments were done. It was also determined that the dietetic technician could have done the kcal counts and the screenings if the dietitian had not been there, and that the foodservice supervisors would have resolved the foodservice issues if the clinical dietitian was not present. The weekend tasks that actually required a registered dietitian averaged 1.2 discharge instructions on Saturday and 0.3 nutritional assessments on Sunday; these tasks required less than 2 hours of RD time on Saturday and about 30 minutes on Sunday. It was also noted that many of the instructions could have been anticipated and done on Friday, had the dietitians chosen to complete them. The staff often delayed instructions that could have been completed on Fridays so that there would be something to keep them occupied on Saturdays.

Based on the accumulated data, the clinical dietitians again requested Sundays off. Again the ADPS agreed, but added that there was an equally compelling argument for scheduling Saturdays off, too. Indeed, clinical dietitians were underutilized on both weekend days. Discussion followed. One dietitian argued that the workload on Fridays and Mondays would increase if they were to take both days off. The ADPS argued that the proposal had to be approved by both the medical staff and the hospital administration and that the request might be only partially granted. Asking for both days off would provide room for negotiation, which would increase the chances of getting at least Sunday off. One clinical dietitian wanted to request every weekend off, one wanted to request only Sundays off, and the other 1.4 clinical dietitians were undecided. The group could not reach an agreement, and the matter was tabled until the next clinical staff meeting.

During the next staff meeting, the question of weekend work was on the agenda again. The arguments were essentially the same, and the group was unable to reach consensus. At this time, one of the full-time clinical dietitians still chose to request every Saturday and Sunday off, and another was uncertain about what position to take. The idea of weekends off was enticing, and the risk of getting neither day off was a problem for her.

Now, however, 1.4 clinical dietitians expressed opposition to having, or even requesting to have, the entire weekends off. The item was tabled again, for lack of consensus. At the following staff meeting, the issue remained unresolved and was tabled again.

The Medical Staff Committee, which oversees clinical nutrition services in this hospital, was scheduled to have its quarterly meeting in three weeks, and it was necessary for the proposed change to be approved by this committee before the matter could be taken to the hospital administration. The ADPS knew about this meeting and informed the staff. She asked them to try once more to reach consensus, but they could not.

Therefore, she announced that she was making the decision to move forward with the request for Saturdays and Sundays off for the clinical dietitians. It was, she said, a management decision based on the productivity figures that they had gathered. The ADPS also told the staff that, if both weekend days were granted by the medical staff and the hospital administration, the issue would be revisited in six months to evaluate how the change was working and to consider changing staffing patterns again if the Friday/Monday workload was too great.

One dietitian protested vigorously that the manager was not being "democratic," because only one of the dietitians wanted the weekends off and 1.4 dietitians wanted only Sundays off. Because the other full-time dietitian was still undecided, she reasoned, the "vote" was 1 to 1.4. She felt that the ADPS should not have a say in the discussion because she did not work on weekends.

The ADPS informed the staff that, despite the protests, the workplace was not required to be a democracy and that the management decision was made. She stated that she was sorry that the group had not reached consensus, but that time did not permit her to delay the decision any longer. She made her recommendation—that clinical dietitians should no longer work on the weekends—to the Medical Staff Committee at their next meeting.

points for discussion

1. Why did the ADPS seek consensus?
2. Was the ADPS being autocratic when consensus was not reached?
3. Did the ADPS have the right to make the decision?
4. Did the ADPS have the authority to make the decision?
5. Did the dietitian who protested have a valid argument when she said the manager was not being democratic?
6. Was the staff being manipulated into reaching consensus on a decision that the ADPS had already made?
7. How do you think things would have evolved if all 3.4 clinical dietitians had reached consensus to request only Sundays off?
8. Should the ADPS have had a voice in the decision although she did not work weekends?
9. Would it have been better for the ADPS to make no decision at this time but continue to seek consensus?

activity 3

Consider the situation described earlier in this chapter: In one very sad situation, a group of clinical dietitians were faced with an RIF in their hospital department. To secure their own jobs, which they needed for a variety of personal reasons, they convinced management to lay off the dietetic technicians and the diet clerks. The rationale was that the dietitians were able to do all three jobs (which was true, though their education usually precluded dietitians doing diet clerk work). Over time, the dietitians found themselves so busy with tasks such as answering the phone, processing computer orders, writing diets, tallying menus, and checking trayline that there was little time for the screening, assessment, and care of patients. After a few years, their clinical skills diminished, and they were no longer able to function as clinical dietitians.

points for discussion

1. Should the manager have agreed to lay off the dietetic technicians and diet clerks?
2. What were the management alternatives at the time the original decision was made?
3. How might the outcomes have been different if an alternative decision had been made?
4. Can the dietitians justify compromising professional standards in order to keep their jobs?
5. What alternatives did the dietitians have when the RIF took place?
6. What alternatives do the dietitians have now?

to study further

These additional sources are recommended for a more comprehensive review of leadership.

- Bennis, Warren, *On Becoming a Leader* (expanded edition). New York: Perseus Press, 2003.
- Bennis, Warren and Robert Townsend. *Reinventing Leadership: Strategies to Empower the Organization*. New York: William Morrow, 1995.
- Campbell, R. *Leadership: Getting It Done*. Columbia, MO: University of Missouri, located online at www/ssu.missouri.edu/faculty/rcampbell/leadership/default.htm
- Coffie, R. and G. Jones. "Why Should Anyone Be Led by You?" *Harvard Business Review,* 78:62–70, 2000.
- Drucker, P. F. "What Makes an Effective Executive?" *Harvard Business Review,* 82:59–63, 2004.
- Eikenberry, K. *Remarkable Leadership: Unleashing Your Leadership Potential One Skill at a Time*. San Francisco: Jossey-Bass, 2007.
- Foltz-Arensberg, M. B., et al. "Transformational leadership of clinical nutrition managers." *Journal of the American Dietetic Association,* 96:39–45, 1996.
- Gregoire, M. B., and S. W. Arendt. "Leadership: Reflections over the Past 100 Years." *Journal of the American Dietetic Association,* 104:395–403, 2004.
- Hunter, M. B. "Constructive Developmental Theory: An Alternative Approach to Leadership." *Journal of the American Dietetic Association*. 111:1804–1808, 2011.
- Katzenbach, J. R., and D. K. Smith. *The Wisdom of Teams: Creating a High Performance Organization*. Boston: Harvard Business School Press, 1993.
- Kotter, John P. *John P. Kotter on What Leaders Really Do*. Boston: Harvard Business School Press. 1999.
- Kouzes, J. M. and B. Z. Posner. *The Leadership Challenge*. 5th ed. San Francisco: Jossey-Bass, 2013.
- Levin, M. *The Gift of Leadership: How to Relight the Volunteer Spirit in the 21st Century*. Columbia, MD: B.A.I., Inc., 1997.
- Mislevy, J. M. et al. "Clinical Nutrition Managers Have Access to Sources of Empowerment." *Journal of the American Dietetic Association,* 100:1038–1043, 2000.
- Parks, S. C. "The Fractured Ant Hill: A New Architecture for Sustaining the Future." *Journal of the American Dietetic Association,* 102:33–38, 2002.
- Useem, Michael. *Leading Up: How to Lead Your Boss so You Both Win*. New York: Crown Business/Random House, 2001.
- Wren, Thomas J. *The Leader's Companion*. New York: Free Press, a division of Simon and Schuster, 1995.

in practice

In any field of dietetics practice, success is possible. For some, success means advancement—moving into management roles, each time with greater responsibility and authority. For others, success means skill enhancement—becoming more confident and adept at solving work-related problems every day. Find successful people, by your chosen definition, and ask yourself: What *skills* do they have? What *knowledge* do they possess? With whom do they *network*? How can I *learn* from them? Whether or not you manage others, define what success means for you, then take steps to achieve it.

who is successful, and why?

Employers say certain traits are common among people in their organizations who have what it takes to succeed. Entrepreneurial skills top the list: thinking for yourself, making good decisions, working independently, demonstrating management thinking, taking calculated risks, and becoming valuable to the organization. Advancement requires staying on the cutting edge. This implies lifelong learning and continuing professional education, keeping up with the world and its many changes. Read both professional and popular journals, attend in-person and distance education classes, participate in seminars, listen to podcasts, and watch relevant videos. Tune in or you will be tuned out!

Remember that you also have much to give. Be a mentor; share your ideas, knowledge, and insights. Often the best way to become successful is by teaching and supporting others.

creative thinking

Successful individuals use creative thinking and problem-solving skills. The ability to identify and solve problems leads to better management of daily work, including the use of precious resources—time, products, money, and even the labor of other people. Here we draw on the emotional intelligence attributes of *conflict management, inspirational leadership,* and being a *change catalyst.*

Conflict management is a learned skill that helps us handle difficult situations more effectively. A more open discussion promotes finding better solutions to a problem. When conflict is likely, try these steps:

- Stop, be calm, and think before you act or speak;
- State the problem(s) clearly and discuss how you feel;
- Set a positive goal together;
- Think of multiple solutions with all possible consequences, intended or unintended; and
- Try the best plan.

Inspirational leaders are able to create or promote a positive vision. They motivate people and set their hearts on fire. They are not only able to perform, but are able to *lead* the performance. Leaders enjoy the thrill of a challenge. But remember, you don't have to be the "manager" to be a leader. You may be the very person in your workplace who sets a positive tone, an environment that inspires others.

You might also be the person who helps implement change. Many situations require a change in process, or a new way of doing business. Thus, a leader can **be the catalyst** for the desired change. When you take on a leadership role where change is imminent, be clear *why* that change is needed. Communicate *what* will happen if change does not take place, what will stay the *same*, and what good things the future holds if change is made. Harness support for your plan from decision makers, resource holders, and those who will be affected by the change. Articulate your goals; make them specific and measurable. Assign responsibilities, encourage and reward teamwork. Eventually, institutionalize the change so that it becomes "just how we do things."

think like a genius

If you always think the way you've always thought, you'll always get what you've always gotten.—Michael Michalko[1]

We can apply the strategies used by geniuses to create a better future. According to author Michael Michalko, we act like geniuses when we look at problems from multiple perspectives.[1] Einstein and Freud, for example, searched for details that did not fit with traditional perspectives, gradually establishing completely new paradigms. In order to solve complex problems, the genius thinker abandons the first or usual solution if it is based on past experiences. Brainstorming with many ideas allows redefinition of the problem, perhaps identifying new ones or leading to better outcomes.

Thus, what are the existing problems at your workplace? Think like a genius. Be inspirational. Challenge the ordinary. Find problems, turn them upside down, solve them, and leave your mark. Success will surely follow.

reference

[1] Michalko M. "Thinking like a genius: Eight strategies used by the super-creative, from Aristotle and Leonardo to Einstein and Edison." *The Futurist*. 1998; 32(4):21–25.

references

1. Kirkpatrick, S. A. and E. A. Locke. "Leadership: Do Traits Matter?" *Academy of Management Executives*, 5:48–60, 1991.
2. Nadler, D. A. and M. L. Tushman. "Beyond the Charismatic Leader: Leadership and Organizational Change." *California Management Review*, 32:77–97, 1990.
3. Commission on Dietetic Registration. http://www.cdrnet.org accessed June 30, 2012.
4. Goleman, D. "Leadership That Gets Results." *Harvard Business Review*, 78:78–90, 2000.
5. Eagly, A. H. et al. "Gender and the Evaluation of Leaders: A Meta-Analysis." *Psychological Bulletin*, 111:3–23, 1992.
6. "She Scores, He Shoots." *Psychology Today*, 25:10, 1992.
7. Pagonis, W. G. "The Work of the Leader." *Harvard Business Review*, 70:118–126, 1992.
8. Stewart, Greg L. and Charles C. Manz. "Leadership for Self-Managing Work Teams: A Typology and Integrative Model." *Human Relations*, 49:747–770, 1995.
9. French, J. and B. H. Raven. "The Bases of Social Power." In *Studies of Social Power,* ed. D. Cartwright. Ann Arbor, MI: Institute for Social Research, 1959.
10. Academy of Nutrition and Dietetics. http://www.adaevidencelibrary.com accessed June 30, 2012.
11. "Ethical Conflicts of Interest." *Journal of the American Dietetic Association*, 103:555–557, 2003.
12. Lynch, L. J. "Keeping the Best." *Association Management*, 55:30–34, 2003.
13. Galford, R. M. and A. Seibold Drapeau. "The Enemies of Trust." *Harvard Business Review,* 81:88–95, 2003.

part two

tools for managers

The next three chapters are devoted to some of the tools that managers use to conduct their activities. Each of these tools—decision making, communication, and marketing—can be used to facilitate the manager's work. The material covered in this text is introductory in nature, designed for the student and the entry-level manager. Each of these topics can be expanded to fill entire textbooks. Experienced managers are likely to benefit from a more in-depth study of these topics.

Although dietetics professionals are not expected to be experts in the fields of decision making, communication, or marketing, they use these tools on a daily basis. The purpose of including this material here is to organize the information for the reader and to validate its use in management practice. Dietitians and dietetic technicians must use these tools with competence in order to be effective managers, whether or not they hold management positions.

As dietetics professionals move into more and more responsible management positions, these tools become increasingly critical. With knowledge and experience, using them with skill becomes second nature. However, for this to happen, there must be a basic knowledge of the underlying theories of decision making, communication, and marketing. Effective use of any one of these tools enhances the dietetic professional's ability to manage with competence. Using them together increases the potential for exceptional managerial performance.

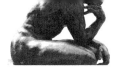

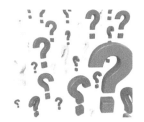

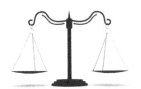

chapter four

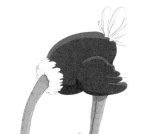

decision making

learning objectives

1. Define *decision making*.

2. Describe how critical-thinking skills are used in decision making.

3. State how decisions relate to problem solving.

4. Describe each step in the decision-making process.

5. Differentiate between structured and unstructured problems, and between programmed and non-programmed decisions.

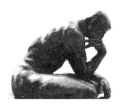

6. Describe the different styles used by managers for decision making.

7. Identify the relationship between decision making and risk.

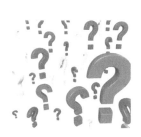

8. List the advantages and disadvantages of group decision making.

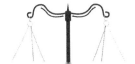

overview

Decision making is the process of making a choice between two or more alternatives. We all make decisions every day. In fact, you are reading this right now instead of playing tennis, surfing the net, or sleeping, because of a decision that you made. Some decisions are so easy to make that we do not usually think of them as decisions. These include such things as how to hold a knife and fork when cutting food or adjusting the car audio while driving. Other decisions, though routine, are made less frequently and require some thought. Such intermediate decisions might include choosing what clothing to wear each day, selecting the route to take to get to work or school, or how to spend a holiday weekend. Big decisions, like the purchase of a house or a car, are not routine for most people. They require considerably more time and effort on the part of the decision maker.

In this chapter, the process of decision making will be analyzed. Each of the eight steps necessary for making good managerial decisions will be discussed. This will be followed by a description of the types of decisions that managers are called on to make at various managerial levels. There will also be consideration of various decision-making styles. The issue of risk involved in decision making will be addressed. Finally, there will be a brief coverage of group decision making.

the process of making decisions

Decision-Making Process. *The logical, stepwise approach that is used to make a choice between options, to solve a problem, or to resolve a dilemma.*

Though the same process could be used for making any decision, the truth is that it is not. In fact, it is hard to identify any **decision-making process** for the most routine decisions, like which hand to write with or how we brush our teeth. Though it is likely that decisions were involved when the skills were being learned, they are no longer relevant; we perform these tasks as a matter of habit, having made the decisions long ago and forgotten the reasoning behind them. However, if a person's dominant hand is injured and that person is forced to operate the computer mouse with a non-dominant hand, for several days a conscious decision must be made each time the mouse is clicked until the new behavior becomes habitual. In fact, this type of habitual decision making is sometimes used in making professional decisions. Most seasoned clinical dietitians will evaluate the sodium and potassium intake of patients with hypertension without consciously recalling the evidence behind the decision that led to this practice.

Contingency Planning. *Anticipation of the need to make a decision sometime in the future and making the decision in advance so that it can be implemented in a timely manner at the time it is needed.*

There are some decisions that do not require the use of every step in the decision-making process, or perhaps, in some situations, two or more steps may be merged. In other situations, the process is not continuous. In other words, decisions are made far in advance of the need for implementation. This is called **contingency planning**. Consider, for example, the choice of which route to take to get to work. The decision maker may know that there are two possible routes: the usual, short route and a

Problem identification

Establishment of decision-making criteria

Weighting of decision-making criteria

Identifying alternatives

Analyzing alternatives

Making the decision

Implementing the decision

Evaluating the outcome

Table 4.1 Steps in the Decision-Making Process

longer, alternate route. If the traffic report on a given day states that the usual, short route is blocked, the driver automatically chooses the alternate route. The decision to use the longer route when the short route is congested may have been made weeks or years ago, but it is not implemented until it is needed. Another example of contingency planning is a hospital's disaster plan. The plan represents an attempt to decrease the response time needed to react to a natural disaster by making as many decisions as possible in advance.

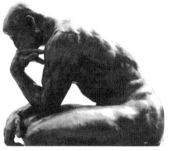

Good decision making, especially for non-routine decisions, requires the use of critical-thinking skills. Critical thinking is the process of employing "purposeful, self-regulatory judgment which gives consideration to the evidence, methods, concepts, context, and criteria on which a judgment is based."[1] The decision maker must be able to identify problems, define objectives for solving the problem, assign weight to those factors, and develop and analyze potential solutions. Only after all of these steps have been taken can a decision be made, implemented, and evaluated. (See Table 4.1.) Each of these steps in the decision-making process requires a great deal of effort and thought. This fact helps to explain why decision making is easier when a problem (or a similar problem) repeats itself for the second or third time. It is because the decision maker has experience with the problem and can move through the process faster by recalling the previous experience. Still, the process is used whenever a new problem arises, or when the required decision is of great importance and mistakes could lead to catastrophe. Decisions involving large amounts of money are usually considered to be very important ones, as are those that have a major impact on the lives of people.

Problem Identification. *The first step in the decision-making process; the act of finding a problem and acknowledging that it exists.*

problem identification

The first step in making a decision is to determine that there is something to make a decision about. This step is called **problem identification**. A **problem** exists when there is a difference between what is and what should be. Though the problems that

Problem. *A difference between what is and what should be.*

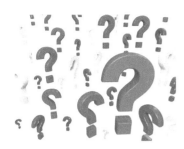

managers face are usually associated with something negative, this is not always the case. A problem may be a dilemma that is neutral, but one that needs resolution. Sometimes the problem requires making a choice among positive alternatives. Consider the clinic manager who has money left over near the end of the fiscal year and has to decide how to spend the excess dollars. This is a problem in that there is excess money that needs to be spent, but most managers would consider it to be positive, not negative, in nature.

The existence of a problem is not enough. The manager must acknowledge that the problem exists. This is easier said than done. Human nature allows people to become comfortable with the status quo and to not want to "rock the boat," so it is easy to ignore problems. Even if a discrepancy between the real and the ideal is noted, it may be dismissed as too trivial to require management attention. One way to facilitate problem identification is to use quality management techniques to compare an organization's performance to internal and external benchmarks. (See Chapter 13.)

In addition, the problem must be real. It is possible to identify something as a problem when it isn't. For example, a decrease in the number of students who participated in the school lunch program one week might indicate a problem with the food quality. On the other hand, the low participation may be the result of an outbreak of the flu that caused a high absentee rate that week. One should not react to the lower level of participation until there is a degree of certainty about what caused the decrease in participation. Identifying the problem correctly is central to the decision-making process; a manager who spends time and energy making decisions to solve problems that are not real is as ineffective as the manager who refuses to make decisions.

In addition to actually perceiving that a problem exists, a manager must feel that there is a need to deal with it. There must be some sense of urgency or pressure to drive the decision-making process. The urgency is sometimes self-generated by the manager who is driven to excel. The pressure may also come from a superior or from subordinates. In any case, the existence of either internal or external pressure will increase the chance that the decision-making process will move forward. Lack of urgency makes it very easy for decisions to be deferred.

Finally, the manager must feel that there are adequate resources for dealing with the problem. If there is insufficient money, labor, or other types of inputs, the manager might determine that nothing can be done and that any decisions made will be inadequate to deal with the problem. If no choice exists, no decision is required.

For the rest of this section on decision making, the following decision will be used as an example. A clinical nutrition manager is planning to upgrade the department's nutrient analysis software. The program that is now in use is not very user-friendly

management practice in dietetics

and was installed on a department computer four years ago. That old computer has a very slow processor, but it is the only one in the department that is compatible with the software. All of the other computers are newer, faster, and have sufficient memory to hold a more sophisticated program. Then, too, the existing program doesn't list enough foods; though there was a way to add new foods to the program when it was purchased, the database is now full and cannot accept more entries. The reason that this program was chosen four years ago is that it listed a wide array of nutrients, including macronutrients (carbohydrates, protein, fats, and kilocalories), fiber, all the RDA minerals, all the vitamins, 20 amino acids, and some of the omega-3 and omega-6 fatty acids. The program is intended to be used in a general hospital's nutrition department, which includes nutritional assessments and Calorie counts. (There is no clinical research center in this hospital.) The program may also be used to analyze the menus for the inpatients and cafeteria and generate Nutrition Facts Panels. The problem at hand is choosing the correct software package to meet the immediate needs of the department while anticipating future needs.

criteria for decision making

Once the problem has been identified, the next step in the process is to **establish decision-making criteria**. In other words, state what factors are important to achieving the best possible outcome or solution to the problem. The criteria might be those that the manager sets independently or those that are set with the help of staff or outside experts. Some criteria might also be imposed on the manager, perhaps by an accrediting agency, through governmental regulations, or because of budgetary constraints. In any case, all of the relevant factors should be spelled out; any other factors are deemed irrelevant and should not be considered in the decision-making process.

In the case of the software program, the manager wants a large database of foods (including processed and fast foods) and nutrients (including at least all the RDA nutrients plus data on omega-3, omega-6, and trans fatty acids, and fiber). The software must be able to accept the addition of additional foods, recipes, and enteral formulae. It is also necessary to have upgrades to the software available through Internet downloads, and a site license so that the program can be installed on all of the office computers. Speed is essential; it would be nice if there was a version that could be installed on the dietitians' handheld devices with a fast interface between those and the desktop computers. The package must be easy for the staff to learn to use with accuracy. Customized report formats would allow different information to be generated for different applications. For example, kilocalories and macronutrients would be reported for patients on Calorie counts, average daily nutrient intake could be reported in bar graph form for nutritional assessments, a spreadsheet format could be generated when doing menu analyses, and a Nutrition Facts Panel used for recipe analysis. The critical limit that is imposed from the outside is

Establish Decision-Making Criteria.
The second step in the decision-making process; determining which factors will have the most relevance in solving a given problem.

the number of dollars allocated for the software by the hospital's administration. These criteria are the factors that should be considered when choosing the nutrient analysis software.

It should be noted that this list is not cast in concrete. It is possible that the manager will learn of other features that are available during subsequent steps in the process. That's OK, as long as the criteria are added to the list and considered for each of the alternatives.

weighting criteria

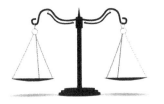

Copyright © 2009 by
Depositphotos/Alexey Bogatyrev.

Weight the Decision-Making Criteria. *The third step in the decision-making process; assigning each established criterion a ranking in terms of importance to the decision that is to be made.*

The identification of criteria will provide the manager with the basic information needed for giving weight to those criteria. Again, this is a task that can be done alone or in conjunction with staff members. **Weighting the decision-making criteria** means ranking them in order of their relative importance. Essentially, the manager is saying what the most important factor is, the second most important factor, and so forth. In the case of the software program, the most important factor might be the number of foods and the number of nutrients included in the database.

Often the two steps just described (identifying and weighting the criteria) are combined into one. That is, the manager may set the criteria and rank their importance at the same time. The exercise may be entirely intellectual, with nothing written down to explain how the decision is going to be made. There are no rules that dictate that the decision-making process requires a paper trail. However, for very complex decisions, it is sometimes helpful to quantify the decision-making process. In addition to clarifying complex decisions for the manager, the quantification makes it possible for others to see how the decision evolved.

In order to quantify the process, the weights are expressed as numerical values. Such weighting allows the manager to score each of the forthcoming alternatives in order to make a decision that is both rational and justifiable to others. Though the actual weighting involves both judgment and intuition, decision making is probably more objective if the process is quantified.

The process of weighting criteria, whether carried out on an intellectual level or quantified and written, is much like a pre-decision. It helps to establish the direction for the remainder of the process. If this part of the process is carried out correctly, then the actual decision will be relatively easy to make.

In the situation related to the purchasing of the software, the manager might determine that the most important criteria are the foods and nutrients in the database, so those criteria would be ranked at the top of the list. The other criteria are also weighted. The weighting that this manager establishes is shown in Table 4.2.

management practice in dietetics

Criterion	Weight
Foods in database	10
Nutrients in database	10
Add foods, recipes, enterals	9
User-friendly	8
Speed	7
Price	6
Upgrades/customer support	5
Site license	4
Customized reports	2
Handheld version with interface	1

Table 4.2 Weighted Decision-Making Criteria

developing alternatives

The next step in this decision-making process is to **identify the alternatives** that are available. Just what choices does the manager have regarding this problem? Remember, if a manager has no choice, then it is unlikely that the problem will be considered solvable. At this point in the process, no attempt should be made to evaluate the alternatives, only to determine what they are. Alternatives can be developed from a number of sources. First, of course, is the manager's own knowledge and experience. In addition, information can be obtained through networking with colleagues and peers. Next, there are various publications and Internet resources that list and evaluate nutrient analysis software. Staff members and supervisors may also have input. If the problem requires a purchase of some sort, salespeople can also be good sources of information about the products that they represent. At the end of this step in the process, a list of all reasonable alternatives for making the decision (solving the problem) has been generated.

analysis of alternatives

Now that the relevant criteria have been established and the possible alternatives identified, it is time to **analyze the alternatives** in light of the criteria. Again, this part of the process can be done entirely without documentation, or the manager may choose to work through the analysis on paper. This step is somewhat subjective, because the analysis will necessarily include the preconceived ideas of the person who is doing the analysis. It should be noted that most decisions have a degree of subjectivity (or intuition) influencing them.

Identify the Alternatives. *The fourth step in the decision-making process; the act of determining the different options available to solve the problem at hand.*

Analyze the Alternatives. *The fifth step in the decision-making process; the process of comparing and examining the alternatives available by measuring them against the same standards, using only relevant criteria.*

The critical element in this part of the decision-making process is to look at every alternative in light the evidence available for each of the predetermined criteria. Just as evidence analysis and evidence-based guidelines are used in providing patient care, evidence must also be evaluated to support the decision-making process in management practice. Data related to each of the alternatives must be measured against the same standards.

On the other hand, factors that are irrelevant *to this particular decision* need to be disregarded, even if they usually have relevance to the decisions that the manager makes. For example, if a clinical nutrition manager usually considers length of time in service when making decisions relative to job status and pay increases for subordinates, it would be natural to think in terms of seniority whenever staffing decisions need to be made. However, if the decision at hand involves promoting one of the clinical dietitians into the position of chief clinical dietitian, seniority should not be considered unless it has been established as a relevant criterion. Extraneous information makes decision making more difficult than it needs to be.

It is important to note that when a wide array of options is available, the decision becomes more difficult to make. In choosing nutrient analysis software, if there are only two programs to choose from, the decision will be very simple, but given the fact that a dozen or more choices are available, the decision could become overwhelming.[2] Sometimes it helps to eliminate those choices that clearly will not be viable before doing the analysis. For example, if the budget for the software is a maximum of $8,000, then any package costing significantly more than that could be eliminated immediately. On the other end of the spectrum, a program that analyzes the macronutrient content of only 100 foods would be deemed inadequate and discarded before spending unnecessary time and energy needed to analyze that option.

For the manager who is looking at nutrient analysis software, the analysis could end up being quantified as depicted in Table 4.3. In this case, the highest scoring program is Option C. Although "C" did not score highest on the two most important criteria of number of foods and nutrients in the database, it did have the best capacity to add foods and it was the top option relative to cost. This type of analysis provides the manager with comparative data about the various software programs on which the decision may be based. Often the appropriate choice becomes apparent during this part of the process.

Make the Decision.
The sixth step in the decision-making process; involves choosing which alternative(s) will best solve the problem based on the analysis that has been done.

choosing an alternative

The sixth step in the decision-making process is actually **making the decision**. If care has been taken in working through the previous steps, the choice may be obvious. If it is not clear, at least the possible options have been narrowed to a manageable number. If the choice is between two or three viable options, it is somewhat easier to make a decision than if the choice is among 10 or 12 options.

management practice in dietetics

Criterion (Weighting)	Option A	Option B	Option C
Foods in database (10)	9 (×10 = 90)	10 (×10 = 100)	8 (×10 = 80)
Nutrients in database (10)	10 (×10 = 100)	8 (×10 = 80)	8 (×10 = 80)
Add foods, recipes, enterals (9)	5 (×9 = 45)	0 (×9 = 0)	10 (×9 = 90)
User-friendly (8)	8 (×8 = 64)	10 (×8 = 80)	9 (×8 = 72)
Speed (7)	10 (×7 = 70)	10 (×7 = 70)	10 (×7 = 70)
Price (6)	5 (×6 = 30)	7 (×6 = 42)	10 (×6 = 60)
Upgrades/customer support (5)	8 (×5 = 40)	9 (×5 = 45)	10 (×5 = 50)
Site license (4)	10 (×4 = 40)	10 (×4 = 40)	0 (×4 = 0)
Customized reports (2)	0 (×2 = 0)	5 (×2 = 10)	10 (×2 = 20)
Handheld version with interface (1)	0 (×1 = 0)	0 (×1 = 0)	10 (×1 = 10)
Total	**479**	**467**	**532**

Table 4.3 Analysis of Criteria for Choosing a Software Program

Up to this point, there is the possibility that other relevant criteria may be identified or new alternatives may arise. Because it is unusual for the decision maker to have access to all of the possible information regarding a topic, care must be taken to make the decision when it is appropriate to do so. It is tempting to use the appearance of new information as an excuse to defer, or to avoid, making a decision. Though there are some occasions when putting off a decision is a reasonable choice for a manager to make, the more likely scenario is that the decision needs to be made in a timely manner to prevent further deterioration of the problem situation. In fact, refusing to make a decision is actually a decision, and often the wrong one.

In the situation with the software program, the manager will choose Option C. The decision will not be deferred, because the need for a new and better nutrient analysis program is more important than having one that is a perfect match to all of the established criteria. In addition, it is interesting to note that Option C was the only option that offered interface with handheld computers, a feature that could make this choice the best to meet future needs as well as present ones.

implementing the decision

After choosing among alternatives, the manager must **implement the decision**. This involves actually doing whatever has been decided. If the decision was to make Fridays a casual dress day in the department, the decision can be implemented with little or no planning. Merely communicating the decision is enough to make it happen. However, implementing the decision may be something that requires some planning and a step-by-step phase-in of the change.

Implement the Decision. *The seventh step in the decision-making process; the act of carrying out the decision that has been made; often involves communicating exactly what is to happen based on the decision.*

The new software program will have to be ordered and received. It is likely that it will require a staff person from the Department of Information Technology to install the program and test it. Someone will have to customize the reporting forms, and the dietitians will need to learn how to use the new program. In this case, implementation of the decision is a process rather than a single event.

Whether the implementation will take one step or many, a very important aspect of implementation is communication. The success of the change that will occur as a result of the decision will be influenced by how it is communicated to the staff, because that will help determine if the change is viewed as negative, positive, or neutral. Consider the decision mentioned earlier about allowing employees to wear casual clothing on Fridays. If the manager gives no other guidance to employees, it is possible that someone will report to work in torn jeans and a stained tank top (which is not acceptable attire for most businesses). On the other hand, if the rules defining casual dress are too explicit, the employees may feel that there is really no benefit offered by the new program, because they are really not free to define what *casual* means to them. The correct method of communication will probably be somewhere in between these two extremes. How the announcement is phrased will have a major impact on how it is interpreted and accepted by the workforce. The multi-stepped implementation for the nutrient analysis program will require communication with different people about different topics over a longer period of time. It is even more critical to communicate effectively in this set of circumstances.

evaluation

Evaluation. *The eighth and last step of the decision-making process; receiving feedback about the decision that has been implemented—that is, was it effective, efficient, appropriate, and adequate?*

The last step in the decision-making process is the **evaluation** of the impact of the decision and using that information. Was the decision effective, efficient, appropriate, and adequate? Did it resolve the problem that was originally identified? If the problem was not resolved, what else is necessary to correct the situation? If the problem was resolved, were new problems identified that need to be addressed? The answer to these and related questions should be considered and used as feedback for the system. The feedback then becomes input that can be considered when future decisions need to be made. Experience is, in many ways, the best teacher.

types of decisions

Decisions are generally classified into two basic types: those that are programmed and those that are non-programmed. Furthermore, it has been observed that different levels of managers tend to make different types of decisions. Just as top-level managers use mostly conceptual skills and frontline managers use more technical skills, the types of decisions vary with management level. Decisions made by top-level managers are more likely to be of the non-programmed type, whereas those made by lower-level managers are more likely to be programmed, or at least programmable, decisions.

structured problems and programmed decisions

Structured problems are routine and predictable discrepancies between what is and what is ideal. It is usually pretty clear what the goal of the decision should be. This type of problem arises in an environment where certain kinds of problems are usual and the decisions that relate to the problem are part of the day-to-day activities of the manager. In addition, the information needed to make the decision is readily available and often complete. Makers of **programmed decisions** can readily transfer information from one situation to another similar situation by invoking a little bit of common sense. Structured problems can usually be handled by making programmed decisions.

Structured problems are likely to occur in established organizations with an institutional history and a stable environment. Often, the outline for making programmed decisions is written down somewhere, perhaps in the form of rules and regulations, labor contracts, internal policies and procedures, or a decision tree. At other times, the decision is based on precedent.

A typical structured problem is faced when a needed employee does not report to work. The problem is to find someone to replace the scheduled employee. There are lots of ways to handle the problem, and the decisions involved will not always be the same. For example, when Bob (a DTR) is ill, the best alternative is to call in Mary (another DTR) to do Bob's job. But if Mary is vacationing in some exotic place, it is not possible to ask her to work. The replacement of absent employees requires a routine decision, but the actual decision about who to use as a replacement is not repeatable in every instance.

The guidelines for replacing employees might consist of the following steps:

1. Make a list of all employees who are able to do the job of the absent employee.
2. Determine the availability of each of these other employees.
3. Narrow the list to those not already scheduled to work 40 hours this week.
4. List the remaining employees in order of seniority.
5. Call those employees, in order of seniority, and offer each the available position.
6. Discontinue the process when the position has been filled.

The manager who is making the decision merely has to follow the guidelines to find a replacement worker; the steps actually take the manager through the decision-making process in a programmed way. Managers who make programmed decisions regularly have an established routine that they use each time a certain type of problem arises.

Structured Problems. *A discrepancy between what is and what should be that is both routine and predictable.*

Programmed Decisions. *Decisions that are made routinely, often relying on precedent, where information can be transferred from one similar situation to the next; usually used to solve structured problems.*

They eventually learn to make these decisions so well that it appears that they are being made automatically. The difficulty, however, is that often the guidelines are not written, so it is difficult for an uninitiated manager to make the decisions as effectively as the seasoned manager.

When a manager is faced with a decision that is unfamiliar, the decision is not programmed; at least, it is not programmed for that manager at that time. If the guidelines for making the decision are written down (like in a union contract, an employee handbook, or a policy and procedure manual), then it will make the process easier for the new manager to work through the decision-making process. Nevertheless, that person will have to make similar decisions several times before it truly becomes programmed. Making programmed decisions is a learned behavior. The new manager, or an experienced manager in a new setting, will require some time before gaining competence at making good decisions with ease.

Consider the supervisor who is replacing the absent worker. The incumbent manager is likely to know each of the employees' job skills, preference for work hours, seniority, availability, and so forth. The new manager will have to figure all this out, basically working from scratch. It may take significantly longer for the new manager to make a decision, and there is a greater chance that the decision will be a poor one. Believe it or not, decision making is hard work.

What makes programmed (or **programmable**) **decisions** unique is the fact that they are repeated frequently, and therefore eventually take on the aspects of a routine. Decisions such as purchasing supplies, dealing with equipment malfunctions, how to handle overproduction and underproduction in foodservice, or what to do when an accident occurs in the workplace are all programmable decisions; how to make these decisions is something that can be learned by the manager. It is the fact that they are predictable and that experience can be readily transferred from one situation to the next that makes it possible to spell out the process on paper.

unstructured problems and non-programmed decisions

Unstructured problems are those that are new, unusual, and often unpredictable. These problems are less readily identified, and the goals of the decision-making process are less clear than with structured problems. In addition, the information that is available for making the decision is often incomplete or ambiguous.

The type of decision that must be made to deal with an unstructured problem is called a **non-programmed decision**. There is, generally, little precedent for such decisions and no written guidelines to follow. The manager who is faced with making a non-programmed decision must use the decision-making process described earlier, for there is no viable alternative. Non-programmed decisions take longer to make than

Programmable Decisions. *Decisions that, though not yet programmed, are of the routine type that can be programmed.*

Unstructured Problems. *A discrepancy between what is and what should be that is new, unusual, and often unpredictable.*

Non-Programmed Decisions. *Decisions that are used to resolve unstructured problems; these decisions require much research and thought.*

management practice in dietetics

programmed decisions. The bigger the decision, the more compelling the need to go through each step of the process that has been described.

Though unstructured problems exist in every organization, there seem to be more of them in start-up operations or in situations without **institutional memory**. Unstructured problems also seem to increase in times of rapid change. In both of these instances, the large number of non-programmed decisions is only partly due to the types of decisions needed. Much of the apparent increase is due to the fact that there are either new managers making the decisions or the managers are making decisions that are unfamiliar to them because of changes in managerial structure or responsibility. Some of these decisions are actually programmable and will eventually be institutionalized in the form of policies, procedures, guidelines, or rules.

Institutional Memory. *The historical precedent of an organization that can be used in the decision-making process.*

managerial levels and decision making

There is a correlation between management level and the type of decision that the manager is called on to make. In general, the bulk of the decisions made by frontline managers are of the programmed (or programmable) type. Upper-level managers tend to make most of the non-programmed decisions in an organization. This does not mean that either type of decision is exclusive to one group or the other, however. It is probable that frontline managers will be required to make some non-programmed decisions and even more likely that upper-level managers will regularly make programmed decisions.

In summary, managers make programmed decisions to deal with routine, structured problems in their organizations. They also make non-programmed decisions to deal with unique, unstructured problems. The more unstructured the problem, the more necessary it is to go through a formal decision-making process. In addition, the more important non-programmed decisions will often be made by upper-level managers, rather than by those at lower management levels. Problem solving and non-programmed decision making require the use of critical-thinking skills to resolve the discrepancies between what is and what should be. (See Figure 4.1.)

decision-making styles

Just as managers have their own leadership styles, they also have decision-making styles that are unique. Some managers seek out problems and thrive on making decisions of all types. Others avoid making decisions if it is at all possible to do so. There are times when each mode of operation is desirable. Sometimes decisions need to be made immediately, and sometimes it is better to delay a decision. Knowing when to make a decision and when to avoid making a decision is an important part of the decision-making process.

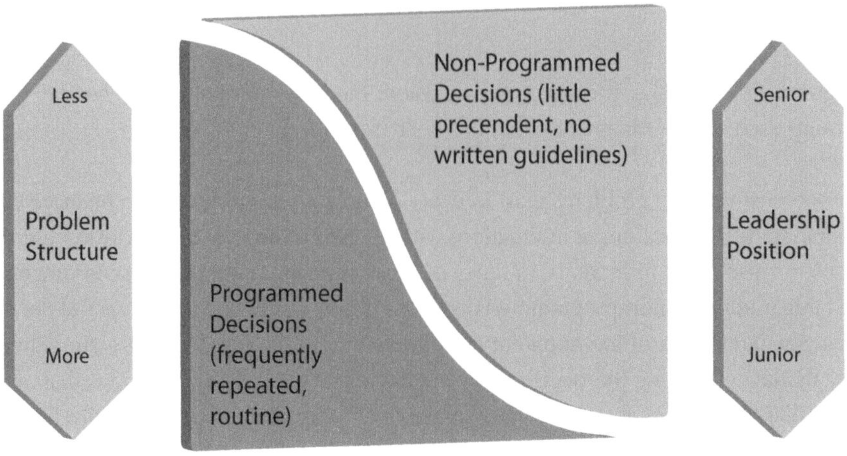

Adapted from: Stephen P. Robbins and Mary Coulter, *Management, 5th ed.* Pearson Education, 1996.

Figure 4.1 Types of Problems, Types of Decisions, and Level in the Organization

Problem Avoider.
A decision-making style in which the person does not recognize a problem or chooses to avoid it; one who may make the choice not to make a decision.

Problem Solver.
A decision-making style in which the person recognizes existing problems and deals with them in a timely manner.

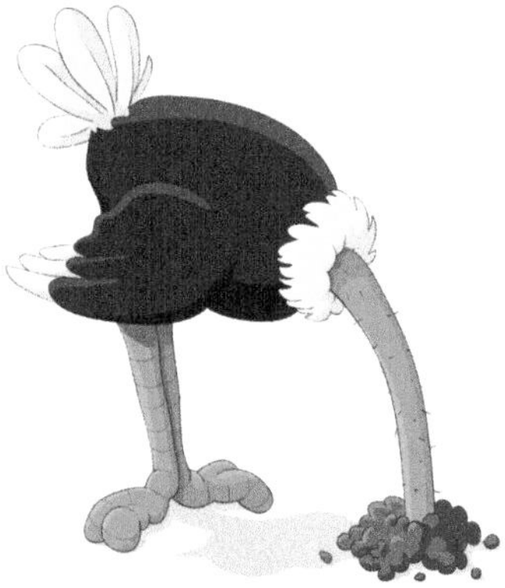

Reactive. *A characteristic of a problem solver who acts on problems after they have become obvious.*

problem avoider

The **problem avoider** is much like the proverbial ostrich that buries his head in the sand in order to evade reality. This person does not recognize a problem, or when one does arise, feels that there is no urgency or no resources for dealing with the problem. This is the type of manager who feels it must be good enough if "we've always done it that way." Another type of problem avoider is the procrastinator, who knows that there is a decision to be made, but puts it off. One author even coined the word *decidophobia*[3] to describe the behavior of problem avoiders.

However, not making a decision is a decision, too. It is deciding to ignore the problem for the moment. Whether or not this is a good decision is dependent on the circumstances, but it is often worse to not make a decision than to make an incorrect one. Obviously, waiting until a problem becomes a crisis is waiting too long, and this can easily happen to the problem avoider. The routine avoidance of decision making causes subordinates to question the manager's effectiveness as a manager.

problem solver

In contrast to the problem avoider, the **problem solver** does not actively withdraw from problems. However, this type of decision maker is **reactive**. As a problem solver, a manager recognizes when a problem exists and deals with that problem in a timely manner, not waiting until the problem becomes a crisis. The cliché that is often used for this type of decision making is "If it ain't broke, don't fix it." Essentially, the problem solver deals with problems as they occur, but does not actively seek problems or anticipate problems that have no urgency.

management practice in dietetics

problem seeker

The **problem seeker** is proactive. This type of problem solver will identify discrepancies between the real and the ideal, even when the discrepancy is minimal. The goal is to make things better, to "tweak" the system in order to refine it. Proactive decision makers seem to thrive on the challenge of making and implementing decisions. They anticipate problems and work on potential solutions before the problems become big ones; often solutions are ready when needed. Problem seekers do contingency planning.

One disadvantage to being proactive is that this manager's subordinates may constantly have to adapt to change. The status quo never really exists in departments with this type of decision maker. If the changes are small, this might not be a problem. However, the proactive manager must regulate the pace of implementing major changes in such a way that subordinates have time to adjust between changes. Too many changes in a short period of time may lead to increased stress in the workplace. This can be detrimental to the health of the workforce.

risk in decision making

When a decision is made, there is usually some degree of risk involved. It is not possible to predict every contingency, or if things will work out as they were planned. Decision makers try to avoid taking unnecessary risks and to make decisions with which they feel secure and relatively certain of a desired outcome. They determine a risk/reward ratio for their decisions, and avoid taking significant risks if the potential for success is low.

However, when the level of risk is high, there is often a commensurate level of reward possible. Where success can yield a high return, either in profits or in the achievement of some other compelling goals, a higher level of risk is more easily justified than when success will yield modest results. A discussion of how managers deal with the risk involved with decision making follows.

certainty

In a perfect world, managers could predict the outcome of every decision that they face. This condition is one that is described as **certainty**. For example, a manager might decide to subscribe to the Academy's *Nutrition Care Manual*. The certainty is that, in exchange for the subscription fee, access to the latest edition of this reference will be available to departmental staff for the coming year. In effect, each decision made under conditions of certainty would be a correct decision because the precise

Problem Seeker.
A decision-making style in which the person is proactive and deals with potential problems before they become obvious.

Certainty.
A situation in which the outcome of a decision is known and expected.

outcome of the decision is known. Though it would be ideal for managers to know the outcomes of all of their decisions before making them, the unfortunate truth is that few decisions are made under conditions of absolute certainty.

risk

Risk. *The unknown or uncertain factors or outcomes involved in making a decision.*

As noted earlier, decisions usually involve some **risk**. Under conditions of risk, sometimes called calculated risk, the manager has information that will help to determine the probable outcomes from each of the alternatives being analyzed. This estimate of probability can come from experience, historical data, networking, or other sources. It is necessary for managers to make decisions that involve risk, but to do so, they should make an effort to gather enough data to be able to predict the outcome with reasonable accuracy. The accurate estimation of risk is so important that an entire management subspecialty is devoted to managing risk. (See Chapter 15.)

Consider the manager who is trying to determine the feasibility of adding WIC (Special Supplemental Nutrition Program for Women, Infants, and Children) services at an existing general medicine clinic. Though there is always risk involved in developing a new service, information is available that can guide the decision-making process. The manager should consider the demography of the clinic's existing clients to determine if this client group needs WIC services. The target clientele should include a significant number of women of childbearing age. Socioeconomic data must also be gathered to determine if the existing clients would be eligible for such a program. In addition, the proximity of other WIC sites in the area should be determined to ascertain if an additional program could be justified. Finally, there must be funding available from the state agency that oversees WIC.

If the data show that there are a large number of WIC-eligible clients in the area who are not currently being served by another WIC program, and that state funding is available, then the manager is justified in developing such a program for the clinic. The major conditions of risk—lack of eligible clients, existence of competing services, and lack of potential funding—have been considered and found to be minimal. In this case, the risk assessment shows that the risk is worth taking because there is the probability that the clinic will be sustainable.

Nevertheless, outcomes are still not certain. The state may reject the proposal. The federal government may withhold funding for new programs. Even if the program is opened, there may be other unforeseen factors that could prevent clients from utilizing the service, like language barriers, poor transportation, or safety concerns. There are no guaranteed outcomes under conditions of risk, though the actual risk is minimized if the decision maker makes the effort to obtain and utilize whatever relevant data are available.

management practice in dietetics

uncertainty

Conditions of uncertainty are those in which the manager is forced to make a decision in a situation where the potential outcomes cannot be predicted with any degree of accuracy. Historical data are unavailable, and the decision maker is faced with making a decision with very little tangible data. Decisions made under conditions of uncertainty are made intuitively and based on hunches, because that is all that is available. Whatever probabilities exist are subjective. The predictions for the success of this type of decision are based on optimism and instinct, rather than on reality.

A decision about whether or not to develop a line of microorganism-free fresh poultry products to enhance food safety would be made under conditions of uncertainty. First, there is no guarantee that a cost-effective process could actually be developed that would result in germ-free poultry. Even if it is developed, it is possible that the process would not be approved by the Food and Drug Administration. Though consumers want safe food, it is unknown if they would purchase such a product if it existed. If they are willing to purchase it, would they be willing to pay a premium price for it so processors could recoup the initial development costs?

If a decision made under conditions of uncertainty were successful, the potential for profit is huge. Consider the introduction of infant formulas to a market where breast-feeding was the norm and alternate infant-feeding systems were used in only the direst circumstances. That decision was made under conditions of uncertainty and has grown into a multibillion-dollar industry. The same is true of supplemental vitamins. Yet, there is also a great potential for failure, as evidenced by the large investment in the development of fat substitutes in the 1990s, of which only a small number have reached the marketplace.

In summary, when little relevant information is available and probable outcomes are unknown, decisions have a high degree of risk. Such high-risk decisions can be wondrously successful or dismal failures. Conversely, a large amount of data helps the decision maker determine probable outcomes and lower the risk involved in decision making. As the chance for success increases, the risk/reward ratio usually decreases.

Uncertainty.
A situation in which the outcomes of a decision cannot be predicted with any degree of accuracy.

group decision making

Often groups are called on to make decisions. Groups that solve problems include committees, task forces, search committees, review panels, editorial boards, focus groups, and total quality management teams. Some groups are transient, meaning that they are put together to deal with a specific problem or set of problems, with the intention of disbanding the group as soon as the work is done. Other groups are ongoing; though the membership of the group may change from time to time, the group itself continues to exist with a stated purpose to direct its activities. These groups may actually make decisions, or they may make recommendations to an individual who is then called on to make a decision based on the input of the group. For example, the clinical nutrition staff may meet as a group to make decisions or to advise the clinical nutrition manager about decisions that are pending.

In the previous chapter, group participation in decision making was mentioned with respect to leadership style. Some advantages to using this technique include obtaining more information with which to make the decision, and group acceptance of a decision in which they were involved. The major disadvantage was identified as the increased time that it takes to go through the group process. This section will look at group decision making from the perspective of the decision, rather than from the perspective of leadership. Besides consensus (mutual agreement, acceptable to all) and democratic ("majority rules") decisions, other considerations in the way that groups make decisions are accommodation, de facto decision making, increased risk, and groupthink. These all have the potential to decrease the value of the decisions that are made by groups.

accommodation

Not all members of a group are equal. More precisely, not all group members are the same. This is one of the major reasons for undertaking group decision making—different types of people bring different ideas to the decision-making process. It has been demonstrated that increased information usually enhances the quality of the decision. However, sometimes groups contain a dominant member who is either more verbal than the other group members or more effective at making a point. At times, the other group members will accept the position of this dominant individual without really agreeing with the decision. This is called **accommodation**.

Accommodation.
A situation in which members of a group feel that they have to accept the position of the dominant member of the group.

This type of acceptance occurs for a number of possible reasons. Perhaps other group members are, by nature, shy and unwilling to verbalize their opinions. The group cannot consider opinions that are unspoken. Another possibility is that a group member's divergent viewpoint is not considered as a viable option because it is poorly articulated. And finally, it may happen that a dominant person either intimidates or wears down the other group members. They eventually give in because the dominant person is unwilling to compromise or just won't "shut up." With accommodation, the outcome may look like consensus has been achieved, but the reality is that the dominant individual has prevailed.

management practice in dietetics

de facto decisions

De facto decisions are those that tend to occur passively. The decision may or may not be a good one, and it may or may not be acceptable to all members of the group. However, the common thread with de facto decisions is that there is no dissent expressed. The lack of dissent is interpreted as agreement, and the decision gets implemented. Group members accept de facto decisions for many reasons. These include disinterest in the problem, a lack of urgency, uncertainty about who is responsible for the decision, being bored with the group decision-making process, lack of assertiveness on the part of some group members, time constraints, and other, less obvious reasons. Again, the process leads to acceptance rather than to consensus.

De Facto Decisions.
Decisions that are made passively with no obvious objections expressed.

groupthink

Groupthink is a characteristic of groups that becomes evident when a group evolves to the point that the cohesiveness of the group is more important than the decision that is to be made. Group members, in this situation, have a vested interest in the group, and in making it work. Members avoid dissent or disagreement because they are invested in the group and do not want to hurt or offend their colleagues. It is more important to maintain the integrity of the group than it is to make a good decision. This is most likely to occur in stable groups, where the membership has been the same for a long time, but can also occur in groups that work together for short periods of time, but with high intensity. The most extreme examples of groupthink occur in cults, where members may completely lose their individuality.

Groupthink.
A characteristic of groups that evolves when the cohesiveness of the group becomes more important than the problem that needs to be solved; in this situation, members feel loyal to each other and may not want to jeopardize this unity by expressing opposing opinions.

risk in group decision making

When groups make decisions, the group is often willing to take greater risks than individual decision makers would be willing to take. Part of the reason for this phenomenon is that the risk is shared, so no one needs to take on the entire burden of responsibility for the decision. Under conditions of certainty, or when risk can be calculated, the willingness of the group to take increased risk may be justifiable. However, conditions of uncertainty create a dilemma. Because a group has more information, which helps the decision-making process, it could be argued that even a high-risk decision is better if made by the group. It will also be easier to implement because the entire group supports it. On the other hand, the group's willingness to incur more risk is not always good. Group decision making may not always be the method of choice, especially for decisions related to unstructured problems with a high degree of uncertainty.

Brainstorming.
The informal process of tackling a given problem by contributing as many ideas as possible without analysis or criticism.

Useful techniques for avoiding the pitfalls of group decision making and ensuring that groups work effectively include brainstorming, brainwriting, the nominal group technique, and the Delphi technique. All of these models are used to solicit the active, equitable participation of all group members.

Brainstorming is an activity in which all participants are called on to respond to a question or a problem in an open forum. Everyone is asked to contribute to the process, which is aimed at getting the largest possible number of ideas. Often these ideas are written down on chalkboards, easels, or overhead slides for all to share. As the ideas are being generated, there is no attempt to evaluate them and no opportunity to critique them. The goal of brainstorming is to develop the largest possible number of creative alternatives. Brainwriting is a variation of this method in which the ideas are written rather than presented orally.[4]

Nominal Group Technique.
A methodical, rational approach to making a group decision in which each member contributes ideas, and alternatives are ranked to deduce a sensible, fair decision.

The **nominal group technique** is a process in which group members meet but follow a formal process for dealing with an issue that is designed to stimulate independent thought. This is a four-step process. Step one is when the problem is presented and each group member is asked to write down ideas, without consulting with other group members. In step two, group members present their ideas to the group, with members taking turns and each member presenting one idea at a time. The ideas are written down as they are described until all ideas are recorded. Step three is a group discussion about the ideas that have been generated. In the final step, each member works independently to rank the ideas that have been generated. The final decision is based on the aggregate ranking.

Delphi Technique.
An approach to coming up with a group decision similar to the nominal group technique except that members do not meet but instead communicate and analyze ideas through written communication until consensus is reached.

The **Delphi technique** is similar to the nominal group technique, except that the entire process is carried out with individuals who never meet as a group. Instead, a questionnaire is sent to group members to generate the ideas. Results are compiled centrally and then redistributed to members who, again, comment in writing. This process is repeated until consensus is achieved. An advantage of this technique is that members do not actually have to meet, which could lead to great savings in time and travel costs. In addition, members of the group do not influence each other to a great degree; therefore, they are more open to independent thinking. On the other hand, lack of verbal interaction may limit the generation of new ideas; the prolonged time involved in completing this process is another major disadvantage.

conclusion

This chapter has provided basic information regarding the decision-making process. Each of the steps in the process has been considered, as have the types of decisions, styles of decision making, risks in making decisions, and group decision making. The information presented in this chapter can be summarized as follows:

1. Decision making is an eight-step process that includes problem identification, establishment and weighting of criteria, development and analysis of alternatives, making the decision, implementing it, and following up.
2. Structured problems require programmed or programmable decisions; unstructured problems require non-programmed decisions.
3. Different levels of managers tend to make different types of decisions.
4. Managers develop personal decision-making styles that can be described as avoidance, reactive, or proactive.
5. There are distinct advantages and disadvantages to group decision making; techniques are available to maximize the group decision-making process.

activities

activity 1

Make a list of at least 10 programmed decisions that you make routinely. These decisions can be related to school, work, or your personal life. For each of these decisions, state the problem that existed that necessitated the decision.

activity 2

Identify a problem that you are facing that will require a non-programmed decision to be made in the near future. (For students who will be applying for dietetics internships soon, the determination of where to apply is a good problem to deal with in this exercise. For those not faced with this decision, select another major decision you are facing, like the purchase of a computer, car, or home; a career choice; a change in family status; or a significant parenting decision.) Use the decision-making process outlined in this chapter to find a solution to the problem. Write a report that:

1. States the problem.
2. Identifies the criteria you will use to make the decision.
3. Assigns weight to each of those criteria.
4. Lists what the alternatives are. (For this exercise, there should be at least three alternatives.)
5. Analyzes each of the alternatives.
6. Identifies the decision.

After you have reached a decision, you may want to repeat the process using a decision-making tool that is available on the Internet at http://www.dannyg.com/javascript/dhnocookie/dhLoad.htm.

activity 3

Groups of five to eight students should work together on this problem. The problem is that students in your dietetics program have too many required courses and not enough electives. Obtain a list of courses that are required for students in dietetics at your school. Assume that your group is the curriculum committee for the dietetics program and that you are charged with eliminating four credits of required courses in order to make room for additional elective courses. Keep in mind that the required

management practice in dietetics

courses are there to meet accreditation standards, so an entire content area—for example, community nutrition, foods, chemistry, or medical nutrition therapy—cannot be eliminated. Work together to reach a decision about how to adjust the curriculum to correct the discrepancy between what is and what should be.

activity 4

For Activity 3, answer the following questions in light of your perceptions about how the group decision-making process worked for your group.

1. Which steps in the decision-making process did your group take?
2. Which steps in the process did your group skip or combine into a single step?
3. Was a decision reached?
4. If the answer to 3 is no, why not?
5. If the answer to 3 is yes, was it by consensus, majority rule, accommodation, or was it a de facto decision?
6. Did you agree with the decision?
7. If you disagreed with the decision, what did you do to have your opinion heard?
8. Do you feel safer presenting this decision to your teacher because it was a group decision, or would you feel better presenting your own personal decision on this topic to your teacher?

to study further

Additional insight into the decision-making process can be obtained from the following sources.

- Browne, Mairead. *Organizational Decision Making and Information*. Stamford, CT: Ablex, 1993.
- Fornari, A. "Approaches to Ethical Decision Making." *Journal of the American Dietetic Association*. 102:865–866, 2002.
- Gladwell, M. *Blink: The Power of Thinking Without Thinking*. New York: Little, Brown and Co., 2005.
- Greenberg, Jerald and Robert A. Baron. *Behavior in Organizations: Understanding and Managing the Human Side of Work*. 8th ed. Upper Saddle River, NJ: Prentice Hall, 2003.
- Guzzo, Richard A., Eduardo Salas, et al. *Team Effectiveness and Decision Making in Organizations*. San Francisco: Jossey-Bass, 1995.
- Hirokawa, Randy Y. and Marshall Scott Poole. *Communication and Group Decision Making*. 2nd ed. Thousand Oaks, CA: Sage, 1996.
- Lehrer, J. *How We Decide*. Boston: Houghton Mifflin Harcourt, 2009.
- Porter, C. and J. L. S. Matel. "Are We Making Decisions Based on Evidence?" *Journal of the American Dietetic Association*. 98: 404–407, 1998.
- Robbins, Stephen P. and Mary Coulter. *Management*. 11th ed. Upper Saddle River, NJ: Pearson Education, Inc., 2012.
- Thaler, R. H. and C. S. Sunstein. *Nudge: Improving Decisions About Health, Wealth, and Happiness*. New Haven, CT: Yale University Press, 2008.
- Turban, Efraim and Jay E. Aronson. *Decision Support Systems and Intelligent Systems*. 7th ed. Upper Saddle River, NJ: Pearson Prentice Hall, 2005.

scholarly journals

- *Decision Analysis*
- *Decision Sciences Journal*
- *Organizational Behavior and Human Decision Processes*

in practice

reality check—decision clusters

In this chapter the discussion was centered on making a single decision at a time, with the realization that most of us make multiple, unrelated decisions during the course of a day. In the real world, it is sometimes inevitable that decisions get clustered around a particular problem, and in many cases, a major decision has a cascading effect that requires that many more decisions need to be made.

Consider the situation in which the following problem has been identified. The nutrition department in a small community hospital/skilled nursing facility is spending too much money on oral and enteral supplements. In order to determine if this is a problem that can be solved, the clinical nutrition manager conducts a study to determine how many supplements are in stock, which ones are normally ordered, what percentage of the product is actually used, and how much is discarded because it has passed its expiration date. The results are amazing. In this facility, physicians can order any product that is available in the marketplace. The products have to be purchased in case lots, so that frequently, a patient is discharged with some of the product still in inventory. If the product is not ordered for another patient, it becomes outdated and has to be discarded. Roughly 15% of what is purchased is being wasted in this manner.

There are also too many different products in stock. For oral supplements, there are five different brands of liquid oral supplements in multiple flavors, two brands of pudding in three flavors each, a clear liquid oral supplement, and some nutrient-dense milkshake-like products. In the enteral category there are three standard formulae without fiber and another two with fiber, a blenderized formula, two others that were designed for use with patients with diabetes, three high-nitrogen formulas, one renal formula, one hepatic formula, a formula with peptides as the protein source, and another with amino acids. Many of these formulae are stocked both in eight-ounce packages for bolus feeding and in one-liter closed systems for use with feeding pumps. The department also stocks modular products that might be added to various formulae or to foods to alter the macronutrient content.

Clearly, little control is being exercised over what is being ordered and what is being used. Until now, there has been no attempt to standardize what is available. It is equally evident that there will be cost savings in the area of waste if the number of products is limited, so that patients requiring similar nutritional support can use the same formula. Moreover, if most of the products are purchased from a single manufacturer, there may be additional savings from negotiated prices that are available with larger purchases.

The decision is made to establish a formulary for oral and enteral supplements. Under this new system, the facility will stock only one product in each product category.

That product will be considered the therapeutic equivalent to all other products in that category, and will be substituted for other products when they are ordered. The decision is an easy one to make and has the potential for saving a great deal of money since the facility will use larger amounts of fewer products. However, determining that a formulary is needed is very different from actually developing a formulary. Lots of additional decisions need to be made to support the initial decision.

The solution to the initial problem was to develop a formulary. The next problem that needs to be resolved is which product categories should be included on the formulary and which should be omitted. With oral feedings, there is also the question of flavors, since flavor-fatigue often occurs in persons taking these supplements routinely. It is decided to limit the oral supplements to three flavors of a single brand of liquid supplement, one clear liquid supplement, and two flavors of a single brand of pudding. The milkshake-like products can still be used as an alternative, since these are purchased through food vendors and not pharmaceutical houses. Once the number of products is determined, criteria for choosing the specific products need to be established. For the oral feedings, the criteria will usually include nutrient composition, flavor, size of the package, and cost. Other criteria can be established as desired, and might include historical data about client satisfaction, waste studies, usage patterns, and so forth. The manager might include both patients and physicians in the taste tests so that they become active participants in the selection process.

In terms of enteral products, clearly, there needs to be a standard "house formula" for the majority of the patients. Criteria for this product should include nutrient density, osmolality, packaging, lactose content, fiber content, viscosity, and price. In most cases there is no need for a hospital to carry more than one isotonic, 1 kcal/cc, nutritionally complete, lactose-free formula. The same formula could be purchased both packaged in a one-liter closed system and in 250cc individual packages for bolus feeding. There is no need to taste-test these products, since they will be delivered to the patient via a feeding tube. The facility may choose to stock two house formulae, one with fiber and one without fiber, to accommodate a greater number of patients.

The determination of the other products to include as enteral feeds should be based on the typical diagnoses seen in the facility. If the facility treats patients with diabetes, renal disease, and liver disease, it may need to have specialized formulae for these patients. However, it may not need products that have been especially designed for patients with HIV/AIDS, burns, or those requiring elemental feedings because of digestive problems. Typically one feeding product for each diagnosis is sufficient for disease-specific formulae. Specific criteria need to be developed for each product category in order to make the best selection.

Weighting and analyzing the criteria makes the decision-making process easier. Though it is unlikely that one manufacturer will have products to meet all of the enteral and oral supplement needs for a facility, it is common that most products

management practice in dietetics

on a formulary will come from a single source in order to achieve the best possible pricing on the majority of products used. Still, there are usually one or two products that will come from a different source. Often it becomes necessary to pay a premium for these products.

Now that the formulary has been determined, there are other decisions to be made. Who will write the new policy to cover the matter of the formulary? What will that policy say? How will the new system be implemented: all at once, or phased in over time? What kind of communication will be used to inform the medical and nursing staff of the change? How should complaints be handled?

As illustrated by this situation, decisions are not always discrete entities that are made and then implemented. Many require multiple layers of decision making that must occur over time. In this case, the manager who made the decision to implement the formulary needed to know the ramifications of that decision and the decision should have included a plan to see the entire project through.

references

1. Facione, P. "The Delphi Report: Research Findings and Recommendations of the American Philosophical Association." *Critical Thinking: A Statement of Expert Consensus for Purposes of Educational Assessment and Instruction.* ERIC Doc. No. ED315-423, 1990.
2. Schwartz, Barry. *The Paradox of Choice.* New York: HarperCollins Publishers, Inc., 2004.
3. Goldsmith, Elizabeth. *Resource Management for Individuals and Families.* St. Paul, MN: West, 1996, p. 103.
4. VanGundy, Arthur B. *Techniques of Structured Problem Solving.* 2nd ed. New York: Van Norstrand Reinhold Co., 1988.

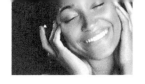

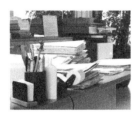

chapter five

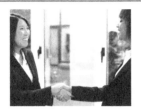

communication

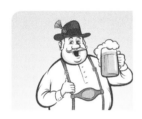

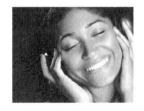

learning objectives

1. Define *communication*.

2. State why communication skills are important ones for managers to develop.

3. Discuss the roles of the senders and the receivers of messages.

4. Differentiate between hearing and listening.

5. Describe the components of a message.

6. Explain how channels, settings, and timing can influence the perception of the message by the receiver.

7. Discuss the role of noise and feedback in communications.

8. Differentiate between the verbal and nonverbal components of interpersonal communication.

9. Describe how the personal characteristics of the sender may contribute to the noise that distorts messages.

10. Differentiate between essential and optional written communication.

11. Discuss how organizational culture affects communication.

12. Outline how computers and other technologies are changing how we communicate.

13. Identify differences between communicating with individuals and with groups.

14. State how to minimize barriers to communication.

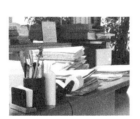

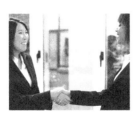

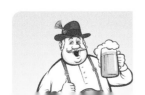

overview

It is assumed that we all know how to communicate. However, good communication between the manager and the employees who report to that manager is crucial to the success of all concerned, so it is an area of management that deserves constant attention. Miscommunication leads to errors and misunderstandings, and can lead to the downfall of an otherwise excellent manager. Effective managers spend more than half of their time communicating with others.[1] They must know how to listen, when to speak, when to write, what modes of communication are effective at reaching different audiences, when to be formal or casual in communicating, and whether to communicate on an individual level or on a group level.

Much communication is spontaneous and routine, so it is easy to take it for granted. It is necessary, however, to think of communication from time to time. This allows the managers to evaluate the skills that they have developed and to identify ways to improve those skills. Wise managers review communications theory every year or so, if only to refresh their memories and to review how they might be able to improve their communications skills. It takes very little effort to go to a continuing education session on communication at a professional meeting or to read a management article on the topic. The benefits of maintaining and improving communications skills are unparalleled by anything else that managers do.

In management, communication is used for a number of purposes. These include information gathering, information dissemination, the sharing of information to coordinate activities, and negotiation. Information gathering occurs in such management tasks as interviewing prospective employees, obtaining data on productivity, conducting market research, evaluating reports from internal and external sources, and determining whether employees should be disciplined or rewarded. Information dissemination takes place during orientation and in-service training; when new programs or products are introduced; to publicize a policy, procedure, event, or change in the organization; and so on. Information sharing is used to coordinate activities between individuals, work groups, departments, and organizations to minimize redundancy and maximize the use of resources. Networking is an example of information sharing. Negotiation is used to determine rights, responsibilities, benefits, liabilities, and contractual issues.

This chapter is designed to be a review of communications theory. Similar material is also found in basic psychology texts, nutrition and other counseling texts, and texts related to education. The material to be covered includes the components of communication and the skills required of successful communicators. Consideration will be given to written, oral, and nonverbal communication. Some of the causes for miscommunication will be identified, along with ways to avoid common communication problems. Considerations for communicating with groups will be included. Throughout the chapter, the use of communications technology such as phones, smartphones, netbooks, and computers will be interspersed as appropriate.

management practice in dietetics

communication

Communication is the interaction between two or more individuals. The interaction allows for information to move from one person to another, either on a person-to-person level or through the use of some type of media. In order for communication to occur, there must be an individual (or group) who sends the message and another (or a group of others) who receives it. Though much of what is communicated is in the form of words, words are not the only factor involved. Other elements of communication include nonverbal images, channels, setting, timing, noise, and feedback.

sending and receiving

It is the responsibility of the **sender** to determine what message is to be sent and to deliver the message in a way that minimizes the chances of the message being distorted, either during transmission or by the receiver of the message. In sending the message, it is the role of the sender to **encode** it in one or more ways, and to **transmit** it to one or more other people. The encoding involves choosing words or other symbols that are clear and unambiguous, and packaging these within a method of delivery that is consistent with the meaning of the underlying message. The package may then be transmitted in person, in print, or through use of other media or technologies.

Care must be taken to avoid sending "mixed messages," in which the verbal message is not supported by the other elements involved in sending the message. For example, if you want to let your employees know that you appreciate their hard work, the message will be more effectively communicated if you speak clearly, with a warm tone of voice and a smile, and have eye contact with the employees while verbalizing the message. Conversely, if you mumble the same message to a group of employees while you continue to work on the stack of papers on your desk, looking at the papers instead of at the people, the words will be less meaningful, or may even take on a distorted meaning.

The **receiver**(s) of the communication must **decode** the message and **interpret** it. They do this by evaluating the various parts of the message they receive and assigning meaning to that information. It should be noted that each receiver will decode the information in a different way, and may apply different interpretations to the message, based on personal experience. This cannot be avoided but can be minimized if the sender is a skilled communicator who has chosen the correct words and has packaged the message well.

Examples of how messages might be received differently follow. Consider the situation in which the clinical nutrition manager commented to a staff dietitian that her assessments of patients with renal disease were "getting better" as she gained experience with this type of patient. The staff member who is pleased with her own progress might take the comment as an affirmation of the hard work that she had done

Sender. *The person who creates and transmits a message to another person or people.*

Encode. *Create a message and determine how it is to be sent.*

Transmit. *Send a message to one or more people (for example, in person, in print, or by using technologies like faxes, modems, phones, and so on).*

Receiver. *The person who gets the message from the sender.*

Decode. *Decipher the message that was received.*

in learning how to work with clients with renal disease, and be motivated to continue to learn more about these clients and their diseases. However, if the clinical dietitian is dissatisfied with her progress in dealing with these patients, she might interpret "getting better" as "still not quite good enough." In this situation, the dietitian could give up and quit trying to improve her skills in dealing with this type of disease.

The interpretation of the message is even somewhat dependent on the current state of mind of the receiver. A cheery "good morning" from the server at a coffee kiosk might get a different reaction from you on a weekday morning when you are late for work than on a weekend morning when you are planning a leisurely visit with a friend over cappuccino.

Though experienced communicators can usually anticipate how a message will be received, they cannot know this with certainty. In mass communications, once a message has been sent, it is difficult to undo any errors in that message. Therefore, this type of message is often pilot-tested on small groups in order to avoid major communications errors when a campaign or advertisement reaches the general public. Test messages or focus groups study the receivers' responses to the communication. Adjustments can then be made in the message or its packaging before the message is distributed on a large scale. Such methods are employed to minimize the potential for miscommunication.

In interpersonal communication, there is little opportunity to pilot-test the message. However, because person-to-person communication is two-way rather than one-way, there is opportunity for adjustment during the interaction. Communicators respond to feedback from receivers and adjust the message in response. Indeed, interpersonal communication is not a series of messages being sent by person A to person B. It is more like a volley of messages being sent by both A and B to each other. Frequently, one or both of the parties is sending and receiving messages simultaneously.

This is as true for the entertainer who responds spontaneously to an audience as it is for the manager who is talking with a single employee. If a musician finds that the audience is falling asleep in the middle of a concert, it is likely that the volume or the tempo of the music will be increased to create more enthusiasm in those attending the event. A comedian may "clean up" the content of his act if he senses that he is offending fans. Speakers use gimmicks, props, slides, voice, movement, and so forth to maintain interaction with those listening to the lecture. Communication is complex and often spontaneous.

listening/hearing

There is a difference between hearing and listening. **Hearing** is a physical sense that takes place automatically, often without thought or attention. It is not possible to turn off hearing voluntarily. People "hear" the music that is played while waiting

management practice in dietetics

"on hold" on the telephone. In this situation, it is not really necessary to pay attention to the music. One notices when the music stops and someone starts to speak, because the spoken word is a signal to begin listening. The voice indicates that person-to-person communication is about to take place; this means it is time to pay attention. Individuals who do more than one activity at a time, like reading a journal while a CD is playing in the background, are likely to be actively involved in the reading and only hearing the music as part of background noise. One notices the background sounds, but may not pay attention to them until there is a change in volume, tone, or some other characteristic of the sound. Athletes running in a marathon will hear the sounds of nature all around them, but may not pay attention to the sounds because they are using their energy and concentration to achieve the goal of completing the marathon. Hearing is often described as passive.

Listening, sometimes referred to as active listening, takes some effort on the part of the listener. It is an active process that requires the individual to decode the message in the context of its package, which includes words, actions, expressions, ideas, and so on. The listener seeks to understand, evaluate, and assimilate the message, and respond to it if necessary. Some listening is done purely for the enjoyment derived from the activity of listening. People play radios and go to concerts for fun, a purely pleasurable use of listening skills. In the workplace, listening is usually done for some other purpose, such as gathering information, or counseling. This type of listening requires that the listener pay attention to the entire message that is being sent.

Some recorded (non-personal) telephone messages, such as those that require a person to "select one of the following six options," require active listening skills even though another person is not involved. That is, the person who is receiving the message must respond in some way for communication to continue. In order to proceed, this person is required to listen to the message, decode it, and then respond, either verbally or by selecting an option on the telephone. To respond appropriately, one must have listened to the instructions in addition to having heard them. If you have ever had to redial a number or replay a list of recorded options because you were unable to make the appropriate selection, it is possible that you heard the recorded message without actually "listening" to it. Thus, active listening may be required even if there is no other person involved.

People who use recorded telephone answering systems for frequent transactions, such as retrieving voice mail messages, know what words are coming and anticipate them by pressing the appropriate button without waiting to hear the recorded message. Active listening is no longer necessary because the transactions have become routine. Though this is acceptable to do when interacting with recorded communications, care must be taken to avoid such temptations when communicating with another person. Recordings send the same message with the same words each time. People are not so predictable. The receiver must be "tuned in" to the sender in interpersonal communication, so active listening takes on an additional dimension.

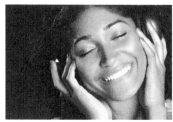

Active listening requires paying attention to what is heard.

Listening.
An active process that requires effort or attention from the listener; used to decode messages.

When communicating with another person, it is necessary for the receiver to decode more than just the words being said. The listener must also interpret the tone of voice of the sender (if the conversation is on the telephone) and the nonverbal communication such as eye contact, body language, facial expressions, and the like if the communication is face to face. Effective listening is hard work that requires concentration and focus. If the receiver does not pay attention to the message that is being sent, it is very possible that the message will be misinterpreted.

components of messages

As stated earlier, the **message** and its **packaging** are the responsibility of the sender. The sender determines both the verbal and nonverbal components of the message. All parts should be consistent. The components of a message are shown in Table 5.1.

content. Communication uses words as symbols. Words are abstract in that it is possible for the same word to have different meanings or interpretations. Consider the message, "Choose healthful snacks." The word *snack* can be interpreted to mean "snack foods," such as cookies or chips, or can be defined as something that is eaten out of the context of a meal, like a piece of fruit or a sandwich. If the receiver of this message uses the former definition and the sender uses the latter, there is room for misinterpretation. The receiver might follow the directive by choosing an oatmeal cookie as a snack, rather than a candy bar. Though this is not necessarily a bad choice, it is not the same as eating a piece of fruit, which may have been the sender's intended message.

language. Words may be delivered orally or in some written form. Either way, care must be taken to choose words that will be understood by the intended recipients of the message. Words that are subject to different interpretations by the receiver should be avoided whenever possible. Scientific jargon may be appropriate when talking or writing to colleagues, but is probably not appropriate when talking to foodservice workers or to people outside of a particular specialty area. Sometimes it is necessary to define words in order to clarify the intended meaning.

The actual content of the message

Level of language/vocabulary used

Other (nonverbal) symbols used to illustrate the message

Delivery style

Complexity of the message

Focus of the message ("I," "you," or neutral)

Table 5.1 Components of a Message

Words, either oral or written, define the content of the message. They also determine the level of the message, how it is delivered, its complexity, and its focus. Words are a major part of the package that is transmitted from the sender to the receiver. They are often supplemented by alternate symbols such as photos, drawings, video, or other graphics that get included as part of the package. Illustrations are used to either enhance the message or to reinforce it. A photo of a well-toned athlete accompanied by words in an advertisement for a sports drink is far more descriptive than the words alone could ever be. Successful public speakers use graphics and photos to enhance and illustrate their presentations. As everyone knows, "A picture is worth a thousand words."

symbols. Sometimes, a message is illustrated with tangible items. These items are intended to extend the message's impact beyond the present. Perhaps the receiver will be given a sample of a product; or a mug, a hat, or a notebook may be imprinted with the message or some key elements of the message (for example, a company logo or a web address). When the receiver takes something tangible away after the initial communication, it is likely that the item will serve as a reminder of the message. Often managers give employees written materials to reinforce their messages. Examples include the employee handbook that is given to an employee upon completion of orientation, or the letter that accompanies a disciplinary action.

delivery style. Delivery styles are as diverse as the message senders, and vary with current circumstances. Examples of delivery styles include warm and friendly, empathetic, calm and collected, businesslike, angry, agitated, overwhelmed, happy, and so on. The style of delivery should be consistent with the message. It is appropriate to smile and be friendly when offering an employee a promotion, but not appropriate to exhibit these emotions when disciplining an employee for poor performance.

complexity. The complexity of the message should be considered, too, as it is an integral part of the message. The message "Don't add fat when cooking" and the message "Consume a diet that contains no more than 30 percent of calories from fat, equally divided among saturated, monounsaturated, and polyunsaturated, and containing an average of no more than 200 mg of cholesterol per day" both speak to the concept of a fat-controlled diet. However, the complexity of the messages is very different. The former message would be appropriate for the cooks in a school lunch program, while the latter would be appropriate for the dietitian who is planning the menu for that program. It is sometimes necessary to sacrifice the precision of the message in order to simplify it enough to achieve understanding by a specific receiver or group of receivers.

focus. The final component of the message is its focus. The message is likely to be interpreted differently if it is focused in a different way. A manager might choose to focus the message on herself ("I see that the report is incomplete"), on the employee ("Your report is incomplete"), or a more neutral focus ("The report is incomplete").

```
Channels
Setting
Timing
Noise
Feedback
Personal Characteristics
    • Verbal
    • Nonverbal
```

Table 5.2 Parts of the Message Package

The first statement expresses the manager's displeasure, the second places blame on the employee, and the latter is a statement of a problem that needs to be corrected. In these examples, the manager might have legitimate reasons to send any of the three different messages. The point is that the focus of the message should be planned as part of the message, not be left to chance.

packaging the message

Channel. *A communication pathway through which a message is transmitted.*

In addition to the message itself (words and other symbols, style, complexity, and focus of the message), the way a message is packaged is also important. The packaging includes the channel through which the message is communicated, the setting, the timing, and other, less controllable conditions listed in Table 5.2.

channels. The **channel** is the pathway between the sender and the receiver of the message. The message travels along this route, which is usually chosen by the sender. Managers have many possible channels for the delivery of messages. These include face-to-face meetings with individuals or groups, telephone calls, voice mail, text messages, e-mail, newsletters, memos, letters, video recordings, and so on. In general, messages that are transmitted through oral channels or electronically move faster than those that are printed and distributed as hard copy.

Direct Channel. *A communication pathway in which the message sent is targeted to a specific group(s) or person(s).*

Indirect Channel. *A communication pathway in which the receiver is not specified.*

Channels may be direct or indirect. Routes are considered to be **direct channels** if specific individuals are targeted to receive the message. When direct channels are used, there is relative certainty that targeted individuals will receive the message. An **indirect channel** is one in which the receiver is not specified. Radio, television, and newspapers are indirect message channels. The "grapevine" is another indirect channel. With these channels, there is no assurance that a designated individual will receive the message. It is best for managers to avoid using indirect channels when the message needs to get to a specific person or people.

management practice in dietetics

It is possible to transmit a single message through more than one channel. In fact, using more than one channel increases the chances of the message being heard. A manager, therefore, might choose to verbalize a message during a staff meeting, follow up with an e-mail or a memo, and post a notice on the bulletin board. Some managers take advantage of the grapevine as a supplementary channel for information dissemination, with good results.

A word of caution is needed when using channels that rely on word-of-mouth transmission of messages from person to person. In such situation, the message is subject to distortion because each person who receives and then transmits the original message interprets it differently. The distortion phenomenon is so predictable that there is a child's game based on it. The more individuals along the route, the more the message will change. Fortunately, advances in communications technology, including group e-mails, instant messaging, automated telephone trees, and robo-calling, have minimized the need for strategies such as the old-fashioned telephone trees that relied on individuals calling other individuals to relay a message by word of mouth.

Setting. *The physical environment in which communication takes place.*

Managers must also be aware that the fact that a message has been received is no guarantee that the receiver has actually read or listened to the message. It is possible to discard unopened letters and memos, to file unread newsletters, or to delete unopened voice mails, e-mails, and instant messages. For critical messages, it may be necessary to include a "return receipt" mechanism in the message channel, so that the receiver is required to acknowledge that the message has been received. This encourages the receiver to attend to the message in a timely manner.

setting. The physical **setting** in which communication takes place is another important part of communication. Consider the meeting room that can be arranged in several different ways, dependent on the purpose of the meeting and the work to be done. If the manager assumes a standing position at the front of the room or the head of the table, the meeting is usually designed to be for information dissemination, in which an individual with authority transfers information to subordinates (Figure 5.1 a). When the manager sits at the head of the table with the group, it indicates that there is openness to two-way communication (Figure 5.1 b). If the manager sits at the table in a position other than the head, it indicates equality among members of the group (Figure 5.1 c). It is appropriate to use different room arrangements for different types of meetings.

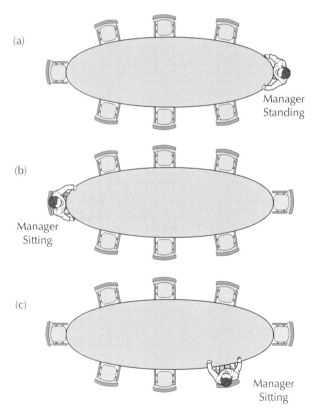

Figure 5.1 Meeting Room Arrangements

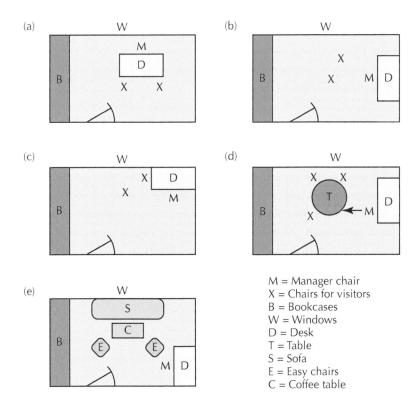

M = Manager chair
X = Chairs for visitors
B = Bookcases
W = Windows
D = Desk
T = Table
S = Sofa
E = Easy chairs
C = Coffee table

Figure 5.2 Office Furniture Arrangements

The arrangement of the room is dictated, in part, by the work to be done. The furniture arrangement in a manager's office also conveys a meaning and should be consistent with the overall message or messages. If a manager sits behind a big desk in the middle of the room (Figure 5.2 a) with the employee seated on the other side of the desk, the manager's power over the employee is a large part of any meeting between them. On the other hand, if the manager's desk is facing a wall, it becomes necessary for the manager to deal with individuals who enter the office by either turning completely away from the desk (Figure 5.2 b) or by working at a closer range across the corner of the desk (Figure 5.2 c). Either of these arrangements indicates a willingness to work together. Another, less intimidating arrangement might be a separate worktable where the parties who are meeting can work together as equals (Figure 5.2 d). An alternate arrangement is no table at all, but seats arranged in the informal fashion of a living room (Figure 5.2 e) where ideas can be exchanged in a relaxed environment. Though the desk is an office fixture in each of the different scenarios, its placement relative to the rest of the furniture sends vastly different messages.

If the content of the communication is sensitive or personal, care must be taken to ensure privacy. For example, it is not appropriate to discipline an employee in a hallway, a general work area, or a cafeteria or restaurant. An office or private meeting

management practice in dietetics

room is a better setting. On the other hand, if the manager and the employee are of different genders, it is probably a good idea to leave the door to the room ajar in order to protect all parties from complaints of sexual harassment. A glass window in the door or in a wall (so that others can see into the office) also provides a degree of protection.

Finally, it should be noted that communication between a manager and an employee sometimes occurs outside of the workplace. It may happen over a meal, during a shared break at the local coffee shop, in a car during travel to an offsite meeting, on public transportation, on the golf course, or in a locker room. Once again, the setting should be in keeping with the underlying message. Proprietary information should be shared in a private setting; general information may be discussed in a more public place. Overall, the setting should be viewed as an essential part of the message package, which should be staged to reinforce the message.

timing. The **timing** of the communication is another important part of the message package. It is not a good idea to announce a major business decision—for example, layoffs or a merger—late Friday afternoon and then send all of the employees home to ponder their fate. Speculation and rumors will run rampant and will not be contained until Monday, when the workforce reassembles. Such major announcements should take place early in the day and toward the beginning of the week. Good timing is also needed on a personal level. If an employee is told of a new assignment the day before a scheduled vacation, it is very likely that the message will be forgotten when that employee returns to work.

Timing. *A strategy for when communication will take place in relation to the present situation and the kind of message relayed.*

Managers often feel the responsibility to pass on information or implement decisions as soon as possible. This allows them to discharge their duties and strike another item off the list. The manager who is also a leader will be sensitive to others in the workplace and may put certain types of communication "on hold" until the time is right. There is a fine line between waiting for the correct time and procrastinating. Care must be taken not to use the former as an excuse for procrastination.

noise. **Noise** is the term used to describe all of the factors that can interfere with the message and distort it. Noise may occur at any point in the communications process. The message may be encoded with words that are not understood by the receiver. The receiver may be otherwise occupied and have insufficient time to decode the message in a coherent way. Noise may come from the setting, from bad timing, or from the communications channel, or may exist because there are incongruities among these factors that dilute the message. External factors like an accident, an illness, or a natural disaster are likely to override the communication and distort the message although they are totally unrelated to the message or its packaging.

Noise. *Interference factors that can affect a message and distort it (for example, physical environment, external factors like illness, bad timing, and so on).*

Another type of noise is technological. With the increased use of electronic devices such as smartphones, netbooks, tablets, and computers, there is the increased potential for noise. Phones ring with an urgency that few people can ignore. Instant messages and e-mail are a constant source of interruption for some individuals. Computers increase our need to sort through more information **now**. The bells, whistles, music, and vibrations produced by these technologies interfere with concentration and decrease attention spans. It is ironic that the very technologies that were designed to improve communication have become a major source of the noise that interferes with that communication.

feedback. Earlier, interpersonal communications were described as a volley of messages being sent back and forth between two or more people. More specifically, **feedback** is the process of responding to messages after interpreting them during two-way interpersonal communication.[2] The message sender can sense whether or not the message has been received and understood. In turn, this information serves as a trigger for further communication.

Feedback goes two ways. The receiver is also a sender in interpersonal communications. If the receiver of a message sends a return message of "I see," the feedback could be a nod or a smile. If the receiver's follow-up message is "I don't agree," the feedback may be a request for more information about the reasons for the disagreement. If the receiver says, "I don't understand," the feedback might be the restating of the basic message in a different package.

The feedback and adjustments in oral communication, whether on the phone or in person, are, in large part, the reason that interpersonal communication is so much faster and more efficient than written or one-way communication. The individuals involved can get immediate clarification that leads to successful communication.

A graphic representation of the communications process is shown in Figure 5.3.

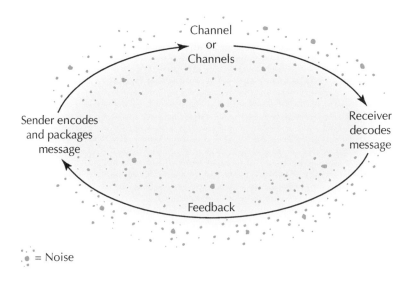

Figure 5.3 The Communication Process

management practice in dietetics

personal characteristics. As discussed earlier, the message sender can exercise a degree of control over much of a message, its content, and its packaging. There are some factors, however, that are out of the sender's control, including decoding, noise, and feedback. In addition, some personal characteristics of the message sender are difficult or impossible to control. Some of these factors enhance communications, some are neutral, and some may interfere with the process. They are factors to be noted, even though it is recognized that it may not be possible to change them. These can be separated into verbal and nonverbal characteristics.

Verbal characteristics include such items as an accent, the speed of natural conversation, tone, pitch, rhythm, and so on. (Accents include both the regional variations of a language and the distinct variations that occur when someone's first spoken language carries over into a second or third language that is learned as an adult.) These characteristics may create noise that distorts the message. This is likely if the receiver is unable to understand the words either because of how they are pronounced or because someone who tends to run words together speaks too quickly. Sometimes these characteristics make it harder to listen to the message. The receiver must concentrate to discern individual words and may miss the concept or the idea being sent.

The nonverbal part of the message also includes some personal characteristics that involve the messenger. These factors are very personal, so it is difficult to deal with them objectively. Non-verbal personal characteristics include artifacts, proxemics, body language, physical characteristics, grooming, and touching behavior.[3] See Table 5.3. Each of these characteristics deserves some elaboration.

Artifacts include the "props" that are used by the message sender. Both the items and their placement send messages. For example, if an employee comes to a manager's office for a scheduled appointment and finds the office organized and a chair available for the employee, it sends the message that the meeting is an important one for the manager. If the work space is cluttered and all chairs are filled with "work in progress" so that a seat has to be cleared for the employee, the message is that the manager considers the meeting to be an interruption. If the manager frequently

Artifacts. *Tangible items and their placement, which are a part of nonverbal communication that can convey an unintended message.*

Artifacts
Proxemics
Body Language
Physical Characteristics
Grooming
Touching Behavior

Table 5.3 Nonverbal Personal Characteristics

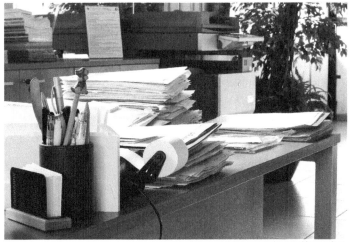

Copyright © 2009 by Depositphotos/Kulikov Andrey.

consults a wristwatch or a large clock that is prominently placed in the room, the employee gets the message that the manager wants the meeting to be over. However, a small clock placed unobtrusively among desk accessories can be checked during a meeting without an employee being aware that the manager is keeping to a time schedule.

In actuality, neither the clutter nor the clock-watching behavior is planned to be a part of the message. In fact, both of these behaviors are probably habitual and unrelated to the communication. However, such behavioral characteristics create noise and may lead to distortion of the message.

Sometimes the artifacts in a cluttered office can interfere with communication.

Proxemics can be described in terms of the spatial relationships between those who are communicating. Usually, small distances between individuals allow for quiet, intimate conversations, whereas large spaces usually require that people speak louder, which results in a loss of privacy. Other factors may influence proxemics, too. For example, if a counseling session must take place in a public area, it may become necessary to use closeness (beyond what is normally considered to be comfortable) as a way to ensure privacy.

Proxemics.
A component of nonverbal communication that defines the spatial relationship between the sender and the receiver of a message.

Individuals require different amounts of personal space to be comfortable. Sometimes the amount of space needed is a matter of individual preference, and sometimes it has a cultural basis. For example, in the United States 1.5–4 feet is considered to be a personal distance. Closer than that is considered intimate; four to 12 feet is called the social zone, and greater than that is the public zone.[5] An attempt by one person to be up close and personal may be interpreted by another to be an invasion of intimate space. Conversely, too large of a distance between individuals may be interpreted by some as avoidance. The spatial preferences of individuals are largely unconscious. Because there is both intercultural and intracultural variation, it is not possible to generalize from a group level to a personal level. Proxemics is, however, a potential source of discomfort and noise during interpersonal communication.

Body Language.
A personal characteristic of nonverbal communication that includes the use and extent of facial expressions and gestures, and may have an impact on communication.

Body language includes gestures, facial expressions, and eye contact. Gestures are important in relationship to proxemics, in that persons who communicate with large gestures require more space around them than those whose gestures are restrained. Broad gestures in small spaces may be threatening. Facial expressions need to be consistent with the message. One should not deliver a serious message with a broad grin, or the message will not be considered serious. On the other hand, a warm smile will reaffirm congratulations for a job well done. Eye contact shows interest and concern.

management practice in dietetics

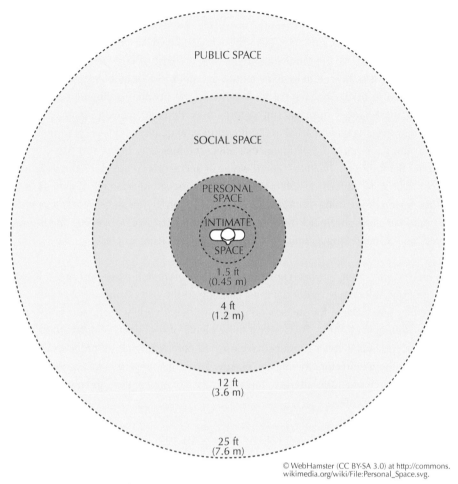

PUBLIC SPACE

SOCIAL SPACE

PERSONAL
SPACE

INTIMATE
SPACE

1.5 ft
(0.45 m)

4 ft
(1.2 m)

12 ft
(3.6 m)

25 ft
(7.6 m)

Figure 5.4 Proxemics[4]

Again, it should be noted that much of what is called body language is actually unconscious, habitual behavior. The inappropriate grin when a serious message is being delivered may be a nervous reaction by the message sender, who is uncomfortable with the task at hand. As with spatial preference and accent, the behavior may not be possible to curtail.

Physical characteristics such as body size and shape are largely predetermined and out of the immediate control of the individual. However, these characteristics sometimes have an effect on how the individual is viewed by others. A large person may be perceived as impressive or intimidating, whereas a small person might be thought to be unimportant or ineffective. Size may also lead to subtle behavioral changes; for example, a small man may routinely use large, dramatic gestures to make his presence felt, whereas a larger woman may use restrained gestures in order to appear to occupy less space. A large person may feel it necessary to sit, so that small colleagues are not intimidated.

Physical Characteristics.
The physical appearance and shape of an individual, which may subtly affect communication.

The **grooming** and attire of the sender are also a part of the message package, albeit frequently an unconscious one. Even though people make choices about what to wear on a daily basis, their individual style is characteristic of the person. If you work in a hospital, it is difficult to imagine a hospital administrator in a tank top and cutoff jeans because that is not typical work attire in the hospital setting. An individual wearing a traditional business suit sends a very different message than the same person in sweatpants and a T-shirt. Furthermore, the quality and level of formality of the clothing are not the only things that affect the message. Color also plays a part, as does flamboyance, neatness, and the type of accessories worn. Such things as hair color, hair style, tattoos, visible pierced body parts, strong-scented cosmetics, and other personal grooming traits also have an impact on the message. A manager with orange hair and long, black fingernails who is wearing twelve earrings might lack credibility when telling a clinical dietitian not to wear jeans to work.

In recent years, there has been much discussion of attire in the business press. Topics range from color, style, and quality of clothing to the use of bows and ribbons on maternity wear. **Dress for success** concepts are being widely used, and not just in the marketing of clothing. There seems to be plenty of anecdotal evidence to support the concept. Social service groups have opened community closet programs, where people without funds for clothing can borrow an outfit to wear to a job interview. The success of such programs attests to the importance of appearance and grooming as a part of communication.

Dress for Success.
The idea that an appropriate appearance and grooming style will create the desired effect during communication.

Appropriate attire and grooming are dependent on the setting. There are no universal rules to follow, and much of what is acceptable is based on current fashion trends. Nevertheless, it is best to exercise prudence where grooming and dress are concerned.

Touching Behavior.
A characteristic of nonverbal communication that describes the extent and ways an individual extends physical contact to others and the kind of message that contact transmits.

The final personal characteristic of nonverbal communication is **touching behavior**. This refers to handshakes, pats on the back, hugs, and hand-holding as well as the touching of clients that may occur during an assessment or a counseling session. These types of behaviors are often spontaneous and unplanned, but do influence the way a message is perceived. For example, it is appropriate to greet a new business acquaintance with a handshake. The firmness or limpness of that initial handshake sends a message of strength and authority or one of weakness and uncertainty. Touching behavior may distort or support the message.

It has been noted that many dietitians do not exhibit touching behavior spontaneously. Indeed, in many clinical roles, dietitians are not required to do much touching, especially when their roles are compared to those of nursing personnel. This is changing as jobs are being enlarged beyond traditional practice roles. For those dietitians who are uncomfortable with touching behavior, it is well to note that some type of physical contact will inevitably become necessary when one assumes a management role.

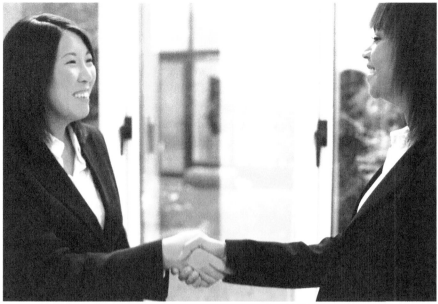

Copyright © 2011 by Depositphotos/Stefano Valle.

Communication includes nonverbal elements such as touching and proxemics.

Because these personal characteristics of message senders are enmeshed in habitual behavior, they are difficult to identify and even more difficult to change. Managers must give some thought to what these personal traits are and how others perceive them. Some of these traits—such as attire, touching behavior, and speech patterns—can be changed, if the individual is willing to work at it. Managers should make an effort to change those behavior patterns that interfere with their ability to manage. A warm smile, a strong handshake, and an expensive suit all have different meanings, but each contributes in a real way to the communication process.

written communication

Within organizations, **written communications** are used for a variety of reasons. Written communications include handwritten, typed, printed, or electronic messages. For a message to be classified as "written" it does not have to be made available as hard copy; written messages can exist exclusively in electronic format. Like oral communication, these methods are used to communicate a message from one or more people to another person or group of people. There are times when written communication is used as a **supplementary channel** to reinforce a message that is sent in other ways as well. Sometimes written messages are used exclusively, without the complementary effect of having the same message sent through alternate channels.

Written Communication.
A type of communication that uses written words to convey the message, either in hard copy or electronic format.

Supplementary Channel.
A secondary pathway used to transmit a message in another way to reinforce the message.

Written communication becomes the preferred method of communication when a message must be imparted to many people who will not all be physically present at the same time. In this situation, repetition is avoided, and there is a degree of confidence that everyone is getting the identical message. Examples of this include the employee handbook, a cafeteria benefits package, or the solicitation for United Way that is included as an insert with paychecks. Some organizations utilize flash drives or DVDs to distribute messages to employees/members. **Websites** are another venue that can be used to provide information to many employees; though graphics are usually included, there is still a great emphasis on the written word in electronic materials.

Websites. *An Internet-based medium that uses electronic, written communication to convey information to many people.*

Written messages are also used when there must be documentation that something happened. In these situations, the written message is the primary channel, and any other channel used is supplementary. Clinical dietitians learn very early in their careers that "if it is not documented, then you didn't do it." If an assessment or the counseling session is not communicated in the medical record, it was not done from the legal viewpoint, and thus cannot be billed or cited for purposes of accreditation or quality management. The medical record is a **legal document**. So are time cards, personnel files, attendance records for in-service training, and minutes of meetings. In all of these cases, the written communication serves as verification that something happened.

Legal Document. *A written record that is required to serve as verifiable evidence that something has occurred.*

There are also optional types of written communication in organizations. These include memos, e-mails, letters, handwritten notes, and so on. These types of written messages are not required, either for legal reasons or for dissemination of the same message to large groups of people. Rather, these types of communications reflect personal and organizational styles. In the following section there is an attempt to differentiate between essential and optional written forms of communication. It should be noted that this division is somewhat arbitrary and varies from organization to organization.

Essential Communications Documents. *Types of written communication that are necessary (fundamental) to carrying out the business of an organization.*

essential communications documents

Some written communications are needed to carry on the business of the organization. These are **essential communications documents**. Included in this category are business letters, reports of all types, strategic plans, and contracts, as well as any legal documentation that is required by an organization. Even the day-to-day activity logs that are used to monitor productivity or temperatures of equipment, telephone logs, and so on are essential to the functioning of the organization. Job postings, advertisements, customer satisfaction surveys, time cards, invoices, receiving documents, and menus are other types of essential business communication.

Longevity of Documents. *The length of time a specific type of written document must be kept.*

Different documents have different uses, so the longevity of documents varies with the document itself. Some documents are transient—that is, used for a short period of time and then discarded. For example, items like satisfaction surveys might be tabulated, and once the aggregated results are reported, the individual surveys are eliminated.

management practice in dietetics

The actual tool or document used need not be kept for long periods of time, because it is the summary of the results that has value to the organization. On the other hand, some documents must be kept for specific periods of time, either because of legal requirements or for accounting purposes. Time cards, cash register tapes, budgets, quality management reports, productivity data, contracts, bids, and other materials have long-term value that requires these items to be stored for prescribed periods of time. The length of time that documents must be stored is determined either by organizational policy or by legal requirements. For example, the Internal Revenue Service requires businesses to keep financial records for a minimum of three years. Medical records are kept indefinitely.

Employee Handbooks and **Human Resource Policy and Procedure Manuals** are other written documents that organizations produce and distribute or disseminate. Both of these documents are essential to the functioning of large organizations, though small ones can sometimes manage without them. Such documents ensure a consistent and evenhanded approach to human resource management and help managers make personnel decisions that are in keeping with organizational priorities. **Departmental Policy and Procedure Manuals** are used to guide departmental activities. In departments that are typically managed by dietitians, these policies might cover such areas as how screenings and assessments are carried out, mealtimes for patients, hours of operation for restaurants and other businesses, how goods are procured, receiving and storage of materials, distribution of food vouchers, and so forth. Even the retention of documents within an organization is usually covered by a written procedure.

optional communications documents

For purposes of this discussion, any written document that is not required for the organization to function is considered to be an **optional communications document**. Such items might include organizational **newsletters**; information about the Red Cross Blood Drive; notes or postings that recognize an individual employee for a job well done, an upcoming marriage, a birth, or another significant life event; and so on. These items are not necessarily related to the business of the organization but have a great deal of value in the realm of employee relations.

Networking is another form of optional communication. Networking is frequently thought of as an oral form of communication (like meeting someone from another department for lunch), but a great deal of networking can also be accomplished through written channels. E-mail to peers in other practice areas or other locations to determine alternate ways to deal with a new challenge is a written form of networking. Sending a letter to recognize a colleague who has published an article in the *Journal of the Academy of Nutrition and Dietetics*, a congratulatory personal note to a local congressional representative who has recently been reelected, or a birthday card to a mentor are also networking. Finally, the **listserve**, designed to allow communication between colleagues about issues of mutual concern, is a very effective type of networking.

Employee Handbooks. *Written or online documents produced by organizations to provide information to employees relating to the organization's mission, policies, rules, benefits, and so on.*

Human Resource Policy and Procedure Manuals. *Written or online documents used as a management tool to direct the actions of management relative to employee relations.*

Departmental Policy and Procedure Manuals. *Written or online documents, specific to a department, that guide the activities and work processes of that department.*

Optional Communications Document. *Any type of written document that is not considered essential to the functioning of an organization.*

All of the examples listed in this section are optional communication because they are not required for day-to-day business purposes. The possibilities for this type of communication are myriad and expanding exponentially as technology becomes more sophisticated. In fact, the use of e-mail and instant messaging is escalating so rapidly that it has replaced many telephone conversations. These formats are shifting the balance of interpersonal business communication from oral to written channels.

organizational culture and written communication

Some managers argue that certain items listed as optional are really an essential part of doing business. It is possible for managers to hold the opinion that networking is a critical part of their jobs and that it is not possible to over-communicate. The more everyone knows, the better. This is true, to a certain extent. In any case, written communication must be viewed within the context of the organization.

It is usually appropriate to withhold **proprietary information** when it is likely that the information will fall into the hands of a competitor. Other types of information may be withheld for a period of time, either to minimize the flow of rumors or to allow for details to be worked out before an announcement is made. Some examples follow. If a company is losing money and needs to lay off a percentage of its workforce, the announcement should be made after the scope of the layoffs has been determined and a plan for the outplacement of those who will lose their jobs is established. It is unfair to the workforce to tell them that "there will be anywhere from 20 to 50 percent reduction in force next year" and then let them worry about their fates for the next several months. That kind of information is fuel for gossip and will lead to dissatisfaction and reduced productivity. In addition, premature announcements will extend the period of turmoil in the workplace that accompanies layoffs. It is far better to make this kind of announcement when there is a plan in place to help workers get through the crisis.

There is sometimes a rationale for withholding good news, as well. If, for example, the organization is growing rapidly and needs a larger facility, it is not necessary to inform all workers of the impending change before a facility is procured and a moving date set. People naturally resist change and may be upset by the prospect of a move. Indeed, when faced with such a change, it is less unsettling to know that the logistics have been worked out. Unscheduled bonuses for workers are another item that should not be announced too far in advance, because anticipation might lower the effect of the bonus program, or an unforeseen downturn in business may lead to a reduction in the planned bonus program.

Finally, there must be a clear understanding of which information is proprietary and which is not. In order to minimize the potential for leaks, individuals must know what can only be shared within the organization and what is acceptable to share externally. Messages that are confidential should be clearly identified so that everyone who has

management practice in dietetics

access to the information knows that the information is restricted. Confidentiality is of special concern when using electronic communication such as e-mail, which may be either sent to the wrong party or intercepted during the transmission.

In health care, confidentiality regarding patient information is considered to be proprietary, only to be shared among authorized personnel and the patient. The law regulating this information and how it is to be used is called the **Health Insurance Portability and Accountability Act of 1996** (HIPAA).[6] Generally speaking, individuals who work with patient information are subject to the requirements of this law with respect to privacy of patient information.

HIPAA.
http://www. hhs.gov/ocr/ privacy/hipaa/ understanding/ index.html.

Outside of the planned withholding of proprietary or other information for planning or verification purposes, the information that is shared within an organization and the methods used to share the information are directly related to the organizational culture. A major variation based on organizational norms is the amount of information that is communicated and who has access to it. In the traditional organization, information flows upward and downward through the organizational levels in a very formal way. Managers are expected to report to their superiors and to disseminate information to their subordinates. The amount of information that is shared is based on how information is viewed. If it is perceived as a source of power, it will be hoarded and shared stingily on a "need to know" basis. If it is viewed as a tool of empowerment, then it will be shared more openly, but still up and down through the normal reporting relationships of the organizational structure.

In less-traditional organizations, information flows more freely and communication is more open without the constraints outlined in the organizational chart. Messages are sent to all potentially interested people. There is very little hoarding of information, because the organizational philosophy is to keep everyone in the loop with the intent that additional information will empower employees and strengthen the organization. It may be difficult to intentionally withhold information in such an organization, because information routinely flows so freely that "leaks" may happen inadvertently.

Another organizational variable is related to the preferred channel of communication. In one organization, it might be routine to write a memo or send an e-mail after a meeting to reinforce any discussions and agreements reached at that meeting. It may even be a standard practice to send copies to everyone in order to disseminate the information as widely as possible. Memos are a part of doing business and are expected. In another organization, one that relies heavily on oral communication, the memo might be used as a last resort when oral communication fails. What is a routine practice in one setting could mean "I don't trust you" someplace else. Though the memo is exactly the same, the way it is interpreted will be dependent on organizational culture. Managers who move from one organization to another would do well to observe how the new organization uses oral and written communication channels before establishing a personal style.

using computers to communicate

There is no doubt that computers have changed the way we handle written communications. Word processing has allowed many managers to prepare their own correspondence, without secretarial support. This has an advantage in that it saves time and duplication of effort. However, it eliminates the "second opinion"—that is, the individual who proofreads and does grammar checks to make sure that the communiqué is correct. Computers can perform this function but do not always do so with precision. Therefore, care must be taken to proofread computer-generated correspondence to eliminate errors in grammar and spelling.

E-mail and instant messaging have a unique set of potential problems. They can be close to real time, in that a volley of messages can go back and forth between individuals in minutes. In addition, one can respond to e-mail in a rote, non-thinking way (much like hearing without listening). It is not uncommon for individuals to have second thoughts about a message after it has been sent. Sometimes a message meant for one recipient goes to a group of recipients instead. As users become more experienced with their own e-mail program, the errors tend to lessen in number. Nevertheless, even the most experienced users occasionally "reply to all" rather than reply to an individual, often with embarrassing consequences.

There is concern that the increased use of e-mail has cluttered the workplace with unnecessary information and that the processing of this increased communication is taking precedence over actually doing work. A variety of e-mail management strategies are evolving to allow individuals to manage the incoming e-mail and still accomplish work. These include only working on e-mail during certain, limited time periods (e.g., 8:00–8:30 a.m. and 2:00–2:30 p.m.), or a specific number of times per day.[7] Of concern, too, is the potential that e-mail has diluted or is replacing face-to-face communication. That is, someone may send an e-mail to the person in the office next door rather walking a few steps to speak directly to that colleague.

When telephones were an emerging technology, the "ring" had a sense of urgency that few people could resist. Phones were answered immediately. As the phone became a common household tool, answering machines and voicemail took some of the urgency out of answering the phone. Call screening and caller ID have effectively allowed "junk" messages to be ignored, just as junk mail is discarded. In the same way, experience with electronic communications allows users to become efficient at sorting through the deluge of mail to identify those items that need attention while being able to screen and discard the junk e-mail (spam). For some tips on using e-mail effectively for business purposes, see Table 5.4.

- Use short subject headings.
- Double-check to be sure that you are sending it to the correct individual/s and not to others inadvertently.
- Use correct capitalization and punctuation.
- Grammar- and spell-check all messages (poorly written e-mails reflect badly on you and your organization).
- Proofread all messages *before* you execute the "send" command.
- Avoid the use of emoticons like ☺ ;-) and :-☐ in business communications.
- Send messages to a group only if everyone needs the information. Do not become a "spammer."
- Keep the message short. Use attachments to send long documents, photos, and other files. Too much information is distracting.
- Don't be reactive; it is not necessary to respond to e-mails immediately.
- Set up and use professional "signatures" to identify yourself to recipients. (Include at least your name, title, and contact information.)
- Use the "return receipt" function if you need to confirm delivery of message that you are sending.
- Keep copies of outgoing mail, if possible. If this is not possible, send copies to yourself.
- Set up a filing system to sort and organize your e-mail.

Table 5.4 Tips for Using E-Mail and Listserves in Business

communication to groups

The discussion on communication has, thus far, made no distinction between individuals and groups. A brief discussion about communicating to groups is necessary, too. As the number of receivers increases, the messages become less personal, even if they are delivered in person. This means there is less tolerance for errors and a greater chance for distortion because each receiver might interpret the message differently. When communication targets groups of receivers, therefore, there must be greater attention to the packaging of the message.

In general, larger audiences require more sophisticated packaging of the messages. In the case of oral communication, if a speaker is conducting a seminar for 12 individuals, the acoustics in the meeting room are of little concern. A PowerPoint projector would probably be sufficient for audiovisual purposes, and the presentation could be planned as a dialogue between the presenter and the audience. However, if the seminar had an audience of 850 people, a public-address system and automatic equipment for projecting presentation materials need to be available. The equipment should be set up and tested beforehand, and an equipment operator should be on hand during the presentation. Furthermore, in this situation, dialogue would probably be replaced with a lecture-style presentation.

Slides and handout materials are useful, but these should be checked for errors and should not be used if they are of poor quality or contain spelling or grammatical errors.

Today's audiences are used to the slick presentations that are entertaining as well as informative. Errors in materials create noise that interferes with the receipt of the message. When slides cannot be read because of small print, or because the focus of the projector is not adjusted properly, whole rooms of attendees become distracted and restless. When equipment fails and the audience becomes distracted, it is preferable for the speaker to abandon the props and rely on the oral presentation alone. Even something that seems trivial—for example, the uncomfortable chairs for the audience or an uncomfortable room temperature—can cause enough noise to distort the message.

Printed materials are costly to produce in large quantities, so care should be taken to evaluate the materials thoroughly before actually printing them. It is expected that printed materials will be free of typographical and grammatical errors. However, these materials should also be evaluated to ensure that they are free of cultural bias and are written at the appropriate reading level for the audience. Printed materials should be gender-neutral and "politically correct." It is not possible to correct an inadvertent slip in a printed document that has been distributed to hundreds of people. Written materials are tangible, permanent, and verifiable.

Politically Correct.
A designation for terminology that is non-offensive or neutral to replace words or phrases in common usage that may be disparaging, offensive, or insensitive.

other communication barriers

A number of barriers to good communications have already been noted in this chapter. Those associated with the message sender include inappropriate channels, poor timing, improper language, unsuitable settings, and distracting verbal or nonverbal characteristics. Receivers create barriers, too. These include selective perception (when they see or hear what they expect to see or hear) and their emotional state at the time the message is received. Finally, noise generated by the sender, the receiver, or the external environment creates a barrier to good communication.

Taking care to encode and package the message properly will minimize some of these barriers, as will making efforts to minimize sender-generated noise. Methods for accomplishing this have been discussed earlier in the chapter. Other techniques that the sender can use to reduce the barriers include using feedback (both verbal and nonverbal), active listening, and constraining one's own emotions when communicating. Some additional communications barriers are described here, along with ways to minimize their negative impact on communications.

regional language

Within the United States and Canada, there are regional variations in language that are well known to locals but may not be understood by those who are not from that geographic region. For example, people from the southern United States use the phrase "tump over" in the same way that Northerners would use "turn over," as in "The cat tumped over the flower vase."[8] In Western Pennsylvania, everyone knows what it means to "redd up the house," but in Oregon the word "redd" is unknown. (*Redd up* means to "make tidy."[9]) If communication is confined to a geographic region, it is acceptable to use regional English. However, if the message is being widely distributed throughout North America, it is best to avoid the use of regional language.

cultural variations

The barriers that occur because of cultural differences among groups are especially apparent for those who work internationally or in places with diverse populations like those found in Florida, New York, California, and Texas. These cultural barriers include language (especially words that do not translate directly), proxemics, body language, touching behavior, and customs.

In Arabic-speaking countries, the word *salaam* is used for hello, good-bye, and peace; *shalom* is a comparable word in Hebrew. However, there is no comparable English word and therefore no way to translate this word directly. New arrivals from Israel or Egypt may have difficulty differentiating between "hello" and "good-bye." Equally confusing are English words with multiple meanings. For example, *hard* might mean difficult, or it might represent the opposite of *soft*. When communicating with individuals who are not fluent in English, words with multiple definitions should be avoided.

It is important to avoid the use of stereotypical terms related to gender, age, body size, ethnicity, etc. For example, not all German men are obese nor do they drink too much beer.

In parts of Eastern Europe, people live in close quarters and are accustomed to having very little personal space. They are comfortable in crowds, and being jostled by others on buses or on the street is perfectly acceptable. Many Americans would feel violated if this happened to them. It is important not to react negatively if you feel that someone from a different culture is invading your personal space.

The ceremony that exists around the exchange of business cards in Japan shows respect and politeness. Westerners often feel uncomfortable when confronted with this situation. They may even feel that it is a waste of time, and unnecessary. However, to the Japanese, it is a way of life, and essential to how business is done.

These and similar differences are prevalent in the United States and Canada, because of the diversity that exists within the populations of these countries, and because of the ready availability of

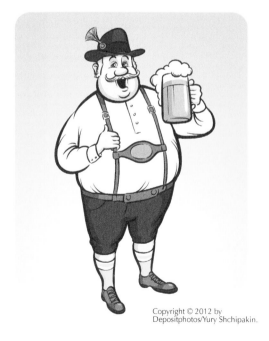

- Expect there to be cultural differences.
- Learn what you can about the other person's culture.
- Become an objective observer of whatever differences exist.
- Do not assume that different means "less" or "worse"; remember that different means "different."
- Don't jump to conclusions.
- Avoid stereotyping.
- Try to take the other person's perspective.
- Appreciate and value diversity.

Table 5.5 Guidelines for Intercultural Communications

international travel. When dealing with cultural differences, it is helpful to follow the guidelines outlined in Table 5.5.

gender

It has been suggested that there are differences in the communication styles of men and women.[10] Men tend to use more "I" messages or "you" messages than do women, who seem to keep their messages more neutral and less judgmental. In doing so, the woman may be attempting to be sensitive and kind, but male colleagues may interpret her words as indirect, or downright sneaky. Men reach conclusions and offer solutions more quickly than do women, who spend more time gathering information before taking action.

Gender differences, while not universal, are apparent in communications style. They also exist in management style and in the decision-making process. Though it is probably not possible (nor desirable) to eliminate the differences related to gender, it is appropriate to be sensitive to them, to respect the differences, and to apply guidelines similar to those outlined for intercultural communication.

One of the characteristics of the profession of dietetics is that it attracts mostly women as practitioners. In fact, 96% of RDs are women.[11] Many dietetics professionals are not assertive, which is consistent with the female style of information gathering and suggesting rather than dictating what is to be done. Women may also be more tentative when dealing with men, than with other women.[12] Dietitians who are considering a transition into managerial roles would do well to assess their own communication patterns and to take steps to develop assertiveness if this skill is lacking.

generational differences

An emerging area of study is the differences between generations and the ways in which they communicate. Four distinct groups have been identified.[13] The Traditionalists (born before 1945) are loyal to an organization and want job security. The Baby Boomers (born from 1946 to 64) are interested in interpersonal communication, want to understand the organization as an entity, and want to work with others to succeed. Generation Xers (born from 1965 to 80) are focused on personal growth, question authority, and embrace change; they have portable careers and are not loyal to any one organization. Generation Yers, also known as Millennials, (born from 1981 to 99) are technologically adept, like to participate in decision-making, seek parallel careers through multitasking, and are comfortable with diversity.

Because of these differences in values and goals, communication between and among these groups is sometimes lacking, sometimes distorted. It is useful to consider these factors when working with individuals of differing ages, or when coordinating the work of such persons. Respect for various viewpoints, flexibility, and trust are critical factors in bridging the generation gap.

politically correct terminology

Much emphasis has been placed on the need to use politically correct (PC) designations for individuals and groups in society. Giving managers the benefit of the doubt, it can be assumed that inappropriate terms are not widely used with the direct intent to harm or disparage those who are different. Still, the use of racial, ethnic, sexual, or other slurs is a common occurrence that hurts and offends people in our society every day. But finding the correct term is a dilemma. Most managers know which terms are taboo but have difficulty choosing replacement words. It is difficult to keep up with the plethora of new PC terms, some of which are cumbersome (*differently abled*) and others of which are even a bit silly (*vertically challenged*).

Within groups, the preferred terminology may also vary. Some people whose heritage is African prefer to use *Black*, whereas others prefer *African American*; people who trace their history to Mexico may prefer *Latino*, *Chicano*, or *Hispanic*, depending on their individual circumstances and ancestry. Asian Americans may favor that term or may prefer a more precise designation such as *Korean-American*, *Vietnamese-American*, or *Chinese-American*. There will be no attempt here to outline PC terminology. The designations are subject to change as society evolves. However, managers need to be sensitive and to use politically correct terminology when communicating. Disparaging remarks and insensitive stereotyping (even positive stereotyping, like "you must be a good cook, you're French") do no one any good and often can do irreparable damage to both business and personal relationships.

conclusion

This chapter has provided a review of communications theory as it relates to management practice in dietetics. The review is not an exhaustive one and does not include therapeutic aspects of communication. The major concepts that have been discussed follow.

1. The message sender encodes and packages the information to be communicated.
2. The receiver is responsible for decoding the message.
3. Listening is an activity that requires concentration and skill; hearing is passive.
4. The message and its packaging should be consistent with each other and geared toward the intended receiver.
5. Feedback and noise are an inevitable part of interpersonal communication.
6. Written communication is tangible, permanent, and verifiable.
7. Communicating with groups requires significant attention to detail.
8. It is important to avoid or minimize barriers to communication.

activities

activity 1

Watch several weather forecasters deliver weather reports on local or national television. Alternately, you may watch a salesperson on a home shopping channel. Analyze the personal characteristics, both verbal and nonverbal, of these people. (Note that you may not be able to evaluate proxemics, but you should be able to make observations about all the other personal characteristics listed in this chapter.)

activity 2

Write a letter to a state or federal legislator on an issue of concern to dietetics professionals. If you are a student, your instructor can give you a list of appropriate topics. If you are reading this text on your own, you may get ideas for this letter by contacting the Academy of Nutrition and Dietetics Legislative Office at 800-877-0877 or visiting the organization's home page at www.eatright.org/ where you can link to Public Policy.

activity 3

You will need the following items to complete this activity:

1 loaf of sliced bread	1 #32 scoop or a 1 tablespoon measure
1 jar of peanut butter	1 spreader for the PB & J
1 jar of grape jelly	1 knife for cutting sandwiches
1 large cutting board	1 serving platter

1. Write down the directions for making ten peanut butter and jelly sandwiches. After the sandwiches are made, they are to be cut in quarters and arranged on a plate. Submit these instructions to your instructor.
2. Your instructor will select one set of directions from among those submitted; the instructor or a designated student will attempt to follow the instructions precisely as they are written.
3. Enjoy your lunch!

activity 4

Look at the arrangement of the furniture in the classroom where you meet for this class. Evaluate the arrangement, and then answer the following questions.

1. Does your instructor rearrange the furniture when different teaching methods are used?
2. If yes, does the rearrangement have an impact on how you learn?
3. If no, could rearranging the furniture change how you learn?

Consider your instructor's teaching methods (for example, lecture, dialogue, discussion, seminar, role playing, use of audiovisuals, in-class exercises, and so on), then answer the following questions.

1. How might these methods change if the class were independent study with only one student?
2. How would you communicate this information to a group of fewer than five students?
3. What changes would be necessary if there were 100 or more students enrolled in the class?
4. How could this information be transmitted entirely though electronic communications?

activity 5

The organization that you work for has a standing policy that prohibits the use of personal smartphones at work. It is your responsibility as the Director of Support Services to enforce this policy. How would you develop and package a message related to this policy for each of the following?

1. An individual employee who was not adhering to the policy.
2. A group of newly hired personnel during their orientation.
3. Generalized noncompliance occurring throughout the entire organization.
4. Employees in one department who chose to ignore the policy.
5. Another manager, who was using a smartphone "because this is an emergency."

to study further

Additional information on communication can be found in the following materials.

- Brown, Damon. "Ways Dietitians of Different Generations Can Work Together." *Journal of the American Dietetic Association,* 103:1461–1462, 2003.
- Bryant, Carol A. et al. *The Cultural Feast: An Introduction to Food and Society.* 2nd ed. Belmont, CA: Wadsworth/Thomson Learning, 2003.
- Buzzanell, Patrice M., ed. *Rethinking Organizational & Managerial Communication from Feminist Perspectives.* Thousand Oaks, CA: Sage Publications, Inc., 2000.
- Chernoff, Ronni. *Communicating as Professionals.* 2nd ed. Chicago: American Dietetic Association, 1994.
- Gross, Kim J. and Jeff Stone. *Chic Simple Dress Smart for Women: Wardrobes That Win in the Workplace.* New York: Warner Books, 2002.
- Gundykunst, William B. *Bridging Differences: Effective Intergroup Communication.* 4ed. Thousand Oaks, CA: Sage Publications, Inc., 2004.
- Gundykunst, William B. and Young Yun, Kim. *Communicating with Strangers: An Approach to Intercultural Communication.* 4th ed. New York: The McGraw-Hill Companies, Inc., 2003.
- Holli, Betsy B. et al. *Communication and Education Skills for Dietetics Professionals.* 5th ed. Philadelphia: Lippincott Williams and Wilkins, 2008.
- Kittler, P. G. et al. *Food and Culture.* 6th ed. Belmont, CA: Wadsworth, Cengage Learning, 2012.
- Lustig, Myron W. and J. Koester. *Intercultural Competence: Interpersonal Communication Across Cultures.* 7th ed. Upper Saddle River, NJ: Prentice Hall, 2012.
- McCaffree, J. "The Generation Gap at Work: Myth or Reality?" *Journal of the American Dietetic Association,* 107:2043–2044, 2007.
- McWilliams, M. and H. Heller. *Food Around the World: A Cultural Perspective.* Upper Saddle River, NJ: Pearson Education, 2002.
- Munter, M. *Guide to Managerial Communication: Effective Business Writing and Speaking.* 9th ed. Upper Saddle River, NJ: Pearson Education, Inc., 2011.
- Peregrin, T., "Clothes Call: Your Professional Image Can Have a Big Impact on Your Career." *Journal of the American Dietetic Association.* 109:395–397, 2009.
- Pinkley, R., "Salary and Compensation Negotiation Skills for Young Professionals." *Journal of the American Dietetic Association.* 104:1064–1068, 2004.
- Reynolds, S. and D. Valentine. *Guide to Cross-Cultural Communication.* 2nd ed. Upper Saddle River, NJ: Pearson Education, Inc., 2011.
- Samovar, L. A. et al. *Communication Between Cultures.* 7th ed. Belmont, CA: Wadsworth, Cengage Learning, 2009.
- Stein, K. "Communication Is the Heart of the Provider-Patient Relationship." *Journal of the American Dietetic Association.* 106:508–512, 2006.
- Stein, K. "Moving Cultural Competency from Abstract to Act." *Journal of the American Dietetic Association,* 110:180–187, 2010.

scholarly journals

- *Communication Studies*
- *Communication Research*
- *Journal of Business Communication*
- *Management Communication Quarterly: An International Journal*

relevant websites

- State of Colorado Employee Handbook http://www.colorado.gov/cs/Satellite/DPA-DHR/DHR/1251573425202
- City and County of San Francisco Employee Handbook http://www.sfdhr.org/index.aspx?page=30

in practice

planned ambiguity

In communication, generally speaking, it is best to be precise. Sometimes, in order to simplify the message for the target audience, some imprecision is acceptable. As an example, the Daily Values are simplified into the Dietary Guidelines for Americans, which are further simplified into ChooseMyPlate in order to meet the needs of the various target audiences for each of these standard tools.

Sometimes the lack of precision in a communication is purposeful for other reasons, and that imprecision is actually a part of the message being transmitted. Consider the following assignment given to students in a dietetic program …

---

analysis of an herb or botanical

(a.k.a. the science behind the claims)

The purpose of this assignment is for the student to complete a critical review of an herb or a botanical supplement that is marketed to the public. Frequently, these products claim many health benefits. Some of these claims are evidence-based, but many are not. Much of what is published is rooted in tradition or folk medicine with no substantiation in science.

You are to complete a critical analysis of the literature related to the herb or botanical that you have chosen using the following general guidelines.

- *Look at the lay literature and websites related to the product and list all the claims that are made regarding the health benefits of the product.*
- *Note the type of supportive evidence cited in this material. Consider if it is science-based, based on testimonials, folklore, or if there is another basis for the claims.*
- *Evaluate materials that are presented on reliable websites like the Cochrane Collaboration http://www.cochrane.org/, the Office of Dietary Supplements http://ods.od.nih.gov/, or the National Center for Complementary and Alternative Medicine http://nccam.nih.gov/.*
- *Check out the questions and controversies related to your product on websites like http://www.quackwatch.com, http://www.ncahf.org, and their affiliated sites.*

- *Do a search on either BIOSIS or PUBMED or your school's library search engine to determine which of the health claims related to your product are substantiated by scientific evidence of effectiveness in **controlled, double-blind human studies**. If there are no definitive human studies proving effectiveness, then you should not indicate that the substance is effective. You will be expected to turn in an assignment that is complete and correct. If you do not substantiate your claims, you will be asked to redo the paper.*
- *Report your findings in a paper that lists bona fide uses for the product as well as those claims that are unsubstantiated. Be sure that you report your findings in scientific or medical terms, not lay terms. For example, if something is effective for digestive problems, state what the specific "digestive problem" is (e.g., nausea, constipation, gastroesophageal reflux, etc.); if something is effective for diabetes, specify type one or type two; if something is used to treat arthritis, specify whether it is used for rheumatoid arthritis, osteoarthritis, or gouty arthritis.*
- *If the physiologic basis for the effectiveness of the product is known, you should include that in your report.*

At first glance the assignment looks clear enough. The instructor was helpful and provided students with a list of resources from which to begin the research. The instructions are very specific regarding how to proceed with the project using a step-by-step approach. Students were even reminded to use precise scientific language when reporting their results.

Once students begin to work on the assignment they find that they have a lot of unanswered questions. How long should the paper be? How many websites should be visited? How many controlled, double-blind human studies are needed to substantiate a claim? How many citations are required? How can the effectiveness of a product really be determined? What if the research data is not conclusive? How should conflicting data be reported?

The instructor's answers to these questions are unbelievably vague. The paper should be long enough to "*complete a critical review of an herb or a botanical supplement that is marketed to the public.*" As to the number of studies needed to substantiate a claim ... "That depends on the total number of studies done." Regarding the number of citations needed ... "As many as you've consulted to substantiate your position, including both scientific and lay literature." How to determine the effectiveness of the product ... "If there is preponderance of evidence in one direction and no real conflicting data, then you probably can say the product is effective." About non-conclusive research data ... "I guess that's why more research is underway."

And questions regarding format … "Present your results in a manner that will be clear to the reader."

Why would an instructor purposefully give such an ambiguous assignment? What could students possibly learn from dealing with this much frustration? The answer has several parts. Doing a critical review is not easy when there are no limits put on the data to be gathered. This leads to the type of confusion that consumers face when trying to make an informed choice about the use of botanicals. One of the lessons for the student, then, is to develop empathy with the consumer. It is easier to reach a conclusion when someone you trust (a teacher) tells you the answer than when you have to figure things out for yourself.

Second, the instructor is trying to help the students to develop critical-thinking and problem-solving skills. This is not possible unless the student is faced with complex problems that they have to deal with on their own. Answering the students' questions more precisely would probably make the instructor more popular, and result in better scores on the end-of-semester evaluations, but the students would not have experienced the same kind of learning.

Finally, the vagueness of the assignment is very much like what happens in the workplace. The public health officer will not tell you to write a proposal to open a new clinic and then tell you what to include in the proposal, how many references you need, and how long the document is to be. If you are a clinical nutrition manager who needs to revise your hospital's patient education materials, no one will tell you what format to use or what diets to include. And the food service director will not be told how to justify the switch from a cook-serve to a cook-chill system. As a professional, the manager is expected to figure this all out, using problem-solving and critical-thinking skills. Essentially, this assignment is preparing students for the future.

In the addition to learning about a botanical, the assignment described above is enabling the student to learn how to locate information, process it, and report it in a coherent way. Problem solving and critical thinking are skills that must be learned by professionals, and it is best done in school, where it is safe(r) to make mistakes.

references

1. Axley, Stephen R. *Communications at Work: Management and the Communication-Intensive Organization*. Westport, CT: Quorum Books, 1996.
2. Holli, Betsy B., Richard D. Calabrese, and Julie O'Sullivan Maillet. *Communication and Education Skills for Dietetics Professionals*. 4th ed. Philadelphia: Lippincott Williams and Wilkins, 2003. p 16.
3. Goldsmith, Elizabeth. *Resource Management for Individuals and Families*. St. Paul, MN: West, 1996.
4. Hall, Edward T. *The Hidden Dimension*. New York: Anchor Books, 1966.
5. Wikipedia. Proxemics. http://en.wikipedia.org/wiki/Proxemics accessed July 6, 2012.
6. Michael, P. and E. Pritchett. "Complying with Health Insurance Portability and Accountability Act: What It Means to Dietetic Practitioners." *Journal of the American Dietetic Association*, 102:1402–1403, 2002.
7. Oklahoma State University. Research in E-Mail Management Strategies http://iris.okstate.edu/rems/index.htm accessed July 8, 2012.
8. Free Online Dictionary. "Tump over." http://www.thefreedictionary.com/tump+over accessed July 8, 2012.
9. Cassidy, Frederic G., ed. *Dictionary of American Regional English*. Cambridge, MA: Belknap Press of Harvard University Press, 1985.
10. Tannen, Deborah. *Talking from 9 to 5: Women and Men in the Workplace: Language, Sex and Power*. New York: Avon, 1995.
11. American Dietetic Association. *Compensation & Benefits Survey of the Dietetics Profession 2011*. Chicago: American Dietetic Association, 2011. p 180.
12. Palomares, Nicholas. "Women Are Sort of More Tentative Than Men, Aren't They?" *Journal of Communications Research*. 36:538–560, 2009.
13. Lancaster, Lynne C. and David Stillman. *When Generations Collide*. New York: Harper Business, 2002.

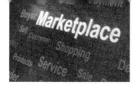

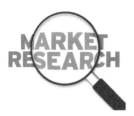

chapter six

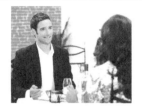

marketing

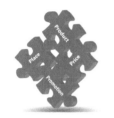

learning objectives

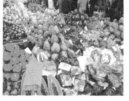

1. Define *marketing*.

2. Describe the various approaches to the marketplace, including production, product, selling, marketing, and social marketing.

3. State why marketing is important to the management process.

4. Identify differences between the nutrition professional's role as a marketer and as a consumer.

5. Discuss the differences between mass marketing and marketing to target populations.

6. List the methods that are used to conduct market research.

7. Identify the components of the marketing mix.

8. Differentiate among the various types of products that are available to consumers.

9. Describe the market channels that are used to get product from producer to consumer.

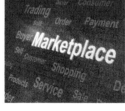

10. Describe the relationship between marketing and price.

11. List several ways to promote goods, services, and combination products.

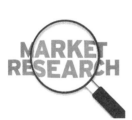

overview

For years, dietitians have been viewed as potential consumers of a variety of food and nutrition-related products. These range from food products to enteral formulas, from commercial kitchen equipment to pumps for delivering nutrition support, from computer systems and books to tableware and disposable napkins. As a matter of fact, every year more than 350 exhibitors market their products to dietitians at the annual meeting of the Academy of Nutrition and Dietetics called The Food and Nutrition Conference and Exhibit (FNCE).

More recently dietetics professionals have been marketing themselves, their profession, and their products. Previous generations of dietitians felt little need for marketing skills because dietetics professionals faced little competition. In foodservice, they worked in the onsite sector with a "captive clientele," so the value of pleasing the customer went unrecognized for a long time. Customers had little choice—they could eat what was served, or they could choose not to eat. There were no nearby restaurants or food trucks in competition with onsite foodservices. In clinical and community settings, the attitude was often that the dietetics professional, using a patriarchal model, determined what the clients needed and delivered it to them. There was little recognition of what the consumers wanted or perceived their needs to be.

Luckily, times have changed, and so have dietetic professionals. In fact, 42% of RDs state that they promote "food/nutrition programs/products/services through interactions with others."[1] In order to compete effectively with other entities that offer nutrition advice, sell questionable supplements, promote ineffective (and sometimes unsafe) diets, and make unsubstantiated claims, dietetic professionals have become more customer oriented. The profession understands that it must meet the needs of consumers if it is to survive. In foodservice, community nutrition, and clinical nutrition, professionals are identifying markets, studying them, and developing products that are responsive to customers' requirements. Onsite foodservices no longer have a "take it or leave it" attitude. Nutrition clinics are leaving the hospitals and opening satellite sites in shopping centers and medical office buildings, where the clients are likely to be. Evening appointments are being scheduled to accommodate the needs of the working person. Mothers who patronize WIC clinics are provided with childcare so that they can attend educational programs. Even the school lunch program provides choices to participants through the "offer versus serve" program. Not only have dietetics professionals learned about marketing, they are also getting pretty good at it!

Marketing.
A management tool that focuses on identifying the needs, wants, and demands of customers and developing products to meet those needs.

Marketing is a management tool that focuses on identifying the needs, wants, and demands of customers and developing products to meet those needs. The view of marketing as a way of satisfying customer needs is a concept that is broad enough to be used as the central focus of the organization. The market-centered organization spends a great deal of time and effort determining who the consumers are and what

management practice in dietetics

they desire, then develops goods or services to meet those needs. Sometimes the organization, either purposefully or accidentally, actually *creates* consumer needs.

This does not imply that, to be successful, an organization must be entirely market-driven. There are plenty of successful organizations that have another type of focus—health care, for example. However, successful organizations are aware of marketing and its impact on the well-being of the organization. Marketing does not have to be the central focus of the organization to have a major impact on enhancing its competitiveness and long-term viability.

This chapter will address how marketing influences dietetics practice from two perspectives—that of the professional in the role of marketer and that of the professional as a consumer. Initially, the various ways that organizations view the marketplace will be described. This will be followed by a look at how various market segments are targeted and a brief description of market research. Finally, there will be a discussion of marketing mix, including product, price, place, and promotion.

Marketplace.
The milieu in which goods are exchanged; can be viewed from the perspective of production, product, selling, marketing, or social marketing.

the marketplace

The way that an organization views its market will have a major impact on how that organization is perceived, both by the organization's staff and by outsiders. There are five classic ways that an organization sees its **marketplace**, and though marketing theory has evolved over time, not all organizations are at the same stage of evolution. In the Americas, various views of the marketplace are held by different organizations. The five ways that companies are oriented toward the marketplace are described in Table 6.1.

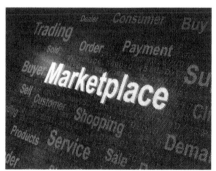

Copyright © 2012 by Depositphotos/Maksim Kabakou.

Production Perspective	The consumer will favor products that are readily available and affordable.
Product Perspective	The consumer will favor the product that has the most value, desirable features, or best performance.
Selling Perspective	Direct promotion to consumers to introduce them to a product that was not being sought.
Marketing Perspective	Determining the wants and needs of the target market and developing products to satisfy those needs.
Social Marketing Perspective	Balancing the customers' needs for satisfaction with the organizational goal of making a profit while acting in the best interest of society.

Table 6.1 Views of the Marketplace

production perspective

The original view of the market developed prior to the industrial revolution. During that time, goods were generally crafted by hand or grown in limited amounts. Demand exceeded production capacity, so most craftspeople had to focus on making the product. Even today, when the demand for the product exceeds the availability of the product, the organization must use a **production perspective**. Consider the introduction of the Amazon Kindle® eReader in 2007. Though it was possible to download books onto phones or computers at that time, it was the first product on the market designed primarily to deliver books. The product sold out in five and one half hours[2] and remained out of stock for the next five months.[3] In the area of nutrition, a parallel can be drawn with the introduction of the PowerBar® energy bar. This product experienced phenomenal (and nearly immediate) success. Soon after its introduction, the independently owned company put much of its energy and resources into learning how to produce adequate quantities of the product.

The other situation in which the production view is taken is when the cost of the product makes it prohibitive for consumers to purchase. The manufacturer needs to find ways to produce the item more efficiently so that costs come down and more consumers can afford the product. Henry Ford revolutionized the automobile industry by reducing production costs. Dietitians, too, use this technique. They have managed to reduce the labor cost involved in nutrition education by offering classes or group counseling sessions as an alternative to individual diet instructions. Thus, the cost of nutrition education to the consumer is reduced.

Along with production issues, the production view of marketing must also include how the product gets to the customer. This is known as **distribution**. It is important to develop ways to get the product to the consumer at the same time that production methods are being established. Otherwise, when the product becomes available in sufficient quantity and at reasonable cost, the customer will have difficulty getting the product, which will undermine the benefits of improved production. Nutrition services and classes are now being offered in shopping malls, health clubs, and satellite clinics, as well as in traditional settings like hospitals. These represent an expanding distribution network. The Kindle is distributed through Amazon.com. PowerBar, Inc. initially opted for retail distribution of its product, including the checkout stands of grocery and convenience stores, and at health clubs, gyms, and spas. Now, PowerBar products are also available on the Internet.

product perspective

During the industrial revolution, it became possible to make large quantities of a specific product at relatively low costs by using mass production and assembly-line

Production Perspective. *A view of the marketplace based on the idea of growing, manufacturing, or creating a product for the marketplace.*

Distribution. *The method of delivering a product to the marketplace.*

techniques. This development led to a different view of the market: the **product perspective**. When the production dilemma is solved and there are ways to get the goods made in an effective and efficient way, time and effort can be put into the development and refinement of the product itself. Organizations begin to look at their products in terms of value, features, and performance.

Among the factors considered are how well the product does what it is supposed to do, the quality and reliability of the product, and how the product might be improved. Variations in product lines came into existence. For example, bowls that had been uniform could now be made in different sizes and colors. The Kindle introduced several new models since its initial product offering. Newer versions include ones with keyboards, ones with on-screen keyboards, ones with larger display screens, and ones with color displays. As PowerBar became a more mature organization and solved its production problems, the product line broadened and new varieties of nutrition bars, gels, and drinks were introduced.

In clinical nutrition, there has been an explosion in the number and variety of enteral feeding products, developed to meet the nutritional needs of various types of patients. (See the "In Practice" feature following Chapter 4.) In healthcare foodservice, one of the areas of product development was specialty foods to be used for clients with dysphasia. For many years, those products were bland and unpalatable and looked like (and sometimes were) baby food. However, new products and cooking techniques have made the production of pureed foods and thickened liquids an art form. These new products are much better than their predecessors and have found a niche market in some upscale healthcare facilities. The major force behind the acceptance of these products is their visual appeal.

selling perspective

Typically, a company with a good product or line of products eventually develops excess production capacity. Therefore, it becomes necessary to adopt a **selling perspective** to move the excess product. This is accompanied by active **promotion** of the product to draw the attention of consumers toward it. Many organizations focus on selling their products, and maintain a large sales force to do just that. This type of promotion and selling is usually used to convince consumers to purchase something that they did not want, or did not know that they wanted. The classic examples are the kinds of goods that are promoted at regional fairs and home shows all over North America. Most consumers do not plan to purchase a new set of cookware, a ring-cleaning solution, or a super-duper all-purpose vegetable slicer when they go to the fair, but are readily convinced by adept salespeople. Promotion is also used to get citizens to support candidates for public office by maximizing the candidates' strengths while minimizing their weaknesses. Ideas, such as the beauty of the emaciated model or the concept that large body size is inherently unattractive, can also be "sold."

The pharmaceutical company representatives who call on dietitians and physicians in healthcare facilities have a primary focus of selling enteral and parenteral nutraceuticals to those institutions. Even though these representatives do not carry products with them to sell directly, they provide information to convince the dietitian to purchase the products and arrange for a reliable method of distribution to get those products delivered. These sales representatives have access to a wide variety of promotional materials to assist them with their work. The selling focus relies heavily on promotion to increase sales. This does not mean that organizations that employ salespeople do no marketing. However, it does mean that, for the sales force, the focus is more on selling than on marketing.

The selling perspective assumes that profits are based on the quantity of goods sold, so the focus is to increase sales volume. Increased production volumes result in better efficiencies and lower costs, which lead to higher profits. It should be noted that some people view selling as marketing. This is not true. As will be demonstrated in the remainder of this chapter, sales is one essential part of marketing, but sales is not equivalent to marketing. Marketing is much broader than convincing customers to buy a product that already exists.

Middlemen. *Individuals or groups who work in the distribution channel, moving the product from the producer or manufacturer to the consumer.*

In areas other than clinical dietetics, the salesperson who calls on the dietetics professional may not be an employee of the manufacturer. For example, someone representing a distributor of several product lines might call on the foodservice director who is purchasing food products or equipment. The salesperson may be employed by a distributor, a retailer, a manufacturer's representative, or other business. The person making the sales call may represent a few product lines and manufacturers, or a wide variety of products. These sales personnel are called **middlemen**, because they bridge the gap between the producer and the end user. Even though this type of sales force is not actually on the payroll of the manufacturer/producer of the product, their role is the same as that of other salespeople—that is, to convince the dietetics professional to purchase a specific product or products.

Marketing Perspective. *A view of the marketplace that considers production, sales, products, and promotion in light of the consumers' needs, wants, and demands.*

Dietitians and dietetic technicians often work for either the manufacturers or the distributors of goods in a sales capacity. They are especially effective in selling foods, foodservice supplies and equipment, and nutraceuticals to other dietetics professionals because the customer and the salesperson speak the same professional language. The collegial relationship between salesperson and customer often adds the perception of value to the goods being sold, and tends to enhance sales for the product.

marketing perspective

Marketing has a much broader scope than the other methods of approaching the marketplace that have been described. The **marketing perspective** looks at production, product, and sales in light of the end users of the products. An organization that is market-driven is also customer-driven. The customer becomes much more than a person with the resources to purchase a product. Marketing also looks at distribution, price, and how the product is introduced and promoted to the customer. These are sometimes referred to as the **four P's of marketing**: product, place, price, and promotion. The thing that is unique about the marketing perspective is that the focus is not on any one of these factors, but how each contributes to the marketing mix.

Marketing theory also differentiates among consumer needs, wants, and demands. **Needs** are those things that are required for well-being, which include physical needs, such as food, clothing, shelter, and safety. Needs also include the social needs for belonging and affection, and the personal needs for knowledge and self-expression. **Wants** are somewhat different than needs, in that wants are socially acceptable ways to meet needs. For example, rice and tofu are socially acceptable foods in Asian countries; beans and tortillas are more appropriate to the culture of Central America. **Demands** are wants that are backed by resources, usually money. In North America, consumers demand a safe food supply, and for the most part, they get it, because they are willing to pay the price for both the food and the technology (irradiation, refrigeration, canning, transportation, governmental intervention, and so on) that keeps the food supply safe. Consumers want the best deal for their money and the most satisfaction for their investment.

To discriminate between needs, wants, and demands, consider the following. A starving man—for example, a U.S. or Canadian pilot shot down behind enemy lines in a war zone—will eat anything that is available to satisfy his "need" for food. Thus, bugs and dog meat, not socially acceptable food sources in North America, may be used as food, if nothing else is available. (Please note that, in some cultures, bugs and/or dog meat are considered to be acceptable foods.) However, when faced with a choice about foods in the safety of his own home, neither bugs nor dog meat would be an option for this pilot because they are not a socially acceptable part of the North American diet. At home, the "want" for food is much more likely to be met with a hamburger, chicken, rice, or bread. Furthermore, as a downed pilot, the man is in no position to demand that the bugs or dog meat be free of pathogens that lead to food-borne illness. The "demand" part of the consumer's profile exists only after the needs and then the wants have been satisfied.

To learn about their needs, wants, and demands, marketing departments study consumers to determine just who they are and what their expectations are. Market research, an integral part of marketing, concentrates on gathering and analyzing data related to consumers and the products that they desire. Marketing takes the view that the products should be developed in response to consumer expectations, and that profits come as a result of customer satisfaction. In turn, satisfaction leads to customer loyalty and repeat business.

Four P's of Marketing. *Product, place, promotion, and price; sometimes called the marketing mix.*

Needs. *Things required for a state of well-being, such as physical (food, safety, and shelter) and mental (belonging, affection, and self-expression) well-being.*

Wants. *Socially accepted ways to meet needs.*

Demands. *Wants that are supported by resources, such as money, that allow the wants to be fulfilled.*

Finally, marketing focuses on the benefits that the product provides, in addition to the product itself. For example, cars are basically a form of personal transportation. However, manufacturers of various automobiles market the car in many other ways. Kia markets fuel-efficient, basic transportation; Jaguar markets luxury and status; Volvo markets safety; and Jeep markets access to rugged terrain and off-road locations. These are benefits that go well beyond personal transportation.

The manufacturers of liquid dietary supplements and meal replacement beverages used to "sell" their product primarily to dietetics and medical professionals; these products were used only at the recommendation of healthcare providers. Now they are marketed directly to consumers on television, in print media, and on the Internet. The focus has gone from "selling" the product to the health professional to "marketing" it directly to the consumer. This transition from the selling to the marketing perspective has also occurred with prescription medications.

Dietetics professionals have learned that their product is more than just food or diet. Their product is nutrition and the good health and the well-being that result from good nutrition. Their customers do not want diets that deprive them of food. Instead, they want approaches that can be used to maximize the use of food to improve health. When dietetics professionals focused on diet, the selling concept prevailed. Dietetics professionals provided clients with a diet to be followed. Now, the attitude of the dietetics professional has changed to health and well-being, in response to the demands of the customers. The focus has switched from what clients should or should not eat to what dietary and other strategies can be implemented to promote and maintain health. Certified Diabetes Educators (CDEs) don't hand out diabetic diets; they give clients the tools to take control of their diseases. Lactation consultants, once primarily concerned with the techniques of breast-feeding, now market concepts such as "bonding," "healthy and natural," and "good for both mom and baby." This marketing view of the products developed by dietetics professionals will continue to develop as the profession moves forward.

Social Marketing Perspective. *A view of the marketplace that balances the needs, wants, and demands of consumers with those of the organization and those of society.*

social marketing perspective

The social marketing perspective carries the whole concept of marketing one step further. It goes beyond meeting the expectations of individual consumers and relates to the good of society; it considers the consumers' welfare in addition to the consumers' wants. The goal of social marketing is to contribute to the common good by balancing the needs of the organization and its customers with the needs of society as a whole. As an example, manufacturers of beer promote the concepts of designated driver and responsible drinking in their advertisements. Quick service restaurants now include messages related to balanced nutrition and increased activity in their promotions, and cereal boxes provide "Nutrition Facts" to consumers each morning at the breakfast table. The Produce for Better Health Foundation (PBH) is doing more than marketing produce when it uses the concept **Fruits and Veggies—More Matters**; it is also promoting good nutrition.

Dietetics professionals are in a unique position to contribute to social marketing programs through organizations such as the **National Dairy Council** and the **International Food Information Council Foundation**. Many of the concepts that dietetics professionals promote are good for both the individual and society. The wellness and health messages associated with social marketing are a natural complement to good nutrition messages, which are marketed by many dietetics professionals. Because there is much growth potential in this area, dietitians, dietetic technicians, and the profession as a whole must develop innovative programs in social marketing.

target markets

Many products are used by the entire population, or by a major portion of the population. Such items as fruits and vegetables, dairy products, **MyPlate**, soft drinks, and quick service restaurants are mass marketed to appeal to these large markets. Mass marketing means that the product is promoted and made available to the population at large, without differentiating one subgroup of the population from another. Mass marketing can be used to promote a single product or several products with different features, such as full-fat dairy products, or low-fat varieties of milk, yogurt, cheese, ice cream, and so on. This type of product-variety marketing is designed to give consumers choice and to allow for changes in preferences or needs over time. Whether it promotes a single product or a variety of products, mass marketing is designed to appeal to wide segments of the population.

It has been noted that marketing is sometimes more effective if products are developed for and promoted to unique subgroups within the population, rather than the population at large. This technique is called **target marketing**. A product, or variations of the product, may be designed for and marketed to small groups within the mass market. Vitamin supplements, for example, are not "one size fits all." For example some of the myriad of varieties available include liquid vitamins for infants, chewable vitamins for small children, vitamins with iron for women, others without iron for men, and those especially designed for and marketed to senior citizens. Target marketing has three parts. These are market segmentation, market targeting, and market positioning.

market segmentation

Markets can be segmented in countless ways. People can be categorized by age, gender, race, ethnicity, social status, income, language spoken, educational level,

Fruits and Veggies—More Matters. *www.fruitsand veggiesmorematters. org*

National Dairy Council. *http:// www.national dairycouncil.org*

International Food Information Council Foundation. *http:// www.foodinsight. org/*

MyPlate. *http://www. choosemyplate. gov/*

Mass Marketing. *The marketing of a product to the population at large without discriminating among population subgroups.*

Target Marketing. *The marketing of a product to a unique subgroup within the population rather than to the population at large.*

geography, and so on. This kind of grouping of potential consumers is called **market segmentation**. The trick is to determine which characteristics would be useful in creating a subgroup that could benefit from a particular product. For example, the manufacturer of cookies could divide the entire population on the basis of hair color, and market its cookies only to brunettes. However, this particular reason for segmentation of customers is meaningless when related to cookies and could alienate individuals with red, black, or blond hair, causing them to boycott both the cookie and its manufacturer. On the other hand, one manufacturer of vitamin supplements has targeted a product to senior citizens, and has successfully marketed it to individuals with "silver" hair. The characteristic or characteristics that form the basis for segmenting the market are specific to the product; what works in one situation may not be appropriate in another.

Traditionally, dietetics professionals working in clinical nutrition have segmented their clients into categories based on medical diagnosis. Different service products have been developed for obese clients, for people with diabetes, for those with cardiovascular disease, for individuals with renal disease, and so on. Segmentation of markets for public health nutrition services is often based on age and developmental tasks, with programs specifically designed for well babies, pregnant women, parents of young children, and the elderly. Food security programs have been successfully marketed to low-income populations.

Nutritionists need to look at new ways to segment markets, in addition to diagnosis, age, developmental tasks, and income. They also need to look at nontraditional market segments. People who have just relocated to an area might want to learn about regional foods and cooking methods. Retired men could benefit from classes on how to negotiate their way through the grocery store. Frequent business travelers need to know about how to eat away from home (and need that information delivered to them when they are "on the road"). Those in the middle income bracket could be potential consumers of fitness or nutrition programs. Those of considerable wealth might be potential consumers of the services of a personal trainer/nutrition consultant, home-delivered gourmet meals, or catering services. Nuclear families with both parents working outside the home need access to take-home meals, or information about how to prepare meals quickly. Grandparents could benefit from learning about the "division of responsibility"[4,5] concept of child feeding. Even within the traditional diagnosis-related segments of the population, there are individual markets, such as African Americans with hypertension, Caucasian women with osteoporosis, and Asian Americans who are lactase deficient. The potential markets for products related to dietetics are limited only by lack of imagination.

market targeting

Once potential target populations have been identified, these market segments must be evaluated to determine if it is feasible to develop a product for, or market a product to, that particular segment. Among the factors to look at are the size of the segment and the anticipated growth of that segment. The prevalence of full-blown celiac disease in the United States was thought to be rare during the last quarter of the previous century. Gluten-free products were difficult to find and often had to be made from scratch at home. However, now that other forms of gluten sensitivity are being diagnosed with increasing frequency, the number of individuals demanding these products is growing rapidly. Manufacturers of products anticipated this growth in the market and increased the number and variety of gluten-free products that are now available.

Steps are already being taken to decrease the sodium content of food products[6,7] in order deal with emerging health problems. Since a significant portion of the population of North America is expected to reach middle age and later years in the coming decades, nutrition programs designed to target the elderly will need to expand. It is also anticipated that additional public health nutrition interventions will be needed to meet the needs of increasingly overweight and obese children and adults.

In addition to size and growth, the segment must be attractive to the producer of the product from other standpoints. For example, consider the effect of competition. It is unwise to enter a market where the competition is firmly entrenched, unless the new product is significantly different from the existing ones in price, features, or availability. If a new product is exactly the same as one that is established in the market, it will be difficult for the new one to gain market share. Brand loyalty and familiarity with a product will keep consumers from trying a new product unless there is some incentive to do so—for example, lower price, additional features, better service, and so on.

The resources required to get a product to market must also be considered. There are costs associated with developing and promoting a product. There must be adequate investment of money, time, and energy if a product is to be successfully developed and marketed. Resource allocation is important because it may force an organization to make a choice from among several potential markets because one is more attractive than another and because there are not enough resources to pursue all potential market segments.

Finally, there is the consideration of return on investment. In most cases, it is not possible to create and market a product without the assurance that there will be some form of revenue generation to offset the costs. In the commercial marketplace, consumers pay, usually directly, for the products that they buy or use. However, in many areas of dietetics, the clients do not pay out of pocket for the goods and services they obtain. Third-party payers sometimes cover the cost of medical nutrition therapy, both in and out of hospitals. Employers may underwrite the cost of cafeteria meals, fitness centers, health club memberships, and wellness classes for staff. The federal government provides free and reduced-cost meals to children under the National School Lunch Program in the United States. Funding may be available through the government or through grants from other sources. It does not matter if the organization is for-profit or not for profit; there must be a way to predict income potential when selecting a target market.

These and other factors are considered when a target market is selected. The goal in target marketing is not to select the largest or the most lucrative market segment, but rather to select one that will need, want, or demand the product that is offered. Targeting and meeting the needs of a well-selected "niche" in the market can be as rewarding as, and sometimes more rewarding than, mass marketing.

market positioning

Market Positioning.
Presenting a product to the target market, emphasizing the characteristics of the product that are most important to those consumers; equating the product with its benefits.

Once the target market has been established and a product has been developed or customized for that market, the product should be positioned. Position is the way that customers perceive the product relative to other similar products.[8] Marketers try to position a product on the basis of its attributes or its use. Low-fat and low-kilocalorie products are positioned to be associated with weight loss; calcium and vitamin D supplements are positioned to promote bone health in post-menopausal women. **Market positioning** entails determining which of the characteristics of the product are most important to the target market, and creating a way for that population to equate the product with that benefit. Examples of market positioning of products that are used by dietetics practitioners include *Computrition®* computer systems designed specifically for hospitals and other onsite foodservices and *Lofenalac®* infant formula for babies with phenylketonuria.

Market Research.
The gathering of information about consumers' wants, needs, and demands to identify target markets and develop the marketing mix for those markets.

It should be noted that the product that is to be marketed to a specific group may be one that has been designed for that group. It may also be a mature product that has saturated the existing market and is expanding into new markets to maintain growth. The classic example of this is the personal computer, which was very costly when it was introduced and marketed to businesses. As prices came down, the market expanded to students and educational institutions, then to the middle class, and then to the elderly. Target markets are not static; they should be reevaluated periodically as society and needs change. Market research is used to identify trends in consumer markets.

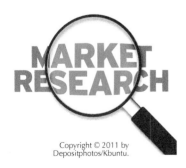

market research

To find out about potential markets, managers often carry out **market research** to learn more about their consumers and what they need, want, and demand. To be effective in market research, the organization must first be able to identify what information it needs. Once the needs have been determined, the data are collected. Finally, the data are evaluated in a way that allows the organization to identify target

management practice in dietetics

markets and develop a marketing mix that meets the needs, wants, and demands of those consumers.

It should be noted that market research may be conducted to identify a target market or to determine the actual needs, wants, and demands of that specific group. There are no hard-and-fast rules about what should come first, the market research or the identification of a target market. The most important thing to remember is that neither activity should put undue constraints on the other. Specifically, targeting one market should not cause another potential market segment to be overlooked. Conversely, market research should not be so broad that it neglects a market segment that has already been identified as viable.

needs identification

In the past, when information was scarce, it was necessary to gather as much data as possible about the marketplace in order to make good marketing decisions. More was better, and it was felt that one could never have too much data. In this age of information technology, it is possible to obtain and process extensive amounts of information. Gathering this information can be costly in both time and money. Too much information can interfere with the development of a sound marketing plan, delay entry into the marketplace, and allow others to get there first. Today's manager can be constrained by either too much or too little data. Managers must be selective about the information they seek. They should identify what information they actually need to make good marketing decisions while avoiding **information overload**.

The types of information that are traditionally used in developing a marketing plan include consumer information such as age, gender, family composition, cultural background, personal economics, lifestyle (including leisure time and activities), occupation, educational level, health, wellness, nutrition, residence, beliefs, attitudes, and so on. These are the same data that are used to identify the target market. Information about the industry is also needed. This includes identifying and studying the competition, including individual product lines, market penetration, market share, growth, market channels, price, and other factors.

The specific information required will be dependent on the product. For example, a private weight-loss camp for teenage girls would need to determine where teenage girls reside, which subgroups could afford a private camp, and how to get information into the homes of the subgroups. There would be no need to gather information related to young children, boys, or the elderly in order to market this product. In addition, it would be helpful to know how many other weight-loss camps for teenage girls exist in the region and the characteristics of these programs, in order to differentiate among programs. (Is the new program more or less costly than the others? How do program lengths compare? Is the program based on diet or lifestyle changes? What results can be expected?)

Information Overload. *Having too much data, which may impede management processes and interfere with decision making.*

information gathering

Once the information needs have been identified, data must be gathered. Several sources are available. Demographic data related to census, population characteristics, and health statistics are widely available in libraries and on websites. Frequently, some market data have been compiled by the industry (The National Restaurant Association compiles data on restaurants; the American Hospital Association gathers information about hospitals). Sometimes the information is free of charge. In other instances, it can be purchased or is made available with membership in a professional organization. If more specific information is needed, data can be collected independently or a market research firm can be hired to gather the necessary information. Market research data are categorized as primary or secondary, depending on how data are obtained.

American Hospital Association.
www.aha.org/

Primary data are gathered solely for market research purposes. As an example, a local restaurateur who is planning to open a second fine-dining restaurant might make personal observations of foot traffic at the noon and dinner hours to determine if a proposed business location is suitable for that business. Alternately, a quick service restaurant chain might hire a consultant to evaluate the flow of automobiles at a particular intersection to determine whether or not to locate a franchise there. Though both examples involve the evaluation of traffic patterns, each demonstrates business-specific data-acquisition methodology. The independent operator could have paid for an analysis conducted by a consultant, but did not need that degree of detail and found a more cost effective way to get the data that were needed. Usually, though, the gathering of primary market research data is more costly than gathering secondary data.

Primary Data.
Information gathered for the sole purpose of the party who requires the information.

Secondary data are data generated by outside sources, or are data that have been gathered for another purpose. It is usually less costly to obtain secondary data because the data already exist in some form or another, though it may not be the exact data desired. Secondary data may come from libraries, business publications, and the Internet. It may also be found in an organization's own records (for example, productivity, sales, production, or shipping records, and cash register tapes).

Secondary Data.
Information that has already been compiled by another source.

The choice about whether to use primary or secondary data, or a combination of these, is dependent on a number of factors. These include the information that is needed, the information that is already available, and the money available for market research. The types of market research tools that are commonly used to gather primary data include surveys (by mail, telephone, and online), personal interviews, group interviews, and focus groups. The research instruments are tested, as they would be for other types of research. Sampling is done using statistical models. Finally, the data are analyzed using the appropriate statistics to draw interpretations and conclusions. Though market research is sometimes viewed as an art, rather than a science, it is actually necessary to impose strict controls to ensure the quality of the results. Market research, when done well, is as rigorous as any other type of research (for example, educational or scientific).

management practice in dietetics

data analysis

The final step in market research involves the compilation and analysis of the primary and secondary data that have been gathered. Data analysis is the step in the decision-making process to determine what an organization's marketing mix will be.

marketing mix

Consumers do not usually purchase a product without consideration of other factors. They generally purchase products in some context. The package (product and context) is known as **marketing mix**.

Marketing mix has four components, the four P's of marketing mentioned earlier: product, place, price, and promotion. More specifically, these are the products that a company makes, the distribution channels for those products, the price that is charged for the products, and the way products are promoted to consumers. (See Table 6.2.)

This section will discuss the four components of marketing mix as they relate to the dietetics profession and some of its products.

Marketing Mix. *A combination of product, price, promotion, and place as they contribute to the marketing of a product.*

products

Most consumers think of a product as something that can be purchased, touched, taken home, and owned. In actuality, products can be anything offered to the market to satisfy the needs, wants, and demands of consumers. Products are not always something that you can hold or see, nor are they always something that can be owned, but they always meet a need, want, or demand of the consumer. Products can be goods, services, places, activities, ideas, and even people.

Product	Goods, services, places, ideas, activities, organizations, and people that are being offered to consumers
Place	Getting the product to a location that is available to the consumer
Price	The cost of the product to the consumer
Promotion	Methods for communicating information about the product to the consumer

Table 6.2 Components of Marketing Mix

Tangible.
*Something that can
be seen, touched,
and felt.*

Durable Goods.
*Products that can
oftentimes be used
and reused repeat-
edly and that have
a life expectancy
measured in years.*

Nondurable Goods.
*Products that get
used up quickly
and that have a life
expectancy usually
measured in days
or months.*

Perishable Goods.
*Products with
a very short
lifespan due to a
high potential for
deterioration or
spoilage.*

goods. One of the ways to characterize products is by their tangibility. The marketing term for **tangible** products is **goods**. Goods are things that can be owned by the consumer and can be seen, touched, and felt. In many cases, the consumers take the product with them. These goods can be eaten, worn, read, used, used up, worn out, discarded, or (sometimes) saved. When customers purchase goods, ownership is transferred to the customers, who are then free to make use of the goods in any way that they choose. Goods are often classified as durable or nondurable.

Durable goods last for a relatively long period of time and are used and reused frequently. Examples of durable goods include foodservice appliances such as ovens and coffee urns, computers, furniture, and vehicles. Durable goods do not have to last indefinitely, and each type of goods has a usual life expectancy, which is usually measured in years, not in days or weeks. These items get used repeatedly. Eventually, they wear out or become obsolete and need to be discarded and replaced.

Nondurable goods are those that are more transient in nature. They have a shorter lifespan and tend to get used up quickly. Examples of nondurable goods include dishes, uniforms, canned goods, soap products, paper products, and fuels, such as gasoline. Some nondurable goods can be reused, but tend to get worn out (uniforms), used up (paper goods), or broken (dishes). These products may have a lifespan of days, months, or a few years, depending, partly, on usage.

Some nondurable goods are perishable. They have an exceedingly short lifespan, which is independent of usage. If unused, they deteriorate and become unsafe to use, or they pass their expiration date. Fresh food products, like meat and produce, are considered to be **perishable goods**. Cooked foods are perishable, too. Other perishable goods that dietetics professionals use are enteral formula and vitamin supplements.

It should be noted that tangible goods sometimes have benefits in addition to the actual product. For example, a microwave oven cooks food, but also offers a degree of speed and energy efficiency not available from a conventional oven, so the micro-wave can be marketed not only as a cooking appliance, but as one that is faster and cheaper to operate than a conventional oven. A 500-kcal weight-loss program may be marketed as one that has "quick results," whereas a program that focuses on lifestyle changes may focus on "long-lasting health benefits." The deli section of a business dining facility may offer both made-to-order sandwiches for the consumer who has distinct food preferences and a "grab-and-go" type sandwich for the consumer who is interested in saving time. Each of these benefits is an intangible component of a tangible product that can be marketed as a complementary feature.

services. Service products have four distinct characteristics. These are intangi-bility, inseparability, variability, and service perishability. It is these characteristics that differentiate services from goods that are tangible and (more or less) durable. (See Table 6.3.)

Intangibility	Service cannot be seen, touched, or heard before purchase
Inseparability	Service cannot be delivered without the presence of the service provider
Variability	Quality of service depends on the individual provider and circumstances
Service Perishability	Service cannot be stored for later use

Table 6.3 Characteristics of Service Products

First, services are **intangible** products. They cannot be held or touched or seen before they are purchased, but are purchased and used nevertheless. Some examples of service products are public transportation and trash collection. Services that dietitians market are diet instructions, nutrition education, nutritional assessments, nutrient analyses, weight-loss classes, and so on. Often, when service is the product, the client will get something tangible to represent that service, either before or after the service is rendered. Just as the airline passenger gets printed confirmation to verify the purchase, the dietitian may hand the client a printout of the nutrient analysis that was done, or a printed copy of nutrition information, to take home. These printed materials are a tangible representation of the service.

Services are also characterized by **inseparability**. This means that the product cannot be separated from its provider. It is not possible to use commercial airline transit without the presence of a pilot and crew to deliver the service. Nutritional services require the presence of a dietetics professional to screen, assess, or educate clients.

Variability in service indicates that service products are not uniform. Goods can be made in such a way that they are reproducible time after time. Restaurants can produce a uniform serving of lasagna, as easily as a manufacturer of Ping-Pong balls can make a standard product. With service, however, there is lack of uniformity due to a number of factors. The provider of the service, the consumer, and the circumstances under which the services take place influence variability. For example, the nutritional assessment done by an entry-level dietitian may be somewhat different from that done by an experienced practitioner. Also, the dietitian's familiarity with the particular type of diagnosis may alter the thoroughness of the assessment. Other circumstances that will cause variability include availability of test results, site of the assessment (outpatient clinic, hospital inpatient setting, emergency room, cocktail party), client readiness to work with the dietetics professional, time of day, background noise, and so on.

Finally, **service perishability** means that the service cannot be stored for later use. Service must be accepted when it is delivered, or it is lost. This characteristic is evident when clients miss scheduled appointments and then cannot be seen later because the dietitian is working with another client. It is not possible to put service into inventory

Intangible.
Something that cannot be held, touched, or seen— like services.

Inseparability.
A characteristic of services in which a product cannot be separated from its provider.

Variability. *A characteristic of services that indicates that services are not uniform, due to factors such as the provider of the service, the consumer, and the circumstances under which the service takes place.*

Service Perishability.
A characteristic of services that implies that a service cannot be stored and used later; the service must be utilized upon delivery.

and then retrieve it when consumer demand increases. Sometimes, however, consumer demand can be predicted and service increased during peak demand times. Local rail and bus systems increase the frequency of their service on workdays and during commute hours. In foodservice operations, increasing staff during lunch and dinner hours accommodates peak service requirements at mealtime. Outpatient clinics may overbook visits (much like airlines oversell flights) to compensate for a certain predictable percentage of "no-shows." However, if this is done, there must be a system in place to deal with the occasion when all of the clients keep their appointments.

other products. There are several other things that can be viewed as products in the world of marketing. These include places (Hawaii), activities (windsurfing or downhill skiing), organizations (American Association of Retired Persons [AARP]), and people (Justin Bieber). In general, dietetics professionals are less involved with these types of products than they are with goods and/or services. But this should not imply that they cannot or should not become involved.

Ideas, too, can be seen as products. An idea may be a discrete product, like a book that is copyrighted or an invention that is patented. More often, though, ideas more closely resemble services. For example, the service given by a consultant when a new computer system is being installed in an office is, actually, the ideas that are provided by the consultant to the office staff. The consultant dietitian who provides menu oversight, guidance on sanitation, and nutritional care in a long-term care facility is dealing with ideas as a product. Other dietitians consult to industry, foodservices, educational institutions, government agencies, and athletic teams, providing insights on the application of nutrition science to particular situations. In other words, the dietitian/consultant is marketing professional expertise.

Foodservice provides customers with two products, the food itself, which is tangible, and the service, which is intangible.

combination products. Unfortunately, products do not always fit into the product categories described here. The fact that an idea might be freestanding or part of a service product is just one example. Another is foodservice itself. Even the word *foodservice* implies two types of products involved: the food, which is tangible, and the service, which is intangible. Nevertheless, it is easy to visualize the service component when one looks at foodservice. It is also easy to see how different levels of service are associated with value as perceived by the consumer. For example, a hamburger and fries at a quick service restaurant are relatively inexpensive, because the consumer waits in line and takes responsibility for the service. On the other hand, many customers are willing to pay more for very similar food in a hotel dining room served (in a leisurely manner on fine china set on linen-covered tables) by well-trained waitstaff.

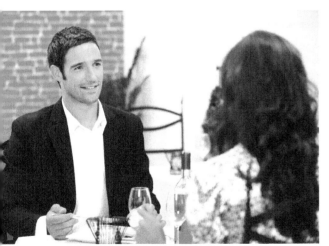

More and more, producers are combining goods and services into combination products. The extended warranties and service contracts on appliances and office equipment are examples of this practice. Another is the provision of product-specific equipment in foodservice. For example, when a foodservice sells a certain brand of soft drink, juice, or coffee, the manufacturers of those beverages will provide (at no cost to the foodservice) the coolers, dispensing equipment, or urns to store and serve these products. The concept is that service can do much to enhance the value of goods. It provides an additional feature that can be used in marketing.

place

Place refers to getting a product to a location where the consumer has access to that product when it is needed. Placement takes advantage of **distribution channels** and middlemen. Retail distribution channels typically put the product in central locations where consumers purchase those products. The channel may be a simple one, where the product goes directly from the manufacturer to the end user. Conversely, it may be very complex, with the goods changing ownership several times along the channel, and with several middlemen playing a part in the movement of goods along the route. Distribution may also be characterized as retail or wholesale depending on whether the goods are being sold to an end user or to someone who plans to resell the goods. Wholesale distribution channels are generally designed for the distribution of products to businesses that plan to resell the products.

distribution channels. The simplest type of distribution channel is one in which the organization, which produces the goods or services, deals directly with the end user of the product, using no middlemen at all. This is called a direct marketing channel; no intermediaries are involved. The Academy of Nutrition and Dietetics uses this type of marketing channel for many of its products. Books, journals, National Nutrition Month materials, national meetings, and so on are marketed directly to members and other interested individuals. Only limited numbers of ADA's products will be sold at the retail bookstore in the local shopping mall. Companies such as Tupperware® and Avon® market products directly to end users, as do organizations that rely primarily on catalog or Internet sales like LL Bean® or Land's End®. Even retail outlets can be considered a direct marketing channel when they are owned and operated by the manufacturer of the products sold there.

A product may go through one middleman between the manufacturer and the end user. This type of distribution generally is reserved for major retailers who purchase large quantities of goods directly from producers and sell those goods to end users. For food products, major grocery store chains like Safeway and Kroger work within this type of system. Such operations purchase directly from growers and manufac-turers, store the products in their own warehouses, and redistribute them to retail

Place. *The location where the product is available to the consumer.*

Distribution Channel. *The route products follow from the manufacturer to the end user; may be direct and simple, or complex with the products changing ownership several times along the way.*

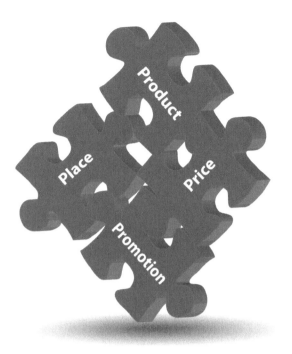

locations as needed. Smaller grocery stores may be unable to purchase directly from growers and manufacturers because their retail sales are lower than those of the major chains. These retailers must purchase from a grocery wholesaler. Thus, the distribution channel for an independent grocery store will be manufacturer to wholesaler to retailer to end user. In this situation, there are two intermediaries between the manufacturer and the end user.

Middlemen are an essential part of many distribution channels. However, it should be noted that middlemen are not all alike. Some take ownership of the product and store it, whereas others act only in a consultative capacity, coordinating transactions between sellers and buyers. Depending on how they perform their roles, middlemen may be called wholesalers, retailers, manufacturers' representatives, distributors, jobbers, brokers, agents, and so on. For the purpose of this text, it is not necessary to make distinctions among the many types of middlemen, but it should be noted that each title describes a specialized function.

In some distribution channels, three or more middlemen are used to get the product to the end user. The number of middlemen involved is often product specific. Fresh food products, like meat and produce, may have three middlemen involved in getting the product to the end user. It should be noted, however, that increasing the number of middlemen might increase the cost of the product and decrease the reliability of the distribution channel. This is why large retailers choose to purchase directly from producers or manufacturers whenever possible.

retail distribution. The sale of products to end users, regardless of the number of middlemen involved in getting the product through the distribution system, is called retail sales. There is a variety of ways for **retailers** to approach the end user. A standard is the retail store, which may sell groceries, clothing, hardware, or a variety of these and other products. Retail stores (sometimes referred to as "brick and mortar" businesses) range in size from the small specialty shop to the superstore. There are also retail service businesses such as hotels, banks, and hospitals. Though the latter are not stores, they are retail outlets where the consumer comes to a specific location to obtain the desired product.

Options available for retailing outside of stores seem almost endless. Some direct marketing is done through mail (magazines, catalogs, or single-purpose mailings), telemarketing (using the phone to sell products directly to consumers), television (shopping channels, or broadcast ads like those that offer solar panels, bathtubs,

Retailers.

An organization or individual who sells products directly to the end user of the product.

management practice in dietetics

kitchen gadgets, and so on), or e-tailing (shopping through the Internet). Other forms of direct selling include door-to-door sales (Girl Scout cookies), demonstration selling (at how-to fairs and in-home parties), vending, and so on. The Academy of Nutrition and Dietetics uses direct marketing channels like mail, e-mail, and its website to introduce and sell its products to members.

Dietitians and other nutritional professionals become involved in retail when they write books or computer software for the public, create food products for sale in grocery stores or restaurants, or offer classes at the local fitness center. They are also involved in the retail distribution of nutrition-related products using electronic media. Even the diet instruction given to a hospitalized patient before discharge or the nutrition class offered at the local community college can be considered in terms of retail, because the service is being provided directly to the end user. When a product or a marketing plan is being developed, it is very useful for nutrition professionals to consider how their products will be distributed.

wholesale distribution. The **wholesaler** buys from the producer or the grower and sells to the retailer, who then sells the product to the end user. This makes the wholesaler a middleman. Dietetics professionals who work in foodservices are likely to purchase from wholesalers. Foodservices then transform those foods into meals, and sell the meals at the retail level to restaurant or cafeteria patrons. The wholesale distribution channels used by foodservices include dairies, prime vendors, restaurant supply houses, warehouse outlets, bakeries, produce vendors, meat vendors, and the like. See Chapter 11, Material Management.

Wholesaler.
An organization or person who buys products from the grower or producer and sells them to the retailer who, in turn, sells the products to the end user.

Dietetics professionals become involved in wholesale operations in other ways, too. It has already been noted that wholesalers sometimes employ nutrition professionals. Also, if nutritional professionals manufacture a food or formula, they will probably deal with the wholesaler as a conduit through which to get the product into the retail market. In most cases, it is more efficient and effective to use an existing wholesale channel than to go directly to the end users, because the wholesaler has a distribution system in place and merely has to add another product. Thus, it is possible that dietetics professionals assume a variety of roles relative to wholesaling, including introducing product into the system, working in the system, or obtaining product from the system. Whenever dietetics professionals deal with goods, rather than pure service, there is likelihood that a wholesale outlet will be involved.

Wholesalers, like retailers, come in a variety of shapes and sizes. Some are full service and offer a range of services to their customers, including large inventories, scheduled deliveries, market information, management services, training of staff, financing, computerized order entry, and so on. Others offer limited service—for example, deliveries provided only on orders of more than $500. Others are cash-and-carry types of operations, which provide little service and very low prices.

service distribution. Finally, one must consider the distribution channels for services. There are usually fewer middlemen involved, because service is perishable and ownership is not usually easy to transfer. (The kinds of middlemen who get involved in the provision of services are event planners and agents for personalities like sports figures or performing artists.) However, some considerations are necessary. One major consideration is the physical placement of services where the consumers are likely to be. Putting a fitness center in a hotel is an example of service placement, as is locating a WIC program in a family medical clinic.

Some service distribution channels use the Internet and other technologies. Universities now webcast classes. Entrepreneurial nutrition professionals are reaching consumers using the Internet. Chat groups for weight-loss clients, continuing-education webinars, online nutrient analysis, and other nutrition services are being offered in this way. The opportunities for dietetics professionals to use the power of the Internet are expanding rapidly.

pricing

Price. *The cost of a product to consumers; the only component in the marketing mix that concerns itself with revenue and profit.*

The third component of the marketing mix is **price**. Price is the cost of the product to consumers. It is the only part of the mix that is associated with revenue, even though product, place, and promotion are all related to price. Determining the price of a product is not easy. It involves a series of decisions that are closely related to the decisions about product, placement, and promotion. The information presented here is only an introduction to pricing strategy and is intended to highlight only a few of the factors that are used to determine price.

One major consideration when making a pricing decision is how the price will fit into the overall marketing program. Indeed, the objectives of the organization relative to the product should be the basis of the pricing decision. An organization that is struggling to survive may set its price relatively low to undercut the competition and increase sales; the organization that wants to earn maximum profits might increase the price to the highest possible level. If increasing sales volume and market share is important, the pricing will probably be different than if the goal is to market quality. The business dining operation with an objective to break even will price its offerings differently than the hospital cafeteria that must make a profit to cover the costs of patient foodservice.

Another consideration that is used when establishing prices is the cost of producing the product. Most organizations need to recover production costs (break even) or to make a profit. Under some circumstances, however, a product may be offered below cost. This may be done for various reasons, including disposing of excess or old inventory, improving cash flow, or passing on subsidies. For example, government funding is available to subsidize school lunches in the United States, so meals can be offered to qualifying students below the cost of producing those meals.

To set prices, the actual costs of producing the product can be calculated. This process is time-consuming, in that the actual costs include raw materials, labor, rent, utilities, insurance, profits, and so on. Frequently, the prices are determined by using one cost (for example, raw material) as the basis for establishing the selling price. Many foodservices use a food-cost basis for determining selling prices. A formula is used to determine the relationship of food cost to selling price. In healthcare foodservices for example, 40 percent food cost is often the basis for setting prices. This means that the foodservice spends 40 percent of its income on food and the other 60 percent on labor, other expenses, and profit. In this situation, a carton of milk that is purchased for 40 cents will be sold for $1.

The formula for determining the food-cost basis for pricing will vary depending on labor costs, type of service, and volume of business done each day. A fine-dining establishment may set a food-cost basis of 20 percent because of the need for high-priced skilled labor and smaller numbers of customers. It may have to sell the milk (probably not in a carton) for $2. In addition, prices may actually be set before a product line is established. For example, a college restaurant that is open to the public may choose to keep its prices in line with the restaurants adjacent to campus, so that it can remain competitive. Thus, the going prices in the neighborhood will help to determine the college restaurant's prices.

The psychology of pricing should also be considered. For example, one expects to pay a high price for a meal at a place where there are clean linens and fresh flowers on the table, especially if the waitstaff are in formal uniforms and are attentive to the customers' needs. It is possible to take advantage of that expectation by pricing the menu accordingly. Customers may also expect to pay more for dinner than for lunch, so it is common practice for some restaurants to charge more at dinnertime. Dining out may be more prevalent on weekends than on weeknights, so some restaurants raise their prices on weekends to take advantage of the supply and demand factor.

The numbers used in the price may be also affected by psychology. Just as a car priced at $29,999 appears to be less expensive than one at $30,000, the $19.95 meal seems less expensive than the one priced at $20. Items may be priced just under an even dollar amount in order to appear less expensive than they really are. Odd numbers in pricing are sometimes associated with value. And finally, some numbers are considered to be "lucky" to individuals of certain ethnicities. In such cases, using those numbers in the pricing strategy may entice particular groups of customers to purchase the product.

Psychology is interesting when it comes to pricing services that are unfamiliar to the customer. In general, when customers know what to expect, they also know what the going rate should be, for either goods or services. Generally, patients know what it will cost to visit a physician. People also are very familiar with what *Weight Watchers* charges for attending a session. However, clients seldom have expectations about what an assessment and counseling session for gestational diabetes should be. When there is no expectation, customers often assume that higher price is associated with better quality. Thus, the dietitian in private practice or in a clinic could, theoretically, charge more for diabetes care than for consultation for an overweight client.

Other external factors may have an impact on pricing, too. Things like the state of the economy, the percent unemployment, and the cost of living in a geographic region could have an influence on how much consumers are willing to pay for a product. Perhaps most importantly, the competition may dictate the price that can be charged. Unless a business is filling a specialty niche, it will have to keep its prices in line with whatever competition exists, or lose its share of the market. For example, for clinical outpatient services, dietitians in private practice may have to charge close to the market rate to remain competitive with the nutrition clinics in hospitals. Prices for nutrition services are also affected by what third-party payers (health insurance companies and health maintenance organizations) are willing to pay.

Dietetics professionals may also encounter price adjustments. When the dietetics professional is a customer, price adjustments may be offered for large-volume purchases, and discounts may be given if payment is made promptly. There may be seasonal specials related to product availability. In addition, there may be allowances given for returned goods or for trade-ins. The latter is usually reserved for durable goods that are being replaced (old mixers have trade-in value, much the same as used cars do). When the dietetics professional is providing the product, it may be necessary to make pricing adjustments for customers. For example, in onsite foodservice, employees of the facility may be offered a discount that is not available to customers from outside the organization. The free and reduced-cost pricing structure for the National School Lunch Program is an example of a type of pricing adjustment.

Other pricing strategies include promotions pricing, options pricing, and product line pricing. Promotions pricing is the pricing that is done for short periods of time, either to introduce a new product, to move existing inventory, or to increase sales during slow periods. It is sometimes known as a "sale" or a "special." Examples include early-bird specials to increase restaurant patronage before 6 p.m., reduced-price memberships in health clubs, and "two for one" offers at weight-management programs.

Options pricing is the type of pricing that allows for increases in price as consumers add options to the basic product. This is well known in the automobile and computer industries. Foodservices also use options pricing—for example, à la carte pricing for individual meal components. Clinical services may also come with options. A nutritional assessment may come with or without a nutrient analysis of a client's usual intake. The client may opt for either alternative, with the components priced separately.

Finally, product-line pricing offers a range of prices for different products. Again, in the automotive world, consider the range of vehicles made by any manufacturer.

Product lines offer different-size vehicles with different prices. Hotels have coffee shops, room service, fine-dining rooms, and banquet services, demonstrating product lines in foodservices. At least one manufacturer of nutritional analysis software offers different packages (product lines) to its customers. These packages vary in the number of foods listed, the number of nutrients analyzed, and the operating systems used. In general, the products with the largest databases and most user-friendly format are more expensive than the smaller, more-difficult-to-use programs.

promotion

Promotion, the fourth of the four P's of marketing, has to do with communicating information about the product to consumers. Ideally, the communication leads the consumer to purchase the product for an initial trial. There are several techniques used to promote products, including advertising, personal selling, sales promotion, public relations, and merchandising. Because communication is considered elsewhere in this text, it will not be presented in detail at this point. However, it is important for dietetics professionals to be able to make a distinction among the various techniques that are used to communicate the product message.

advertising. Advertising is a form of promotion that carries the message about the product to wide segments of the population. It may be targeted to a specific market by careful selection of where the ad is placed. For example, if one is targeting elderly citizens, one could advertise in the publications of the AARP. This would be a good place to promote remedies for constipation, but not a good place to promote prenatal vitamins.

Advertising has many positive attributes. Because the advertiser pays for the promotion, the content and placement of the ad are under the total control of the advertiser. Depending on budget, the organization can dramatize its product through the use of print, text, sound, color, and image. An advertiser can choose to use print, radio, television, the Internet, or other media. It is also possible to determine ad placement (the Super Bowl or late-night TV, right or left page of a magazine or newspaper, during the news or the music segments of radio programming, and so on). In essence, the advertisers are in control because they are paying for advertising and can demand to get whatever they can afford to purchase. Though advertising is expensive, the cost per exposure is often very low because of the size of the audience reached by an ad. Also, ads can be repeated, and repetition leads to familiarity and interest in the product.

Ads also have some negative aspects. The major one is that they tend to be impersonal. Another is that ads offer only one-way communication, which is less effective than two-way communication. The final pitfall is that advertising can be very expensive, especially if one chooses to target a large market through a national televised advertising campaign. It should be noted that advertising is usually priced on the basis of circulation of print materials and audience size for radio and television ads. Theoretically, the cost rises as more people are exposed to the advertisement.

personal selling. If you have ever been told by a member of the waitstaff at a fine-dining establishment that "The salmon is excellent this evening," you have experienced personal selling. Often, chefs or managers will preview the current day's menu with the waitstaff and provide information about what product should be "sold" tonight. The same philosophy is behind the one-on-one sales of clothing in a full-service department store, or the provision of product information to a foodservice from a full-service wholesaler. Personal selling is the most effective form of promotion because it is the only form that encourages two-way communication. Customers listen, sometimes because it is impolite not to do so.

Personal selling, however, is much more expensive than advertising. This is due to the fact that it involves a long-term commitment to hire and train a sales force. It cannot be turned on and off as advertising can. Personal selling is the most productive as well as the highest-cost promotional tool available.

sales promotion. Sales promotion is the use of tools to attract the consumers' attention. These include games, prizes, coupons, premiums, reduced-price sales, and so on. Sales promotions are usually used to boost sales for the short term, or to introduce customers to new products. They focus on immediate sales. Though they exist all the time, they may become more prevalent during downturns in the overall economy, when people are less likely to purchase discretionary items.

Merchandising can be an effective method of promoting a product.

public relations. Public relations is unpaid publicity. Often, it takes the form of a news story or a photograph. It is more believable than advertising, because it is not paid for by the organization that is promoting the product. However, this is a disadvantage in that there is no control over what is being said in the piece, nor can one determine its placement. However, a well-planned public relations campaign is a very useful and cost-effective way to promote a product.

merchandising. Merchandising is sometimes considered to be a promotional tool, and sometimes considered to be more related to placement than to promotion. Merchandising involves the physical display of the product to the customer. It includes placement on a shelf, in store window, or in another type of display. As an example, consider the cereal aisle at the grocery store where pre-sweetened "children's" cereals are placed on low shelves at a child's eye level, and where adult-type cereals are placed on shelves that are several feet higher. Another example of merchandising is the artistic arrangement of produce in upscale supermarkets.

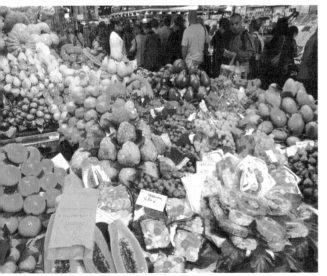

Foods in cafeterias and dessert trays in restaurants are ways in which prepared food is merchandised. Books may be merchandised in prominent, front-forward positions in bookstores, rather than being hidden on a shelf with only the spine showing. Vendors who bring samples of their products to trade shows, professional meetings, or fairs usually display them in enticing ways that are considered to be merchandising.

conclusion

This chapter presents an overview of marketing as it affects dietetics practice. There are many aspects of marketing that have not been covered. Marketing is a discipline in its own right. Like dietetics, it can take years of education and practice to master. Effective marketing requires that the components of the marketing mix be based on the organization's marketing philosophy, backed by market research, and focused on meeting the needs of a target market.

Marketing can be the primary focus and driving force in an organization, as often occurs when the product is tangible. Sometimes, when the product is a service—like entertainment, education, or health care—the organization sees the service as the focus of the organization. However, even in such situations, it is impossible to ignore marketing, because that is the function that synchronizes the product of the organization with the consumers of that product. It is difficult for an organization to succeed in today's environment without recognizing the value of marketing theory and using market research to develop its marketing mix. The major concepts that have been discussed in this chapter follow.

1. Marketing is a process that enables an organization to meet the wants, needs, and desires of consumers.
2. The marketplace can be addressed from five perspectives: production, product, selling, marketing, and social marketing.
3. A target market is identified as potential consumers for a product.
4. In order to design products for a market, or for a target market, it is necessary to learn about characteristics of the consumers as well as to identify and analyze the competition in the marketplace. This is done through market research.
5. The development of the marketing mix should be based on an organization's approach to the marketplace, the target market it has identified, and the research data that it has acquired, molded together in a way that will reach consumers.
6. The marketing mix includes product, placement, price, and promotion.

activities

activity 1

Look a recent copy of one of the following periodicals:

- *Food Management*
- *Journal of the Academy of Nutrition and Dietetics*
- *Today's Dietitian*

From this publication, select one advertisement and complete the following exercise:

1. Describe the ad.
2. Where was it located?
3. Who is the target audience?
4. Was the placement of the ad likely to reach the target audience?
5. Describe any social marketing in this ad.
6. If there is no social marketing message, could one be added?
   If yes, what would it say?
   If no, why not?

activity 2

Choose a public relations article from one of the following periodicals:

- *Food Management* http://food-management.com/
- *Nutrition Action Healthletter* http://www.cspinet.org/nah/index.htm
- *Today's Dietitian* http://www.todaysdietitian.com/

Based on this article, answer the following questions:

1. Describe the public relations component of the article.
2. What product did it promote?
3. Was the article favorable?
4. Was the article fair and balanced?
5. Are you likely to purchase this product as the result of reading this article?

activity

Working in groups of four to six people:

1. Create an idea for a product related to food, nutrition, or dietetics. (Your instructor may choose to assign a product to the group.)
2. Evaluate potential target markets for your product.
3. Select a target market for your product. Explain your rationale for the selection.
4. Determine that target market's needs as related to your product.
5. Tailor the product to the target market.
6. Describe how you would market the product to the target market. Include the four components of marketing mix in your discussion.

to study further

The following sources provide more in-depth treatment of marketing.

- Aaker, D. A., V. Kumar, G. S. Day, and R. Leone. *Marketing Research*. 10th ed. New York: Wiley, 2009.
- Baker, M. J., ed. *The IEBM Encyclopedia of Marketing*. Boston: International Thomson Business, 1999.
- Boyce, B. "Making Menus Friendly: Marketing Your Food Intolerance Expertise." *Journal of the American Dietetic Association*. 111:1809–1812, 2011.
- Francis, C. L. and M. L. Taylor. "A Social Marketing Theory-Based Diet: Education Program for Women Ages 54 to 83 Years Improved Dietary Status." *Journal of the American Dietetic Association*. 109:2052–2056, 2009.
- Hackley, C. E. *Doing Research Projects in Marketing, Management and Consumer Research*. New York: Routledge, 2003.
- Kotler, P. and K. L. Keller. *Principles of Marketing*. 12th ed. Upper Saddle River, NJ: Prentice Hall, 2006.
- Lovelock, C. H. and J. Wirtz. *Services Marketing: People, Technology, Strategy*. 7th ed. Upper Saddle River, NJ: Prentice Hall, 2010.
- Lovelock, C. H. and L. Wright. *Principles of Service Marketing and Management*. 2nd ed. Upper Saddle River, NJ: Prentice Hall, 2002.
- Machalczyk, D. "MNT Works: Marketing Resources Spread the Message." *Journal of the American Dietetic Association*. 101: 740–741, 2001.
- Marconi, Joe. *Future Marketing: Targeting Seniors, Boomers, and Generations X and Y*. Lincolnwood, IL: NTC Business Books: in conjunction with The American Marketing Association, 2001.
- McDaniel, C. D. and R. Gates. *Marketing Research*. 9th ed. Hoboken, NJ: Wiley, 2011.
- McDonald, M. and H. Wilson. *Marketing Plans: How to Prepare Them, How to Use Them*. 7th ed. New York: Wiley, 2011.
- McGivern, Y. *The Practice of Market and Social Research: An Introduction*. 3rd ed. New York: Financial Times, 2011.
- McKay, E. S. *The Marketing Mystique*. New York: Amacom, 1994.
- Meredith, G. E., C. D. Schewe, and J. Karlovich. *Defining Markets, Defining Moments: America's Seven Generational Cohorts, Their Shared Experiences and Why Businesses Should Care*. New York: Hungry Minds, 2002.
- Nagle, T. T., J. E. Holden, and J. Zale. *The Strategy and Tactics of Pricing: A Guide to Growing More Profitably*. 5th ed. Upper Saddle River, NJ: Prentice Hall, 2012.
- Perlmutter, C. A., D. B. Canter, and M. B. Gregoire. "Profitability and Acceptability of Fat- and Sodium-Modified Hot Entrees in a Worksite Cafeteria." *Journal of the American Dietetic Association*. 97:319–395, 1997.

- R. Lane, K. King, and T. Reichert. *Kleppner's Advertising Procedure*. 18th ed. Upper Saddle River, NJ: Prentice Hall, 2010.
- Smith, D. V. L. and J. H. Fletcher. *The Art and Science of Interpreting Market Research Evidence*. Hoboken, NJ: John Wiley, 2004.
- Stopke, T. J. et al. "An Innovative Community-Based Approach to Encourage Breastfeeding Among Hispanic/Latino Women." *Journal of the American Dietetic Association*.102:766–767, 2002.
- Van Wave, T. W. and M. Decker. "Secondary Analysis of a Marketing Research Database Reveals Patterns in Dairy Product Purchases over Time." *Journal of the American Dietetic Association*. 103:445–453, 2003.

scholarly journals

- *Journal of the Academy of Marketing Science*
- *Academy of Marketing Science Review*
- *Journal of Foodservice Business Research*
- *Journal of Hospitality Marketing and Management*

relevant websites

- American Marketing Association http://www.marketingpower.com/Pages/default.aspx
- Advertising Age http://www.adage.com

in practice

the marketing of nutritionjobs.com
by Stacey Dunn-Emke, MS, RD; Owner, NutritionJobs

When I launched the website NutritionJobs.com, it became immediately apparent that I was not only in the business of being an online job-board service for nutrition professionals. I was really in the business of marketing. I quickly became aware that the business existed in a vacuum unless I found a way to get the word out to my customers. Spreading the news about the newly created website became my first priority as a small business owner.

With the website launched and running, it was time to develop a formal strategic marketing plan. I decided that four major steps needed to be taken: research the market for the business, identify the market segmentation, define the marketing mix, and then develop the appropriate promotional plan that met the operational objectives and goals of NutritionJobs. I also knew I needed some help!

Being armed with two degrees in nutrition, and not one in marketing, meant I needed to learn new skills. As a small business owner, I didn't have the funding that a larger company has to hire a professional marketing and branding team. Instead, I engaged friends and family who worked in marketing and invested in books on the topic, such as Jay Conrad Levinson's *Guerrilla Marketing*. I also leveraged websites geared to small business owners, such as www.entrepreneur.com, that offered primers on the fundamentals of marketing, downloadable forms, and motivating stories about the steps other successful entrepreneurs have taken to grow their business.

market research

Developing a business model based on a needs assessment of the market is the first crucial step to marketing any business. It turned out that I had already done that step. As a dietitian looking for a new job and surveying the job market, I felt frustrated. The large, diverse, top-rated online job boards had few, if any, job postings for dietitians or other nutrition professionals. I knew that there were jobs available in my field but I couldn't find them online. I also knew I wanted to avoid traditional methods for finding jobs, such as advertising in print media, because it seemed I was always responding to the notice after the job had already been filled. It was then that I decided that dietetic professionals needed a website to suit our own niche needs for online job hunting. The subsequent success of NutritionJobs proved that the initial needs assessment was right on track.

My market research also included a review of the competition, including online businesses and traditional recruiting businesses. This helped me to identify best practices, threats, and opportunities to the business.

Researching the market, however, isn't a one-time effort. The market information is constantly evolving and needs to be evaluated regularly to stay competitive. We now check in with the employers (job posters) regularly to make sure NutritionJobs is still meeting their needs. We conduct phone surveys, e-mail surveys, and personal interviews. The job posters are surveyed about the quality and quantity of job-seeking applicants as well as the functional aspects of the job posting process. We also routinely conduct general user surveys either online or via direct e-mail to assess satisfaction, users' needs, and existing knowledge of our many features offered for both job seekers and job posters. The advantage of running a small business is that adjustments to the process and functionality can be made quickly in response to feedback from the users.

Regular reassessment of the market is built in to the marketing objectives. Analysis of the market is aided with the use of an online analytical tool. This tool provides us with data on demographics, traffic flux, traffic targets, target sources, and page usage. Specific functionality, such as job categories that employers and job seekers use for filtering and the navigation routes that they employ, are modified to better meet user needs.

market segmentation

"Who are my customers?" was the next big question. All subsequent marketing activities would be geared toward this defined audience. It turned out that an online job board actually has two target populations. These are the job seekers and the job posters. The job posters are the employers, human resource hiring managers, or professional recruiters. The job seekers include registered dietitians, dietetic technicians, dietetic students, and other nutrition-related professionals. It is essential to attract a balance from both target populations. Having one population visit without the other visiting wouldn't be of value to either and it just wouldn't drive the business. I needed to focus on the two distinct target audiences so that marketing and promotions could be tailored accordingly.

marketing mix

Determining what to charge the users became the next important step. This defined both the product and the pricing structure in the context of the competitive environment. The product in this business model is the job posting.

promotional plan

A systematic plan was needed to communicate the brand and the value of NutritionJobs to the target markets in a clear and consistent manner. The promotional plan needed to have a high impact with a modest budget. It also had to meet the short-term and long-term goals of the business.

Prior to the inception of NutritionJobs, dietitians and other nutrition professionals found jobs by traditional methods, such as job hotlines hosted by local dietetic associations, job announcements in newsletters and other publications, or through networking. Most dietitians, and especially recruiters, were not yet online for the job-hunt process. The audience needed to be convinced that online job recruiting and job hunting was the way of the future and NutritionJobs was there to provide the service.

A tag line, or brand message, was developed for the promotional items. This message also spoke to the advantages of online recruiting for nutrition professionals.

*nutrition***jobs.com**

The following tactics are employed to communicate the message and spread the word about NutritionJobs:

Social Media—Twitter, Facebook, and a professional group on LinkedIn, titled Nutrition and Dietetic Jobs, are used to communicate job listings, career discussions, our original Dietetic Career Spotlight Blog entries, and our original Dietetic Career Articles to our social media community.

Electronic Newsletter—A newsletter is sent to registered NutritionJobs users who have opted in to receive periodic communication highlighting our Featured Hot Jobs, Dietetic Career Spotlights, and Dietetic Career Articles from our Blog. The e-newsletter strives to keep the brand fresh in the mind of the users and to communicate recruiting and job-search related content.

Promotional Offers—Special offers by way of direct e-mail marketing or on the website are extended to new job posters, infrequent job posters, or as seasonal offers. Promotional discounts on new services are also offered to bring awareness to site services. Typically, free or significantly discounted job postings or branded advertising are offered. Large-volume discounts are also offered to frequent users to instill brand loyalty and satisfaction.

E-Mail Confirmations, Business Stationery, and Invoices—All customer correspondence from NutritionJobs, including welcome e-mails, e-mail confirmation of transactions, business stationery, and electronic invoices sent to job posters for services, carry the consistent brand message, tag line, and identity. All correspondence sent to customers is an opportunity to acknowledge their business and to thank users for choosing NutritionJobs.

Presence at Professional Meetings—Making myself available for professional dietetic meetings, either by staffing a product booth or speaking on the topic of dietetic careers and recruiting, communicates the message of NutritionJobs to potential users.

Freebies—The business model has a built-in system for propagating the jobs database by allowing non-profit organizations, such as Women, Infants, and Children's Programs, to post jobs without a fee. This eliminates barriers to database growth for job seekers while enlisting job posters who would not have otherwise been able to afford the service. This, in turn, helps spawn brand loyalty.

NutritionJobs has become an established brand and a successful business. Through the trials of developing and executing the marketing plan, I learned that marketing is a process and not just a one-time event. That means that the plan is constantly being revisited and revised to reflect the market situation and the business goals. This is essential in order for the business to stay competitive and to achieve long-term viability in the market. While some of the growth NutritionJobs experienced was organic and spread by word of mouth, the crux of its success can be attributed to a strategic and systematic marketing process.

references

1. Rogers, D., B. L. Leonberg, and C. B. Broadhurst. "2000 Commission on Dietetic Registration Dietetics Practice Audit." *Journal of the American Dietetic Association*. 102:270–292, 2002.

2. Patel, Nilay (November 21, 2007). "Kindle Sells Out in 5.5 Hours." *Engadget.com*. http://www.engadget.com/2007/11/21/kindle-sells-out-in-two-days/. Archived from the original on November 23, 2007. Accessed July 13, 2012.

3. Sorrel, Charlie (April 21, 2008). "Amazon's Kindle Back in Stock." *Wired.com*. "Gadget Lab" blog. http://www.wired.com/gadgetlab/2008/04/amazons-kindle/. Archived from the original on April 22, 2008. Accessed July 13, 2012.

4. Satter, Ellyn. *Child of Mine*. 3rd ed. Palo Alto, CA: Bull Publishing, 2000.

5. Satter, Ellyn. *Secrets of Feeding a Healthy Family: How to Eat, How to Raise Good Eaters, How to Cook*. 2nd ed. Madison, WI: Kelsy Press, 2008.

6. Health Canada. "Guidance for the Food Industry for Reducing the Sodium in Processed Foods." http://www.hc-sc.gc.ca/fn-an/legislation/guide-ld/2012-sodium-reduction-indust-eng.php. Accessed July 14, 2012.

7. Home Page for the Food and Beverage Industry. "Challenges of Lowering Sodium: Consumers Want to Be Assured that Lower Sodium Does Not Mean Less Taste." http://www.foodprocessing.com/articles/2010/salt reduction.html. Accessed July 14, 2012.

8. Lamb, Charles W., Joseph F. Hair, and Carl McDaniel. *Marketing*. 7th ed. Mason, OH: Thomson/South-Western, 2004.

part three

human resources management

People are important to any organization. Without them, work does not get done. Human resources are one of the more valuable assets—some would argue the most valuable asset—that an organization has. It is certainly true that employees can make or break an organization. Their attitudes can attract business or repel it. When employees are treated fairly and equitably, it is likely that they will pass this type of treatment on to their "customers."

The focus of the next four chapters is to introduce the reader to some of the areas of human resource management that managers confront. These include characteristics of the workforce, types of jobs available, and how jobs relate to staffing patterns and to the work that needs to be accomplished. The relationship between the employee and the employer is considered from the beginning—recruitment and hiring—to the time when the relationship ends. The emphasis is on working with employees in a supportive way, so that the relationship is mutually beneficial.

Human relationships, though challenging, can be quite rewarding to all participants. It is hoped that information provided in these pages prepares the manager to view workers as valuable resources who should be supported, as opposed to viewing them as "hired hands" who need to be controlled.

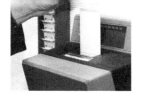

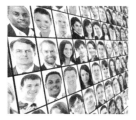

chapter seven

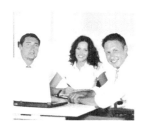

the workforce

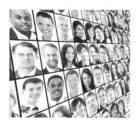

learning objectives

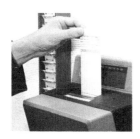

1. Describe different categories of workers.

2. Differentiate between regular employees and contingent workers.

3. Define *full-time, part-time, short-hour*, and *casual employees*.

4. Discuss the advantages of job sharing.

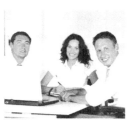

5. Differentiate between exempt and nonexempt employment status.

6. Describe differences in the payment of hourly workers and salaried workers.

7. Describe compensatory time.

8. State when and how differential wages are calculated.

9. Perform calculations about full-time equivalents (FTEs).

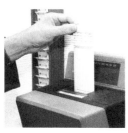

10. Define *diversity in the workplace*.

11. Differentiate between affirmative action and equal opportunity.

12. Discuss the advantages and disadvantages of workplace diversity.

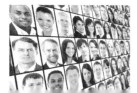

overview

If you've ever worked, you probably know that all jobs are not created equal. Each job and each work environment is different. The terms and conditions of employment vary, too, as do the salaries, the benefits, and the "perks" offered to workers. This chapter will cover the major categories of employees and the typical conditions of employment encountered by the dietetics manager. The challenges and opportunities of working with a diverse workforce will also be discussed.

The material presented here is not meant to be an exhaustive coverage of these topics. Some differences will occur because of the legal requirements of the state or country in which the work is done. The collective bargaining agreement that covers the employment relationship is another reason for variation. Policies and procedures set up by the employer account for other distinctions. Finally, differences occur because the employment relationship is flexible and individual contracts may be negotiated between the employee and the employer to suit the needs of either or both parties. It would be impossible to describe all the possibilities. When hiring managers offer positions to prospective employees, it is the managers' responsibility to be familiar with the rules and regulations that govern employment in the particular setting so that job seekers are not misled about the jobs. Conversely, an individual seeking employment should learn as much as possible about the position before making a commitment.

types of workers

In dietetics practice, four types of workers predominate. These are professionals, supervisory, skilled, and unskilled workers. Note that the terms are not mutually exclusive. Overlap may occur among the categories. For example, a registered dietitian is considered to be a professional but may function as a supervisor for dietetic technicians in a hospital's clinical nutrition office. A manager in a family restaurant might bus tables during a peak period, even though this is usually considered to be work for an unskilled employee. The skilled computer technician might assume an additional role as the supervisor of a group of colleagues in the state health department's nutrition section.

The descriptions of the various types of workers that follow are meant to describe the groups, not individuals within a group. One must be careful not to use this information to stereotype members of a group. Still, to understand the types of workers whom dietitians manage, it is appropriate to be aware of some of the overriding factors that characterize the groups.

professional staff

According to Hatch,[1] a *profession* is an occupation based on three criteria: first, a definable body of knowledge requiring extensive academic training; second, a commitment to public service; and third, relative autonomy in professional life. During the course of their careers, dietitians come into contact with many professionals, including other dietitians, physicians, nurses, engineers, pharmacists, lawyers, and others. The dietitian manager will certainly be called on to manage other professionals, usually within the fields of dietetics or health care, but sometimes from other fields as well. For example, the legal counsel for the Human Resources Department may report to a dietitian who is working as a corporate vice president.

Professionals, by virtue of their education, should have the knowledge and the skills to make independent judgments and to work on their own with a minimum of supervision. Given the facts that each profession has its own "body of knowledge" from which to draw, and that individuals within a given profession have specific areas of expertise, it is assumed that the manager will allow each professional a great deal of latitude in performing assigned tasks. Consider **entry-level** dietetics professionals who have basic skills in the areas of nutritional assessment, medical nutrition therapy, community nutrition, and foodservice systems. They should be able to work independently as generalist dietitians, requiring a minimum of supervision. As these professionals gain experience, they become more competent in their specific areas of practice. This acquisition of additional knowledge and skill leads to specialization in a practice area.

Specialization has two distinct effects. First, the practitioner becomes even more proficient and independent in the selected area of practice. Yet, some of the skills needed for generalist practice may be dulled, or even lost, from lack of use. Thus, the specialist who is more proficient in one task may become less skilled in doing other tasks.

It is not necessary for managers to have the same skills as the professionals who report to them. Indeed, management requires its own set of skills. It is inevitable that managers whose management skills are well honed will have lost some "practice skills" as they developed the necessary management skills. This should not be a concern when managing a professional staff, because by their nature, professionals are expected to act independently. Still, managers need to have a conceptual awareness of the professional roles of subordinates so that realistic performance expectations are set for staff. Managers are not expected to have the same proficiency level as the professionals who report to them, and it doesn't matter if the staff are in the same field as the manager or in another professional field.

Professionals. *Individuals who have extensive formal education in a field and have acquired the knowledge and skills to make independent judgments and to function in that field with minimum supervision.*

Entry-Level. *A beginning position in a profession (for example, an entry-level dietitian).*

Specialization. *The process of acquiring in-depth knowledge and skills in a narrow area of a profession.*

It is important to note that basic knowledge and skills are not synonymous with proficiency.[2] One needs experience with both the task and the setting in order to be truly proficient—that is, able to perform more routine jobs with less detailed forethought than the beginning professional would need. Professionals work most efficiently in a familiar setting where there is a comfort level with the physical environment, the clientele, the staff, and the policies and procedures of the facility. When one or more of these factors change, there is an adjustment period during which a degree of proficiency may be lost.

Consider those dietitians whose area of specialization has been in WIC. They will be proficient in providing nutrition services to women, infants, and children who are, for the most part, healthy. Despite this level of proficiency, they might have to "go back to the books" to plan the care for a pregnant woman on hemodialysis or to complete a sanitation check in the local senior citizens' feeding site. This does not reflect negatively on the skills of the dietitians; it merely indicates that they are responding to a need that is outside of their area of proficiency.

Professionals need time to learn new tasks that are assigned to them. It helps to have an experienced colleague to guide them through a task the first time it is done, but this is not required. For the professional, on-the-job training decreases the time spent on the learning curve and minimizes the mistakes made while learning is occurring. However, new tasks can be mastered without additional training, because professionals come equipped with the basic knowledge and skills necessary to learn to perform tasks outside of their areas of expertise.

Generally, it is assumed that professionals prefer participative management. (See Chapter 3.) They have opinions about the workplace and the jobs being done that merit the attention of management. Often, they make suggestions that can enhance the work environment for themselves and others. Many professionals feel that it is their duty to express opinions and that it is their right to be heard. A management style that encourages participation or consensus management may be very effective when dealing with professional staff. Conversely, an autocratic management style may create discontent among professional employees.

Supervisors.
Individuals with authority to oversee and direct the work of subordinates as well as having responsibility for their own work.

supervisory personnel

A person in a supervisory position oversees the work of one or more other individuals, with responsibility for the output of a work area or a work group, or for a particular time period or shift. **Supervisors** are accountable for their own work and also have responsibility for the work of others; they should also have the authority to direct subordinates in the work process. Often a supervisor is a frontline manager.

At any level, supervisors should have enough information about their positions to be able to identify the limits of their responsibility and authority. The level of authority of each supervisor should be sufficient to allow for the fulfillment of the assigned responsibility. For example, the supervisor who is responsible for the operation of the breakfast trayline must have the authority to reject a food product that tastes bad, is not at the proper temperature, has a wilted appearance, or is otherwise not up to standard. If that supervisor cannot reject a substandard product, then the responsibility exceeds the authority, making the supervisor unable to perform the assigned job effectively.

As supervisors take on new responsibilities, they must be given an opportunity to acquire the necessary knowledge and skills before being asked to perform the task. If, for example, supervisors are to perform the task of schedule-writing for the first time, it is essential that they be given information regarding institutional policy, legal constraints, union contracts (if any) that relate to work hours, work schedules, seniority, shift work, shift differentials, use of overtime, holidays, weekends, and so on. It should not be assumed that the supervisor would know what information is needed or how to obtain that information. (That is a characteristic of a professional, and not all supervisors are professionals.) The supervisor should also be allowed to perform the new task several times before being given full responsibility and should be supported through the transitional period. The work, in the case of the employee schedule, should be checked before it is posted by whoever will take ultimate responsibility for errors throughout the transition. This type of on-the-job training, optional for the professional, is essential for the supervisor who is not a professional.

skilled workers

A **skilled worker** is one who can perform jobs that require special training or ability. Cooks are usually classified as skilled workers, as are secretaries, equipment repairmen, exterminators, and individuals who code dietary intake data. A skilled worker learns the particular job skills through on-the-job training or by participating in technical training in a more formalized (for example, school or classroom) setting. The skilled worker is adept at the "how to" of the task but does not always have the knowledge base to address the "why" of the job. The training/educational process for the skilled worker does not usually require a baccalaureate degree; indeed, it frequently does not require any formal credentialing.

The manager or supervisor of skilled workers is usually capable of performing the tasks that skilled workers perform, though the manager may not have the same degree of proficiency with every task. It is often the manager/supervisor who conducts the on-the-job training for skill development. Skilled workers differ in the amount of supervision needed. Some require little oversight. They are aware of the responsibility inherent in the job and of the limits of their particular training or skill level. These

Skilled Worker.
An individual who has special training or skills to perform a specific job (for example, cooks, secretaries, exterminators).

skilled workers can be expected to identify potential problems and seek help as necessary. It is common that supervisors will check in with these personnel several times during the day to verify progress and to be available to take appropriate actions as needed. Usually, skilled workers do not need "**micromanagement**." However, a skilled worker who is new to the job may need more intensive supervision, and the supervisor must maintain high visibility and be available to support the employee as required.

unskilled workers

Unskilled workers are those who bring no marketable skills to the job. The tasks they perform require only skills that are taught in the work setting. The trainer may be an experienced peer or the supervisor. Often, these people earn minimum wage, though this is not always true. Unskilled workers include receptionists, cashiers, data entry personnel, housekeeping staff, foodservice workers, and so on.

Sometimes unskilled workers come to the job without basic literacy or math skills. This may occur because of educational deficits or because the primary language of the employee is not English. In this situation, the employer may provide these workers with literacy training or remedial math classes in order to increase their skills and enable them to be cross-trained to do additional jobs.

Participative management techniques are not always appropriate when the workers are unskilled. These workers may view their role as being followers, not leaders. They may not want the responsibility of decision making, viewing that as a function of management. Many unskilled workers prefer to be told what and how to do the job, and then to do it.

This does not mean that the unskilled worker cannot or will not contribute to the management process. These workers usually know more about their jobs than their supervisors and can contribute to the management process by providing information and ideas without participating in the decision-making process. It is appropriate to solicit input from this constituency when making decisions that affect their jobs, even if the manager will make the final decision.

There are no clear boundaries between professional, supervisory, skilled, and unskilled workers, nor are there precise definitions for the terms. These job categories are not mutually exclusive, and the characteristics described here are not universal. There are professionals who are unable or unwilling to act independently outside of their area of specialization. Conversely, there are unskilled workers who are eager to contribute to management decisions and who take an active role in a structure that encourages participative management. It is the manager's job to assess the workforce to determine the characteristics of each worker, without stereotyping individuals into groups. An effective manager will support each individual employee in a way that respects the individuality, needs, and potential of that employee.

full and partial employment status

The various terms used for employment status in the following section are typical terms. However, there are no standard definitions for many of these terms, which may have different meanings from region to region or from employer to employer. The reason for attempting to define the major categories of employment is not to provide an exhaustive list of the variations, but to give the reader a concept of the types of employment statuses that may be encountered in practice. The terminology will vary in different settings.

Before going on, it should be noted that it is expensive to hire and train a new employee. The cost is related to many factors, including the position, the labor market in the geographic region, if an outside recruitment firm is used, if there are reimbursed relocation costs, and so on. There is also the cost of the time and energy expended by the hiring manager and the human resources staff. The minimum cost associated with hiring and training a new employee is around $3,500 and the range can extend beyond $150,000 for upper-level executives. It is cost-effective to retain employees whenever possible.

full-time

A **full-time employee** is an individual who is expected to work that number of hours each week that the employer or the government designates as "full time." The usual number of hours designated as full time is 40; in some settings, 37½ hours per week is considered to be full time. For purposes of this text, the 40-hour figure will be used. Full-time workers may work more than the regularly scheduled 40 hours, but these individuals are guaranteed a minimum of 40 hours of work each week. An employer can expect to pay a full-time worker for 2,080 hours of work in a year (40 hours per week × 52 weeks = 2,080 hours). Full-time employees probably do not actually work 2,080 hours, because the employees are usually entitled to some paid time off—for example, vacation, holiday, sick, or personal leave.

Typically, the full-time workweek is eight hours per day, five days per week. Alternate schedules are sometimes followed to accommodate the needs of the employer or the employee. For example, a worker may opt to work four 10-hour days instead of five 8-hour days. In cases where this is a part of the employment agreement, the employee is not usually entitled to overtime pay for the longer days worked. Such alternate employment agreements may be negotiated between an individual and an employer under the general term of *flextime* or may be included as part of a contract between an employer and a labor union—for example, between a hospital and the local nurses' union.

Full-Time Employee. *An individual who is designated to work a certain number of hours a week who is considered "full time" by the employer (typically 40 hours/week).*

part-time

Part-Time Employee. *An individual who works a certain number of hours a week that is less than what is considered "full time" by the employer (usually less than 40 hours/week).*

A **part-time employee** also works a predetermined number of hours a week, but that number of hours is less than 40. The predetermined number of hours can be any number that is less than full time. A typical part-time employee may work 24 hours each week. Part-time employees may work more than the predetermined number of hours but are guaranteed only the predetermined work hours (in this case, 24 hours each week).

short-hour

Short-Hour Employee. *An individual who works a predetermined number of hours a week that is less than half time (typically less than 20 hours a week).*

Some employers also have a category of worker called "short-hour." A **short-hour employee** is defined as one who has a predetermined number of hours to work each week, but that number of hours is less than half time—that is, less than 20 hours per week. People in this classification may work more than their scheduled number of hours but are guaranteed only the predetermined number of hours each week.

Short-hour workers are usually not entitled to benefits such as health insurance or retirement programs. Some employers use short-hour employees in order to save on the cost of providing benefits (such as health insurance) to workers. In this case, the definition of *short-hour* may be any number of hours that is less than the number at which benefits are mandated by state or federal labor law. Other employers share with the short-hour employee the savings associated with not providing benefits by giving the employee increased pay. This increase is termed "pay in lieu of benefits"; it is frequently calculated as a percentage (perhaps 10 or 12 percent) of base pay. Not all employers make a distinction for this category of employment. In many cases, *part-time* is the only term used to designate any employee who is employed any predetermined number of hours that is less than 40 per week.

casual

Casual Employee. *A worker who is not guaranteed any set number of hours each week but who is scheduled for work as needed.*

A casual employee is a worker who is not guaranteed any set number of hours each week but who may be scheduled to work as needed. Casual workers do not receive benefits and, depending on the employer, may or may not be entitled to "pay in lieu of benefits." Another term used for this category of employee is *on call*, because the employee can be called in to meet an unscheduled need. *Casual* is a better term, because it recognizes the fact that these employees are frequently scheduled in advance, perhaps to cover for another employee who is on vacation. They are not just "called" to work when extra workers are needed at the last minute. (The term *on-call* also has another meaning that will be discussed later in this chapter.)

job-sharing

Job-sharing is a relatively new concept in the workplace. It occurs when two or more individuals work in tandem to perform a full-time job. The job may be divided in a variety of ways. For example, one employee may work mornings, and the other may work afternoons. Another situation might be that the first employee works Monday, Tuesday, and every other Wednesday, while the other employee works alternate Wednesdays and every Thursday and Friday. A third model for job-sharing could be when one employee takes half the caseload, and the other deals with entirely different cases. This latter model more closely resembles two part-time positions than job-sharing. (As an example, a full-time dietitian in a public school system might have covered nutrition education programs in ten elementary schools, but two dietitians who job-shared could each take full responsibility for the programs in five schools.)

The employer benefits from job-sharing in that there are two individuals who bring their ideas, talents, and skills to the job. Frequently, the individuals sharing the position have been full-time employees in the past and therefore have a short learning curve. On the other hand, the disadvantages of job-sharing can be lack of continuity and decreased productivity. The individuals who are sharing the position have to spend a significant portion of their time communicating with each other to avoid duplication of effort or omission of essential elements of the job.

At this time, most job-sharing arrangements are worked out on an individual basis. There are no set patterns that determine how benefits are allocated, how vacations are scheduled, and so on. These factors are determined by the employers. If job-sharing is widely used in a particular work setting, there should be published human resources policies and procedures to assure that all workers are treated equitably. Employers are not required to provide opportunities for job-sharing.

probation

A **probationary employee** is one who is newly hired into a position. For a set period of time, often 60 or 90 days, the worker is learning the job functions and getting acquainted with the work environment. During this period of probation, it is the manager's prerogative to dismiss the worker "**without cause**." If an employee is unable to learn the tasks required, or demonstrates behaviors that are problematic (for example, persistent tardiness), dismissal should take place during the probationary period. Employees who continue to work beyond the probationary period cannot usually be fired unless there is **cause**, which is a time-consuming and difficult managerial process. In some cases, the probationary period may be extended beyond the usual time limit. If a manager wishes to extend the probationary period, the employer's human resources policy should be consulted to determine the proper procedure to be followed.

Job-Sharing. *The concept of having two employees share one full-time job.*

Probationary Employee. *A newly hired employee who has not yet demonstrated that he can successfully perform the job for which he was hired. The employee is given a set period of time, often 60 or 90 days, to learn the job.*

Without Cause. *The case in which a probationary employee may be dismissed for whatever reason the manager feels is appropriate.*

Cause. *A documented, legitimate reason for terminating a non-probationary employee.*

temporary

Temporary workers may be needed for a specific project, to cover a leave of absence, or when there is a transient need for extra employees. These workers may or may not be placed on the payroll of the employer. Examples of temporary workers who are hired by the employer are students who cover the summertime vacations of permanent workers. These employees typically work without benefits, though some employers offer pay in lieu of benefits to them. Usually they will work for several months, which justifies the cost of hiring and training them.

Temporary workers who are not on the payroll of the employer are hired through a temporary employment agency. All types of workers, from unskilled to professional, can be hired in this way. These include waitstaff, secretaries, computer engineers, dietary managers, and even Registered Dietitians. The temporary agency provides the workers for a published fee. The workers are employed and paid by the agency. The employer, in turn, pays the agency. This type of arrangement is typically used in situations in which the shortage of staff is unexpected (secondary to an illness) or anticipated to be short term (the accounting clerk takes a two-week vacation, and there is no other staff member who can perform the job functions). Obtaining staff through a temporary agency is expensive, because the employer is paying for both the employee and the agency's fees for providing the service. However, the cost is usually offset when the time and financial costs of hiring and training a new employee (and possibly the cost of employee benefits) are factored into the equation.

contract

A contract employee is one who is hired to do a job that is finite in nature. Examples include the computer engineers and data entry personnel who are hired to install and bring a new computer system online or a Registered Dietitian who provides a series of weight-loss classes for the patients of a group of physicians. Though it is possible to put these people on the employer's payroll, this type of work is frequently contracted out as a one-time job. It is possible to hire contract personnel from a contract agency (in the computer start-up situation, this might be the manufacturer of the computer system), or one might hire an independent (freelance) contractor or a consultant. In the case of the contract agency, the arrangement is similar to that with the temporary agency described earlier.

An independent contractor may be paid a fee for the project, or may be paid an hourly (or monthly) consultant fee. The fee will be higher than the rate that would be paid if the contractor were on the payroll. Again, the costs will usually be offset by the savings of not having to hire, train, and provide benefits to an employee. Independent contractors and consultants must provide their own benefits and pay taxes on the **consultant fees**.

contingent workers

Both temporary and contract employees may be grouped together under the term *contingent workers*. The term differentiates these workers from career employees. **Contingent workers** know that their positions are not permanent, whereas **career employees** fully expect to have a job as long as their work performance is adequate.

salaried and hourly compensation

Distinction is also made among workers based on how they are paid. Some employees are paid for the number of hours worked, whereas others are paid a salary to do a job. In many situations, hourly workers are also called *nonexempt* employees and salaried workers are called *exempt*. Once again, these terms do not have universal definitions and are subject to interpretation by the employer. Managers should become familiar with the precise meanings of these terms in their workplaces.

the hourly worker

An **hourly worker** is paid a set rate for each hour worked. This amount is at least the minimum wage set by the federal government. States may have a legal rate that is higher than the federal rate; where such law exists, the higher rate prevails.

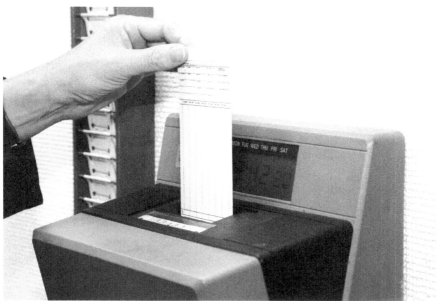

Copyright © 2011 by Depositphotos/Alexey Stiop.

A time clock may be used to track the time spent on the job by hourly workers.

Contingent Workers. *Employees, such as temporary and contract employees, who know that their work positions are short-term or temporary.*

Career Employees. *Workers who expect to continue working in a job as long as their work performance is adequate.*

Hourly Worker. *An employee who is paid a set rate for each hour worked, which is at least the minimum wage set by the government.*

The hourly rate for an individual is also known as that worker's **base rate**. It is from this rate that differential rates of pay are calculated. For example, if a short-hour worker has a base rate of $9.00 per hour and is to receive pay in lieu of benefits of 10 percent, the actual rate of pay for this worker would be $9.90 ($9.00 × 10% = $0.90 + $9.00 = $9.90) per hour.

Employers must keep track of the time worked by hourly employees, either by using a time clock or by keeping time sheets. Electronic systems are available in which time is automatically recorded when an employee uses an encoded identification badge to enter and exit the workplace. If the employees are involved in the record keeping, as with a self-reported time sheet, they are expected to be honest and accurate. Falsification of these documents can lead to disciplinary action.

Hourly workers are not guaranteed a minimum salary each pay period. A full-time hourly worker is guaranteed to be scheduled to work 40 hours each week, but if the employee is late for work, fails to report to work, or leaves early, the employer can "dock" (not pay) that employee for being absent. On the other hand, an hourly worker who works more than the guaranteed number of hours will be paid for those additional hours. Hourly status is common for unskilled and skilled workers; it may also be used for supervisorial and professional employees.

Because hourly employees are paid for the number of hours worked, they may be willing or even anxious to work beyond the guaranteed number of hours in order to earn additional money. If there is a pay differential for working overtime or for working on weekends or holidays, it is relatively easy to recruit volunteers to work the extra hours. A manager must be careful to be equitable in the assignment of extra hours and should not unduly burden (or reward) one or two employees. The primary concern should always be the employee, who has health and safety needs as well as the desire to earn additional pay. Employees who are tired are more likely to have accidents on the job. Managers should exercise prudence when assigning overtime work to employees.

differential wages

Differential wage rates are a method to reimburse hourly workers for work that is performed either outside of the normal work hours or for extraordinary types of work. The most commonly used differential rate is for overtime. Differential rates of pay, if they exist, may be mandated by law, by union contract, or by institutional policy. Managers need to be aware of procedures for calculating wage differentials for workers whom they employ. (See Table 7.1.)

Part-time or short-hour employees who work more than the guaranteed hours are paid for additional hours worked at the base rate of pay. If an hourly employee works more

management practice in dietetics

than 40 hours in a week (or eight hours in a day if the state law or union contract mandates it), the worker will be entitled to "time-and-a-half" for the hours that exceed those stated above. This is equivalent to the base rate multiplied by 150 percent. If the base rate is $9.00 per hour and the employee worked 48 hours in a week, the gross pay would be $468.00. This is calculated as follows:

$9.00 × 40 hours = $360.00 (base salary for week)
$9.00 × 150% = $13.50 per hour (overtime rate)
$13.50 × 8 hours = $108.00 (overtime pay)
$360.00 + $108.00 = $468.00 (gross pay for week)

The example given here is straightforward. The calculation of pay rates is not always so simple. Some contractual agreements use differential wage rates for variations in the work performed, the time of work, holidays, weekends, split shifts, excessively long work days, and so on. Examples of conditions that alter the base rate are shown in Table 7.1.

Double-Back	Additional pay earned if less than a minimum period of time (for example, 10 hours) elapses between the time an employee completes a shift and begins the next shift
Double-Time	Pay earned at twice the base rate; used if an employee works excessively long hours (for example, more than 12 hours in a day) or for many consecutive days (for example, eight); sometimes used for overtime on a holiday
Hazard Pay	Additional pay given to an employee for hours worked performing a particularly hazardous or distasteful task
Holiday Pay	Premium pay for time worked on an employer-designated holiday
Overtime	Additional pay for hours worked in excess of full-time; often this is more than eight hours in a day or 40 hours in a week
Pay in Lieu of Benefits	Addition to the base pay rate earned by employees who are not eligible for benefits
Shift Differential	Additional pay for employees who work evenings or nights or who come to work very early in the morning; may be paid for all or part of a shift
Split Shift	Additional pay for working a shift that is non-continuous or "split" into two distinct blocks of time
Time-and-a-Half	Pay rate of 150 percent of base rate for overtime (for example, more than 40 hours in a week or eight hours in a day)
Work in a Higher Job Classification	Employee is paid at the rate for the job performed rather than at that employee's usual base rate
Work in a Lower Job Classification	Employee earns the usual base rate, even though a lower-rated job is performed

Table 7.1 Types of Differential Wages

the salaried employee

A **salaried worker** is paid for doing a job. This employee is expected to work as many hours as it takes to get the job done. The underlying assumption is that a full-time, salaried position is roughly equivalent to a 40-hour workweek *on average;* however, the work may be subject to fluctuations from week to week. Individuals in salaried positions may work 50 or more hours one week, and then have a lighter workload the next. An example of a salaried employee with a variable workload is a clinical dietitian who usually works between 40 and 45 hours each week in a community hospital. Toward the end of December, patients do not choose to have elective medical procedures done, so patient census drops, as does the workload. The clinical dietitian may find that the weekly work during the holiday season can be completed in 30 hours rather than the usual 40 hours.

Salaried individuals are also called exempt, since they are "exempt from overtime pay provisions" of the Fair Labor Standards Act.[3] Employers might be tempted to take advantage of these employees by expecting them to work a *minimum* of 40 hours each week. The corporate culture may be such that individuals feel compelled to be at work before the boss arrives and stay until the boss leaves at the end of the day. If this is, in fact, a condition of employment, the employee should be made aware of the expectation prior to employment. A job should not be offered under the pretense that the employee will be expected to work 40 hours a week if the job actually takes 50 hours to do.

Though long hours are common in exempt employment situations, it is well for managers to consider the consequences before encouraging this practice. Employees who work long hours will become tired and will have to give up personal time to put in the additional hours at work. Though this can easily be done for short periods of time, the expectation of extended hours as a job requirement will lead to resentment and job dissatisfaction. This is especially true if prospective employees are not told in advance and the expectation comes as a surprise after they begin to work in the new positions. Employees who are tired, dissatisfied, or angry do not perform as well as other employees. Allowing this behavior to persist over time might seem appealing to managers because they think that they are getting more for their money, but in the long term, the costs of illness, **burnout**, and **attrition** may well outweigh any short-term cost benefits. Employees who habitually put in longer-than-necessary hours at work should be discouraged from continuing this behavior.

Telecommuting is an option for some individuals with salaried, exempt positions. The burden of long hours in the work setting is offset by the decreased time that they spend getting to and from the workplace. It is becoming necessary to find alternate ways to measure the performance of salaried employees other than the number of hours spent on the job. As new methods for performance evaluation are developed, the actual number of hours worked will become less important. These emerging techniques for measuring productivity should level the playing field for individuals who work at differing speeds or with different degrees of efficiency and effectiveness.

management practice in dietetics

In order to calculate the hourly pay rate for the salaried employee, it is necessary to know the total number of hours to be paid. For most employees, this number is 2,080 hours per year (40 hours per week × 52 weeks = 2,080 hours). Thus, the hourly rate is calculated as the annual salary divided by 2,080. For the employee who makes $50,000 each year, the hourly rate is $24.04. If the employee actually works 50 hours each week (2,600 hours per year), the hourly rate drops to $19.23. Note that 2,080 is the number that is usually used to calculate the conversions between hourly rates and annual salaries.

compensatory time

Some employers allow salaried employees to take time off for the hours they work that are greater than 40 in a week. Thus, the employee who worked 42 hours on the first week of the month, 45 hours the second week, and 41 hours the third week would be entitled to a full day (eight hours) off the fourth week of the month.

There is potential for abuse when this system is in place, so the policy governing compensatory time off should be uniform for all employees and should be written and published so that both management and employees are aware of what it is. For example, the policy may be written so that the employee must use the compensatory time within 60 days or lose it. This type of restriction would prevent the accumulation of large numbers of hours that the employee could later claim as an extended period of paid vacation, which could interfere with the smooth functioning of an organizational unit. Alternately, the policy may allow the employee to take the "comp" time or relinquish the right to that time off and be paid for the extra time worked at a specified rate, perhaps the hourly rate as determined by the gross annual salary divided by 2,080.

There is no requirement for an employer to offer compensatory time off to salaried employees. Comp time is an employee benefit that is given at the discretion of the employer. The critical factors to be addressed when employees have this benefit are that the policy must be clearly written and uniformly administered.

on-call

Some positions require that an employee be available to be called in to work in the case of an emergency. This requires that the individual be available during off-hours via a beeper, a smartphone, e-mail, or other electronic means. This is a typical condition of employment when the employer is an acute health care organization. Physicians, pharmacists, dietitians, and managers are among those who are scheduled to be **on-call** during specified hours.

Compensatory Time Off. *A method used to give salaried employees who work long hours some extra time off to compensate them for unpaid overtime worked.*

On-Call. *A position that requires the employee to be available to come to work on short notice during unscheduled hours, if needed.*

If a job requires that an employee will be responsible for being on-call, this should be stated in the job description as a condition of employment. In addition, employees should know how frequently they will be scheduled to be on-call; this type of obligation should be scheduled equitably among all eligible employees. The employer may set up a pay structure to compensate individuals for the time that they are on-call, or for the hours that they actually work if they are called in to work when they are on-call. In some situations, on-call time is paid back in compensatory time off; in other circumstances, it may be considered to be part of the job and there is no additional pay or time off.

calculating full-time equivalents

Full-Time Equivalent (FTE). *A standard term used to describe the number of full-time positions worked by all employees, including full-time, part-time, short-hour, and casual. One FTE is usually equal to 40 hours per week or 2,080 hours per year.*

The number of full-time equivalent employees managed measures, in part, a manager's span of control. A full-time equivalent (FTE) is equal to 40 hours per week or 2,080 hours per year. FTE is a term used to compare the management responsibility of a manager who directs the activities of regular, full-time career employees with that of a colleague who manages part-time and short-hour employees. It is the customary method used to count the number of employees who work for a manager, an employer, or an organizational unit. The calculation of FTEs is an integral part of the budgeting process, too.

Consider the local community hospital's foodservices department. There are 20 employees who work 40 hours each week, mostly Monday through Friday, day shift. In addition, there are 10 employees who work 20 hours each week and 8 employees who work 16 hours per week to cover the evening meal and weekends. The total number of employees in the department is 38 (20 +10 + 8 = 38). The number of FTEs is based on the number of hours scheduled rather than on the number of people who work. The number of FTEs is computed as follows:

> 20 employees × 40 hours = 800 hours
> 10 employees × 20 hours = 200 hours
> 8 employees × 16 hours = 128 hours
> 800 + 200 + 128 = 1,128 hours per week
> 1,128 / 40 = 28.2 FTEs

Thus, the foodservice department has 38 employees but only 28.2 FTEs.

It is sometimes important to look at FTEs from the opposite point of view. Consider the urgent-care center that operates eight hours per day seven days each week with nine nurses needed to staff the services offered. It is obvious that more than nine nurses will be needed if any of them is to get any time off. To determine the number of nurses who need to be hired, one must first calculate the total number of hours to be worked by all nurses. In this case, the total number of hours is 504 per week (8 hours × 7 days × 9 nurses). Assuming that the positions are interchangeable, and that each of the nurses can work any of the nine positions, it will take a minimum of 12.6 nurses to staff the clinic (504 total hours / 40 hours per nurse = 12.6 FTE nurses). In reality, more than this number of nurses will be needed because the full-time nurses will earn and use vacation days, holidays, sick days, and other paid time off. Some casual or contingent nursing staff could work to cover the clinic positions when the full-time nurses are taking time off. Another option would be to hire some part-time staff whose hours could be increased when the full-time nurses are not working.

FTE figures can be used in other ways, too. For example, the number of FTEs who work in a week could be monitored as part of a productivity measurement, where FTEs are compared with work output. If it takes two 8-hour shifts and one 4-hour shift per day for diet clerks to process menus, that is equivalent to 3.5 FTEs (20 hours per day × 7 days per week / 40 hours per FTE = 3.5 FTEs) per week. Assuming that the average daily census of the hospital is 300, those 3.5 FTEs are needed for each 2,100 patient days (300 patients × 7 days = 2,100 patient days). This amounts to one FTE for every 600 patient days (2,100 / 3.5 = 600). Tracking these data over time helps the manager to control staffing by adding tasks when the patient census drops, and approving overtime when the patient census increases. Experienced managers know that records documenting these kinds of data over time are essential to identify potential labor problems and take corrective action in a timely manner.

Another reason to monitor FTEs actually working is to determine the effect of change within the operation. If the diet clerks mentioned above needed to begin using a new menu, the change will slow work processes for a period of time. Tracking the number of FTEs used in a week helps the manager to know when the change has been accomplished and things have returned to normal in the diet office. It will also provide data regarding the labor costs involved in making the change.

Historical FTE data are also useful in determining appropriate staffing levels. In a WIC clinic, the number of FTEs is usually related to the caseload of the clinic. For example, if it takes 2.5 FTEs to carry a total clinic caseload of 1,200 clients, staffing should increase by 0.5 FTE when the caseload increases to 1,440 clients. The calculation is as follows:

    1,200 clients / 2.5 FTEs = 480 clients per FTE
    1,440 clients − 1,200 clients = 240 new clients
    240 new clients / 480 clients = ½ FTE (0.5)

It is the responsibility of the dietitian manager to become familiar with the calculations pertaining to FTEs and to be able to use the information in the management process. It is a useful tool to measure the manager's span of control. It is even more valuable for the ongoing monitoring of the workforce and is critical in helping the manager measure job performance, determine staffing needs, and manage labor costs.

diversity in the workplace

Diversity. *In the workplace, this refers to ethnic, racial, gender, age, and other differences among workers.*

The issue of **diversity** in the workplace is not a new one. America's workforce has been changing and adapting for generations as the demographics of the country have evolved. Each wave of immigrants has brought changes that have, in time, enhanced the work environment, though each transitional period has been difficult. The new workers have brought new ideas, new skills, new problems, and solutions for these problems into the workplace.

Xenophobia—that is, fear of strangers or foreigners—on the part of those who are already in the workforce may contribute to the anxiety and discomfort that inevitably accompany change. Nevertheless, change has been accommodated in the past and will be accommodated again. The remainder of this chapter is designed to provide the manager with the information needed to facilitate the integration of diverse workers into the workplace in a way that is unifying rather than divisive. The goal of fostering a diverse workforce is to strengthen the organization.

Before exploring diversity further, it is important to note that dietetics professionals are not reflective of the community in which they work. Ninety-six percent of RDs

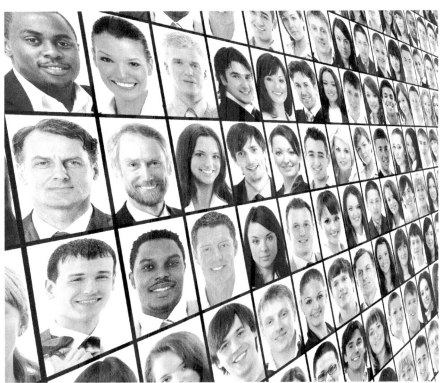

Ideally, the workforce should reflect the community that is being served.

management practice in dietetics

and DTRs are women and 83% of them are white.[4] Though the profession has worked diligently to increase its diversity over the past two decades, it has been an elusive goal.

diversity defined

The cultural background of an individual, primarily reflective of that person's country of origin, has been discussed in the diversity literature as one of its major issues. Indeed, with each wave of immigration into this country, new ethnic groups have been gradually integrated into the workforce. In the past, people from Ireland, Italy, and other European countries were regarded with suspicion when they first entered the workforce. Today, these groups have become so well integrated that they make up the dominant segment in the workplace: the white worker. Still, multiculturalism remains one of the goals for diversity, with the inclusion of a higher number of different ethnic groups than ever before. Fine[5] differentiates between a culturally diverse organization (one in which the workforce has representatives from different groups) and a multicultural organization. The latter is defined as "an organization that:

1. values, encourages, and affirms diverse cultural modes of being and interacting;
2. creates an organizational dialogue in which no one cultural perspective is presumed to be more valid than other perspectives;
3. empowers all cultural voices to participate fully in setting goals and making decisions."

Today, people of different ethnicity (for purposes of this discussion, *ethnicity* refers to country of origin) continue to enter the workforce, but cultural diversity is no longer the only factor included under discussion. Other subgroups of the population are entering the workforce in large numbers and must be considered when discussing diversity. These include people of various races, women, age groups, and those who have differing physical abilities, in addition to people of different ethnic backgrounds. Baytos[6] calls these five characteristics the primary dimensions of diversity because they are "inborn and immutable." In addition, he adds examples of secondary dimensions, which include education, work experience, marital status, religion, and functional specialty. These secondary dimensions are innumerable, so no attempt is made to list them all here. However, it should be noted that these dimensions include such characteristics as sexual orientation and body size, the latter often being an issue for health professionals, especially for dietetic professionals. It is important to value all types of diversity, not just that related to culture.

changing demographics and legislative initiatives

The population of the United States is changing, as is the workforce. In order for an organization to maximize its opportunity for success, it needs to reflect the community

Culturally Diverse Organization. *An organization that has a workforce representative of many different cultural groups.*

Multicultural Organization. *An organization that values, encourages, and affirms diverse cultural modes, in which each point of view is valid and different cultures contribute to decision making.*

that it serves. The more precisely an organization's workforce reflects the community, the better chance it will have to provide goods and services that the community wants and will purchase and use. In order to understand and manage diversity, there is a need to understand the changes that are occurring in the population at large and, more narrowly, changes in the workforce. Demographics and legislation affecting the workforce make a significant impact on organizations in relationship to some of the primary dimensions listed above. These data can help managers to position the organization for the future.

gender. Women started entering the workforce in large numbers during the final three decades of the last century. In 1994, 46% of the 132.5 million workers in the U.S. were women. At that time, their salaries still lagged significantly behind those of men. By 2005, 48% of 147 million workers were women. This represents an increase of nearly 10 million additional women in the workforce. It is projected that by 2050, half of the U.S. workers will be women. That's somewhere between 85 and 91 million workers, depending on the projections used.[7] As the percentage of women increases and that of men declines, the "glass ceiling" that has characterized the emerging feminization of the workplace is giving way as more women gain the requisite tenure and experience to qualify for advancement.

Employers and organizations are changing to meet the needs of women by making jobs more flexible and by providing access to services that women, especially those with child-rearing responsibilities, need. These include telecommuting, job-sharing, day care, family leave, and more adjustable benefit packages. As women advance in organizations, more of their needs are being identified and addressed.

age. As the baby boom generation moves through the life cycle, the age of the workforce is increasing, partly because their numbers are large and partly because the following generation is small in proportion. The projections from *Workforce 2020*[8] show that older Americans will keep working longer than they have in the past. Some of this is due to the improved health and well-being of older individuals who feel that they still have a contribution to make, but another major factor is the increased age at which workers from this group can collect Social Security benefits. It has also been projected that these benefits will not be as great as they were in the past. People will have to work longer to make ends meet, and may continue to work some after retirement.

U.S. Dept. of Labor. *http:// www.dol.gov/*

Older workers have some special needs that must be accommodated, including better lighting, larger print, and equipment that requires less dexterity and less strength to operate.[9] On the other hand, older workers reflect the aging of the population at large, and their presence in an organization will help the organization to react more appropriately to external customers who are also aging. The most current data on the workforce can be obtained from the **U.S. Department of Labor** and its **Bureau of Labor Statistics**.

Bureau of Labor Statistics. *http:// www.bls.gov/*

management practice in dietetics

culture. Both racial and ethnic minorities in the workplace are changing. To date, the majority of the workforce has been white non-Hispanic (that is, those with European backgrounds). In 1994, they made up 77 percent of the workforce. The percentage of the whites in the workforce is declining while the growth of other groups of workers is increasing rapidly. The percentage of non-whites and immigrants in the workforce is expected to continue to grow. Though non-Hispanic whites will remain the largest group in the workforce, they will hold only 53% of jobs in 2050. Further, it is projected that the percentage of African Americans in the workforce will only grow to about 14%; Asians and Hispanics are expected to double their numbers in the workforce.[10] Organizations and all individuals within those organizations will have to become sensitive to the needs of the nonwhite and foreign-born workers as this transition progresses. These workers are an integral part of the workplace of the future.

As with female and older workers, racial and ethnic workers represent an associated market potential. Inclusion of them and their diverse viewpoints directly influences the business's ability to respond to external market forces.

differences in physical ability. People with differing physical abilities (sometimes called people with handicaps, disabilities, or physical challenges) are entering the workforce in greater numbers since the implementation of legislation known as the **Americans with Disabilities Act** in 1990. Organizations are required to make reasonable accommodation for these individuals, such as accessible parking, lavatories, and workstations. As accommodation is made for these employees, coworkers develop sensitivity in dealing with colleagues with differing physical abilities. It follows that the organization will become more user-friendly for external customers who have physical challenges as well.

equal opportunity/affirmative action. Legislation that mandated **equal opportunity** for Americans grew out of the civil rights movement of the 1960s. Until that time, many workers, most especially women and racial minorities, were denied access to certain segments of the workplace; many jobs were out of reach to them. The creation of the **U.S. Equal Employment Opportunity Commission** changed such overt discrimination, though discrimination still exists in subtle (and sometimes not-so-subtle) forms. With the passage of this legislation, many career opportunities, which had been the exclusive domain of white males, opened to other groups.

Though the changes were good, progress was slow. Groups who had been excluded in the past found that they lacked the necessary training and skills to take advantage of the opportunities now available. Thus, **affirmative action** became mandated in venues where past discrimination was shown to have decreased the competitiveness of population subgroups. Affirmative action legislation gives hiring preference to traditionally disenfranchised workers. It has facilitated the advancement of women and minorities.

Americans with Disabilities Act. *A federal law that enables people with different physical abilities to enter the mainstream with greater ease by mandating that organizations and businesses provide the appropriate accommodation (for example, accessible lavatories, parking, and so on) for all.*

Equal Opportunity. *A federal law that prohibits discrimination against certain groups, such as women or minorities, in the workforce.*

U.S. Equal Employment Opportunity Commission. *http://www.eeoc.gov/*

Affirmative Action. *A federal law that requires giving hiring preference to previously disenfranchised workers.*

There is national debate over whether or not affirmative action legislation has outlived its usefulness. Some factions believe that it will take many more years for disadvantaged groups to have a level playing field in the area of job opportunity. At this writing, contractors on federally funded projects in the U.S. are required to take affirmative action. Some states have similar laws. Many employers have this type of policy in place. Others believe that the goals of affirmative action have been achieved and that the continuation of this policy will result in discrimination against other population groups. It is likely that the reality is somewhere between these two opposing points of view. However, if the goals of a truly diverse workforce are met, the question will become irrelevant. A workplace that reflects the community will provide opportunity for all workers.

benefits of diversity

The benefits of diversity are myriad. In addition to having a larger pool of potential workers from which to draw, the organization benefits because it has access to a broader variety of viewpoints and ideas. The breadth and depth of the experiences of each member of the workforce can be tapped to develop products and services for the diverse markets that each represents. For example, a weight-control program that employs only older white women may find that it is most effective in dealing with clients who are also older white women because the clients can easily identify with the provider of service. However, this program may be ineffective in working with men, with adolescents, or with women of color. It will be harder for these groups to identify with the service provider, and they may also find it difficult to adhere to a program designed for people whose lifestyles are very different from their own. As the target markets for a product broaden, the need for a diverse workforce to understand and meet the needs of the various market segments increases, too. In the meantime, dietitians need to develop **cultural competence** in order to work effectively with groups who differ from them.

Cultural Competence. *The ability to provide linguistically and culturally appropriate services.*

Institutions and businesses that ignore these opportunities and continue to avoid fostering diversity will find themselves lagging behind other companies that have embraced diversity. In fact, it has been demonstrated that fostering diversity in the workplace increases the diversity of customers in the marketplace, and is good for business. It is good for the bottom line.[11]

The employee who works in an environment that is committed to fostering diversity also benefits. The environment is a safe one that values the uniqueness of the individual and provides opportunity for growth and the development of self-efficacy.

Finally, the external customer benefits from a diverse workforce. This occurs because the organization that fosters diversity is able to be responsive to the greater community in which it operates. It will be well equipped to satisfy the needs of the diverse community it serves.

management practice in dietetics

drawbacks of diversity

There are drawbacks inherent in introducing diversity into the work environment, too. When initial attempts are made to integrate new workers into an existing workforce, xenophobia becomes apparent and sometimes takes control of otherwise rational individuals. Employees may feel threatened and sabotage the new workers or the system that brought them into "our" workplace; this may be an intentional or an unconscious reaction. It will take time, energy, and money to implement a program that helps workers to overcome their biases and deal with the diverse people in a sensitive and fair way. There will probably be some losses along the way, as long-term employees refuse to change or new employees refuse to put up with subtle forms of discrimination. The volatility that accompanies change often makes the workplace an unpleasant place to be for a period of time.

goals of diversity in the workplace

The goal of diversity in the workplace is to provide a work environment where everyone is a contributing member of the organization. Every person is respectful and respected. Each individual is treated equally and fairly, but also as an individual and in a manner that is sensitive to that person's uniqueness. All individuals feel secure enough to speak openly, knowing that they will not be penalized for doing so. In short, the organization is a benevolent and humane place to work, and every worker pitches in to further the goals of the organization. And all of this is done because people want to do it, not because they are forced to do it. The concept is somewhat idealistic, but the nearer a workplace gets to reaching these goals, the better (and the more successful) the overall organization will be.

compliance versus commitment

Diversity strategies work best when the entire organization, institution, or business is committed to the program. This means that all levels of staff and management must be aware of the program and determined to make it work. Everyone must model behaviors that demonstrate sensitivity to each member of the workforce, regardless of that person's "status." It is admirable for one or two managers to foster diversity within their particular area of influence, but if either their superiors or their subordinates do not demonstrate similar values, there will be a lack of credibility in the program.

This is indicative of the difference between compliance and commitment. It is part of the reason that neither equal opportunity nor affirmative action has been as successful as it could have been. As long as the "letter of the law" is being followed, it is unlikely that there will be any penalty for noncompliance. To go the extra step and demonstrate commitment requires an investment of time, money, and self.

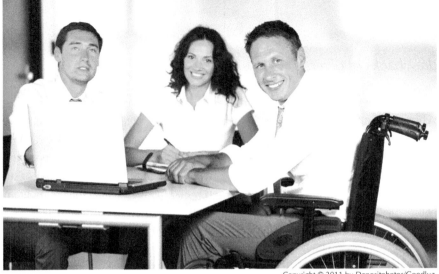

Copyright © 2011 by Depositphotos/Goodluz.

Sensitivity training can help managers become aware of different needs of individuals.

It is only after these investments have been made that the benefits of diversity, which translate to the bottom line, can be realized. It is not enough to appoint an affirmative action officer who plans and implements affirmative action programs and monitors the results of such programs. To get optimal results, the program must belong to everyone, from the chief executive officer to the frontline worker. Everyone must know the value of diversity and must have a vested interest in achieving it. As Walters stated in 1996, "Yes, we do it because it is morally right. But we also do it because it is smart."[12]

diversity training

To achieve true diversity in the workplace, the individual workers must be aware of their prejudices and be willing to suppress these in order to be sensitive to the needs of their coworkers. It is probably not possible to overcome all of the life experiences and prejudices that are brought into the workplace. Awareness leads to tolerance, which can foster the nonjudgmental acceptance of differences. Sensitivity training, however, allows workers to learn how to deal with differences that are encountered in the work environment in order to make the workplace non-threatening to everyone there.

Consider the situation in which two colleagues, one seated in a wheelchair and the other standing, are having a lengthy conversation. The person who is seated would be in the uncomfortable (both physical and psychological) position of having to look up for an extended period of time. Because conversations between peers are usually conducted at eye level for both parties, it would be appropriate for both parties to be seated. However, that behavior may not be spontaneous for the individual who is

232   *management practice in dietetics*

standing. Sensitivity training can teach awareness of differing perspectives that will lead to a more equitable workplace for all. Similar examples can be found throughout the workplace whenever differences exist between workers.

It is the responsibility of management to develop and implement programs that explore the diversity issues in the organization and deal with them in a constructive manner. For a closer look at managing diversity, further readings are listed at the end of this chapter.

conclusion

This chapter has outlined the basic characteristics of the workforce that dietetics managers will encounter as they practice in the arena of management. Categories of workers and worker status have been described, and common types of programs for employee compensation have been discussed. This information should help the manager to perform competently in today's workplace.

Of greater importance, however, is the issue of diversity that was discussed in the latter part of this chapter. Diversity will characterize the workplace of the future. Successful managers will deal with these issues effectively throughout their careers. The terminology may change as new buzzwords are created to draw attention to workplace issues, but the concepts will remain. Managers must foster diversity if their organizations and institutions are to thrive in the twenty-first century. The materials in this chapter can be summarized in the following manner.

1. Dietetics professionals manage several types of workers, including professionals (who range from entry-level to specialists), supervisory personnel, skilled workers, and unskilled workers.
2. Employees may work full-time or may be partially employed in a number of different categories, with or without guaranteed numbers of hours.
3. Employees may work directly for an organization as a career employee, expecting to hold a position there for a long period of time, or they may be contingent workers.
4. Compensation will be on either an hourly or a salaried basis; hourly workers may be entitled to differential wages at some times.
5. One FTE is equal to one full-time workweek, usually 40 hours.
6. Diversity in the workplace includes the embracing of differences among workers, which include, but are not limited to, race, culture, gender, age, and differences in physical abilities.
7. As society transitions into achieving the goal of a truly diverse workforce, the problems encountered will be overshadowed by the enrichment of the workplace that diversity brings.

activities

activity 1

The three time cards shown here belong to diet office personnel. Joan and Craig are full-time diet clerks, whose base salary is $9.50 per hour. Joan has just passed the registration exam and is now a Dietetic Technician, Registered (DTR); she sometimes works as a DTR, which is a higher job classification. She wants to move into a full-time DTR position as soon as one becomes available. DTRs make $11.25 per hour. Sueling is a DTR who is in a casual position and receives pay in lieu of benefits. During the week illustrated on the time cards, she is working more hours than usual because another DTR is on vacation.

For each of the three employees, calculate the gross pay for the week, using the following information about wage differential in this institution:

a. Pay in lieu of benefits is 12.5 percent.
b. Weekend shift differential is $1.50 per hour.
c. Holiday pay is time-and-a-half (150 percent).
d. Overtime pay is also time-and-a-half.
e. Shift differential for hours before 6 a.m. or after 6 p.m. is $1.25 per hour.
f. Temporary work in a higher classification gets paid at the rate for the higher classification.

Name: _Craig_

Pay Period From: _____ to _____

Date	In	Out	In	Out	In	Out	Total	
S								off
M	11:00	2:30	3:00	7:30				
T								off
W	5:30	10:00	10:30	2:00				
T	5:30	10:00	10:30	2:00				
F	5:30	10:00	10:30	2:00				
S	5:30	10:00	10:30	2:00				
S	5:30	10:00	10:30	2:30	3:00	7:30		
M								off
T								off
W	11:00	2:30	3:00	7:30				
T	11:00	2:30	3:00	7:30				Thanksgiving
F	11:00	2:30	3:00	7:30				
S	11:00	2:30	3:00	7:30				

Employer's Signature _____

Supervisor's Signature _____

Name: _Joan_

Pay Period From: _____ to _____

Date	In	Out	In	Out	In	Out	Total	
S	5:30	10:00	10:30	2:00				
M	5:30	10:00	10:30	2:00				
T	5:30	10:00	10:30	2:15				
W								off
T	8:00	11:30	12:00	4:30				worked as DTR
F	8:00	11:30	12:00	4:30				worked as DTR
S								off
S								off
M	5:30	10:00	10:30	2:30				
T	5:30	10:00	10:30	2:00				
W	8:00	11:30	12:00	4:30				worked as DTR
T	5:30	10:00	10:30	2:30				Thanksgiving
F	5:30	10:00	10:30	2:30				
S								off

Employer's Signature _____

Supervisor's Signature _____

Name: Sueling							
Pay Period From: _____ to _____							

Date	In	Out	In	Out	In	Out	Total	
S	8:00	11:30	12:00	4:30				
M	8:00	11:45	12:15	4:30				
T	8:00	11:30	12:00	4:30				
W	8:00	11:30	12:00	5:15				
T								off
F								off
S	8:00	11:30	12:00	4:30				
S	8:00	11:30	12:00	4:30				
M	8:00	11:45	12:00	4:30				
T	8:00	11:30	12:00	4:45				
W								off
T	8:00	11:30	12:00	4:45				Thanksgiving
F	8:00	11:30	12:00	4:30				
S	8:00	11:30	12:00	4:30				

Employer's Signature _____

Supervisor's Signature _____

activity 2

As the manager of a health and fitness club, you have done a market survey of your clientele and determined that you should keep the facility open 24 hours a day. Because you are the manager, you will have flexible hours. You have also decided that you want to staff the club as follows:

a. One receptionist on duty 24 hours per day, 7 days per week.
b. One housekeeper on duty from 6 a.m. to 10 p.m. Monday through Friday.
c. Two housekeepers on duty from 6 a.m. to 10 p.m. Saturday and Sunday.
d. One RD on duty from 6 a.m. to 10 a.m. and from 2 p.m. to 10 p.m. daily.
e. Two personal fitness instructors on duty from 6 a.m. to 10 p.m. Monday through Friday.
f. Three personal fitness instructors on duty from 6 a.m. to midnight Saturday and Sunday.
g. One business manager who works 9 a.m. to 5:30 p.m. Monday through Friday.

Calculate the number of FTEs needed in each job category (receptionist, housekeeper, RD, personal fitness instructor, and business manager). How many FTEs, total, are needed to staff the facility?

activity 3

You are the manager of nutrition services in a clinic that serves a multiethnic clientele, which is 70 percent Hispanic and 20 percent Vietnamese. Only 10 percent of the clients speak English comfortably. You are fortunate in that you have been able to hire staff who reflect the population subgroups, so that 70 percent of your staff speaks Spanish.

When you had a staff meeting, you noticed that the Spanish-speaking staff were using that language to speak to each other when you entered the room. Later, the English- and Vietnamese-speaking staff members commented that this "always happens" and that they feel "left out." The only common language spoken by all members of the group is English. As manager, how should you deal with this situation?

activity 4

As manager of an obesity program, you pride yourself on having staff who are empathetic and effective in working with clients. They foster a philosophy of size acceptance, and work with clients to achieve healthy lifestyles. Weight loss is encouraged but is not essential. The program has a high success rate as measured by improved health outcomes but is slightly less successful with weight loss.

A new client comes into the program and is to be evaluated by Terilyn Fujitsu, RD. Terilyn is slim and relatively young. The client weighs more than 250 pounds and is 5'5" tall. She is middle-aged. After meeting the dietitian, the client storms into your office. She is extremely agitated as she tells you that she doesn't think she would benefit from being treated by "a skinny child" who couldn't possibly understand her struggle with weight and weight control. How would you deal with this situation?

to study further

In addition to the websites noted in the margins of this chapter, these additional sources are recommended for a more comprehensive review of the workforce and diversity in the workplace.

- Bucher, R. D. *Diversity Consciousness: Opening Our Minds to Peoples, Cultures, and Opportunities.* Upper Saddle River, NJ: Prentice Hall, 2010.
- Carnevale, A. P. and S. C. Stone. *The American Mosaic: An In-Depth Report on the Advantage of Diversity in the U.S. Work Force.* New York: R.R. Donnelley and Sons, 1995.
- Fitz, P. A. and B. E. Mitchell. "Building Our Future: A Summary of the ADA Diversity Mentoring Project." *Journal of the American Dietetic Association.* 102:1001–1007, 2002.
- Harvey, C. P. and M. J. Allard. *Understanding Diversity: Readings, Cases and Exercises.* 4th ed. Upper Saddle River, NJ: Pearson Prentice Hall, 2009.
- Jarratt, J. and J. B. Mahaffie. "Key Trends Affecting the Dietetics Profession and the American Dietetic Association." *Journal of the American Dietetic Association.* 102:1821–1939, 2002.
- Moran, R. T., P. R. Harris, and S. V. Moran. *Managing Cultural Difference: Global Leadership Strategies for Cross-Cultural Business Success.* 8th ed. Oxford: Butterworth-Heinemann, 2011.
- O'Sullivan Maillet, J., B. U. Dykes, and M. M. Yadrick. "The Changing Face of America—and ADA." *Journal of the American Dietetic Association.* 102:1384, 2002.
- Page, S. E. *The Difference: How the Power of Diversity Creates Better Groups, Firms, Schools and Societies.* Princeton, NJ: Princeton University Press, 2007.
- Stein, K. "The Balancing Act of Diversity Initiatives." *Journal of the American Dietetic Association.* 111:1110–1117, 2011.
- U.S. Department of Health and Human Services, "What Is Cultural Competency?" *Office of Minority Health.* 2005. http://minorityhealth.hhs.gov/templates/browse. aspx?lvl=2&lvlID=11.
- U.S. General Accounting Office. *Human Capital: Key Principles for Effective Strategic Workforce Planning.* Washington, DC: U.S. General Accounting Office, 2003. http://purl.access.gpo.gov/GPO/LPS42139.

scholarly journals

- *Journal of Cultural Diversity* http://tuckerpub.com/jcd.htm

other relevant periodical

- *Profiles in Diversity Journal* http://www.diversityjournal.com/

relevant websites

- The Diversity Training Group http://www.diversitydtg.com/
- Cultural Diversity Hotwire http://www.diversityhotwire.com/
- Equal Opportunity Advisory Council http://www.eeac.org/

in practice

pregnant women in the workplace

The dietetics profession is disproportionately female; it is only natural that issues arise regarding the rights of women during and after pregnancy. Employers also have questions about their rights and responsibilities when working with women of childbearing age. The following is reproduced from the US-EEOC website. This website is updated periodically, so interested readers may want to visit the site for recent changes.

The U.S. Equal Employment Opportunity Commission http://www.eeoc.gov/laws/types/pregnancy.cfm

---

pregnancy discrimination

Pregnancy discrimination involves treating a woman (an applicant or employee) unfavorably because of pregnancy, childbirth, or a medical condition related to pregnancy or childbirth.

pregnancy discrimination & work situations

The Pregnancy Discrimination Act (PDA) forbids discrimination based on pregnancy when it comes to any aspect of employment, including hiring, firing, pay, job assignments, promotions, layoff, training, fringe benefits, such as leave and health insurance, and any other term or condition of employment.

pregnancy discrimination & temporary disability

If a woman is temporarily unable to perform her job due to a medical condition related to pregnancy or childbirth, the employer or other covered entity must treat her in the same way as it treats any other temporarily disabled employee. For example, the employer may have to provide light duty, alternative assignments, disability leave, or unpaid leave to pregnant employees if it does so for other temporarily disabled employees.

Additionally, impairments resulting from pregnancy (for example, gestational diabetes or preeclampsia, a condition characterized by pregnancy-induced hypertension and protein in the urine) may be disabilities under the Americans with Disabilities Act (ADA). An employer may have to provide a reasonable accommodation (such as leave or modifications that enable an employee to perform her job) for a disability related to pregnancy, absent undue hardship (significant difficulty or expense). The ADA Amendments Act of 2008 makes it much easier to show that

---

Americans with Disabilities Act Home Page. *http://www.ada.gov/*

a medical condition is a covered disability. For more information about the ADA, see http://www.eeoc.gov/laws/types/disability.cfm. For information about the ADA Amendments Act, see http://www.eeoc.gov/laws/types/disability_regulations.cfm.

pregnancy discrimination & harassment

It is unlawful to harass a woman because of pregnancy, childbirth, or a medical condition related to pregnancy or childbirth. Harassment is illegal when it is so frequent or severe that it creates a hostile or offensive work environment or when it results in an adverse employment decision (such as the victim being fired or demoted). The harasser can be the victim's supervisor, a supervisor in another area, a co-worker, or someone who is not an employee of the employer, such as a client or customer.

pregnancy, maternity & parental leave

Under the PDA, an employer that allows temporarily disabled employees to take disability leave or leave without pay, must allow an employee who is temporarily disabled due to pregnancy to do the same.

An employer may not single out pregnancy-related conditions for special procedures to determine an employee's ability to work. However, if an employer requires its employees to submit a doctor's statement concerning their ability to work before granting leave or paying sick benefits, the employer may require employees affected by pregnancy-related conditions to submit such statements.

Further, under the Family and Medical Leave Act (FMLA) of 1993, a new parent (including foster and adoptive parents) may be eligible for 12 weeks of leave (unpaid or paid if the employee has earned or accrued it) that may be used for care of the new child. To be eligible, the employee must have worked for the employer for 12 months prior to taking the leave and the employer must have a specified number of employees. See http://www.dol.gov/whd/regs/compliance/whdfs28.htm.

pregnancy & workplace laws

Pregnant employees may have additional rights under the Family and Medical Leave Act (FMLA), which is enforced by the U.S. Department of Labor. Nursing mothers may also have the right to express milk in the workplace under a provision of the Fair Labor Standards Act enforced by the U.S. Department of Labor's Wage and Hour Division. See http://www.dol.gov/whd/regs/compliance/whdfs73.htm.

For more information about the Family Medical Leave Act or break time for nursing mothers, go to http://www.dol.gov/whd, or call 202-693-0051 or 1-866-487-9243 (voice), 202-693-7755 (TTY).

references

1. Hatch, Nathan O. *The Professions in American History*. Notre Dame, IN: University of Notre Dame Press, 1988.
2. Chambers, D. W. et al. "Another Look at Competency-Based Education in Dietetics." *Journal of the American Dietetic Association* 96 (1996): 614–617.
3. U.S. Department of Labor, Fair Labor Standards Act Advisor. *Exemptions*. http://www.dol.gov/elaws/esa/flsa/screen75.asp. Accessed July 17, 2012.
4. American Dietetic Association. *Compensation & Benefits Survey of the Dietetics Profession 2011*. Chicago: American Dietetic Association, 2011.
5. Fine, Marlene G. *Building Successful Multicultural Organizations: Challenges and Opportunities*. Westport, CT: Quorum Books, 1995.
6. Baytos, Lawrence M. *Designing and Implementing Successful Diversity Programs*. Englewood Cliffs, NJ: Prentice Hall, 1995.
7. Judy, Richard W. and Carol D'Amico. *Workforce 2020: Work and Workers in the 21st Century*. Indianapolis: Hudson Institute, 1997.
8. Ibid.
9. Labich, Kenneth. "Making Diversity Pay." *Fortune* 134:177–179. 1996.
10. Toossi, Mitra. "A Century of Change: The U.S. Labor Force 1950–2050." *Monthly Labor Review*. Bureau of Labor Statistics, May, 2002. http://www.bls.gov/opub/mlr/2002/05/art2full.pdf. Accessed July 17, 2012.
11. Flynn, Gillian. "Do You Have the Right Approach to Diversity?" *Personnel Journal* 74 (October 1996): 68–74.
12. Walters, Farah M. "Successfully Managing Diversity: Why Doing the Right Thing Is also the Smart Thing to Do." *Vital Speeches* 61:16 (1995): 496–501.

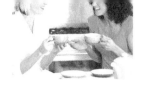

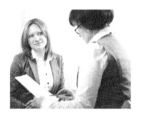

chapter eight

the employment process

learning objectives

1. Cite factors that must be considered when determining staffing needs.

2. Differentiate among job specifications, job descriptions, and job analyses.

3. Write a job specification, a job description, and a job analysis.

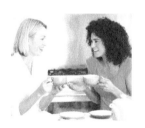

4. Discuss how such factors as regional workforce, financial resources, and other environmental conditions might influence staffing.

5. Describe various recruitment methods available.

6. Determine which recruitment methods are best for each of several different positions.

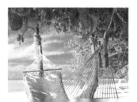

7. Differentiate between an unstructured, a semi-structured, and a structured interview.

8. Write an interview schedule for a specific job.

9. Discuss the pros and cons of the group interview.

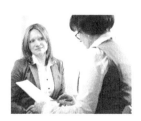

10. State the factors that should be considered when making a hiring decision.

11. Describe how to check references.

12. Discuss how compensation levels are set.

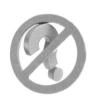

13. State how benefits and benefit packages can relate to the employment process.

overview

Personnel, the *workforce, manpower, staff,* and *employees* are all terms that could be better defined as human resources. **Human resources** are more dynamic than fiscal and material resources. They are people who can choose what, when, how, and how much they will contribute to an organization or business. Like other types of resources, they should be treated as valuable assets, not to be wasted or misused. Unlike those other resources, human resources are made up of individuals who react to their environment and have a high potential to influence the level of productivity that an organization achieves (or doesn't achieve). To be successful, the manager must learn to deal with people as valuable resources. It is often said that people are the most valuable resource within any system, ranging from the family unit to government, from a mom-and-pop neighborhood store to a multinational corporation.

In small or start-up businesses, individual managers deal with human resources activities. This means that the human resources functions are as good (or as bad) as each manager is. As organizations grow, they can no longer deal with employees in such a haphazard way, so **Human Resources Departments** are established to administer personnel issues. These departments are used to monitor the organization to ensure that the needs of all employees are being met and that their rights are being respected and protected, from their initial contact with the organization until the employment relationship ends. Most aspects of human resources are very positive. Among these are the staffing and hiring functions, which provide the organization access to the type of personnel needed to carry out its work. This chapter will describe how to determine staffing needs, how to recruit candidates for available positions, how to screen these candidates, and how to interview them. The process continues with a discussion of how hiring decisions are made, which includes determining the compensation level (and sometimes the benefits package) for the prospective employee. Finally, the employment offer is discussed, along with the alternatives available to the hiring manager if the offer is declined.

It is usual for the Human Resources Department (HR) to support managers as well as employees. The rationale is that if the manager knows how to deal with human resources effectively, problems in this arena will be minimized, employee morale will improve, and productivity will increase. Even more, managers who are knowledgeable about HR management will make fewer mistakes when dealing with their staff members. Such mistakes can be costly in terms of litigation and public relations. HR is responsible for training managers in human resources functions, which include determining staffing needs, recruitment, screening, interviewing, and hiring. Depending on the size and complexity of the organization, the HR staff will participate in some or all of these steps in the employment process. At the very least, they are there to act as a resource to the hiring manager. Sometimes HR actually does the staffing studies, the recruitment, and the screening functions, leaving only the final interview and the actual hiring to the manager. In either case, the process works best when all parties

management practice in dietetics

are competent and confident in their roles, knowing both the organizational objectives and the legal requirements of the employment process. It is important that this management function be viewed as an opportunity to maintain and improve the organization.

determining staffing needs

Staffing is the determination of the type and number of employees that are needed to carry out the work of an organization. On very rare occasions, a manager is asked to open a new business, start a new department, or develop a new program within an organization. These situations are the most challenging, from a staffing perspective, because the manager must rely on external sources, personal experience, and instinct to make staffing decisions. Though the opportunities for building an organization from the ground up are nearly limitless, the chance for error is great because of the lack of organizational history and institutional memory.

Staffing. *The determination of the type and number of employees that are needed to carry out the work of an organization.*

More typically, a manager makes staffing decisions because of attrition, growth, or **reductions in force** (RIFs). In the first situation, an employee is being hired to replace one who has left the organization, either voluntarily or involuntarily. In the second, the hiring is done to meet increased needs in an organization. The third example is one in which the workforce is reduced in size and the manager is forced to decide which of the current employees to keep on the job and which to transfer into other positions or terminate. RIFs are sometimes called layoffs. Because these decisions are often made one at a time, on a person-by-person basis, the manager may not view this process as staffing, which is often described as encompassing the workforce rather than individuals. This type of thinking is probably a mistake. Opportunities to strengthen the organization occur each time there is turnover among employees, even if only one employee is replaced. The manager must always think of both the short-term and the long-term staffing goals when making decisions regarding the workforce. It is imperative that any hiring decision be made with the entire organization, not just the individual position, in mind.

Reductions in Force (RIFs). *A decrease in the workforce, also called layoffs. Employees may be either transferred or terminated.*

When looking at staffing, it is important to determine what work needs to be done. If the work is making cookies, the staffing requirements will be different than if the work is the care of sick children. Next, the skills needed to do those jobs must be established, along with the determination of which members of the workforce are likely to have those skills. Among the workers who may have the appropriate skill sets, one must determine what level of worker is best suited to the specific job. If one employee, such as an RD, can do all the jobs in a small WIC clinic, it might be a good idea to hire the RD, rather than hiring a short-hour clerk, a short-hour nutrition aide, and a short-hour dietitian. On the other hand, in a larger site, one might hire a dietitian, a nutrition aide, and a filing clerk, rather than paying more to hire three dietitians. (Note that it would be inappropriate to hire only the filing clerk for the smaller site, because that person would not have the requisite skills to do the entire job.)

When an employee has left a job, the manager usually replaces that employee with another who has the same qualifications. This is not always the correct thing to do. For example, if a clinical dietitian (with lots of seniority and at the top of the pay scale) retires, it seems logical to hire another clinical dietitian into that position. However, if inpatient census is dropping and catering business is increasing, it might be better to hire a catering manager to meet the increased need, and a dietetic technician to assist the clinical dietitians who remain on the staff. It might even be possible to hire both of these people for close to the same salary as the senior dietitian was earning. Every time an employee needs to be replaced, the manager is provided with an opportunity to consider staffing. Each decision requires serious consideration.

Once the jobs have been identified, it becomes necessary to describe them. This is done with job specifications and job descriptions, and sometimes with a job analysis, too. Finally, it is imperative to look at the workforce to determine if the appropriate workers are available, and to determine if the budget is adequate to pay the going rate for their services. If these factors interfere with the ideal staffing for the organization, compromises will have to be made. In such circumstances, the compromises must be made with deliberation and awareness of the ramifications of such decisions, both in the short and long term.

the jobs

The concept of designing jobs is not a new one. In the past, there were attempts to design every job to the smallest detail. This is not necessary in all situations and can serve to inhibit productivity and creativity on the job. Thus, the guidelines offered here are just that—guidelines. It is equally important to be flexible enough to take advantage of unforeseen opportunities as they present themselves. This includes allowing some employees to have a degree of autonomy related to their jobs. (The sections in Chapter 12 on job enrichment and job enlargement cover this topic in greater detail.)

Job Specification.
A list of requirements for a specific job, which can be evaluated objectively and that apply to all candidates for that job.

job specifications. A **job specification** is a list of the requirements that must be fulfilled by the candidate who is to be considered for a specific job. It should include anything that is necessary to perform the job and that can be tested objectively, including minimum levels of education, skill, and experience. These specifications should be uniformly applied to all candidates for the job. The job specification might include a credential, like RD or DTR, or it may specify a college degree in a specific field of study.

Different jobs have different requirements. When hiring for a clerk to process the paperwork related to purchasing, inventory, accounting, and payroll, the requisite skills might include proficiency with data entry. If the inventory were automated, then data entry is not the critical skill, but competence with a certain type of accounting software may be. Jobs that require a great deal of typing might require mastery of a specific word processing program, or the ability to keyboard at a certain rate. Foodservice workers may be required to be able to lift or bend in the performance of their jobs, so this should

246   *management practice in dietetics*

be included in the job specifications. Some jobs require the ability to read and speak a specific language (English, Spanish, or Mandarin, for example); some require that the incumbent be able to write legibly. All of the items above can be tested objectively, either through verification of credentials, a physical exam, or a performance test.

Sometimes certain personal characteristics are desirable for certain positions. These include, but are not limited to, an ability to perform under stress, good telephone manners, interpersonal skills, assertiveness, good judgment related to job activities, or clinical judgment on the part of RDs. These characteristics may or may not be stated on the job specification, depending on the organizational culture. If they are not stated, it may be because they are difficult to measure objectively. If such characteristics are noted, there should be a way to measure all candidates for the desired trait. Sometimes this is done with a psychological test, sometimes with the questions in a structured interview. The former can be more accurate (if the test is reliable) but is not widely used; the latter method is highly subjective but is generally thought to be a more acceptable way to evaluate these characteristics.

job descriptions. A **job description** lists the duties that the employee will have to perform on the job. Like the job specification, it is an HR tool that is used in the recruitment and selection of employees. It is also used when employees are being oriented to the new position. The job description provides an overview of the job duties that are to be performed. It does not specify each individual task that is to be performed or outline how the task is to be done. For example, the job description for the morning cook in a hospital could include such items as "prepares breakfast for the cafeteria and patients" and "prepares entrées for the cafeteria's noon meal."

> **Job Description.** *A listing of the general duties related to a job or job classification.*

As the skill level of the employee rises, the list of job duties often increases. This is related to the fact that upper-level jobs are less routine and more subject to day-to-day variation than are lower-level jobs. Sometimes, for example, managerial jobs have cyclical variation. Perhaps at the beginning of an accounting period, a manager will have to do a budget variance report on year-to-date financial performance. Near the end of the fiscal year, it will be necessary to prepare a budget for the next year. In the spring, it may be necessary to hire staff for vacation relief. Occasionally, a major capital acquisition might be needed, so the manager will have to write a specification for the piece of equipment. Therefore, the job description of the manager may list a significant number of duties that are done occasionally, in contrast to the cook, who has fewer duties but is required to perform each duty on a daily basis.

Most job descriptions have an additional statement added to the bottom of the actual list of duties. It often reads "performs other duties as assigned." This is there to allow management to ask employees to do things that are not listed on the job description; for the cook, it might be something like develop a new recipe for a special event or prepare a special meal for the board of directors' luncheon. This type of "escape clause" protects a manager from being denied a request because "it's not in my job description." However, managers must not abuse this item by making unreasonable or too-frequent additional requests of an employee. The "other duties" clause should be used judiciously. If an additional duty becomes a routine part of a certain job, it should be added to the job description.

This terminology ("performs other duties as assigned") may be appropriate when dealing with those jobs in which the employee has daily contact with the supervisor. However, for managerial and professional positions in which the employee works independently, it is better to make the statement more self-regulatory. Perhaps the better terminology would read "performs other duties as needed." In this case, the employee is given permission to make judgments and act independently. It allows either the manager or the employee to define the word *needed*.

In many organizations, the job specifications and job descriptions are listed on the same document, which is part of the permanent records in the HR department. Other items might also be included in this document. These include job title, the employment grade or pay range, the number of positions authorized under this job title, and so on. Reporting relationships are sometimes listed, too. This is a statement that describes what position the job reports to and what positions report to the individual in this job. Figure 8.1 illustrates a job description that also contains specifications for the job.

In addition to being useful in the process of selecting and hiring new employees, job descriptions serve as a management tool for other functions. They are used for on-the-job training for new employees. They can serve as the basis for performance appraisals as will be discussed in Chapter 9. And, finally, job descriptions can provide the basic criteria for the initiation of the disciplinary process for poorly performing employees. These are among the controls put in place to assist the manager.

Job Analysis. *A detailed description of the daily duties to be carried out in a specific job, often including time frames for each job activity.*

job analysis. The **job analysis**, sometimes called a task analysis, is a more detailed description of the job to be carried out on a daily basis. For the breakfast cook in a hospital, it would include statements such as:

> 5:30 Begin shift. Preheat ovens and grill.
> 5:35 Pick up production schedule from supervisor's office; review menu items.
> 5:40 Assemble ingredients for breakfast menu.
> 5:50 Start breakfast preparation.
> 6:25 Deliver hot foods to patient trayline.
> 6:55 Deliver hot foods to cafeteria line. …

It is very useful to have this type of detailed analysis available when training a new employee to do a job, or when orienting a new manager about what each position is supposed to do each day. Another use for this document is in situations in which several individuals hold the same job classification and work interchangeably in various positions. This ensures that each individual doing the job knows what is expected for that particular shift.

management practice in dietetics

```
Position:              Clinical Dietitian
Salary Range:          $50,000–$63,000 per year
Reports to:            Clinical Nutrition Manager
Responsible for:       Diet Technician/Diet Clerk
Job Specifications:    RD Credential, State License, Bilingual English/Spanish required.
                       Three years' acute care clinical experience desired.
Job Description:       The Clinical Dietitian is responsible for the care of patients on
                       assigned hospital care units. This includes screening, assessment,
                       planning, implementing, and evaluating care, or overseeing others
                       who complete some aspects of the care process.
Job Duties:
     The clinical dietitian will:

                       •  Schedule patient care activities for the day.
                       •  Assign patient care tasks to diet clerks and diet techs as appropriate.
                       •  Assess all patients who are on nutrition support.
                       •  Assess all high-risk patients.
                       •  Plan care for, and chart on, all patients assessed.
                       •  Monitor high-risk patients.
                       •  Evaluate effectiveness of care plans.
                       •  Conduct meal rounds at least twice a week.
                       •  Evaluate one test tray each week.
                       •  Oversee menu preparation by clerks and techs.
                       •  Manage the patient-satisfaction survey process on unit.
                       •  Develop education materials for patients in specialty area.
                       •  Update diet manual for this specialty area.
                       •  Participate in monthly clinical staff meetings.
                       •  Participate in weekly patient care rounds.
                       •  Attend Grand Rounds when relevant.
                       •  Perform other duties as required.

Revised 3/12/2013
```

Figure 8.1 Sample Job Description (Including Job Specification)

The detail that is built into a job analysis will depend on the job and the deadlines associated with the job. In contrast with the cook's job, the clinical dietitian's job analysis might have fewer tasks listed. For example:

8:00 Check in.

8:00–9:00 Review changes since end of last day worked. Set patient care priorities for day.

9:00–12:00 See highest-priority patients; carry out patient care activities.

12:00–1:00 Conduct meal rounds.

1:00–1:30 Lunch.

1:30–4:25 Continue patient care activities.

4:20–4:30 Taste test for dinner trayline. End of shift.

In this analysis, the tasks that must be done at specified times are delineated, but the tasks related to patient care are stated in very general terms, because the dietitian's work style and the characteristics of her individual caseload would make it impossible to outline these activities with precision. If the dietitian's position is hourly, with designated start and stop times, this type of analysis is probably appropriate.

Job analysis is not required for all positions, because some positions are so variable and flexible that it would be impossible to write an accurate job analysis. In addition, a written job analysis for some positions would probably serve to limit the employee. Indeed, if the position is exempt with no designated hours and variable tasks, a task analysis might even interfere with an employee's ability to do the assigned job. For managerial and professional positions, it is acceptable to forgo a written job analysis. In fact, it is probably desirable to do so. In these positions, the staff often perform best when given an area of responsibility and empowered to carry out those responsibilities in the way that works best for them.

From this discussion, it may seem that the requirement for a job analysis is based on the level of the position. This is not entirely true. It is more related to deadlines that must be met. In positions where deadlines are few, job analyses are less necessary than in positions with multiple deadlines. Positions that involve routine tasks are more easily analyzed and written down than those that are less routine. These factors cross all levels of employees, from the unskilled worker to the president of a large organization. Job analyses should never be written in such a way that they limit employees and keep them from performing to the best of their ability.

Incumbent. *The person who currently holds the position.*

There is one thought to be considered before leaving the topic of job specifications, job descriptions, and job analysis. The best source of information about each job is the **incumbent** who actually performs the job. It might be appropriate for the manager to be given the task of writing these documents, to assure that the format is consistent and that the writing is clear and correct, but it is the employee who knows what the job is all about. It is imperative that the employee be consulted when these documents are being prepared so that useful HR tools are developed. Without employee input, the accuracy of these documents is compromised. The needed information may be obtained in writing, via interview, or through observation. It is a mistake for the manager to attempt to prepare these documents without input from the people who actually do the work.

As careful as a manager is about writing job specifications and accurate job descriptions, having these documents does not guarantee success in staffing. Jobs and incumbents in those jobs change with time, variation in incumbents, and advances in technology. It is not reasonable to expect that job descriptions will have a life expectancy of more than two or three years. Ideally, they should be reviewed and edited whenever changes are made in the way jobs are done, or at least once a year if no changes are obvious. The date of the last review should be noted on the document that is filed in the HR department. In reality, however, this is not usually done. It is more likely that the documents are reviewed and updated every three to five years. The disadvantage of waiting so long between reviews is that the jobs have usually changed so much in that period of time that an update generally is not sufficient and it becomes necessary to rewrite the entire job description and analysis.

the issue of flexibility

No matter how well the job specifications and job descriptions are written, these documents do not guarantee that staff members will be found who exactly meet the stated needs. These tools help managers narrow their search and increase the possibility of success in staffing, but there are a number of circumstances that require flexibility in staffing. These include the lack of candidates who meet the job specifications; budgetary considerations that may interfere with the ability to hire the most qualified candidate; qualified candidates who need accommodation regarding scheduled hours, days off, physical limitations, and so on; overqualified candidates; and candidates who are not available to begin the job for a period of time. Hiring managers must be willing to reevaluate their staffing goals and make whatever adjustment circumstances require.

These adaptations may be either positive or negative. For example, an overqualified individual, perhaps someone with a bachelor's degree in nutrition but with limited keyboarding skills, may apply for the position of a clerk in a school district's food-service. Even though the skills do not match the job precisely, having such a person on staff could be good because it would allow the manager to do some **succession planning** and prepare that individual to take on a managerial role when a future vacancy occurs. If a vacancy is foreseen in the near future, perhaps because a senior supervisor is retiring at the end of the school year, it would be good to anticipate the future need by hiring the overqualified clerk. On the other hand, if no such vacancy was anticipated, it would probably be unwise to hire the overqualified candidate, because he or she might get bored and quit very soon. Though it is never possible to predict the future with precision, it is a good idea to adjust one's staffing plans to accommodate those circumstances that are somewhat predictable, like retirements or planned career moves.

Succession Planning. *A staffing strategy that anticipates what jobs will open due to retirements and promotions, and prepares other individuals to be eligible to move into these positions.*

Another circumstance that requires some flexibility could be the hiring of a DTR. If the hiring facility is located in a part of the country where there are no accredited educational programs for preparing Dietetic Technicians, the likelihood of finding a candidate with that credential is minimal. The job specification might need to be rewritten to state, "DTR, or an individual with a bachelor's degree in nutrition."

the recruitment process

Once the staffing needs have been determined, some sort of recruiting must begin, to announce that positions are available. Recruitment might be as simple as word of mouth, or it might be complex enough to justify the hiring of a professional recruiter to find qualified candidates for an open position. Recruitment may be facilitated by advertisement, paid or unpaid, or by public relations efforts. The type of recruitment efforts made will be dependent on the types of jobs that are available, and the characteristics of the workforce from which candidates will be drawn. In some cases, incentives are needed to attract qualified candidates.

advertisement

A characteristic of an **advertisement** is that the person or the organization that generates the ad has complete control over what the ad says, where the ad is placed, and the time frame for running that ad. Some advertising is local or internal to an organization, with little or no associated cost. For example, most large organizations have a bulletin board or intranet web page that is available to the HR department for the purpose of listing available jobs to internal candidates. In fact, some organizations require that all jobs be posted internally for a period of time before they are advertised externally, so that current employees have adequate opportunity to compete for the vacant positions. Jobs may also be posted in a company newsletter, on an Internet site, or on a job "hot line." The newsletter is usually available only to an organization's employees and their families and close friends; the latter two methods of advertisement are available to larger potential audiences.

Paid advertisements are targeted more directly at specific groups outside of the organization. If, for example, a clinical nutrition manager for a large teaching medical center was needed by an organization, it is likely that the organization would purchase advertising space in a nationwide professional publication such as the *Journal of the Academy of Nutrition and Dietetics* or *Today's Dietitian*. A research center might place an ad for a nutrition researcher in *The American Journal of Clinical Nutrition*. National organizations have employment advertisements posted on their websites as well. Some online job search sites are targeted specifically to dietetics and nutrition professionals. See "In Practice" feature, Chapter 6.

If the position to be filled is for a typist, a foodservice worker, or a bookkeeper, it might be more appropriate to advertise in a local or regional publication such as a newspaper. These classified ads may also appear on the newspaper's website. Again, it should be noted that, when an advertisement is paid for, the advertiser has the right to expect that the ad will appear exactly as written, on the correct date or dates. Sometimes the advertiser can even specify the ad's placement on the page. Care must be taken to be non-discriminatory in advertising. That is, the ads should encourage

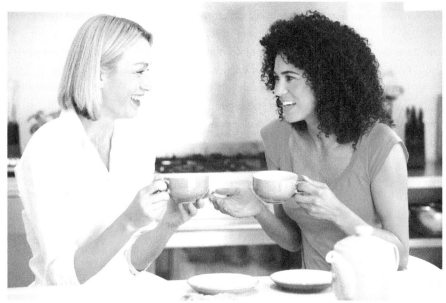

Many dietetics professionals find their jobs through "word of mouth."

all qualified applicants to apply, and should take care not to eliminate candidates by using media that would not be accessible to certain ethnic or age groups.

It is possible to use other media, like radio or TV, to advertise for employees as well. However, these expensive methods are generally reserved for hiring large numbers of qualified people, not just one or two workers.

There are places where jobs can be listed at no cost to the hiring party. These may include bulletin boards in public places like grocery stores, churches, or schools. Technically, these are not advertisements, because the hiring party cannot necessarily control the content of the job posting. The content often depends on available space or time constraints. Open listings may also be available from state or local professional associations. These are free to the employer because the association provides the service as a courtesy to its membership. Another way to inform the community of available jobs is through public relations initiatives, usually most effective when large numbers of jobs are available, like when a new business is opening or an existing one is planning significant expansion.

networking

One of the clichés related to employment activities that is often cited is, "It's not what you know, but who you know." In fact, networking and **word-of-mouth** dissemination

Word of Mouth. *An informal method of information exchange that relies on verbal communication between individuals.*

of information are two of the main ways that people find their jobs. Either they know someone who works at …, or they went to school with someone who …, or a friend told them that. … Because this type of information exchange is a fact of life, employers should not overlook it. In fact, use of networking to fill vacancies should be encouraged. Employees should be told about job openings and asked to share the information with colleagues outside of the organization. Employees can spread the word through listserves to which they subscribe, at professional meetings, on community bulletin boards, and so on. It is a low-cost way to get the word out about available positions. This informal method takes advantage of existing networks and helps both the employer and the job candidates. It is not intended to replace more conventional methods, but to supplement them.

recruitment agencies

Recruiting Firms.
Agencies that specialize in matching qualified candidates to available jobs.

There are a number of **recruiting firms** or agencies that make a business out of matching candidates to jobs. Commonly called *headhunters*, these firms usually specialize in certain types of positions and certain classifications of jobs. They earn their money when an individual is hired by an organization. These companies usually operate one of two ways, with some minor variations. Either the employer pays the fee for their services, or the fee is paid by the job seeker.

Hiring managers are most likely to deal with a recruiting firm that gets paid by the hiring organization. The specific firm is chosen for its expertise in recruiting candidates for a certain type of job, such as health care, accounting, engineering, manufacturing, banking, and so on. Firms that specialize in health care often have one staff member who specializes in the placement of dietetics professionals. There are a few firms that deal primarily with dietitians and dietetics professionals, and do not have major involvement in other areas of health care. These firms might be used for finding candidates for positions in education, community nutrition, and non-healthcare foodservices. Large contract foodservice organizations may use this type of specialty recruiter to locate both nutrition managers and clinicians.

The professional recruiters described in the previous paragraph usually operate on a national or international basis. As such, they have access to a database of available professionals, which includes information on their area of specialization, their willingness to relocate, their ability to travel as part of the job, salary and benefit requirements of the candidates, and so on. A major advantage of using this type of recruiter is that it speeds the hiring process by providing a nationwide list of qualified candidates in a very timely way. (It may take as long as three months to get an adequate response from an ad placed in a professional journal that is published monthly.) For this type of recruiter, the fee is paid by the hiring organization and is frequently calculated as a percentage of the annual salary of the candidate who is hired. Another fee structure is based on a flat fee per job filled or for each candidate referred. Alternately, the recruiter may work on

management practice in dietetics

a retainer, whereby a monthly fee is paid to the recruitment company to ensure that it will be available to recruit for the organization whenever a vacancy occurs.

The recruiter who is paid by the job seeker is more likely to be used on a local level, in a situation where there are few jobs and many candidates (that is, in times of high unemployment). The candidates pay the recruitment agency for assistance with resume preparation, job interviewing skills, and so on. The recruiter may or may not refer candidates to hiring organizations. The fee for this type of service is paid by the candidate seeking employment, sometimes as an up-front fee to the recruiter, and sometimes payable when the candidate finds a job.

hiring incentives

Hiring incentives are used in times of low unemployment and when qualified job candidates are scarce. A relocation package to assist with moving expenses, an enhanced benefits package, a company car, or a generous expense account could all be viewed as hiring incentives. Such perquisites ("perks") are usually considered to be part of the employee's benefits package but can also be used effectively in the recruitment process. The type of hiring incentive available will be related to the employment market, the kind of employee needed, and the creativity of the HR department in creating a package to attract qualified candidates. It should be noted that, in times of economic downturns, when unemployment is high and qualified workers are readily available, the use of hiring incentives usually decreases.

Hiring Incentives.
Rewards or bonuses that are given to job candidates to entice them to accept a position.

Another type of hiring incentive is called a "signing bonus." This is a lump sum payment to the candidate who accepts a position with a company. It may be given when the employee starts the new job, or when that person has been working in the position for a specified period of time. The signing bonus may be used to lure an individual away from a current position, or as an incentive when recruiting outstanding students into their first positions. (In the latter case, the money is frequently used to pay off or reduce education loans.) Signing bonuses used to be reserved for executives, managers, and professionals. However, when the economy is strong, and good employees are hard to find, some companies extend the idea all the way down to their frontline and hourly workers. It is thought that the use of this type of tool may increase loyalty and decrease turnover among employees at all levels.

A similar technique, not technically a hiring bonus because it is not given to the new employee, encourages an organization's employees to use their networking skills to recruit others to come to work for the organization. For example, a dietitian may have good contacts from being an active member of a dietetic practice group. If she recruits a qualified colleague into her own organization, she could earn a bonus, also called a "finder's fee." Typically, the bonus is paid when the new hire continues in the job beyond the probationary period.

interviewing

As a result of recruitment efforts, a number of applications from candidates seeking employment may be received. The applications will be screened by a **paper review**, which is done to exclude candidates who do not appear to meet the job specifications. In large organizations, the HR department does this screening so that the applications from unqualified candidates never reach the hiring manager. Sometimes the HR department will administer a test—for example, a typing test—to verify what is written on the application. Because this is a preliminary screening process, it may not include checking references or giving the candidate a physical exam.

If the applicant pool is a large one, and the available jobs are few, some additional screening techniques will be necessary to determine which candidates will be interviewed. Conversely, if there are few candidates, or there are many jobs to be filled, it might be appropriate to interview all qualified candidates. The secondary screening process is an attempt to select the best possible group of candidates to progress to the interview.

Once the final candidates are determined, interviews should be scheduled to help the hiring manager determine which candidate to hire. Care must be taken to ensure that the manager has time to review the applications before the interviews, and that the candidates have enough notice to prepare for the interview. Sometimes the manager does the hiring independently, sometimes a work group is established to interview and select new employees, and sometimes several constituencies are involved in the hiring decision. For example, representatives of hospital administration, the medical staff, and the clinical dietitians might interview a candidate for the clinical nutrition manager position in a large healthcare facility. If a group interview is to be conducted, it is necessary to plan where and when the meeting will be held, especially if meeting space needs to be reserved. Whichever of these models is used, there needs to be a degree of consistency in the interviews to clearly distinguish among the candidates.

The employment interview should be designed to exchange information with the candidates. Interviews should all follow a similar pattern, which starts with introductions and rapport building, followed by the information-seeking phase. This provides the interviewer/s with data about the candidate's qualifications for the job. At some point during the interview, the candidate is given the opportunity to get information about the job and the organization from the interviewer. Finally, there is closure, which includes a plan for follow-up so that both parties are clear about what will happen next.

Employment interviews should be well planned, be equitable, and protect the rights of both the candidates and the organization. Everyone involved in interviewing needs some basic information about how to conduct themselves and how to interview candidates. Documentation of the interviews may be required by some organizations. Ultimately, the hiring manager must use the information obtained during the interviews, make the final decision, and follow up with a job offer.

unstructured interview

An unstructured interview is one in which there is a free-flowing conversation between the candidate and the interviewer. This is *not* an appropriate tool to use when interviewing candidates for employment because the information obtained is haphazard, making it difficult to compare one candidate with another. The interviewer does get some superficial information about the candidate and usually can determine if the candidate is likable, but that is about the extent of the usefulness of the information. Any other information gleaned—for example, skill level, experience, career goals, and so on—will be serendipitous; without this kind of information on every candidate, it will be useless for comparative purposes.

Even though unstructured employment interviews are not recommended, they are commonplace. Persons who have little experience conducting interviews usually use them. There are two reasons for describing an unstructured interview in this section. The first is to characterize the type of interview that can take place when the process is too casual and to note that this type of unproductive conversation can be avoided if interviewers receive some training regarding the employment interview. The second reason is to serve as a warning that this type of employment interview may undermine the position of the hiring organization in the view of the candidate. Candidates may justifiably feel that such an interview has been a waste of their time, and may decline an offer of employment on the basis of the unstructured interview. Seasoned hiring managers approach the hiring process in a much more organized manner.

semi-structured interview

The **semi-structured interview** takes on a conversational tone but is structured in the sense that the interviewer has planned for the interview by determining the topics to be covered ahead of time. Like all good interviews, the beginning should be the rapport-building stage, when the candidate and the interviewer get comfortable with one another and the interviewer outlines the format of the interview for the candidate. An interviewer might say something like, "First we'll talk about the job duties of the position you are applying for, then I'll ask you some questions about yourself and your special talents, and finally, there will be time for you to ask me questions. I expect this discussion to take about 45 minutes."

For the semi-structured interview, the interviewer will have an outline of the topics to be covered and some examples or ideas of how the questions will be asked. However, the exact questions will not be written out in advance, because the semi-structured interview allows for some spontaneous conversation. This type of interview is comfortable for the candidate but is more difficult for the interviewer than is the structured interview because it is very easy to get "off track" and not

Unstructured Interview. *An interview that resembles an informal conversation.*

Semi-Structured Interview. *A type of interview that takes on a conversational tone but is somewhat organized by an outline of topics to be covered and an idea of how questions will be asked.*

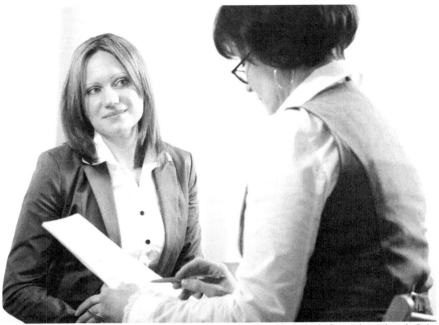

Experienced managers use the semi-structured interview to exchange information with candidates in a non-threatening way.

cover all of the topics outlined. Experienced interviewers who do a relatively large number of employment interviews tend to use this method. This method also has to do with the personal style or preference of the hiring manager. When the manager is skilled at the process, the semi-structured interview can be as productive as its more-structured counterpart.

structured interview

The usefulness of the information obtained in the employment interview is dependent on the interviewer's ability to get the same type of information from each candidate. For beginning interviewers, the best way to do this is to write an **interview schedule**—that is, a list of questions to be covered in discussions with every candidate. Essentially, it is the agenda for the interview. Each candidate is asked the questions in exactly the same way and in the same chronological order. This is a commonly used format for a **structured interview**. It may be less comfortable for the candidate because it puts an additional stress into an already stressful situation when the interviewer has to break eye contact in order to read the questions. When using this method, the interviewer should explain the process to the candidate during the opening (rapport-building) phase of the interview so that the candidate knows what to expect.

Interview Schedule. *A list of all of the questions that will be asked of each candidate in an employment interview; the agenda for the interview.*

Structured Interview. *An interview that follows a predetermined agenda.*

management practice in dietetics

Some of the questions should relate directly to the job tasks. It is useful to use the job description as the basis for preparing an interview schedule. This increases the likelihood that the questions asked will actually relate to the job. Questions may be related to the technical aspects of the specific job. For example, a cook might be asked what could be done to repair a sauce that has separated. A clinical dietitian might be required to calculate a parenteral formula or plan enteral support for a client described in a case study. A purchasing manager might have to describe how inventory is valued. A clinic manager might be asked to discuss how to find and obtain grant funding.

Some questions are designed to deal with less-tangible characteristics rather than with knowledge. If one were hiring a foodservice supervisor for the morning shift, a possible question is, "What would you do if you came to work in the morning and found that the main refrigerator registered a temperature of 45 degrees?" The answer would give the interviewer information about the candidate's knowledge of safe food temperatures *and* would provide some insight into the candidate's decision-making skills. Foodservice management positions are often characterized by many simultaneous activities, so individuals who can handle multiple tasks at one time would be ideal candidates. To obtain this type of information in an interview, one could say, "Tell me about a time when you had more to do than you thought could get done. How did you handle the situation, and how did it turn out?" A query used to determine assertiveness in a clinical dietitian might be, "What would you do if a physician ordered a diet for a pregnant diabetic woman that severely limited her Caloric intake?"

Structured interviews give the hiring manager a more objective way to compare candidates with one another, since the variability in the way the interview approaches the meeting is eliminated. All candidates are faced with a controlled situation. Structured interviews take more planning on the part of the manager, and tend to be more stressful for the candidate.

group interviews

If the interview is a group interview, the structure of the interview takes on even more importance. Group interviews require considerably more planning than do individual interviews. There should be some preliminary discussions within the group before the first candidate is interviewed. The purpose of this is to determine what questions need to be asked in relationship to the job to be filled, who will ask each of the questions, and the order that the questions will be asked, so that all candidates have a similar experience in the interview. Questions must be related to the job; those not related to the candidate's ability to do the job should be avoided. All members of the interview team must know what subjects should be avoided, especially from the legal perspective. (See Table 8.1.)

Group Interview.
An interview in which more than one person interviews the candidate.

Subject	Questions Not Recommended	Recommended Questions
Name	What is your maiden name? Have you ever used any other name? Have you ever worked under another name? Have you ever changed your name?	Have you ever worked for this company under a different name? Is additional information relative to a change in name, use of an assumed name, or nickname necessary for us to check your work record? If yes, please explain.
Address	Do you rent or own your own home? How long have you lived at this address?	What is your address? Where do you live?
Age	How old are you? What is your date of birth? Are you between 18 and 24, 25 and 34, etc.?	Are you above the minimum working age of _____?
Physical Appearance	How tall are you? How much do you weigh? What is the color of your eyes and hair?	None
Citizenship and National Origin	Of what country are you a citizen? Where were you born? Where were your parents born? Are you a naturalized or a native-born citizen? What is your nationality? What kind of a name is _____?	Are you a citizen of the United States? If you are not a U.S. citizen, do you have the legal right to remain permanently in the United States?
Marital Status	What is your marital status? Have you ever been married? Divorced? Do you wish to be addressed as Mrs., Miss, or Ms.?	None
Children	Do you have any children? How many children do you have? What child care arrangements have you made? Do you intend to have children? When do you plan to have children? If you have children while employed, will you return to work?	None
Police Records	Have you ever been arrested?	Have you ever been convicted of a (crime? felony? crime greater than a misdemeanor?) Please explain. (NOTE: Applicants may not be denied employment because of a conviction record unless there is a direct correlation between the offense and the job, or unless hiring would constitute and unreasonable risk. [Correction Law Article 22-A Sec.754])
Religion	What is your religious background? What religious holidays do you observe? Is there anything in your religious beliefs that would prevent you from working the required schedule?	None

Table 8.1 Pre-Employment Inquiries

Subject	Questions Not Recommended	Recommended Questions
Disabilities	Do you have any disabilities? Have you ever been treated for any of the following (list of diseases and illnesses)? Do you now have, or have you ever had, a drug or alcohol addiction? Do you have physical, mental, or medical impediments that would interfere with your ability to perform the job for which you are applying? Are there any positions or duties for which you should not be considered because of existing physical, mental, or medical disabilities?	Can you perform the tasks required to carry out the job for which you have applied, with or without accommodation?
Photographs	Any question requiring that a photo be supplied before hire.	None
Languages	What is your native language? How did you learn to speak _____?	What is the degree of fluency with which you speak/write fluently any language, including English? (Ask only if job-related)
Military Experience	Have you ever served in the armed forces of any country? What kind of discharge did you receive?	What is your military experience in the armed forces of the United States?
Organizations	What clubs, organizations, or associations do you belong to?	What clubs, organizations, or associations, relative to the position for which you are applying, do you belong to?
References	A requirement that a reference be supplied by a particular kind of person, such as a religious leader.	Please provide the names, titles, addresses, and phone numbers of business references who are not related to you other than your present or former employers.
Finances	Do you have any overdue bills?	None
Education	Are you a high school or college graduate? When did you attend high school or college?	Questions about the applicant's academic, vocational, or professional education, including the names and locations of the schools, the number of years completed, honors, diplomas and degrees received, and the major courses of study.
Experience	Any question regarding experience unrelated to the job.	Any questions regarding relevant work experience.

Table 8.1 (Continued)

Group interviews may be either semi-structured or structured. Oral **civil service examinations** often use the structured group interview format, as do some foodservice management companies. Telephone and Internet-based interviews (using Skype™ or Go-to-Meeting® software), which may be used for candidates who are located far away from the interview site, are also highly structured.

On the other hand, there are often some interviewers on **search committees** (often used to hire upper-level managers, administrators, and academic personnel) who resist structure. Their presence during an interview makes the interview process semi-structured rather than structured. In fact, when large groups are involved in interviewing candidates for a position, the level of structure will be variable, depending on the individual group members' styles.

Sometimes during group interviews, one member of the group is assigned to be an observer/note-taker. In other scenarios, each member of the group takes notes individually. In either case, a few moments should be allowed for group discussion between interviews, so that the interviewers can formulate their thoughts and share their perceptions with each other before the next candidate arrives.

taking notes

It is usually wise to take some notes when interviewing, whether in a group or in an individual session. This is especially important if there are a number of interviews scheduled in a short time span. The notes can be taken during the interview or can be jotted down (or tape-recorded by the interviewer) between interviews. The notes do not have to be extensive, but do need to capture the salient points of the information given by the candidate. In fact, taking extensive notes during the interview may actually lessen the quality of the interview by slowing its pace. Comprehensive note taking can also interfere with the interpersonal aspects of the interaction, such as observance of body language, eye contact, smiles, nods, and so on.

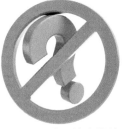

Copyright © 2011 by Depositphotos/3dfoto.

Interviewers should avoid asking questions that are not related to the job.

Some managers prefer to record the entire interview, so that it can be reviewed at a later time. If an audio or video recording device is used, the candidate should be informed of its use. Candidates have a right to decline to be interviewed if they have an objection to being recorded. The practical value of recording interviews is questionable when interviewing for most positions, because reviewing the tapes is very time-consuming and seldom yields more information than the interview itself did. There are few situations in which recording interviews is justifiable.

As noted earlier, in group interviews, there may be an individual designated to take notes during the interview, or notes may be taken by each group member. For the results to be consistent, it is suggested that the same method of note taking be used during each interview conducted by the group. In the civil service exam process,

management practice in dietetics

it is not uncommon for one member of the interview panel to ask the questions and another to take notes. Though it is not absolutely necessary to inform the candidate if notes will be taken during the interview process, it is common courtesy to do so. Giving the candidate as much information about the process at the beginning of the interview decreases the stress and increases the likelihood that the interview will go well for all parties involved.

what not to ask

There are some questions that are clearly too personal to be used in a job interview, and others that are considered to be potentially discriminatory and therefore prohibited from a legal standpoint. Questions related to age, sexual orientation, marital status, parental obligations, and so on have nothing to do with an individual's ability to do the job and should be avoided. Table 8.1 lists topics that should be avoided. The rule of thumb, however, is that the questioning should be limited to job-related issues, and other topics should be avoided. If the candidate volunteers personal information, it is best to inform the candidate that the information is not job-related and then to redirect the discussion back to the topics on the interview schedule.

the content of the interview

The main part of the employment interview consists of information sharing between the candidate and the interviewer. In addition to gathering information from the candidate, the interviewer should provide information about the job and job-related duties. Sometimes, especially in the semi-structured interview, this information giving is interspersed throughout the interview; sometimes it is held until the candidate has answered all the questions on the interview schedule. The candidate should be provided with information like the scheduling requirements, whether the position is hourly or salaried, what the job duties are, the potential for promotion, and so on. Much of this can be given in printed form, if it is available, as can information on the organization, benefits packages, and so on.

The candidate should be given the opportunity to ask questions, and the interviewer should allow adequate time to answer them. If an answer is not available—for example, for a question such as, "If you hire me, how much can I expect to earn?"—the manager should answer as truthfully as possible. For this question, a good answer could be, "The salary will be determined based on the candidate's experience and education. The bottom of the salary range is $X.XX, which is the minimum we expect to pay the person we hire." One could also answer this question by enumerating the salary range for the position, but this may lead some candidates to expect to be hired at the top of the range. It is tempting to enhance the answers to a candidate's questions in order to entice a candidate into taking a job. This is ill-advised, because in doing so the interviewer creates expectations that may not be met in the workplace. This is likely to lead to employee dissatisfaction and increased turnover. If the candidate's question is not appropriate, the manager should decline to answer the question.

closing an employment interview

In closing an employment interview, the interviewer should make sure that the candidate knows what to expect next. Here, the interviewer should make every attempt to be truthful, without being overly optimistic. It is appropriate for the hiring manager to tell the candidates that a hiring decision will be made by a certain date, and that the candidate will be notified of the outcome of the interview by that time. Managers should be cautioned, though, about the pitfalls of providing the candidates with an unrealistic date. If a candidate expects to hear "by Friday," it is the manager's responsibility to contact the candidate by Friday, whether or not a decision has been finalized. It is unfair to the candidate and represents the organization poorly if the manager does not honor a time commitment that has been made. By Friday, however, the manager may be able to say only that a decision has not yet been reached. On the other hand, candidates who expect to hear "by Friday" will begin to call the organization that day to find out if the position has been filled. Either scenario is an avoidable waste of time for the hiring manager, the HR department, or both.

Often, it is better to give the latest possible date as the follow-up date to the candidates. For example, if a hiring manager intends to make a hiring decision on Friday, it might be best to tell all candidates interviewed that "I hope to have this all wrapped up by Wednesday of next week." Then, if the lead candidate is offered the job on Friday and asks to have the weekend to decide whether or not to accept the offer, the manager has some time before the other candidates expect to be contacted. If the lead candidate declines the offer, the job can be offered to another candidate on Monday. In the meantime, no bridges have been burned, because no alternate candidates were told that someone else was offered the job. The organization and the manager are seen as credible, because all commitments were honored.

the hiring decision

Hiring Decision.
The selection of the best candidate for the position.

The final part of the employment process is the actual **hiring decision**. It is generally made by the manager. If other constituencies have been involved in the interviewing process, their input is considered before the decision is made. If the manager uses a consensus style of management, the decision may be a group one, but it should be noted that the manager still has to take the ultimate responsibility for the decision that is made. If the group cannot reach consensus, then the manager must decide whether or not to interview more candidates, or to select one without group consensus.

management practice in dietetics

The hiring decision is not merely a matter of picking the best candidate for the job. Many other factors have to be considered. First is the checking of references to validate what was learned in the interview. Then there is the issue of compensation. Another is diversity. It is both appropriate and desirable for an organization to reflect the diversity of the community in which it is located so that it can better understand and meet the needs of that community. Other items include start date, scheduling requirements, relocation allowance, benefits, and in some cases, passing a physical examination. Some of these items are negotiable; the negotiations should be completed during the hiring phase.

checking references

The checking of references is done according to organizational policy. Some organizations prefer to check references on all candidates prior to the interviewing process in order to eliminate unnecessary interviews for unqualified candidates. Others wait until close to the end of the employment process in order to check references on only the final one or two candidates. This latter method has the added benefit of maintaining confidentiality for candidates who may not want current employers to know that they are actively seeking other employment. However, once a candidate is selected, references must be checked before an offer of employment can be made. Sometimes the HR department does the reference check for the hiring manager, but often the manager prefers to perform this task. In general, the manager knows more about the job and can ask more relevant questions than the HR staff are able to ask.

There are three possible types of references that a candidate may provide to a prospective employer. These are employment, educational, and personal references. It is appropriate to check educational references if the corresponding education is a requirement of the job. Otherwise, it is best to check employment references. If employment references are not available or turn out to yield insufficient information, then the education references may be used in lieu of employment references. Personal references are likely to be biased and should be used only as a last resort.

Candidates may request that a current employer not be contacted regarding reference verification. This is a legitimate request because some employers penalize employees who seek work elsewhere. If a candidate makes such a request, it should be honored. Checking other references and withholding the verification of this last source of information until after an employment offer has been made are appropriate, as long as the offer is contingent on verification of this final reference check.

When checking references by phone, a manager should be certain that the person on the other end of the phone is qualified to give a reference. If possible, the manager should use a switchboard or secretary, rather than a direct line, to verify who the person is. Alternately, the phone number can be checked through the telephone company's information service. Merely dialing the phone number a candidate gives you is no guarantee that the person on the other end of the line is the person you need to contact. (Conversely, if you are asked to give a reference, it is prudent to decline to do so until you can verify who the caller is. This may entail returning a call after you have been able to verify the identity of the caller.)

There are some other thoughts to keep in mind when checking references. The first is to realize that many managers are not very willing to provide detailed references. In fact, all that is required of a former or current employer is verification that the candidate did, indeed, work there, and whether or not the candidate is eligible for rehire. The previous employer may also give the dates of employment and the salary (or salary range) of the employee. If the recommender states that the candidate is not eligible for rehire, it is prudent to follow up with the question, "Why not?" However, the recommender may not be willing to answer that query for either legal or for policy reasons.

The abbreviated reference described above might be given because it is a matter of policy to give out only this much information. It also may be an indication that the former manager has nothing good to say about the candidate or that something was amiss that the previous manager is unable to talk about. In such cases, it is best to check several references instead of just one. If all recommendations are equally terse, it could mean that this person is a problem employee.

On the other hand, if the employee was a good employee and if the organization does not prohibit it, the previous manager may be willing to give more than the basic information. In fact, some managers want to give more information than is necessary. Like interview topics, questions used for the purpose of reference checks should be job-related.

Recently, there has been a developing trend to outsourcing the checking of references. Some of the companies involved are requesting that the person doing the recommendation fill out an electronic form regarding the job candidate. If this type of system is used, it the hiring manager's responsibility to inform the candidate of the process so that individual is able to inform those doing the recommendations. Otherwise a potential recommender may decline to respond to a "blind" request for a reference from an unknown source.

compensation

Compensation.
The salary given for work performed.

Several factors must be considered when determining the **compensation** for a new employee. In many cases, there is a pay range that has been published for the particular position, and the offer must be within that range. Some managers prefer to hire candidates at the bottom of the range to save on their labor budget. Others prefer to hire at or close to the top of the range to attract the very best candidate. There is a problem with this latter strategy. If an individual is hired at the top of the range, there is little room for growth. Future raises will be minimal, and employee dissatisfaction could result. It is prudent to hire new employees between the bottom and the middle of the range, if that is possible.

If the candidate is currently working, it is advisable to set the salary level at or above the individual's current salary level. It is rare for an applicant to accept a decrease in pay unless the work conditions or geographic location of the new position are far superior to those of the current job. If the benefits are unequal, the salary may need to be adjusted. For example, if the benefits are superior, a candidate might be willing to make a lateral move, with respect to pay.

Another consideration is that of equity among similar employees. If five clinical dietitians work in an organization and a sixth is hired at a higher salary, there is bound to be some resentment among the senior staff who earn less. (Even though salaries are supposed to be confidential, they seldom are.) On the other hand, the new hire does not necessarily need to be paid the least amount of money. If, for example, the new hire has eight years of experience and one of the incumbent dietitians has only six months of experience, then it is probably OK to hire the new person at a salary above that of the entry-level dietitian. The salary for the new employee should not be greater than that of another dietitian with equal or more experience.

Other issues involve economics. It may be necessary to hire someone at a lower rate than desirable because of budgetary limits on dollars available for salaries. Then, too, salaries are market driven. If the candidates for the job are few, it may be necessary for an organization to pay more money in order to employ someone who is able to do the job. On the other hand, if there are many qualified candidates and few jobs, the salary rates may be lower.

For some candidates, money is not the most important issue. Someone may be willing to negotiate a lower salary if the benefits are exceptionally good. Alternately, if insurance benefits are available through another family member, the candidate may prefer a higher salary and fewer benefits. A classic example of the trade-offs involved in salary negotiations is in foodservice. Some foodservice managers give up lucrative positions in commercial foodservice, which requires working many weekend and evening hours, to work at lower-paying jobs in the onsite sector. They do this because they are less likely to need to work as many holidays, weekends, and evenings.

equal opportunity/affirmative action

Equal opportunity is a fact of life in the United States. The basic premise is that candidates should be judged on their ability to do the job rather than on other factors such as race, gender, ethnicity, religion, and so on. Affirmative action is an attempt to correct past injustices by giving preference in hiring to members of various under-represented groups. Requirements for employers to implement affirmative action programs vary from state to state in the U.S.

Nevertheless, it is good business to have a staff that reflects the community in which it operates. Members of a group may be more readily accepted by other members of that same group. It is also appropriate that members of each group are dispersed throughout the organization. It is not acceptable for all the hourly workers to be of one subgroup of the population and for all the management to represent another group. Sometimes it is inappropriate to hire the best qualified candidate if that individual widens the discrepancy between the organization and the community. Individual decisions must be made, weighing the qualifications of the candidates against other factors.

At times, it is not possible to find qualified dietetics practitioners who reflect the diversity of the community. For example, the profession has traditionally attracted women, so that it has a distinct gender bias. Efforts are being made to correct this and other biases within the profession, as well as in the programs that educate dietitians and dietetic technicians. However, it will be some time before the population of dietetics professionals truly reflects the communities in which they serve. Meanwhile, attempts should be made to keep the workforce as diverse as possible, given the limitations that are inevitable in today's market.

the offer

The final step in the employment process is the job offer, which includes the level of compensation. The offer is made to the candidate by either the hiring manager or the HR department. This should be done in person or on the phone. Usually, if the hiring manager has done the job correctly, the offer will be one that the candidate can accept. If some details remain to be settled, this is the time for those negotiations to take place. One issue to be considered is that of benefits. Another is the start date. The hiring manager may also need to check the one final reference, and it may be necessary for the candidate to pass a physical exam.

benefits

Benefits include such items as insurance (health, life, disability, and so on), paid time off (holidays, vacation, sick time), employee assistance programs, wellness programs, and the like. Perks include items like expense accounts, cars, company credit cards, mobile telephones, and so on. Sometimes relocation packages or signing bonuses are made available to assist people in moving to a new location. The generosity of these various benefits and perks varies with the organization and the job market.

Some organizations offer their employees a **cafeteria package** of benefits. This is, essentially, a list of the available benefits from which employees can choose those that meet their individual needs. For example, a single young worker might choose a catastrophic-illness type of health insurance (which is relatively inexpensive) and membership in a health club or a weight-loss program. An older worker with family responsibilities might choose a more comprehensive (and more expensive) health insurance policy for the entire family and forgo the health club membership. Older workers are often more interested in

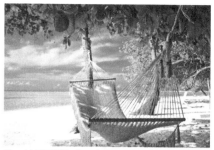

retirement programs, whereas younger workers might prefer to take home larger paychecks. The options in these cafeteria packages are somewhat regional in nature and are also dependent on the job market. Offerings are usually more generous during times of economic growth and low unemployment.

Employee benefits usually include paid time off that can be used for vacation or for personal reasons.

leave. Paid time off is the amount of time that employees can be absent from work and still take home their usual compensation. There are several types of paid time off; the major ones are listed in Table 8.2. In addition, there is also the potential for unpaid time off. For example, if an employee has planned a vacation prior to taking a new position, a condition of employment might be that the employee takes the prearranged time off without pay. Other time off without pay is the time that military reservists in the United States are called to active duty. Because the military service pays the employee during that period, the employer is not required to pay the employee, but must grant the time off without penalty to the employee.

Cafeteria Package. *A selection of benefits offered to employees from which they can pick and choose according to individual needs.*

Usually, there are a certain number of employer-designated holidays each year, when employees traditionally are paid but do not work. This number of paid holidays is up to the employer, but it usually ranges from 5 to 10 days each year. Some typical paid holidays are Christmas, Thanksgiving, and the Fourth of July. If the business—for example, a bank—can close on those days, no one works. If the business—for example, a supermarket—stays open, those who work on the holiday usually get paid a premium to work that day. The designated holidays may be part of a contractual agreement with a union.

Employer-designated holidays
Personal days
Vacation
Sick time
Bereavement leave
Jury duty

Table 8.2 Types of Paid Time Off

Some employers designate only a few holidays and, instead, give the employees a set number of personal days each year. Personal days can be used whenever the employee wants time off, rather than on days that the employer designates. There is no requirement to give employees personal days. However, the use of personal days in lieu of designated holidays is advantageous to both the employer and the employee. Because employees choose which days they will take off, it is unlikely that everyone will be off on the same day. Therefore, the employer does not have to close down or pay overtime, as would have to be done for a designated holiday; this saves labor dollars. The advantage to the employee is one of personal choice. The individual chooses when to use the time off, perhaps to accompany a friend on a skiing or camping trip, or to chaperone a child's school field trip.

Vacation and **sick time** are usually handled in similar ways. Employees earn a certain number of sick days and vacation days each pay period. They can use whatever sick days are accrued when they become ill, and they can request vacations when vacation time has been accrued. In this model, sick time can be used for illness but cannot be used as personal time or vacation time. Occasionally, if an employee has used up all available sick time, vacation time can be used so that pay will continue uninterrupted during an extended illness. Sometimes an organization will allow an employee with lots of accrued sick time to donate that time to a colleague who has a catastrophic illness.

Bereavement time is to be used if an employee experiences a death in the family. When it is offered to employees, it is usually limited to two or three days each year. There is no requirement for an employer to provide this benefit to employees.

A newer method that is gaining acceptance is the model in which employees earn **paid time off (PTO)**, rather than personal days, vacation, and sick time. The amount of time is roughly equivalent to the combination of vacation, personal, and sick time that would normally be accrued. The difference is that the employee is not told how to use the time. The accrued time can be used for illness, for bereavement, for vacation, as personal days, and so forth. With this system, the employee who seldom misses work for illness can use the time as additional vacation or as personal time.

Jury duty is mandated by statute in the United States. If an employee is called for jury duty, the government usually pays that individual a minimal amount to serve on the jury. The employer is expected to pay the difference between what the employee earns as a juror and what would have normally been earned during that time. The employee does not use any accrued time (sick, vacation, personal, or PTO) while on jury duty.

A final word about paid time off. Some organizations put a cap on the amount of time that an employee may accrue. This is true for both PTO systems and systems that give vacation, sick, and personal days. Setting this type of cap often causes employees to develop a "use it or lose it" attitude, in which they take time off when they do not need or want to in order not to lose what they have earned. This is a real problem in

---

Vacation Time. *Paid time off from work designated for leisure activities or rest.*

Sick Time. *Paid time off to be used for illness or injury.*

Bereavement Time. *Paid time off when there is a death in the family.*

Paid Time Off (PTO). *The time an employee can be absent from work with pay.*

an organization that has many long-term employees who are near the cap of accrued time. An equitable solution that can be implemented is one in which employers **buy back** the paid time off. In essence, the employee with lots of accrued time sells it back to the organization for cash. This rewards the employee who does not use excessive time off, while not punishing those who use all the time they accrue.

insurance. Another benefit that employees get is insurance coverage. Some of the coverage is statutory—that is, required by law. Examples include Social Security, Unemployment Insurance, and Workers' Compensation. Beginning in 2014, the Patient Protection and Affordable Care Act of 2010, mandates that certain employers offer health insurance to workers and their families.[1] Other types of insurance are not required by law but may be offered to employees as benefits, either partly or entirely paid for by the employer. Among the types of voluntary insurance coverage that may be offered are life insurance, dependent life insurance, a retirement program, dental insurance, vision insurance, disability insurance, accidental death insurance, and legal insurance. Some or all of these may be available in a cafeteria package of benefits. Insurance coverage is not necessarily free. The employee may be asked to make a contribution toward his coverage, just as both employees and employers in the United States contribute to Social Security. Even when employees pay a significant amount for insurance coverage, it is usually cheaper to be a member of a group plan than to purchase the same insurance as an individual.

other. Employees may earn other benefits through their jobs. Often, they can buy products made by the organization at a reduced price (for example, cafeterias may offer employee discounts). Some employers pay for dues to professional organizations, for subscriptions to journals, for registration and travel to meetings, and give paid time off for educational activities. Others offer tuition reimbursement for employees who take job-related courses at local colleges and universities. In addition, employees may participate in companywide profit-sharing programs, or they may earn bonuses when business is good.

acceptance or rejection

Once an employment offer has been made, and details of that offer negotiated, the prospective employee should be allowed a reasonable period of time to make a decision about the offer. A family member may need to be consulted, or research into housing and living costs in a new location may need to be completed. The operative word is *reasonable*. There are no set rules, but for someone who is being recruited from another internal job, or for someone who is out of work, reasonable is usually less than a week, perhaps two weeks if relocation is involved. For a student who may not be graduating and available for several months, a reasonable period of time could be up to a month. The candidate should not keep the hiring manager waiting for very long; in such situations, the manager may have second thoughts and withdraw the offer.

Buy Back. *An option in which the employer pays the employee for accrued time off that was not used.*

Social Security Administration. *http://socialsecurity. gov/*

If the candidate declines the employment offer, there is seldom any real benefit in trying to renegotiate with that candidate. This is especially true if the offer was a thoughtful and honest one. The factors that existed when the offer was made seldom change dramatically in a matter of days. Though there may be exceptions, it is usually best to terminate the relationship and make an offer to an alternate candidate.

After a candidate has accepted the offer, a start date needs to be arranged. If the prospective employee is currently working, it is likely that some notice needs to be given to the current employer (usually one month for exempt employees and two weeks for hourly workers). If the employee is working for a competitor, the competitor will want to minimize any chance of information leakage and may dismiss the employee immediately, without penalty. Otherwise, it is likely that person will have to work through the notice period. It is also reasonable for the candidate to want to take a few days off before starting a new position. If all has proceeded smoothly, the candidate will start work on the designated date and the relationship will change. It is at this point that the employment process ends and the employer/employee relationship begins.

One final word about the employment process. Once the offer has been made and accepted by a candidate, it is courteous to notify other candidates that the position has been filled. This is usually done in writing, a personal letter if the candidate pool was small, or a form letter or postcard if the candidate pool was large. Though this is not always done, when it is, rejected candidates feel better about the experience and are more likely to reapply to that organization in the future. It is a good public relations strategy.

conclusion

This chapter has included an overview of the employment process, from the identification of staffing needs through hiring. The key concepts that can be found in this chapter include:

1. Staffing should be undertaken in a planned, deliberate manner, whether it involves hiring a single employee or building an organization from the ground up.
2. The jobs to be done are outlined in job specifications, job descriptions, and, sometimes, job analyses.
3. A variety of recruitment tools are available to HR departments and to hiring managers to publicize available jobs.
4. The employment interview should be planned in such a way that candidates can be compared with one another.
5. The hiring decision is made based on the qualifications of the candidates and other factors such as compensation, diversity goals, reference checks, and so on.
6. An employment offer often includes benefits such as paid time off, insurance, and the like.

activities

activity 1

Write a job specification, a job description, and a job analysis for a job that you have held.

activity 2

List three recruitment methods that would be appropriate to use when seeking employees in each of the following positions:

a. Foodservice director for a school district with 200,000 students.
b. Foodservice supervisor for a 35-bed skilled nursing facility.
c. Clinical dietitian for a 150-bed community hospital.
d. Dietitian for a tertiary care facility's neonatal intensive care unit with 78 beds.
e. WIC administrator for a large state like New York, California, or Texas.
f. Registered dietitian to work eight hours a week in a private obstetrician's office.
g. Foodservice worker in an adult day care center with 80 clients.
h. Cook for a summer camp for children with diabetes.

activity 3

Write an interview schedule for a structured interview (at least 10 items in length) for one of the jobs listed in Activity 2. State what information you are seeking from each question.

to study further

More comprehensive coverage of the employment process and the employment interview can be found in:

- Arthur, D. *Managing Human Resources in Small and Midsize Companies*. New York: American Management Association, 1995.
- Arthur, D. *Recruiting, Interviewing, Selecting, and Orienting New Employees*. 5th ed. New York: AMACOM, 2012.
- Cascio, W. F. *Managing Human Resources: Productivity, Quality of Work Life, Profits*. 9th ed. New York: McGraw-Hill/Irwin, 2012.
- *Fundamentals of Employee Benefits Programs*. 6th ed. Washington, DC: Employee Benefits Research Institute, Education and Research Fund, 2009.
- Gryna, F. *Work Overload! Redesigning Jobs to Minimize Stress and Burnout*. Milwaukee: ASQ Quality Press, 2004.
- Holli, Betsy B. et al. *Communication and Education Skills for Dietetics Professionals*. 5th ed. Philadelphia: Lippincott Williams and Wilkins, 2008.
- McCaffree, J. "Clinical Staffing: Determining the Right Size." *Journal of the American Dietetic Association*. 106:25–26, 2006.
- Milkovich, G. T., J. M. Newman, and B. Gerhart. *Compensation*. 10th ed. New York: McGraw-Hill/Irwin, 2010.
- Morgan, R. B. and J. E. Smith. *Staffing the New Workplace: Selecting and Promoting for Quality Improvement*. Milwaukee: ASQC Quality Press, 1996.
- Pinkley, R. L. "Salary and Compensation Negotiation Skills for Young Professionals." *Journal of the American Dietetic Association*. 104: 1064–1068, 2004.
- Pynes, J. E. *Human Resources Management for Public and Nonprofit Organizations*. 3rd ed. San Francisco: Jossey-Bass, 2009.
- Shell, Richard L. *Management of Professionals*. 2nd ed. New York: Marcel Dekker, 2003.
- Statt, David A. *Psychology and the World of Work*. 2nd ed. New York: Palgrave Macmillan, 2004.
- Stein, K. "Staying Current in the Job Search Arena." *Journal of the American Dietetic Association*. 108: 1290–1292, 2008.
- Switt, J. T. "Hiring the Right Person the First Time: Tips on Conducting a Job Interview." *Journal of the American Dietetic Association*. 108:1118–1120, 2008.
- Volkema, Roger J. *The Negotiation Toolkit: How to Get Exactly What You Want in any Business or Personal Situation*. New York: American Management Association, 1999.
- Zackin, F. M. "Employment References—Giving and Receiving." *Journal of the American Dietetic Association*. 108: 1053–1055, 2008.

scholarly journals

- *Industrial and Labor Relations Review*
- *Journal of Insurance Issues*

other relevant periodical

- *Benefits Quarterly*

relevant websites

- Employee Benefit News http://ebn.benefitnews.com/
- Public Service Employees http://www.pse-net.com/
- U.S. Department of Labor, Employment and Training Administration http://www.doleta.gov/

in practice

the national search

It will probably be a few years before anyone reading this text will be recruited for a position of major responsibility through a national search. However, many will have the opportunity in their careers to serve as a member of a search committee. The following is a summary of the way a national search may be conducted, and the roles that various individuals play in such an undertaking. This type of recruiting is expensive, so it is generally reserved for senior management positions, academic appointments, or highly specialized/skilled workers. This is not the type of search that would be conducted for a foodservice worker, or even for a clinical dietitian.

The first step is to determine that someone is needed to do a particular job. Typically, a position is open because someone has moved on (or soon will be moving on). On rare occasions, a new position is created. This is the time to write or update the job specification to outline the minimum credentials, skills, and education needed for the position. A current job description is also needed to delineate the duties that the person who takes the position must be willing and able to perform. Based on these documents, a search is organized seeking qualified candidates from across the nation.

Assume, for purposes of this discussion, that the vacant position is for the director of campus dining for a major university. The manager for such an operation needs to have upper-level management experience in campus dining, and in operating a department with a very large budget (e.g., revenues of >$20 million per year) and a large number of employees (>150 FTEs). A background in the culinary arts and an MBA might also be deemed necessary, as well as a history of active participation in a professional organization, in this case the National Association of College and University Food Services (NACUFS). Because of the specificity of these qualifications, it is assumed that the pool of qualified applicants will be limited and that many qualified people may not be interested in changing jobs. The search will have to be conducted nationwide.

Based on the job specification and the job description, an advertisement is placed through NACUFS. In addition, a local foodservice management recruiter is engaged to locate any qualified applicants from the region. This alternative was added in the hope of including an individual with local connections who might not be looking for a job and, therefore, might miss the NACUFS ad. Once the advertisement is placed, there is a waiting period during which resumes are submitted. For purpose of this illustration, assume that 40 resumes are received.

Now, it is the job of the Human Resources Department (HR) to sort through the resumes and complete the paper review. Some applicants can be eliminated immediately because they do not meet the basic qualifications (MBA, professional affiliation, experience). Though these individuals are effectively eliminated from the search, their resumes are kept on hand. This is done for two reasons. First, it may be that none of the qualified candidates are hired and the organization needs to change its decision-making criteria. Second, even if a manager is hired, additional management staff may be needed in the near future, and these resumes may prove valuable at that time. Assume that 25 of the 40 applicants did not make it through the paper review and their resumes were put aside.

Fifteen qualified candidates have now been identified. This is still too many to be brought in for in-depth interviews, so additional screening must be done. At this point, HR may share the credentials of the 15 with the hiring administrator, who also completes a paper review and may possibly eliminate another candidate or two. The remaining candidates are then scheduled for either a phone or a video-phone interview. Note the word "scheduled." This type of interview should be planned far enough in advance that the candidate has the opportunity to arrange a time and place where there will be privacy and freedom from interruptions. The interview will be conducted by HR personnel with an interview schedule developed using the job specification, the job description, institutional values, and input from the hiring administrator. This process should serve to eliminate more candidates. For purposes of this example, the pool of applicants is now pared to four.

The final four candidates will be brought to campus for a final round of interviews. This time, the interviews will be conducted by "search committees" representing various campus constituencies. In this large university, there are several groups who need to be represented. These include:

- Students
- Foodservice managers
- Foodservice workers
- Other customers (faculty, staff, and catering customers)
- Peers (managers from resident services, marketing, information systems, facilities planning, etc.)

Though it would be possible to appoint a committee with one representative from each of these groups, it is better to have several small groups, each representing one of these constituencies. Remember that when more people participate in the decision-making process, support for the decision is enhanced.

Each group then meets to determine what they feel are important characteristics for the director of campus dining to demonstrate. Each group develops an interview schedule to seek relevant information, and each group assigns an order to its questions and sets an agenda for the forthcoming meetings to ensure that they are as consistent as possible among the candidates. Some sort of score sheet may be developed that will allow members of each search committee to rank the candidates after all have been interviewed.

Next, each candidate is scheduled to visit campus for two days, during which each candidate meets with each of the above groups, tours the campus, and meets the staff, administrators, and students. During this time there are structured interviews with each group. At the end of all of the visits, the scores are compiled by HR and submitted to the hiring administrator to assist in decision making. If the choice is clear, the offer will be made and the specifics of employment negotiated. If the choice is not yet clear, the administrator might need to visit the final two candidates in their workplaces to further evaluate their qualifications before making the hiring decision. Once everything has been finalized, all other candidates should be thanked for their interest and informed that the position has been filled.

The national search process is long and arduous, but certainly worth the time and money that it costs. (The cost for this search, including advertisement, recruiter, HR manpower, administrator time, time for group members, travel expenses, and communication expenses could exceed $100,000.) The new manager will have a major influence on the direction, productivity, finances, and long-term stability of campus dining. In the long run, it is better to invest the resources needed to make a good hiring decision than to have to correct a bad decision in the future.

reference

1. United States House of Representatives, Legislative Council. *Compilation of the Patient Protection and Affordable Care Act.* 2010. http://housedocs.house.gov/energycommerce/ppacacon.pdf. Accessed July 22, 2012.

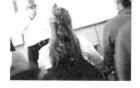

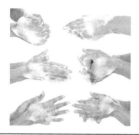

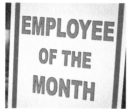

chapter nine

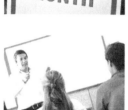

developing and motivating employees

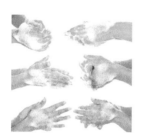

learning objectives

1. State the reasons for having a structured orientation program for new employees.

2. List the components of new employee orientation programs.

3. Describe the purpose of using an orientation checklist.

4. Differentiate between organizational orientation and orientation to the job.

5. Describe the purpose of in-service training programs.

6. Differentiate between in-service training and continuing education.

7. Describe ways in which employees are supported in continuing education endeavors.

8. State the reasons for conducting performance appraisals.

9. Describe how performance appraisals are conducted.

10. List the characteristics of effective compensation programs.

11. Identify the relationship between motivation and compensation.

12. Differentiate among components of compensation packages including merit increases, cost-of-living adjustments, single pay rates, and pay for performance.

13. Discuss non-monetary methods for motivating employees.

14. Describe the relationship between motivation and job mobility.

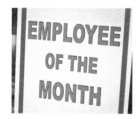

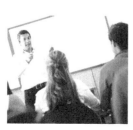

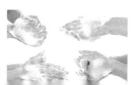

overview

Have you ever walked into a new situation—social, school, or work-related—where no one was there to greet you, to introduce you to others, or to show you where things were located? How did it make you feel? Did you feel frightened, unwanted, unappreciated, lost, disoriented, or angry because you were ignored? It is common courtesy to greet and welcome newcomers, but this type of basic kindness is often lacking in today's rushed society. People are left to fend for themselves and make their own way in new situations.

The workplace is no different from any other setting in our society in this respect. In fact, it may be worse. Managers are busy people and may not make the time to greet new employees and get them started on the right foot. However, when new employees are left to their own devices, valuable time is lost to trial and error. Motivating and developing employees has a major impact on job performance, job satisfaction, and the retention of staff. It begins the moment a new employee enters the workplace for orientation. It continues throughout a person's employment, with individualized training programs and appropriate performance incentives.

This chapter begins with a discussion of the orientation for new employees. This is followed by a summary of the types of training and development programs that are essential to keep the workforce up to date regarding technologies and other work-related matters. Finally, motivational factors such as performance appraisals, types of compensation programs, pay for performance, and nonfinancial rewards will be addressed.

employee orientation

The orientation process begins the moment newly hired employees enter the workplace. How they are greeted and made to feel welcome, the information provided about the job, whom they meet, whether or not their workstations are prepared for them, and other factors will provide the basis for how they feel about the job and about the employer for a long time to come. A positive introduction to the workplace, as demonstrated by making the new employees know that they were expected and some effort had been put into preparations for their arrival, will greatly influence long-term job satisfaction, commitment to the organization, and retention by the organization.[1]

Orientation.
The process of introducing a new employee to an organization, job, and work unit.

Orientation of new employees has two distinct parts. One part is the orientation to the organization. The second is the orientation to the job. Though it might be ideal to start all new employees with an orientation to the organization as a whole, and then introduce them to their individual jobs, this is not always practical, given the variation of hiring and starting dates. The important part is that both parts of the orientation occur within a reasonable period of time after the employee begins work.

orientation to the job

In many cases, the new employee is introduced to the job prior to being introduced to the larger organization. This orientation should not be left to chance. It should be a planned and scheduled series of events. The hiring manager should plan to meet with a new employee early on the starting date and conduct the initial part of the orientation in person. If this is not possible, someone should be assigned this duty well in advance of the start date, so that the person who is orienting the new employee has time to prepare and to be free of other tasks that would interfere with the orientation process.

The orientation to the job should start with an outline of the day so that the new employee knows what to expect. This is to be followed by an introduction to all of the people with whom the new employee will work on a daily basis. The introduction should include both the name of the colleague and a brief description of that person's job. This gives the new employee an idea of who performs each of the various functions in an organization. The introductions should not include any judgmental statements about the staff members being introduced. Care should be taken to allow the new hire to develop independent opinions about colleagues.

In addition, there should be a tour of the immediate workplace. It is essential to remember to include seemingly mundane things like restrooms, fire extinguishers, bulletin boards, water fountains, elevators, exits, and stairways. The employee should be shown where to store personal belongings. If there is danger of theft in the workplace, security issues should be discussed. If the newly hired individual has an assigned workstation, desk, or office, this should be pointed out. If these spaces are shared with others, the usual arrangements for sharing should be discussed as well.

New employees may not be familiar with the equipment that is used in the workplace. Though most people can use home telephones with no difficulty, a phone console with multiple incoming lines, many answering options, and multiple functions may take some special skills. The new employee may need to learn how to operate this and other equipment, like copiers, faxes, printers, and so on. Access to frequently used telephone numbers should be made available, if the job requires it. Guidelines for making personal phone calls and for the personal use of faxes, computers, and copiers should be reviewed. If computer or copier access requires clearance or passwords, these should be arranged. Where equipment or supplies are kept in storage, the employee needs to be shown where the storage is and how to get materials from that area. It is helpful to provide this information in written form, if available.

If there is a job analysis for the position, the employee should be given a copy of it. This will introduce the tasks and the deadlines associated with the job. It can also act as a note sheet for writing down the "tricks of the trade" that are picked up during the orientation. Remember, though, that job analyses are not available (or necessary) for all jobs. If there is no job analysis, the current job description will serve a similar purpose. It is also helpful for the employee to be given access to departmental policies and procedures and be given time to review those pertinent to the job. For a clinical dietitian, the procedure for charting might be appropriate to review. A DTR might need to review the screening policy, and a cook should review the policies related to using recipes. The policy review serves two functions—first, to describe how things are done in this setting, and second, to introduce the employee to the resources that are available for future reference.

Mentor. *A person whom one with less experience may consult for advice and guidance.*

Frequently, the newly hired employee is assigned to "shadow" an experienced employee for the first few days of work. This provides the new employee with a **mentor** to consult while learning the job. Sometimes the newly hired employee may work with several individuals in several different positions for a week or so, until the basic knowledge and skills needed for the job are acquired. Orientation may vary in length from a day to several weeks, during which time the employee is expected to become more independent in carrying out the routine tasks of the job.

Breaks and meals during the first day of work should not be left to chance. The manager should make sure that the new employee has someone to talk to during meals and breaks. That someone may be the manager, who can use the opportunity to answer any questions that may have arisen. Alternately, it may be a colleague, the employee who is being "shadowed," or a group of other employees.

Orientation Checklist. *A document that lists all of the items that are to be accomplished or introduced during a new employee orientation.*

The orientation process may be facilitated through the use of an **orientation checklist**. This document is a list of all of the items that are supposed to be accomplished or introduced during the new employee's orientation period. It can be designed to be general or all-inclusive. For example, it can list a "tour of the department" as one item on the list, or it can specify the individual items that need to be pointed out, like restrooms, lounges, and water fountains. The specificity of the list will depend, in part, on the number of new employees hired each year, and whether one individual or a variety of people carry out the orientations. Generally, when more people are involved in orienting employees to a department or a work group, the checklist needs to be more specific, so that nothing is missed or left to chance. If one person does all of the orientations for a department, that person is accountable to ensure that the process is uniform and complete. Still, the checklist is a useful tool that can be used by others to orient new employees when the designated individual is absent.

Some employers also use the orientation checklist for formal documentation. The checklist is used as a guide for orientation, as stated above, but the items on the list are actually checked off or initialed as they are completed. When the entire list is checked, the employee and the supervisor (or the individual responsible for the orientation) sign the sheet to document that the various items have been covered. The document then becomes a part of the employee's file and can be reviewed if there is disagreement about what was covered during that time. In addition, these documents

management practice in dietetics

may verify that content required by oversight agencies has been discussed with the employee. This content may include such topics as fire safety, cardiopulmonary resuscitation, principles of safe food handling, and so on. An example of an orientation checklist is shown in Figure 9.1.

orientation to the organization

The introduction to the organization is carried out to familiarize the employee with the overall organization, its philosophy and mission, and the relationship that exists between the organization and its staff. Typically, someone from the human resources department carries out this part of the orientation, with assistance by others as required. The content and length of the orientation will vary with the size and complexity of the organization and the number of persons that are hired during a typical week or month.

Employee _____ Supervisor _____

Position: Dietetic Clerk

_____ Physical exam
_____ Name tag/ID Badge
_____ Computer password
_____ Personnel paperwork (federal, state, employee benefits, etc.)
_____ Orientation to the organization
_____ Employee handbook
_____ Tour of department/introduction to coworkers
_____ Review of policies
_____ Review of menus, forms, guidelines, etc.
_____ Use of computer systems
_____ Use of telephones
_____ Use of copiers
_____ Time cards
_____ Heading menus
_____ Diet changes
_____ Checking trayline
_____ Processing late trays
_____ Fire safety
_____ CPR
_____ Disaster Plan
_____ HACCP training
_____ Body mechanics

Hire date: _____   Date completed: _____

Signature of Employee: _____

Signature of Supervisor: _____

Figure 9.1 Orientation Checklist

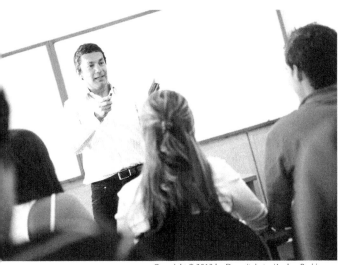

In large organizations, the orientation to the organization is often scheduled so that a group of new employees can participate in the program together.

During recruitment and hiring, it is natural for both candidates and hiring managers to "over sell." To present themselves in the best possible lights, candidates may neglect to inform the prospective employer of gaps in knowledge or experience. The hiring manager, anxious to attract the best-qualified candidates, may also paint a picture that is not entirely accurate. Part of the purpose of organizational orientation is to reconcile these perceptions and to present a realistic view of the workplace.

Small organizations may conduct the organizational orientation on an individual basis as employees are hired. This can be very personal and positive. For this type of one-on-one meeting, the orientation checklist is helpful. When more than one person is to be oriented at a time, a more structured orientation program is usually used. Some large organizations do this type of orientation on a regularly scheduled basis—for example, every Monday or the first and third Thursday of each month. Some large organizations even require new employees to start on a day when the orientation is scheduled; it is the first thing that they do when they arrive on the job. It is helpful to limit the size of these organizational orientations to 20 or fewer people so that there is ample opportunity for individuals to ask questions and to get immediate responses.

The same basic content should be covered for either individual or group orientations. It should include a welcome and an introduction to the overall mission or philosophy of the organization (often presented to groups by an executive in the organization). There should be an explanation of the benefits package, including time off, insurance, employee assistance programs, and so on. Organization-wide policies and procedures, like parking, dress code, and smoking regulations should be addressed. The orientation should include a tour of the entire facility, not just the new employee's workstation, pointing out such areas of interest as the executive suites, cafeteria, mail room, payroll offices, human resources, meeting rooms, libraries, and so on. This type of orientation usually takes from four to eight hours and may include time to fill out paperwork related to taxes, insurance, and the like. Several speakers may be scheduled to address topics related to their area of expertise. It is helpful if their presentations are conducted in a professional manner, using appropriate teaching aids to hold the interest of the new staff.

Sometimes the orientations are tailored to specific types of employees. This allows additional information to be provided to subgroups of new employees who need it. For example, managerial staff could attend a different orientation than clerical workers. Management programs might include information on how to do administrative tasks that hourly workers are not required to do, such as budget preparation, procedures for personnel management, and so on. The clerical staff might be oriented to the office software suite that is being used by the organization.

management practice in dietetics

Large organizations often provide an **employee handbook**, which addresses the various items covered in the orientation and can serve as a reference to employees after the orientation is completed. It is usually designed to cover those topics that generate questions from employees. In the past, this tool was used primarily by large companies who could afford the printing costs associated with its production. Now, with the use of computers, even the smallest company can provide this type of uniform information, either in print or on a page on the company website. In addition to the employee handbook, other items that may be included in the **orientation packet** are information on benefits, a map (if the facility is large), a list of commonly used telephone numbers and Internet addresses, a copy of the organization chart (described in Chapter 2), and so on.

During the initial period of employment, employees are frequently classified as *probationary*. This means that, for a period of about 90 days (variable among organizations) from the start date, they are subject to termination without due process if their performance does not meet expectations. This may occur merely because the employee does not fit in with the organization's culture. It is not necessary to justify termination during the probationary period. Employees should be made aware of their probationary status. It often provides the impetus for good performance, a habit that could carry through for the long term if the employee is retained.

Some employees experience a "honeymoon period" during the initial phase of employment. This is a common phenomenon for professional and managerial personnel. Though it has not been definitively characterized, it is a period when new staff are encouraged to ask questions and not expected to achieve peak performance. Often, new ideas are generated by new employees during this time, because they enter the organization with fresh perspectives. These ideas contribute to the development of the organization. It is also during the honeymoon period that concessions may be made that were denied in the past, or that will not be made when the new employee achieves seniority and should "know better" than to ask. Like the employment process, this is a period during which the organization (both management and subordinates) is trying to impress the new employee and will be more forgiving than during most other phases of the employee's career in that organization. A perceptive employee will note that this is the time to implement change and request accommodation, as necessary.

in-service training

Orienting the new employee to the organization and the job does not mark the end of the training process. Orientation is not enough to sustain an employee throughout an extended career in an organization. Staff, at all levels, need to review or be updated on various issues from time to time. Some updates are mandated by accreditation or oversight organizations, others are needed because of changes within the

Employee Handbook. *A publication, either print or web-based, that can serve as a reference manual to employees after the orientation process is completed. It usually reiterates material covered during the orientation and addresses other frequently asked questions.*

Orientation Packet. *An information packet handed out during an orientation that may include such items as information on benefits, a map of the facility, a list of commonly used telephone numbers and Internet addresses, a copy of the organization chart, and so on.*

In-Services. *Educational activities that are designed to update and introduce employees to new issues or topics pertinent to their jobs and organization, or to review and refresh employees on material that is already known. They usually occur at the workplace and during work hours.*

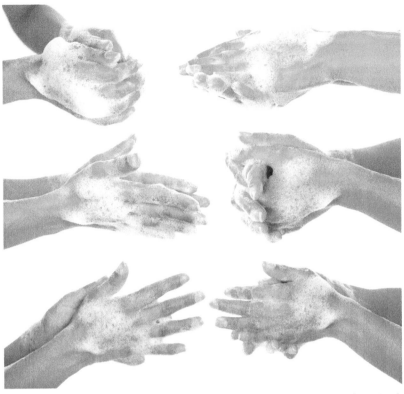

Proper hand washing techniques are a topic for in-service education sessions in food service departments and healthcare organizations.

organization, and still others are required because new technologies are introduced. In-services are educational activities that are sponsored by the employer and usually take place during regular work hours.

In-services can be broadly classified into two distinct types. The first is the work-related training that is relatively brief and carried out in the immediate work setting. In foodservices, topics for these training sessions might be related to fire safety, sanitation, hand washing, body mechanics, or the proper use of a specific piece of equipment. In the inpatient clinical setting, the topics might include isolation techniques, cardiopulmonary resuscitation, or methods of anthropometric assessment. Often, this type of training is designed to review and refresh employees on material that is already known but not talked about frequently. The in-services are designed to increase knowledge and skill and to give the topic a degree of immediacy, especially if it is something that has become routine, like hand washing.

These short in-services should be considered routine and should be carried out on a regularly scheduled basis. For example, fire safety should be reviewed annually for every employee who works in a health care foodservice. Employees' attendance at these classes is usually documented in one (or both) of two places. An in-service training book is usually kept as part of official documentation for a department. This book contains outlines of each class that was presented and a list of personnel who attended each class. The date of attendance is also recorded. The in-service may be given several times during the course of a month if employees work staggered schedules. This ensures that everyone has an opportunity to attend at least one of the sessions. In addition, a record may also be kept in the employee's file. This record allows a manager to quickly determine if individual staff members have specific information, and who still needs training on a topic.

The second type of in-service training is more extensive and requires that the individual attending the training session be freed from normal work activities for extended periods of time. This type of session is often conducted offsite so that individual staff members cannot be called back to their regular duties. This kind of event may go by a number of different names, such as retreat, management seminar, computer training, sales meeting, and so on. The name of the event may also indicate the topic to be presented at the meeting, such as performance appraisal, team-building, sensitivity training, sanitation, or customer relations. Though such educational sessions may be offered to employees at any level in an organization, it is more likely that professional or managerial staff will be in attendance. Sometimes, when succession planning has identified candidates for promotion to managerial positions, this type of training may be given in anticipation of the promotions. In such cases, the in-service can be used as a tool to motivate the candidates to accept the challenge of a new position.

Organizations often use these sessions to introduce new ideas into the organization. These "new" things may range from new products to new policies and procedures. Because the training sessions are held on an organization-wide basis, individuals in attendance have the opportunity to network with colleagues outside of their own departments. Sensitivity for individual and departmental differences increases, and relationships are built that have the potential for enhancing an organization's overall performance. Sometimes these sessions are used to reinforce the organization's mission and goals, or to brainstorm for ideas that can be used to further these goals. In any case, team-building is a usual outcome of this type of event, whether or not that topic was covered as a specific content area.

Furthermore, these events provide information that increases the knowledge base of those who attend. Professionals may even gain some continuing education units for the topics that were addressed. This is an incidental benefit that enhances the entire concept of in-service training. This type of event can also be used to allow staff to reexamine the skills they need on a daily basis, such as communication, leadership, decision making, and so on.

Finally, it should be noted that offsite training events are often more successful if they are carried out by professionals who are trained in conducting such events. Some large organizations employ a training manager who evaluates the educational needs of staff in light of organizational goals, and plans the events on a corporate level. Other organizations use consultants to carry out this function. Regardless of who is responsible, it is generally understood that the people who present the material need to be experts in their fields, and that it is generally not wise to use the same person for the same audience on a repeated basis. The messages are usually more effective if they are varied and come from diverse perspectives. However, it is acceptable to use the same speaker if the members of the audience change. For example, one speaker could travel to different areas of the country to present a seminar to employees at each of five regional sites. This type of program is used by the contract foodservice management companies to keep local operators in touch with the parent corporation.

continuing education

Continuing Education.
Educational activities that are conducted by an external organization and that take place outside of the workplace. Examples include trade shows, educational workshops or seminars, college or university courses, and so on.

Continuing education differs from in-service training in that the content is not under the control of the employer. Continuing education may be offered by a professional association at a trade show or an annual meeting. It may also be offered by a private organization whose business is conducting training sessions and seminars. Webinars are mini-courses offered by either of these groups. Frequently one or two hours long, these often take place during regular business hours. Though employers are not required to do so, many choose to subsidize continuing education for their professional staff, usually on the condition that it is job-related. It is another tool for motivating employees to keep current in their respective fields.

Continuing education can be subsidized in a number of ways. It may be part of an employee's benefit package that a specified number of days are allowed for the employee to engage in continuing education activities each year. The employee then selects events that are of interest and gets permission from management to be freed from regular duties on those days in order to attend the event. The dates are always subject to management's approval. In this situation, because the employee is paying for the continuing education event, the manager does not usually pass judgment on the worthiness of the event. Management may, however, request verification of attendance at the program prior to paying wages for the day or days the employee was absent.

A second method of subsidy involves the employer actually assuming the costs for the employee attending an educational session. The employer may underwrite all or part of the costs. A department may budget a set dollar amount for each employee each year, or there may be a departmental budget item that the manager distributes among staff. The employer pays the employee's salary plus part or all of the costs of attendance, including registration, housing, if applicable, transportation, and meals. Under these circumstances, because the employer is actually paying for the employee to attend the event, the employer makes a judgment about the potential value of the continuing education program to the organization. In many cases, the continuing education event must have a direct relationship to the individual's job. For example, a clinical dietitian could get funding to attend a workshop on the Nutrition Care Process, but be denied funds to pay for attendance at a workshop on quilting. Often, the employee is asked to report back to the organization by giving a presentation about the event at a staff meeting or sharing program materials with colleagues.

Another type of subsidy provided by some employers for the continuing education of employees is tuition reimbursement for taking college or university courses. Because this type of subsidy can be costly (especially if the employee enrolls at a private institution), and because the employee is committed for longer periods of time than a day or a week (the usual schedule for meetings or seminars), the procedure for tuition reimbursement is often complex. Typically, the employee enrolls in a course and pays the tuition out of pocket. The employer is informed of the enrollment and how it is related to the employee's job. At the end of the course, the employee must submit the course grade to the employer, who will reimburse the enrollment fee if the employee completed the course and earned the minimum grade specified in the tuition reimbursement policy. This type of tuition reimbursement may be used repeatedly. Many employees find it attractive to complete their bachelor's degree or earn a master's degree while working full time and using this type of funding from their employers.

It is beneficial to both the employer and the employee when the latter continues to learn and to grow while on the job. The staff member benefits by developing more skills that can be brought into the workplace, which, in turn, benefits the organization. Internal education programs (in-services) make sense to keep the employees heading in the same direction and equipped with knowledge about the latest advances in the workplace. External programs also benefit the organization by bringing fresh ideas into the workplace and by providing networking opportunities to staff members. Though the latter can be costly, and may have to be curtailed when budgets are limited, many organizations understand that investing in the continuing education of employees is one way to motivate employees to achieve and maintain a competitive edge.

Continuing education is currently required to maintain the RD and DTR credentials and, in some states, the license to practice as a dietitian. Practitioners develop a personalized learning plan based on their professional needs and goals. Then, over a five-year period, they take advantage of educational opportunities that will assist them in meeting those goals, and document these continuing education activities in a professional portfolio. Many employers find that providing financial assistance to aid individuals in maintaining their credentials is another strong motivator for their professional staff.

performance appraisal

Performance Appraisal. *A tool used by managers to evaluate personnel and to help employees identify their strengths as well as areas that need improvement.*

Employees need to know how they are doing. Too often, managers neglect this aspect of personnel management, and employees are left to figure it out for themselves. The self-assessment may not agree with the manager's evaluation of the employee. It is imperative that managers understand that employees will not be able to improve in problem areas unless they know what the problems are, nor will good behavior be reinforced if employees are not told that they are doing a good job. It is the manager's responsibility to evaluate personnel and to communicate the results to the employees so that they know what their strengths are and where they need to improve. **Performance appraisal** is the tool that is usually used to achieve this end. This tool can be a detailed tool designed to evaluate individuals in a specific position (e.g., dietetic clerk) or it can be more generic, like the one shown in Figure 9.2. No matter which type of form is used, the performance appraisal needs to relate to the specific job the employee is doing, using the job description for the position as its basis.

Figure 9.2 Performance Evaluation

Performance Appraisal – TLC Hospital

Employee Name_____ ID Number_____ Date_____
Position_____ Department _____
Supervior_____ ☐ Annual Review
☐ Other (please specify) _____

Rating scale is as follows:
5 – Exceptional
4 – Exceeds expectations
3 – Meets expectations
2 – Needs improvement
1 – Unsatisfactory

Part I – Core Competencies

Competency	Rating	Supervisor's Comments
Communication – Demonstrates clarity of expression in oral and written work; exhibits good listening skills		
Problem Solving/Decision Making – Identifies problems; includes the views of others in making decisions; acts with integrity		
Inclusiveness – Is respectful of individual differences; promotes fairness and tries to understand other points of view		
Teamwork – Is collaborative; works in partnerships with others		
Environmental Stewardship – Shows integrity and accountability in the utilization of resources		
Leadership – Accepts responsibility for own work; develops trust and credibility		
Customer Service – Understands the needs of internal and external customers and responds appropriately to those needs		
Other (please specify)		

Figure 9.2 Performance Evaluation (continued)

Part II – Goals for Review Period

Goals for this evaluation period	Rating	Supervisors Comments
1.		
2.		
3.		
4.		

Part III – Goals for next review

Goals for upcoming year	Comments
1.	
2.	
3.	
4.	

Part IV – Employee Comments

Signatures:

Employee:_____ Date: _____

My signature indicates that I have received a copy of this review.

Manager/supervisor: Name:_____

Signature: _____ Date: _____

The employee being reviewed is to receive a copy of the completed form

and one copy shall be placed in the personnel file.

To review performance since last review

To evaluate the achievement of goals set at the last review

To identify strengths and areas for growth

To serve as the basis for pay increases, for some, non-contractual employees

To set goals for the next review period

Table 9.1 Purposes for Performance Appraisals

The timing of performance appraisals is often institutionalized. For example, an employee may be evaluated at the end of the probationary period, six months after the hire date, on the first anniversary of employment, and yearly after that. Each scheduled evaluation is a forum to discuss the employee's performance from the time of the previous review. (Performance prior to the previous review is history, and for the most part, not relevant to the discussion.) Strengths and areas for growth, both from the perspective of the supervisor and from that of the employee, should be considered. The performance appraisal is also a time to set goals for the next appraisal period.

Conducting a performance appraisal is similar to conducting any other structured interview. (See Chapter 8.) There are a couple of differences in the preparatory work, however. Usually a performance appraisal uses a standard form that is filled out according to an organization's guidelines. The form will vary from organization to organization; sometimes an organization will have different forms for different classifications of employees. Though the format of the tool is important, it will not be addressed here because it almost always organization-specific.

The form is a tool that may be used in a number of ways. A manager may prepare the form and then meet with the employee to discuss its content. If used in this way, the manager should be prepared to alter the form during or after the discussion, if the employee had substantive comments to add, or disagrees with the manager's assessment. If both the manager and the employee come to an agreement, the form may be revised or amended before it is submitted to human resources. If there is disagreement with what the manager has written, the employee's comments should also be noted on the form.

Some managers use a technique that gives the employee a more participative role in the appraisal process. Both the employee and the manager complete the form independently. (In addition, both parties may write a short statement about the employee's performance and future goals.) The manager then uses these documents to prepare for a meeting with the employee. By having access to both documents in advance, the manager can be prepared to discuss the differences (either positive or negative) that

management practice in dietetics

exist in perceptions. The employee also has the chance to remind the supervisor of things that have been achieved since the previous review.

The goals that were established during the last review are also addressed. Are the goals still valid, or have they changed in light of changes in the workplace? For example, if the employee had a goal to help train three new colleagues during the year, but no new personnel were hired, the goal was not one that could possibly have been achieved. The employee should not be penalized for not meeting the goal. If the goals are still appropriate, progress toward meeting those goals should be identified.

Once all of the documents have been prepared, the manager and the employee sit down and discuss them, reconciling differences and setting goals for the coming year. As with other interviews, the session should begin with positive comments by the manager. This is followed by a review of the employee's performance since the last review, in the form of a dialogue, not a lecture. If the manager has done a good job of communicating with the employee throughout the year, the information in the performance appraisal will not come as a surprise to the employee. Next, goals should be set individually for each employee; these should be negotiated, rather than imposed by the manager. Employees are more apt to work to achieve goals that they have agreed are plausible. On the other hand, an employee may give up if someone else mandates the goals, especially if they are considered to be unreasonable or unachievable. Finally, both the manager and the employee should sign the final document, as amended during the discussion. The interview should end with positive comments by the manager such as "Keep up the good work" or "I know you will continue to improve." A copy of the final document should be placed in the employee's file and another given to the employee for future reference.

When performance appraisals are handled properly, they provide a strong motivational tool for managers to use with employees. Unfortunately, some managers dislike conducting performance appraisals and view this process as a time-consuming task, rather than as a useful tool. Managers are more diligent in keeping up with performance appraisals if some real incentive is attached. This may be a pay increase for the employee that is tied to the completion of the performance appraisal document. In such a case, the employee will actively seek the appraisal in order to become eligible for the raise in pay. Managers who do not conduct timely evaluations of employees under these circumstances are likely to find themselves faced with unhappy and uncooperative subordinates.

It is easier for a manager to evade conducting performance appraisals for employees who work under the umbrella of a contractual labor agreement, or in production jobs where all employees in a certain job classification earn the same rate of pay. These employees are not usually eligible for incremental wage increases related to performance appraisals, so there is little motivation for the employee to actively seek one. However, it is unfair for a manager to avoid doing individual performance assessments for employees just because there is no pay increase associated with the review.

To counter the lack of urgency sometimes associated with performance appraisals for this type of worker, some organizations base the manager's pay increases or bonuses on the timely completion of performance appraisals for their subordinates. This may provide the necessary incentive for the manager to perform this task in a timely manner.

The importance of the performance appraisal should not be underestimated. It opens lines of communication between the employee and the manager. It gives both individuals a chance to discuss successes and problems and to generate ideas about improving how they work together. If the manager creates a non-threatening environment, the employee may express ideas and opinions that help the manager as well. Overall, it is one of the more useful tools that the manager can use. It should be used regularly, in a timely manner, with all employees.

compensation issues

One of the best ways to motivate employees is to increase their wages, or to give them the opportunity to earn more money either as salary or in the form of bonuses. This is outlined in an organization's compensation package. The most important consideration related to compensation is that there needs to be an organized plan for establishing pay rates and for administering the plan uniformly. Well-designed compensation packages are competitive, are internally equitable, and allow for employee growth. The package should recognize the performance of individuals and groups within the organization, giving management some latitude in making decisions related to compensation. However, it should also be structured enough to be presented to employees in a way that is understandable and reflects impartiality. Employees can, and do, share information about compensation. Any attempts to play games with salary administration will be quickly identified and could lead to legal challenges.

Several types of compensation packages are widely used, either alone or in combination. Some organizations have different packages for different types of workers. Salaried workers may be treated differently from hourly workers. Workers represented by one labor union may have a different compensation package from those represented by another. Management personnel may be seen as distinct from non-management professionals. In this section, four basic types of compensation plans will be described: merit, cost of living, single rate, and pay for performance. Though the list is not exhaustive, it does present an overview of the common practices in North America.

merit increases

In addition to providing employees with data about how their performance is viewed by management, the performance appraisal is often used to initiate the paperwork for a pay increase in a system that bases raises on performance. This type of increase is generally called a **merit increase**. When the paperwork for the appraisal is filed, a recommendation is made regarding a suggested pay increase for the employee, based on performance since the last review. Under the merit increase system, in which raises are based on an employee's performance, the performance appraisal serves the dual purposes of communication and of generating pay increases. The percentage of increase in pay is often associated with the overall rating. The terminology and the rates of salary increase will vary from organization to organization, and within the same organization over time. An example is that an employee who does an outstanding job might get a 5 percent raise, one who performs adequately might earn 3 percent, and an employee who is rated as a poor performer might get no raise at all.

It is generally thought that merit increases that are related to performance provide greater incentive for individuals to improve performance than are raises that are based on seniority or cost of living. Thus, many employers have based their compensation packages on salary grades with increments within the grade based on how well an individual performs on the job. For example, consider that the pay grade for a diet clerk has a range of $9.50 to $13.00 per hour and that the employee is earning $10.00 per hour. It might be possible to give that employee a 2 percent raise if performance is adequate or a 5 percent raise if performance is outstanding. A 5 percent raise would bring the salary up to $10.50 per hour. It should be noted, however, that the employee earning $12.50 per hour could not earn a 5 percent raise, because that would bring the hourly pay rate to $13.12, which is above the top of the range. The most a diet clerk can earn in this scenario is $13.00 per hour. Because of this, periodic adjustments are made to the ranges, which allow the people who have reached the top of the scale to earn more money. People at the top of the scale do not usually earn increases as fast as those lower on the scale. Under this type of system, there will be some employees who are not eligible for raises either because they have "maxed out" or because their performance is substandard.

cost-of-living adjustments

Merit increases may stand alone as the organization's compensation package, or may be given in conjunction with cost-of-living increases. **Cost-of-living adjustments (COLAs)** are increases based on inflation rates and are used to keep an employee's purchasing power intact over time. It should be noted, though, that in times of economic downturn, when inflation is negligible, COLAs may not be given at all. When the COLA system is used, the increases are given to everyone in the organization. In the past, cost-of-living compensation programs were sometimes the only (or the primary) compensation system for an organization. This is no longer the norm. When it is used, it is usually in conjunction with a merit or a pay for performance compensation program. Under the combined COLA and merit-based compensation system, the individual employee may be given an automatic adjustment in pay on an annual basis (cost of living), perhaps at the end of a company's fiscal year, and a merit increase on the anniversary of the hire date.

Merit Increase. *Pay raises that are based on employee performance. These raises change the base pay rate permanently.*

Cost-of-Living Adjustments (COLAs). *Pay raises that are based on inflation rates and are used to keep an employee's purchasing power intact despite economic changes over time. These raises change the base pay rate permanently.*

Single Rate. *Pay raises that are universal and given to all employees either on an anniversary date or on an annual basis. It rewards employees equally, as long as their work falls within the standard range. This pay increase results in a permanent adjustment in the base pay rate.*

Pay for Performance. *Incentive-pay programs that may be used alone or in combination with other compensation plans to reward employees based on performance. These are one-time incentives that do not change the base pay rate.*

Annual Bonus. *One type of pay for performance that is earned at the end of the year for outstanding performance during that year. It usually results from meeting a pre-established goal. This is a one-time bonus that does not change the base pay rate.*

In such situations, the merit increase may be less than that which might have been awarded if there had been no cost-of-living increase. For example, the employee with outstanding performance might get a 3 percent cost-of-living increase and a 3 percent merit increase. In this type of program, even an employee who does not perform well is eligible for the cost-of-living increase. This allows poor performers to maintain their purchasing power, while outstanding performers have the potential to make substantial gains over time.

single rate systems

Some employers give no merit increases at all, but rather rely on across-the-board increases to all employees, either on an anniversary date or on an annual basis. There may be a separate starting rate that is used until a new employee reaches the same level of productivity as more seasoned peers. This compensation system is referred to as **single rate**. The raises are universal and have nothing to do with individual performance. This type of compensation package is most appropriate in situations in which many employees have similar jobs and there are clear standards for both the quality and quantity of performance. It rewards all employees equally, as long as their work falls within the performance requirements. This type of compensation program should not be used in situations in which worker productivity can vary significantly. Single-rate systems are frequently used in unionized settings, where the compensation package for all union members is negotiated by the union and guaranteed by contract. When this type of compensation system is used, the increases apply to everyone in the organization. This is a permanent increase to the base pay rate.

pay for performance

Pay for performance is an umbrella term that covers a number of different programs that may be used, either alone or in combination with other compensation plans. When they are used for individuals, they allow for individual workers to be compensated at different levels than others, depending on the achievement of pre-established goals. However, the financial gains are not always cumulative, as are the types of increases previously described.

One type of pay for performance is the **annual bonus** that some personnel earn at the end of the year if performance meets or exceeds expectations. It is usually based on meeting a measurable goal—for example, financial, productivity, or quality related. For example, if a sales representative exceeded the projected sales volume for the year, a bonus might be awarded that is equivalent to 30 percent or more of that individual's annual base pay. The theory behind this type of program, sometimes called

variable pay, is that 30 percent is more motivating to an individual than 2 percent would be. When this type of program is in place, the base salary is often lower than it would be if there were no bonus program. A major advantage is that the employee can earn large bonuses for outstanding performance.

The bonus programs may cover only executives, may be extended to all managerial levels, or may be extended to all employees. If it covers a large number of employees, the program provides the organization with a degree of protection during years when business is not good. Because base salaries are lower, the organization can still pay the usual wages and eliminate bonuses during bad years, rather than having to lay off experienced workers. This type of bonus program is being used in all types of organizations, including hospitals and other health care facilities. With this type of bonus plan, however, the employee is not guaranteed more money each year—that is, total compensation for each employee is variable from year to year depending on performance.

Performance bonuses are sometimes applied to work groups or departments within an organization instead of to individuals. Under this type of system, the entire group earns additional pay when the group meets certain goals. The downside of this type of program, especially when it is used throughout an organization for teams of workers, is that it may alienate individual achievers and may lower their productivity to the level of the group. There is greater motivation for an individual to perform well when results can be directly linked to the work that the individual performs, rather than to the group.

A second type of pay for performance is a one-time **cash award** for outstanding performance, for a significant contribution that an employee made to the organization, or for earning recognition through a program such as employee of the year, employee of the month, and so on. Such programs are varied and may range from a small check for helping out a colleague, to a finder's fee for bringing a new employee into the organization, to a percentage of the first year's savings for the employee who develops a money-saving procedure for the organization. This type of award may range from small to very large. Such awards provide motivation for employees to extend themselves beyond the requirements of the job to be creative, innovative, helpful, or just a good citizen. Rewarding this type of behavior in a substantial and public way motivates the employee to continue this type of activity and encourages others in the organization to become aware of the potential for such recognition.

Other pay-for-performance programs are related to skill development. Individuals are compensated, not on their productivity at any one time, but on the basis of the skills that they have acquired and the number of tasks that they are able to perform. This type of program rewards individuals who are cross-trained, by paying them more for their versatility. To be effective, this type of program must be supported by adequate in-service training opportunities for staff, so that there is ample opportunity for them to learn how to do various jobs in the organization.

Variable Pay. *A compensation plan in which an employee receives a base salary or hourly wage and then an added bonus based on performance.*

Cash Award. *A pay-for-performance plan that awards cash to employees for being creative, innovative, helpful, or just a good citizen. It is usually a one-time award.*

In this section, a few types of pay for performance programs have been described. This list is not exhaustive. Options for pay-for-performance programs are only beginning to be identified. However, like other types of compensation programs, these programs must be well defined, clearly communicated, applied equitably, and evaluated periodically to determine their effectiveness.

nonfinancial incentives

Sometimes it is not possible for an organization to give financial rewards to employees who perform well. This is often the case in start-up organizations, where all excess dollars must be reinvested to support growth. It also occurs when companies are in financial difficulty (which may or may not be associated with a poor economy). When this type of situation prevails, other types of incentives can help to motivate individual employees. These types of tools may not be as effective as financial rewards, but they are something that can be used by managers to recognize good performance when money is tight. They can also be used in conjunction with financial rewards, as an additional motivational tool, when adequate resources are available.

One way to reward good performance is by naming an "Employee of the Month" and awarding that individual a designated parking space.

The types of recognition that can be implemented at little or no additional cost to employers include such things as a specially designated parking place (for example, reserved for the employee of the month) close to the entrance to the building. Another might be a news release to the local newspaper by the public relations department, recognizing an achievement, an award earned, or an increase in responsibility. Plaques or trophies, or a framed certificate that can be displayed in or near the work area, also provide public recognition for a job well done.

These methods can be used to recognize group as well as individual achievements. Several examples follow. The number of days without an accident at the work site can be posted to encourage safety in the workplace. Productivity numbers, like the number of meals that a foodservice produces each week, can be posted so employees can see how much they accomplish. Sales figures are often represented on a drawing of a thermometer, which shows how the sales force is performing in relation to the goal. It is nice for the manager to be aware of such data, but if the employees are also made aware of it, then they can work with management to improve performance, set records, and achieve goals.

Sometimes just a pat on the back and a public compliment from the manager are enough to motivate employees. Even though it is important to discuss problems with employees in

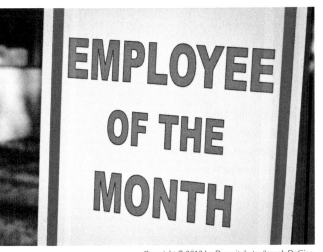

management practice in dietetics

private, sometimes managers "slip" and show their dissatisfaction with an employee's behavior or performance in public. That is not appropriate. However, it is appropriate to praise an employee for a job well done where the praise can be heard and recognized by others. It is important that the praise be genuine and be administered equitably. Employees are motivated to perform well if they know that what they are doing is being noted and appreciated by their superiors.

Other nonfinancial rewards are those that can give the employee a sense of accomplishment or satisfaction. Employees can be offered additional training in an area that interests them. Clinical DTRs may wish to gain some supervisory experience so that they can become eligible for promotion to higher levels of management. A foodservice worker may want to apprentice to a cook to gain new skills in that area. A dietitian might be encouraged to use some work time to do some committee work for the local dietetic association. Even if a manager cannot afford to pay expenses for continuing education meetings, an internally administered journal club can be organized to keep staff current on professional topics. Departmental subscriptions to journals or newsletters (preferably chosen by staff members) will allow dietitians to feel that their professional needs are being supported by management. Listening and following up on staff suggestions can go a long way to keeping staff members motivated.

job mobility

The last issue to be addressed in this chapter is that of job mobility. This is an area that can be highly motivating or it can be very counterproductive, depending on how it is handled by the manager. It is natural for a manager to want to develop a productive workforce with high standards of quality. However, once that is achieved, managers like the comfort level that has been reached and often try to maintain the status quo. It takes an astute and secure manager to understand that many employees need to feel that there is potential for upward mobility. Otherwise, they may become frustrated and unhappy in what they perceive as "dead-end" jobs. There is little motivation to continue to perform at a high level if one cannot identify some sort of reward at the end of a certain period of time. Not all employees feel the need for advancement to the same degree, and individuals may be more apt to seek advancement during some periods in their lives and not in others. When significant changes are going on in people's personal lives, they are likely to want stability in the workplace.

Job mobility does not necessarily mean upward mobility within an organization. Many moves are lateral, rather than upward. Such moves can be justified if the individual wants or needs to learn new skills to become eligible for promotion at some later date. Moves can also be outward—that is, movement to a different

Job Mobility.
The ability of an employee to change jobs. Moves can be downward, upward, or lateral within an organization, or can be a move to another organization.

Downward Mobility. *When an employee reverts to a previous or lower position in an organization.*

organization—if the current organization offers little opportunity for growth. On occasion, individuals may opt to decline an upward move or opt for **downward mobility** in order to lessen their responsibility or workload. The latter may occur when a person wants to spend more time on family matters, needs to recover from an illness, chooses to lower the level of personal stress, or feels the need for more balance in life. When individuals seek to remain in a role or revert to a previous and perhaps less-prestigious position, their wishes should be respected and honored, if possible.

Upward Mobility. *When an employee is promoted to a higher position in an organization.*

Providing for **upward mobility** does not necessarily mean that a manager should train all staff members to take over the boss's job. Still, it is necessary for a manager to be able to identify when someone has stopped growing in his or her job and give that person new opportunities for growth. As mentioned earlier, the individual may make a **lateral move** in order to learn new skills. It may mean that the manager trains a replacement so that both individuals can move upward. It may mean that the manager is willing to let (or even help) the employee move out of the organization, even though that means that the status quo will be disturbed and the flow of work disrupted for some time. An effective manager understands that there is a time for some employees to move on; if there are no opportunities within an organization when that time arrives, the employee must be encouraged to seek opportunities elsewhere. Even the very best employees should not be cajoled into staying for the convenience of the organization, especially if the job they are doing is no longer satisfying to them.

Lateral Move. *When an employee takes a new position at the same organizational level as the former position. This is sometimes done so the employee can learn new skills.*

conclusion

In this chapter, several of the tools for employee development and motivation have been presented. The materials presented include the following key concepts.

1. New employees need to be welcomed into an organization with an orientation to both the job and to the organization itself.
2. Employee development includes internal programs, called in-services, and continuing education opportunities outside of the organization.
3. Performance appraisals are an effective tool for managers and employees to evaluate performance and to set goals for future development.
4. Organizations use different kinds of compensation programs to motivate employees to perform well and to reward them for good performance or longevity.
5. Compensation programs should be competitive, allow for employee growth, be well defined, and be equitably administered.
6. Nonfinancial motivational tools, though not always as effective as financial ones, can be used as a substitute for, or in conjunction with, financial incentives.

activities

activity 1

Design an interview schedule that focuses on issues related to performance appraisal and employee motivation, including at least three queries on each of these topics. Interview a manager in your geographic region using the interview schedule as a guide to direct your interaction. Write a brief paper comparing what you learned from the manager with what is discussed in this chapter.

activity 2

Brainstorm to create a list of methods that can be used by managers to motivate employees. You may come up with some creative ideas if you consider what makes you perform well in school. Estimate the cost of each of the methods listed. (For example, a pay raise of $1.00 per hour for a full-time employee will cost $2,080.00 per year for as long as the employee continues to work for the organization. A one-time bonus could cost a lump sum of $1,000.00 with no long-term consequences.) It is likely that all of the methods listed can be used in times when an organization is in good financial health. Determine which of the methods on the list can be used during periods of austerity when budgets are tight. These will be the methods that have a relatively low cost.

activity 3

Look through journals, in professional newsletters and websites, on departmental bulletin boards, in college catalogs, and so on, to find out what kind of continuing education activities are available in your area. Assuming that you are a dietetics professional, write a proposal to your manager describing the activity you want to participate in, stating the cost of the activity, and providing a rationale for the organization to pay your expenses for this activity.

to study further

The following materials are useful in developing a more in-depth knowledge of employee development, performance appraisal, and compensation issues.

- Armstrong, M. *Armstrong's Handbook of Reward Management Practice: Improving Performance Through Reward*. 4th ed. Philadelphia: Kogan Page, 2012.
- Arthur, D. *The First-Time Manager's Guide to Performance Appraisals*. New York: AMACOM, 2008.
- Arthur, D. *Recruiting, Interviewing, Selecting, and Orienting New Employees*. 5th ed. New York: AMACOM, 2012.
- Cascio, W. F. *Managing Human Resources: Productivity, Quality of Work Life, Profits*. 9th ed. New York: McGraw-Hill/Irwin, 2012.
- Chingos, P. T. *Paying for Performance: A Guide to Compensation Management*. 2nd ed. New York: Wiley, 2002.
- Falcone, P. and R. T. Sachs. *Productive Performance Appraisals*. 2nd ed. New York: AMACOM, 2008.
- Gryna, F. *Work Overload! Redesigning Jobs to Minimize Stress and Burnout*. Milwaukee: ASQ Quality Press, 2004.
- McKenzie, R. B. and D. R. Lee. *Managing Through Incentives: How to Build a More Collaborative, Productive, and Profitable Organization*. New York: Oxford University Press, 1998.
- Milkovich, G. T., J. M. Newman, and B. Gerhart. *Compensation*. 10th ed. New York: McGraw-Hill/Irwin, 2010.
- Shell, Richard L. *Management of Professionals*. 2nd ed. New York: Marcel Dekker, 2003.
- Statt, David A. *Psychology and the World of Work*. 2nd ed. New York: Palgrave Macmillan, 2004.
- Steers, Richard M., Lyman W. Porter, and Gregory A. Bigley. *Motivation and Leadership at Work*. 6th ed. New York: McGraw-Hill, 1996.

scholarly journals

- *Journal of Applied Psychology*
- *The Journal of Social Psychology*
- *Healthcare Management Review*
- *Labor Studies Journal*

other relevant periodical

- *HR Magazine*

relevant websites

- Society for Human Resource Management http://www.shrm.org/pages/default. aspx
- Archer North's Performance Appraisal: The Complete Online Guide http:// www.performance-appraisal.com/home.htm
- Employers of America http://employerhelp.org/

in practice

motivation in a union environment

Many nutrition professionals manage employees who belong to a labor union; some dietitians and dietetic technicians are represented by labor unions as well. Labor unions first arose in the late 1800s during the industrial revolution. They were established to protect workers from unsafe work conditions, poor wages, and unreasonably long hours. Individual workers could hardly make an impact on these practices, but organized groups of workers could effect strikes and work slowdowns designed to disrupt productivity and profitability of businesses that have unfair labor practices. In North America, labor unions have had a major effect on the work life in general, not just for union members. Many of the reforms that have occurred in all work settings are rooted in union activities. Issues like minimum wage, the 40-hour work week, overtime pay, and worker's compensation were addressed by unions before they were mandated by federal or local laws.

In a perfect world, labor unions would not need to exist, because all businesses would be fair and honest with their workers and all labor practices would be humane. There would never be favoritism or harassment, discrimination or bias. But since this is not always the case, labor unions are still a part of the American workplace.

The body of law that regulates labor unions and their relationship with the parent organizations is complex. In the United States, the National Labor Relations Act is administered by the National Labor Relations Board, an independent federal agency established in 1935. See http://www.nlrb.gov/.

In today's workplace, labor unions represent their membership in many areas. They negotiate wages and differential wages, work hours, insurance benefits, worker's compensation, paid time off, and working conditions for those they represent. The union may also negotiate other conditions of employment, like paid release time for continuing education. Another responsibility of the labor union is to define what constitutes the worker's jobs, which can be done only by union members, and what constitutes management jobs that cannot be done by represented employees. In general, managers should not do union work and union members should not participate in management.

The results of these negotiations between management and the labor union are set forth in a contract, usually covering a specific period of time (say three years). It should be noted, too, that representatives of workers are involved in the negotiation process and that labor contracts are ratified by a vote of union members. That contract between the organization and the labor union is binding. All employees doing a specific job and having the same seniority get a set rate of pay. Jobs are predefined. Benefits are set, as are opportunities for continuing education. Even layoffs are prescribed in the contract. When RIFs occur, the employees that are retained are those with the most seniority, not necessarily those with the best performance.

In some cases, there may be multiple unions involved in a single work setting. For example, within a foodservice, the cooks may belong to one union, the foodservice workers to another, the dietetic technicians and clerks to a third, and the dietitians to a fourth union. This makes for a fairly complex management environment, since each union will negotiate different contracts with the parent organization, which means that each group of workers is subject to negotiated wages and benefits, which may differ from those of the other groups of workers. This causes confusion for both employees and managers, because things like pay differential and benefits may differ on a contract-by-contract basis. It is important to be cognizant of the intricacies of each contract when working in a multi-union environment so that contractual obligations are met for all.

One of the outcomes of working with union contracts is that many of the motivational tools that are available to management in non-contractual settings are not particularly useful when there is a labor contract to be followed. Management does not have the authority to give pay raises based on merit or performance because pay rates are preset. Supervisors cannot preferentially assign overtime hours to those who request it, since this too is defined by contract, and is usually based on seniority. It may not be possible to promote individuals from one position to another because of provisions in the contracts.

That being the case, managers must become more creative at motivating their employees. One of the best ways to do that is with well-thought-out, timely performance appraisals. It was mentioned earlier that managers in contractual settings may not do performance appraisals on time since there is no pay increase associated with the evaluation, and thus employees may be indifferent to the process. This is a mistake. The performance appraisal serves as a formal tool that can be used to praise the employee for tasks done well and to identify areas where performance can be improved. It is a strong motivational tool.

Other employee recognition programs like "Employee of the Month" or monetary incentives for suggestions that are implemented by the organization encourage unionized workers to participate at the organizational level. It is also important to recognize good performance on a day-to-day basis with smiles, a pat on the back, or a sincere "Job well done" from the manager. When managers take notice of how individuals are doing their jobs and what contributions they are making to the organization, the opportunities for positive reinforcement and motivation are myriad.

Many managers feel that it is burdensome to work in a unionized setting and that the mere fact of the union's existence sets up an antagonistic relationship between managers and employees. This is counterproductive. A good manager/leader will treat employees with fairness and empathy whether a union is present or not.

references

1. Wanous, John P. "Newcomer Orientation Programs that Facilitate Organizational Entry." In *Personnel Selection and Assessment, Individual and Organizational Perspectives,* Heinz Schuler, James L. Farr, and Mike Smith, eds. Hillsdale, NJ: Lawrence Erlbaum Associates, 1993

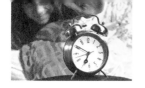

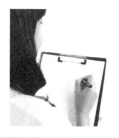

chapter ten

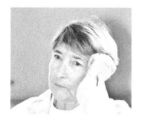

employee discipline

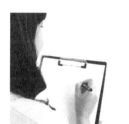

learning objectives

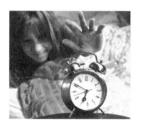

1. State the purpose of employee discipline.

2. List common reasons that employees are disciplined.

3. Identify the reasons for having a written disciplinary policy and procedure.

4. Describe the components of a disciplinary policy.

5. List the steps included in the disciplinary procedure.

6. Discuss the importance of timeliness in employee discipline.

7. Define *progressive discipline*.

8. Describe how to conduct each type of disciplinary action.

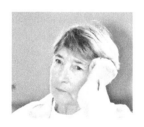

9. List situations in which the employee may be terminated without following progressive discipline.

10. Describe the types of documentation necessary during progressive discipline.

11. Define *positive discipline*.

12. Discuss employee assistance programs in conjunction with discipline.

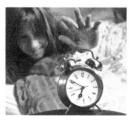

13. Identify the employee's rights when there is a conflict with management.

14. Discuss the grievance process in a nonunionized workplace.

15. Write a policy and procedure for employee grievances.

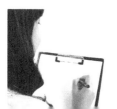

overview

The disciplining of employees is not the most pleasant part of being a manager. Nevertheless, it is an important part of the management role, included under the staffing function. Every manager needs to have the basic skills involved in employee discipline. Discipline is a process that must be used as necessary, and not avoided by the manager. However, the use of discipline must be tempered with compassion and understanding. It is not a tool to be used vindictively or as a way of displaying power. In fact, when it is well done, it is another management tool that can be used for employee development.

In this chapter, guidelines for the appropriate use of discipline will be described, starting with the need for a written disciplinary policy and accompanying procedures. The components of the policy will be discussed, as will the steps that are usually included in the procedure and the documentation that is necessary to support the process.

The final step in the disciplinary process is termination of the employee. Because it is a costly proposition, emotionally and financially, it may sometimes be necessary to explore other options. Alternatives to termination will be discussed, along with the positive and negative aspects of these alternatives. The chapter will close with consideration of what employees can do if they feel that they have been treated unfairly. This section describes the grievance procedure.

the purpose of employee discipline

The underlying concept behind the disciplining of employees is to improve the work environment for all by eliminating or minimizing the chance for unsafe, abusive, or disruptive behavior in the workplace. It can also be used to improve the performance of an employee, in terms of either the quality or the quantity of work done. Generally it is used after coaching or performance appraisals have failed to elicit desired behavioral changes.

Employee Discipline. *A tool used by managers to improve poor performance and enforce appropriate behavior to ensure a productive and safe workplace.*

Employee discipline, sometimes called "corrective action," is generally thought of as something negative. It is perceived as the use of coercive power to punish an individual who has done something wrong. Although the disciplinary process is sometimes perceived as punishment, that should not be its purpose. The purpose of discipline is to encourage a worker to replace an inappropriate behavior with a more appropriate behavior, which contributes to a safe, pleasant, and productive workplace for staff and for management, too. A list of the types of behaviors and performance issues that warrant disciplinary action can be found in Table 10.1.

Issues Related to Conduct	Tardiness
	Absenteeism
	Insubordination
	Negligence
	Fighting
	Stealing
	Falsification of documents
	Abusiveness
	Harassment
	Use of obscene language
	Possession of a controlled substance
	Reporting to work under the influence of alcohol or other controlled drug
	Substance abuse
	Infractions of published work rules (for example, dress code, safety procedures, and so on)
Issues Related to Performance	Low productivity
	High error rate, overall
	Repetition of a specific error

Table 10.1 Typical Reasons for Disciplining Employees

Consider, for example, the employee who is chronically late in arriving for work. The lateness may affect the employee's compensation (if hourly wages are paid), and it will also have an effect on the productivity of the work group and on the morale of other workers who must "pick up the slack" until the tardy employee arrives at work. But the tardy employee is trained to do the job and, in that sense, is an asset to the work group. It is far better to work with the individual to find ways to solve the tardiness problem than to punish the worker for being late. The real goal is to eliminate the inappropriate behavior and create a win-win situation for the whole group.

Not all managers see discipline in this way. There are some managers who try to use the disciplinary process to "get even with" or to "get rid of" problem employees. This is imprudent for a number of reasons. First, the time and energy involved in going through the disciplinary process is substantial. One has to participate in numerous meetings with the employee and produce a seemingly endless amount of paperwork to get to the point of termination. When termination does occur, there is no guarantee that it will be sustained through a series of appeals. In addition, the replacement worker may not perform any better than the one being replaced. Finally, there is significant dollar cost for recruiting, hiring, and training the replacement worker.

There are managers who prefer to avoid conflict at all costs and who do not use discipline when it is appropriate or necessary. This is also problematic. Though it may be less stressful to the manager to ignore the negative behavior (for example, chronic tardiness) and pretend that it is not a problem, the consequences relating to work-group morale and productivity can be devastating. In the long run, the problem will intensify until something has to be done. However, lack of precedent in enforcing work rules over time will make it difficult for the manager to discipline the employee. Sometimes the only way to deal with long-term but ignored behavioral or performance problems in employees is to replace the supervisor with someone who is willing to enforce work rules and set performance standards.

It is inevitable that some employees will end up being terminated for inability or unwillingness to correct poor performance or improper behavior. This is seldom easy to do, and most managers feel little sense of accomplishment after terminating an employee (even a notably difficult one). It is unsettling to the work group to lose a colleague in this way. Furthermore, because a manager must respect the confidentiality of the terminated worker, it is not possible to justify the action taken in order to placate the rest of the staff. Some effective leaders even view the termination of an employee as a failure in themselves, because they were unable to help the employee work through the problem successfully.

Disciplinary Process. *A step-by-step method of dealing with performance problems in employees.*

Thus, employee discipline should be viewed as a necessary part of the manager's staffing function. It should be carried out as required to improve performance or to correct inappropriate behavior, but it should never be used with the sole purpose of punishing a particular employee. Managers should approach the **disciplinary process** as they do any other management function, with consistency and fairness for all employees.

organizational policy and procedure

Policy and Procedure (P&P). *A written standard used within an organization to describe what is to be done and how to do it. Usually policies and procedures are written for tasks that are done repeatedly and by more than one individual.*

Large organizations have a human resources department, which is responsible for personnel issues, including recruitment, hiring, employee benefits, compensation, and employee discipline. It is traditional for the human resources department to develop a policy and procedure manual to direct managers on the processes involving these and other personnel matters. This manual will have at least one **policy and procedure (P&P)** governing employee discipline and termination. An organization may actually have more than one disciplinary P&P if the process differs for different groups of workers. For example, there may be a different method for dealing with discipline for hourly workers than there is for salaried employees. Unionized employees are usually subject to guidelines that are different from those used for nonunionized groups. It is also possible that an organization may have one P&P for employee discipline and another for termination.

Often a small organization does not have a human resources department and may function without written human resources policies (sometimes known as personnel policies). These organizations may have few discipline problems and do not feel the need to have written policies. At a minimum, all organizations must comply with federal and state regulations that govern the termination of employees. They are required to follow whatever legal mandates are in place. (In California, for example, the employee must receive a final paycheck at the time of termination.)

As companies grow, the human resources function expands and the number of managers increases. It usually becomes necessary to put a P&P manual in place. Small companies can acquire a generic human resources policy and procedure manual, and adapt the individual P&Ps to match the organization's needs and philosophy. These tools are available in hard copy, in software packages, and on the Internet. Often these manuals are posted on the organization's website.

importance of a written disciplinary policy and procedure

As with other P&Ps, the one related to employee discipline is written to ensure some degree of consistency among the various managers who use it. It builds in protection for the organization and the manager, and at the same time guarantees the rights of the employee. Every manager has access to the same information and must follow the stated procedure. Similarly, the employee will have access to this information (perhaps in a different format) in the employee handbook. If there is no employee handbook, the employee should be allowed access to the disciplinary P&P upon request.

In addition, the written P&P is a guide that teaches managers how to administer discipline. If followed, it ensures that the manager will function within the law and in concert with the stated philosophy of the organization. The disciplinary P&P can be thought of as a preventive tool in that it helps organizations and managers avoid making costly mistakes.

components of policies and procedures

Each policy and procedure should be formatted to include certain components. The policy section of the document should include a clear statement of the policy and the purpose for the policy. These two items may be included as part of one statement, or stated as two distinct entities, but both need to be stated in one way or another. The policy may also include a listing of who is covered by the policy. The procedure section of the document includes a step-by-step description of what is to be done. A discussion of each of these components follows.

policy statement. The **policy statement** is a declaration of what the organization's official position is on the topic. The policy may be: "In order to provide a safe and positive workplace for all, employees are expected to comply with standards of conduct and performance while on the job. When standards are not met, **progressive discipline** will be used as a way of encouraging an employee to meet the standards." Note that the policy statement is presented in a positive, nonthreatening manner.

purpose. The policy also includes a **statement of purpose** explaining the intended use of the policy. It may also include an indication of the organization's philosophy as it relates to this policy. The statement of purpose for the disciplinary policy stated above could be: "This policy serves as a means to deal with problems related to poor performance or inappropriate conduct. It is to be administered equitably and consistently, with emphasis on correcting the problem rather than on punishing the employee." Depending on the format chosen by the organization, the policy statement and the statement of purpose may be presented as a unified whole, or as two separate entities.

scope. The **scope** is an optional part of the policy. It is a statement or list of individuals or groups that are impacted by the policy. If there were only one disciplinary policy for an organization, the scope would be "all employees." If there are differing disciplinary policies or procedures for different subgroups of employees, the scope could be "all unrepresented employees." This implies that a different policy and/or different procedures have been established for unionized employees. If the scope lists "hourly workers," then it is assumed that there are alternate methods in place to deal with exempt employees.

It is not always necessary to state the scope of a policy. This is usually reserved for use in very complex organizations. A privately owned health club with 50 employees would probably not need to include the scope for a policy, because it has a small number of employees doing similar types of jobs. On the other hand, an urban teaching medical center with multiple unions, several levels of management, and many different kinds of professional staff might find it helpful to list the scope as an addition to a policy. See Figure 10.1, Example B.

procedure. The **procedure** is a step-by-step outline of what should happen, the order in which events will occur, and the timelines to be followed, if any. Its specificity will be determined by the organizational needs. In general, larger organizations with many managers at different levels will need to have a more detailed policy than a smaller company whose few managers are all at the same level. It should be noted that procedures should be stated as simply and concisely as possible. Procedures that are too detailed and complex may interfere with the managers' ability to respond differently to different situations, thus interfering with their ability to manage. On the other hand, the procedures should be clear and complete enough to serve as guidelines for use in most circumstances.

management practice in dietetics

```
┌─────────────────────────────────────────────────────────────────────────────┐
│  Example A                                                                    │
│                         Employee Discipline                                   │
│                                                                               │
│  Policy:       In order to provide a safe and positive workplace for all,     │
│                employees are expected to comply with standards of conduct     │
│                and performance while on the job. When standards are not met,   │
│                employee discipline will be used as a way of encouraging an     │
│                employee to meet the standards. Managers are to administer      │
│                discipline equitably and consistently, with emphasis on         │
│                correcting the problem rather than punishing the employee.      │
│                                                                               │
│  Procedure:    1.                                                             │
│                2.                                                             │
│                3.                                                             │
│                4.                                                             │
│                                                                               │
│  ───────────────────────────────────────────────────────────────────────     │
│                                                                               │
│  Example B                                                                    │
│                         Employee Discipline                                   │
│                                                                               │
│  Policy:       In order to provide a safe and positive workplace for all,     │
│                employees are expected to comply with standards of conduct      │
│                and performance while on the job. When standards are not met,   │
│                employee discipline will be used as a way of encouraging an     │
│                employee to meet the standards.                                │
│                                                                               │
│  Purpose:      This policy serves as a means to deal with problems related     │
│                to poor performance or inappropriate conduct. It is to be       │
│                administered equitably and consistently, with emphasis on       │
│                correcting the problem rather than punishing the employee.      │
│                                                                               │
│  Scope:        All non-supervisory staff.                                     │
│                                                                               │
│  Procedure:    1.                                                             │
│                2.                                                             │
│                3.                                                             │
│                4.                                                             │
│  ───────────────────────────────────────────────────────────────────────     │
└─────────────────────────────────────────────────────────────────────────────┘
```

Figure 10.1 Formats for Disciplinary Policy and Procedure

Another consideration when writing or implementing a disciplinary procedure is that discipline must take place as soon as possible after the problem occurred. (Note that not all P&Ps need to include time as a point of reference—for example, there will usually not be a need for time frames in a policy related to the type of attire to be worn at work.) It would be unfair to take disciplinary action against an employee in December for an occurrence that happened three months earlier. Time frames are included in those human resource P&Ps when it would be inappropriate or unsafe to delay action for a significant amount of time. (Time frames may also be needed in operational policies. For example, the policy on nutritional screening will include how soon the screening is to occur in relationship to the patient's admission to the hospital; the policy on how to determine kilocaloric needs for a patient would not need to have a timeline included.)

The procedure that is specific to employee discipline and termination usually has a minimum of four steps. These are verbal warning, written warning, suspension, and termination. Thus, a basic procedure for employee discipline might read:

1. The manager will meet with the employee to discuss the behavioral or performance problem that has been identified. This interview will take place within five days of the most recent event.
2. If this problem recurs within 90 days, the manager will have a second interview with the employee, during which a written warning will be issued and placed in the employee's file. The written warning will be issued within five days of the event described in the written warning.
3. If there is another occurrence of this problem within six months of the date of the written warning, the manager will suspend the employee for two to four days without pay. The suspension must be initiated within five days of the incident that led to the suspension.
4. If this problem recurs within a year of the date of the suspension, the employee will be terminated. Termination must occur within five days of the incident that led to termination.

There are some items of note in the procedure outlined here. First, all steps in the process refer back to the same underlying behavioral or performance problem. For example, if a **disciplinary action** was taken because of tardiness, the discipline can progress to the next step only for additional incidences of tardiness. If the same employee exhibits a different behavioral problem—for example, making a verbal threat to a coworker—a separate disciplinary process would have to be initiated. One cannot escalate through progressive discipline to the next level for different problems. Therefore, it is possible that an individual employee could be the subject of more than one disciplinary process at a time.

Second, the disciplinary process stops when a prescribed period of time has elapsed without repetition of the same behavioral or performance problem. Generally, the elapsed time is dependent on how far the process has progressed before the behavior was corrected. In the procedure outlined, any record of progressive discipline will be voided if 90 days pass after a verbal warning, but not until one year has passed from the date of a suspension.

Finally, the procedure shown here is very basic and outlines the minimum number of steps needed for employee discipline and termination. A disciplinary process for another organization or for a different group of employees within the same organization may include a second written warning before the process escalates to suspension. In the "In Practice" feature located at the end of this chapter, a more-detailed disciplinary procedure is presented. It is a policy that is used for a large academic institution, which includes both a traditional campus and a teaching medical center. Note that two options in addition to verbal warning, written warning, suspension and termination are included in this policy.

Employee discipline is necessary in some situations. In organizations with many managers who may be administering discipline, it is useful to have a published P&P related to employee discipline. This is done to ensure consistency in how the process is administered and to safeguard the organization from the improper use of discipline. It also protects the employee from arbitrary action by management. Once a P&P is in place, it can be implemented as needed for the purpose of improving employee performance. The following section describes how to go about carrying out employee discipline by using the procedure described earlier in this section.

the disciplinary process

Progressive discipline is usually carried out after a problem behavior with an employee has been identified and the manager has attempted to coach the employee about the problem. Often this coaching is enough to resolve the problem. The problem may also have been addressed during the employee's annual performance appraisal. If the problem has not been resolved with these tools, the disciplinary process should be initiated. When this is the case, discipline is easier to carry out if there is a written policy and procedure to guide a manager than when no such procedure is in place. A manager who has never conducted a disciplinary action before, or who does so infrequently, would benefit from consultation with an experienced colleague, a superior, or a human resources specialist before initiating such an action. Similar consultation is also warranted if the circumstances or event leading to the initiation of the disciplinary action is unusual.

The discussion that follows is meant to serve as a guide for managing the disciplinary process. It is not intended to be an exhaustive explanation of all of the issues that might be anticipated, but an overview of those that are frequently present during the process.

verbal warning

The **verbal warning** is usually the formal first step in employee discipline. It entails meeting with the employee and stating that the problem has been identified and then listening to the employee's perspective of the situation. In most organizations, documentation of this meeting is kept by the manager, but it does not become an official part of the employee's personnel file. (Occasionally, an organization may require that a copy of the documentation on verbal warnings be forwarded to the human resources department.) The meeting is more of an information exchange interview than it is anything else. The employee learns that a problem has been identified by management and is given a chance to explain what happened from his perspective. Together, the manager and the employee discuss potential solutions, and the manager informs the employee of possible consequences if the problem is not resolved.

Verbal Warning.
The first step in employee discipline, which includes identification of the problem and information sharing between the manager and the employee.

Employees cannot be disciplined for something that they do not know about. For example, if employees were never told that wearing nail polish while working on trayline was against the departmental dress code, they can not be disciplined for wearing polish. In the case of an individual employee wearing nail polish, the interview will be used as a training session, to review the dress code with the employee. This informational interview would not be considered to be a disciplinary action, but it would be noted that "the dress code was reviewed with the employee on December 12th." This is an example of coaching.

The verbal warning should not take place until some other things have happened. First, there must be awareness that a behavioral or performance problem exists, followed by verification that it is real. Using the example of a tardy employee, it is unlikely that a single instance of tardiness will lead to disciplinary action. It is likely that a coworker will "cover for" a tardy colleague if the tardiness is a first or an occasional event. Many managers are forgiving of occasional tardiness, knowing that transportation problems, minor emergencies, problems related to childcare, and so on are inevitable. Thus, it is unlikely that arriving late to work on a single occasion will justify a verbal warning. Such occasions are, however, opportunities for coaching the employee about the importance of arriving to work on time.

When the tardiness becomes a real disciplinary problem, it may already be a persistent one. The manager may learn of the problem by direct observation, from other staff members, or through another route, such as reviewing payroll or productivity reports. Whenever the manager becomes aware of the probable existence of a problem, it becomes necessary to investigate to determine if it is an actual problem or merely a matter of perception. The number of instances of tardiness over a specified period of time must be documented. If the employee is one whose work time is monitored automatically (for example, through the use of a time clock or an electronically coded badge to enter and exit the building), the problem can often be confirmed by checking the records that have been generated by the automated system. This method is not foolproof. An employee may "punch in" before changing into a uniform and starting the workday or may let someone else use the ID badge. Still, in many cases it is possible to verify a problem with tardiness for some employees using historical data.

For employees whose time sheets are altered, as well as for those who generate manual time sheets and for salaried workers, the verification process is more difficult. The manager might actually have to rearrange her own personal work schedule so that the employee in question is observed at the start of the workday to determine if the designated start time is being routinely ignored. In any case, no disciplinary action should take place until the manager has verification that the employee is actually arriving late for work on a regular basis. The manager has then identified and documented the existence of a specific problem—in this case, persistent tardiness.

management practice in dietetics

With the preconditions met, the actual disciplinary action can take place between the manager and the employee. It usually is in the form of an interview, which should be initiated by the manager in a nonthreatening manner. After a few moments of general (rapport-building) conversation with the employee, the manager should state the problem that has been identified and relate that the behavior is not appropriate in the work setting. The reasons that the behavior is not acceptable should also be presented. (For example, "The tardiness makes it impossible for the diet clerks to get the lunch tally to the cooks on time.") Though difficult to do, the manager needs to separate the behavior from the employee. It should be very clear to the employee that the problem is the behavior, not the employee.

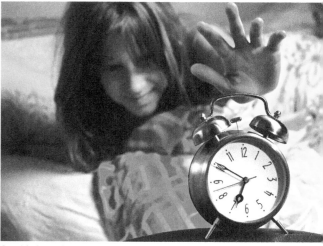

Copyright © 2011 by Depositphotos/Nermin Smajic.

Sometimes chronic tardiness can be corrected simply by getting a new alarm clock.

Next, the employee is given the opportunity to reply. The reply might take the form of a denial, an apology, an excuse, or an explanation of the problematic behavior. The manager needs to be an active listener throughout the reply, encouraging the employee to be as open as possible. The manager should also understand that the actual reasons for the tardiness must be identified and addressed before the problem will be solved. If the tardiness is occurring because the employee's alarm clock is broken, the solution could be as simple as getting a new alarm clock. If the problem is transportation, the manager and the employee might explore alternate transportation options. Often the problem can be easily solved once it is identified and discussed openly.

This disciplinary action should always end on a positive note. This is difficult because it is the manager's responsibility to let the employee know that failure to correct the problem will lead to further disciplinary actions and could ultimately result in suspension or termination. The meeting has served as a reminder of what is expected. In addition, the employee needs to know that a record of the meeting will be kept but not placed in the employee's permanent record. In order to return to the positive, the manager must express confidence that, now that the problem has been identified, the employee will be able to correct it. The employee should leave the meeting with a feeling of hope that the problem can be solved.

written warning

A **written warning** is the next step in the disciplinary process. In the policy noted earlier, it is specified that discipline will progress to the next step if the problem recurs within 90 days of the verbal warning. Again, the manager must use judgment and compassion when moving forward through progressive discipline. If the employee is tardy on multiple occasions during the 90-day period, these events should be documented and progressive discipline should be escalated to the next step. However, if

Written Warning. *The second, more formal step in employee discipline, which includes stating the problem and noting repetition over time. Information sharing between the manager and the employee is also part of this step.*

the employee was late only once, and there had been a major snowstorm that day, it would be prudent not to escalate the process to a written warning. The manager needs to exercise good judgment in all matters of employee discipline.

The interview accompanying the written warning follows the same general pattern as that which took place with the verbal warning. It should start on a positive note, if possible, stating that a decrease in the frequency of tardiness had been observed, but that on-time arrival at work was still not 100 percent. Dates and times when the employee was tardy since the verbal warning was issued should be listed for the employee, and these should be related back to the verbal warning. The negative effects of the tardiness in the workplace should be enumerated once again. Next, the employee should be allowed to explain the situation. This is followed by a joint discussion of potential solutions to the ongoing problem.

With a written warning, however, a formal document must be placed in the employee's file. The employee needs to know that this will happen. Usually, the manager prepares three copies of the warning—one for the manager, one for the employee, and one for the employee's file. The employee will be asked to sign the document, attesting to having seen and discussed the content of the document with the manager. The employee's signature does not mean that there is agreement with the content of the document, merely that there is an awareness of its existence. Occasionally, an employee will opt not to sign the document. In that case, a witness should be called on to sign that the employee is aware of the document's existence. The witness need not be aware of the contents of the document, nor will the witness be involved in the disciplinary interview.

Finally, the interview should be concluded with similar comments as in the earlier interview. That is to say, the employee will be made aware of the specific consequences of failing to correct the behavior. All of this information will be included in the written document, too. The manager should close the interview by expressing confidence that the employee will be able to correct the problem. If progressive discipline has reached this point, the employee needs to know that the problem must be solved, that potential solutions really do exist, and that it is still possible to correct the problem. The closure of this interview should be as positive as circumstances permit.

Suspension.
The third step in the employee disciplinary process, in which the employee is given time off, usually without pay, to demonstrate the seriousness of the problem.

suspension

The next step in the progressive disciplinary process outlined earlier is **suspension**. If, within the time designated, the problem occurs again, the employee will be given one or more days off without pay, as a strong reminder that the problem is very serious and could lead to the loss of employment. Again, new managers should be reminded to seek advice from more-experienced managers before they suspend an employee, especially if they have never taken this type of disciplinary action before.

management practice in dietetics

A senior colleague will provide insight into how the specific situation might be handled and will provide new managers with the support they need to get through this very difficult task.

The actual meeting with the employee will not be as positive as the previous two meetings have been, because the manager must actually penalize the employee by requiring that the employee take time off without pay. This has the potential for causing hardship for the employee and for the rest of the staff as well. However, the other parts of the interview will be very similar to the previous meetings. The employee will need to know the specific details about the latest occurrence of the problem and how this event (or these events) relates back to the previous disciplinary actions. Then the employee must be given a chance to explain the situation to the manager. The employee must be told that failure to correct the problem will lead to further disciplinary action and possible termination.

Next, the manager must review the supporting written document with the employee, who will be asked to sign the document, acknowledging that it has been discussed with him or her. If the employee refuses to sign the document, a witness may be used as described earlier. The employee is then asked to leave work and told when to return to work, after having missed the designated number of days without pay.

Again, there are some pitfalls that should be avoided. First, the suspension must take place in a timely manner. This may cause some hardship in the workplace if a substitute worker is not available. However, if the manager waits to suspend an employee until it is "convenient" for staffing purposes, the opportunity of making a strong statement to the employee could be missed. If the employee is suspended during a busy time, it reinforces the message to that employee that he or she is dispensable. Finally, the manager must be sure not to allow the employee to make up the lost wages by calling the employee in for extra shifts after the suspension is over.

termination

The ultimate disciplinary action is the **termination** of the employee. This, too, should occur as soon as possible after the next incident—for this example, tardiness. The manager, especially one who is new to the managerial role, should verify that the infraction occurred and should then review the matter with a superior or with a human resources staff member before initiating this final disciplinary action. Because termination is so drastic, it is in the best interest of the organization and all of the parties involved that this action be reviewed by two or more individuals to make sure that all of the guidelines and procedures leading to this event have been followed and documented. If due process has not been followed, the employee should not be terminated at this time, but a less severe disciplinary action should be taken instead. If all parties agree that the termination should proceed, then the manager must carry out the process.

Termination. *The final action in the employee disciplinary process, which leads to the end of employment and results after repeated failure of the employee to correct the problem.*

Do:	Don't:
Get all necessary approvals	Terminate someone on Friday
Complete the paperwork first	Terminate on the day before a holiday
Keep the message brief	Terminate someone who is on vacation
Schedule the termination in the morning	Phrase the reason for termination in personal terms
Allow yourself time to recover	Expect the employee to behave rationally

Table 10.2 Guidelines for Terminating an Employee

Termination is very unpleasant for both of the parties involved. The manager must inform the employee that failure to correct the ongoing problem has led to the need to end the employment relationship between the individual employee and the organization. There will be a number of items that must be discussed with the individual, including the employee's rights in this situation, discontinuation of benefits, final compensation, and so on. Then the employee must be allowed to gather personal belongings before being escorted out of the workplace. It is disruptive for others in the workplace to permit the terminated employee to stay in the setting for any significant amount of time following termination. There are some other "do's" and "don'ts" of how to handle the termination of an employee[1,2]. These are shown in Table 10.2.

special circumstances

Certain events may occur that could warrant the termination of an employee without following the disciplinary process as specified in the organizational policy and procedure. Some specific behaviors that could lead to immediate termination are the physical endangerment of coworkers, theft, falsification of documents, reporting to work under the influence of alcohol or controlled substances, or using such substances while at work. (See Table 10.3.) As with other disciplinary issues, the manager must use good judgment and investigate the specific details of the event before taking any action.

For example, one employee might have "helped" a coworker who was tardy once by "punching in" for the late worker. Technically, this is "falsification of documents," one of the types of behaviors that could lead to immediate termination. Another example of falsification of documents might involve an employee who is working 40 hours per week at $12.50 per hour. (Assume that this income is high enough to make the employee ineligible for federal rent subsidy.) If this employee stole letterhead and

Usually Leads to Immediate Termination	Physical endangerment of others
	Consuming alcohol while on the job
	Using controlled substances while on the job
	Willful destruction of property
	Possession of firearms while on work premises
	Unauthorized disclosure of confidential information
	Viewing pornography on work computers/work time
May Lead to Immediate Termination if the Magnitude of the Offense Is Large	Stealing
	Falsification of documents
	Reporting to work under the influence of alcohol or controlled substances

Table 10.3 Grounds for Immediate Termination

wrote a letter to a public housing agency claiming wages of only $9.00 per hour for an average workweek of 20 hours, and signed the manager's name to the document, this offense would also be "falsification of documents." The two offenses are technically the same, but very different in magnitude. The former would probably lead to a verbal warning and the initiation of the disciplinary process; the latter could lead to immediate termination.

Another variable to be considered when making such managerial judgments related to employee discipline is the prior work record of the employee. If the offense is a major one (perhaps theft of $300 from the petty cash drawer), but also the first for a long-term employee, the manager may opt to suspend the employee for a period of time without pay. Another employee with a history of behavioral and performance problems would probably be terminated for such a theft.

There are few absolutes when dealing with employee discipline. Staying within the policy and procedural guidelines, while recognizing the need for fairness and consistency to employees, requires the manager to exercise a considerable amount of judgment. One of the dangers is that judgment can be used to justify the behavior of a favorite employee while simultaneously being used to find fault with the behavior of a less-favored one. Therefore, it is imperative that the manager be able to separate the behavior from the individual and look at the behavior objectively, as well as subjectively.

It should be noted that the process described thus far is typical but not universal. Managers must consult the human resources P&P manual in their organization to be sure that they are following the process described there when disciplining unrepresented employees. The process is usually different for the employee who works under a contractual agreement between the employer and a labor union. In this circumstance, the disciplinary process described in the labor contract will supersede the organizational procedure. Quite often, a unionized worker will request that a representative of the union be present for any disciplinary action. This is a request that should be honored. One of the roles of the union is to protect its workers from arbitrary actions by management. Thus, whatever representation is mandated by the contract must be followed for any disciplinary action that is taken in order to ensure that the employee's rights are not violated.

Progressive discipline is a step-by-step process that is designed to help the employee to correct his or her inappropriate behavior or poor performance. It usually has four or more steps. These include the verbal warning, one or more written warnings, suspension, and termination. The series of disciplinary actions should relate to a specific behavioral or performance problem, not to problems in general. Time frames regulate the administration of progressive discipline.

It is important that the manager administer discipline in a non-arbitrary manner. Fairness and compassion are of utmost importance. A good disciplinary P&P will allow managers to exercise their judgment in individual cases and will ensure that both the employees and the managers are protected. The steps outlined are used to impose order on what is a difficult process for all of the parties involved.

documentation

Documentation.
A written record of the disciplinary actions taken.

The disciplinary process must be supported by **documentation** at each step in order to achieve the goal of correcting inappropriate behavior or improving performance. Some of the documentation is a formal part of the employee record and must be written in precise language. Other documentation consists of unofficial notes kept by the manager to serve as reminders of previous interactions with staff. Each type of information is useful and has value relative to employee discipline, but such information may be used for other purposes, too.

anecdotal information

Anecdotal Information.
Optional informal notes that are sometimes kept by a manager as a reminder of things that have occurred.

The notes that managers keep for their own use are not intended to be a part of an employee's formal employment record. This **anecdotal information** includes notes made after meetings or encounters with employees. These are used to remind the manager what has transpired, either positive or negative. Such information is not deemed official, nor is it necessary for a manager to keep such information on file. These notes are optional. Still, some managers find it useful for them to have a system for keeping track of their interactions with employees. If they exist, however, such notes can be subpoenaed for legal purposes.

For managers who choose to keep anecdotal information, there are some issues to consider. The first is that the information system should be uniformly applied to all employees, not just to those who are subject to disciplinary action. Thus, a note sheet might be made for each employee who reports directly to a manager. The information that is recorded on such notes should be factual and nonjudgmental. It may be positive, negative, or neutral. For example, such notations might include statements like:

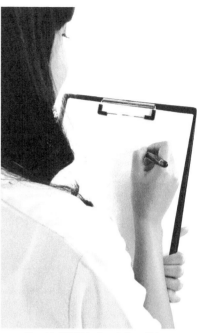

- 12/26—Susie has set her wedding date for July 17.
- 1/14—James wrote an article on the department renovation for the newsletter.
- 1/16—Max announced that his wife is expecting a baby in six months.
- 1/16—Sonia and I discussed the budget for continuing education for next year.
- 1/17—John was 25 minutes late to work this morning.
- 1/22—Lisa asked if I would write a letter of recommendation for grad school.

These notes are more useful if they are dated. The tone of the notes should be neutral and nonjudgmental.

Managers who keep anecdotal information should do so for all their employees, not just those with disciplinary issues.

The anecdotal information has many uses. A manager may use these notes to review what has happened with an employee during the past year in order to write the annual performance appraisal. The notes may also be used to aid in schedule writing (perhaps to ensure that Susie has adequate time for a honeymoon) or to plan for staffing to cover leaves of absence (Max plans to take family leave when his child is born). The information may serve to remind the manager of promises made or goals set (I told Sonia that I would send her to the State Dietetic Association Meeting in June if she completed the revision of the screening and assessment policy by May 1). Finally, the anecdotal notes may remind the manager of behavioral or performance problems.

The point is that these notes have many uses and should be used to meet a variety of needs, not just the one related to employee discipline. If only problems are noted for troublesome employees, the manager risks being accused of not treating all employees equitably. Disparate treatment of employees could have negative effects if a disciplinary action is challenged. Therefore, some managers make notes on a regular schedule (perhaps weekly or monthly) for every employee who reports to them. Others make notes each time something significant transpires between the manager and the employee. This informal record is used in the various ways described above, and then the notes are discarded. Once the information has been transferred to an official document, such as a performance appraisal or a disciplinary action form/letter, the notes are no longer needed. It is seldom necessary to keep anecdotal records for more than a year.

official documentation

Those documents that become an official part of the employee's file must be written in accordance with the organization's policy and procedure, often on a prescribed form. If a standard institutional form is used, it will contain all of the elements described in this section; there may be more information required as deemed necessary by the organization. If there is no prescribed form, then the disciplinary action is formatted in the form of a letter or an interoffice memorandum.

The critical components to be included in the documentation of a disciplinary action include:

- The employee's identifying information (name, employee ID number, position);
- The manager's identifying information (name and title);
- Behavioral or performance problem for which the action is being taken;
- Description of events and discussions preceding this action;
- Description of the specific events leading to this action;
- Possible consequences if this behavioral or performance problem is not corrected;
- Duration of the warning;
- Signature of the manager; and
- Signature of the employee, with a disclaimer regarding agreement.

There may also be a space for the employee's comments and space for the signature of a witness, if this is necessary. A sample of a disciplinary action memo for a written warning is shown in Figure 10.2.

As with other documentation made by dietetics professionals—like charting in the medical records, keeping records on productivity, or monitoring financial performance relative to budget—the message is universal. If you didn't write it down, you didn't do it. Trying to reconstruct information for use in employee discipline without having recorded the data in the first place is time consuming and difficult (if not impossible) to do. Recall alone is not enough to warrant taking action. The intent of record keeping is not to make the dietetics manager a slave to documentation and unnecessary paperwork but to record data that are likely to serve a useful purpose in the future. If done in a routine way, documentation will take very little time and has the potential to be very useful to the manager.

employee assistance programs

Increasingly, employers are finding that it is beneficial to provide workers with a supportive work environment. Flextime, family leave, employer-supported childcare, job-sharing, onsite fitness centers, and cafeteria-type health care options are innovations that employers are now offering in order to retain a loyal and a diverse workforce.

July 31, 20xx

To: Jane Doe
           Dietetic Clerk
           ID# 83427821

From: Janice Sparks
           Chief Clinical Dietitian

Re: Persistent Tardiness

In accordance with the job analysis that you were given when you started working here, you are expected to report to work at 9 a.m. On July 16, we discussed the fact that you had been late six times in the previous month:

6/20	10 minutes late	7/5	20 minutes late
6/24	18 minutes late	7/8	14 minutes late
6/30	25 minutes late	7/12	12 minutes late

During that meeting, you acknowledged that the tardiness has occurred because parking was difficult for you. You agreed to leave home earlier to allow time for you to make it to work on time, even if you had to walk several blocks from the parking area to the office.

Since July 17 you have been late twice:

| 7/23 | 15 minutes late | 7/28 | 22 minutes late |

Failure to correct this behavior will result in further disciplinary action, which could include suspension without pay or termination.

A copy of this written warning will be placed in your employment file. If there are no further instances of tardiness in the next six months, the warning will be removed.

_____   _____

Manager's Signature   Employee Signature (indicates
                                            understanding of the warning,
                                            not agreement with it)

Employee comments:

Figure 10.2 Sample Written Warning

Organizations are also offering **employee assistance programs** (EAP), sometimes as part of the insurance package available to employees, sometimes as a freestanding program, and sometimes by using a combination of both strategies. Employee assistance programs are designed to support individual employees through personal crises[3] (such as mental health issues, a divorce, or the death of a loved one) that could have a negative impact on their work performance and could lead to the loss of employment. It is becoming common to deal with disciplinary problems that might have led to termination by referring an employee to an EAP, with the expectation that the employee will learn how to cope with the situation and remain a productive member of the organization.

Employee Assistance Programs. *Plans that provide employees with support in dealing with personal crises that could negatively impact work performance.*

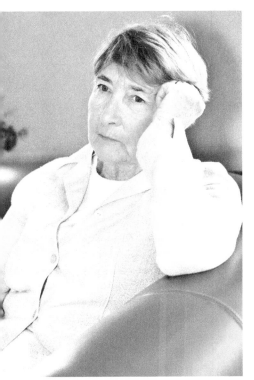

EAPs help employees deal with problems such as depression, addiction, and loss.

For example, some employers will enroll employees who have problems with alcohol abuse in a treatment program, rather than terminate them.

EAPs are extremely helpful for employees who must find effective ways to deal with stress, grief, family/marital problems, financial concerns, mental health issues, legal questions, and so on.[4] These programs are developing in new directions as trends emerge and attitudes change, both within the organization and in society at large. It is exciting to see the expansion of such programs, because it demonstrates that employers value staff and are willing to help them through difficult times.

Employee assistance programs are commonly used for the employee who has a problem with, or is at risk for, substance abuse. This specific type of EAP evolved from concerns centered on workers in some types of jobs (for example, airline pilots and bus drivers) in which substance abuse could have a significant effect on the health and safety of the public. Routine or random drug testing is used for these and other types of workers, for athletes, and for some people with a history of substance abuse. The justification for this testing in the workplace is to identify problems early and to intervene before the problem gets out of control. Rehabilitation of individuals who abuse alcohol and drugs is the ultimate goal. The legal issues involved in the testing of employees for drug and alcohol use and the issue of privacy versus public safety are evolving through the legislative and the court systems. Absolute rules do not apply for many situations.

Employees with problems that are identified early are likely to benefit most from these programs and will often have a less disruptive effect in the work setting. Therefore, supervisors and managers are trained to identify changes in behavior that may indicate such a problem.[5] They are taught to make referrals to the EAP in a non-diagnostic manner. For example, it is better to say, "You seem to not be able to concentrate on your work lately; maybe you should talk to ..." rather than, "You must get treatment for your alcoholism if you want to continue to work here." It is imperative that the managers not betray the confidentiality of employees who are referred to an EAP for substance abuse or for any other personal problem.

If the employee's problem has progressed to the point that disciplinary action is needed, participation in the EAP may be required as a condition of continued employment. This is typical for the employee who abuses alcohol or drugs. Depending on the type of work that the employee does, and its impact on the health and safety of others, it may be mandatory that the employee complete the program and earn the right to return to work. Because each case is individual, the requirements for returning to work are not usually formally spelled out in policy and procedure format. However, it is appropriate that the employee have an individualized, written contract with the employer that clearly states what is required for continued employment.

EAPs may be run by the employer or may be contracted to an outside provider. An internal (self-operated) program works well for large organizations that can afford to support their own staff of counselors and are large enough to guarantee anonymity. Very large organizations with thousands of employees can usually provide the services onsite. An organization that is large enough to provide the service, but too small to ensure privacy for the employee, would probably opt for an offsite location for the program. Smaller businesses usually contract for the service from an independent, offsite provider. The contract may be a general one covering all employees, all the time, or may be negotiated on a case-by-case basis.

Employee assistance programs are beneficial to both the employer and the employee. The employer is able to keep an employee on the payroll and retain (or regain) productivity. The time and energy involved in progressive discipline may be avoided, and negative repercussions may be minimized. In addition, there is often a cost savings, because it is usually more cost-effective to support a seasoned employee through a crisis than it is to hire and train a new employee. In some cases, the availability of an EAP may contribute to enhanced employee loyalty. The employee benefits by getting the help that is needed to deal with the crisis while maintaining income, job security, dignity, and self-esteem. It is a method for confronting a problem in a manner that provides the least disruptive solution for both parties, sometimes described as a "win-win" situation.

employee grievances

Because organizations are not perfect and managers are human, most organizations have a mechanism in place for conflict resolution between an employee and his or her manager. This mechanism may take the form of a policy and procedure on **employee grievances**. A grievance P&P uses the same basic format as the P&P covering progressive discipline in that it states the policy, the purpose of the policy, the scope (if needed), and the step-by-step process for dealing with conflict. Time frames are included as an important part of the grievance procedure.

Employees use the grievance process when they feel that they have been treated unfairly in the workplace. Typical reasons for filing grievances are listed in Table 10.4. Employees have the right to challenge their managers when they perceive that they are victims of unfair treatment. The procedure for dealing with grievances is set up to delineate how the conflict is to be resolved. Employees are encouraged to utilize this internal process before taking their complaint outside the organization, to the court system, or to the media.

A typical grievance procedure will direct the employee to first discuss the problem with his or her supervisor or manager. This is often difficult for the employee to do, because the manager has power over the employee, who may fear that any form of criticism toward the manager may lead to retaliation. In the ideal world, this would not occur.

Employee Grievances.
A method for employees to use to resolve conflicts when they feel they have been treated unfairly by management.

Table 10.4 Typical Reasons for Employee Grievances

The manager would listen to the description of the problem, and then discuss the issue from the manager's perspective. If the problem was inadvertent or a matter of oversight, the manager's awareness might be enough to solve the problem. For example, if the employee was offended by the manager's habitual use of the phrase "you people" when talking to staff members, having insight into the negative reaction of the employee could lead the manager to use a different form of address. If the problem was a transient one—for example, asking an employee to work excessive overtime because there was a job vacancy that had not been filled—this, too, might be discussed so that the employee became aware of what was being done to solve the problem.

Unfortunately, the world is not always an ideal place; managers do things that are inappropriate or discriminatory. The manager may be acting with negative intent or, perhaps, inadvertently. In the real world, managers do become defensive and react poorly to criticism from employees. Some managers really do seek retaliation against employees who question or criticize them. Thus, it is important for the employee to have a way to deal with the conflict if bringing the issue to the immediate manager does not resolve the conflict.

If resolution is not achieved when the conflict has been brought to the manager's attention, the next step is usually to present the issue to the manager's superior. Beyond that, the steps in the procedure are somewhat dependent on the size and complexity of the organization. Large organizations may have a grievance committee, made up of staff and managers, who "hear" the case and propose a resolution. If the employee is still not satisfied, the matter may be referred to the CEO or to an independent arbitrator whose decision is final. Smaller organizations usually refer such issues directly to the CEO, bypassing the "hearing" before a committee.

Employees who are covered by a collective bargaining agreement will follow the procedure outlined in the union contract rather than follow the organization's P&P for employee grievances. Unions have paid staff and legal counsel who help an employee with the grievance process. It is their job to determine if the worker has a legitimate grievance and, if so, to represent the employee in all meetings and negotiations concerning that matter. In addition to those reasons listed in Table 10.4, contractual workers may file grievances if they are asked to do non-union work, if non-union workers perform union jobs, or if other terms of the union contract are not followed. It is not unusual for union grievances to be settled either through **arbitration** or by **mediation**.

In summary, the employee grievance policy and procedure is designed to provide a framework for conflict resolution between the employee and the manager. It outlines the process available for employees to use if they feel that they have been treated unfairly in the workplace. Though it is not used frequently, it is essential that employees have such a tool at their disposal.

conclusion

In this chapter, the purpose for employee discipline and the processes used for discipline have been discussed. Both the traditional and alternative methods of dealing with employee problems were presented. Consideration was also given to how an employee might deal with conflict with management in the work setting.

The key concepts presented in this chapter are outlined here.

1. Employee discipline should be used for the purpose of helping the employee to correct behavioral or performance problems that have a negative impact on the workplace.
2. A disciplinary policy and procedure should be in place that includes a policy statement, the purpose for the policy, and a step-by-step procedure (with specific timelines) for the process.
3. The usual steps in a disciplinary procedure include the following disciplinary actions:
   * verbal warning
   * written warning
   * suspension
   * termination
4. Managers must use judgment, empathy, consistency, and fairness when administering employee discipline.
5. All disciplinary actions should be documented in a factual, nonjudgmental way.
6. Alternatives to the traditional disciplinary process include the use of employee assistance programs.
7. Employees can use the grievance procedure to resolve conflicts with management.

Arbitration. *A hearing before someone empowered to resolve the dispute.*

Mediation. *Negotiation between two parties, using a neutral intermediary to assist in settling a dispute.*

activities

activity 1

You are the patient services manager for a hospital's food and nutrition services department. You have received reports that the lunch meals that are delivered to the obstetrics unit in the facility are arriving about 30 minutes later than the scheduled time. This has been happening for about a month. You have also heard that the employee whose job it is to deliver the trays is dealing in illegal drugs. You have observed that the employee in question carries a mobile phone at work. This is not usual, but there is no departmental regulation that deals with employees carrying personal phones. The employee had approached you last year when she got the new phone and informed you that it was intended "to allow my children to text me if there is an emergency at home." At the time, you did not object to the use of the phone for that reason, as long as it did not interfere with the employee's work.

1. What is the problem?
2. What did the employee do that was wrong?
3. Should the employee be terminated for this offense?
4. If you answered "no" to question three, do you have enough information to initiate progressive discipline?
5. If yes, what would the disciplinary action be? If no, what additional information do you need?
6. Should the department have a policy about the use of personal phones for employees?

activity 2

Using one of the formats illustrated in Figure 10.1 and the information that you have learned regarding how a P&P is written, write a policy and procedure dealing with employee grievances. You may use additional references to complete this activity, such as the sources cited in the "To Study Further" section at the end of this chapter.

activity 3

case study. Marilyn Hayes is a nice woman, a widow and grandmother who struggles hard to make ends meet. She completed a training course at the local community college and became a Certified Dietary Manager nine years ago. At that time, she was hired by Metro Hospital and worked as a Foodservice Supervisor for four years. In this position, she performed adequately. She was neither a "superstar" nor was she a "problem."

She did her job in a reliable and acceptable way. Marilyn sustained a back injury during her fifth year of employment and took a three-month medical leave. When she returned to work, it was with the stipulation that she could not lift anything heavier than three pounds. That meant that she could no longer work as a Foodservice Supervisor.

The Clinical Nutrition Department (a separate department in Metro Hospital) had an opening for a Diet Clerk when Marilyn returned to work. Marilyn met the basic requirements for this position (high school diploma and the ability to read and write in English). Though the position was a demotion for her, the hospital agreed to pay her at her previous hourly wage, so she accepted the job.

The Diet Clerk position required that Marilyn process diet orders that arrived in the Clinical Nutrition Department via a centralized computer system. In addition, she answered the telephone, headed selective menus for patients, generated the order (forecast plus tally of special items) for patient foods for the Foodservices Department, and checked the breakfast trayline. As with all newly hired Diet Clerks at Metro Hospital, Marilyn received five days of training prior to being expected to do the job on her own. She was scheduled to work from 6:00 a.m. until 2:30 p.m. In her first few days alone on the job, she did well with the forecasting, the phones, and the heading of menus, but had difficulty with processing the orders on time and with checking the trayline accurately. Marilyn was given an additional three days of training, which focused on the computerized order system and on trayline accuracy. Then she was again on her own.

Marilyn did the job in an acceptable manner for about a year and was given a performance evaluation at the end of this time. The evaluation indicated that her strengths included the positive way in which she handled problems over the telephone and the accuracy of her forecasting and tallies. She needed to continue to improve in the areas of tray accuracy (Marilyn averaged 84 percent accuracy, whereas the department standard was 95 percent) and in meeting deadlines (often breakfast trayline started late when Marilyn was on duty). She was still slower that other Diet Clerks in processing computer-generated diet orders. This made the breakfast trayline late because she both processed the orders and checked the trayline; it did not affect the timing for lunch trayline because Marilyn could continue to process orders while the afternoon clerk (who arrived at work at 11:00 a.m.) checked trayline.

Six months after the performance review, Metro Hospital was faced with a need to reduce costs, so a reduction in force (RIF) led to layoffs in all departments. Marilyn was not laid off because of her seniority, but the job that she was doing changed. Prior to the RIF, the Clinical Nutrition Department had 16 Diet Clerk hours each day; this was reduced to 12. The afternoon clerk was now scheduled to start work at 3:00 p.m. Prior to the RIF, Marilyn processed orders for breakfast and lunch and checked only the breakfast trayline. Now she was required to process orders for and check trayline at both breakfast and lunch. To facilitate these changes, new computer software was purchased that generated the forecast and headed the menus, and a voice mail system was installed to deal with phone messages during peak times. Marilyn was now left with tasks that were difficult for her, while the tasks that she did well were automated.

Marilyn's difficulties began almost immediately after the RIF took place. Not only were the breakfast traylines late in starting, but now the lunch traylines were late on a regular basis. Marilyn and her manager discussed the problem, and Marilyn agreed to try harder to meet the lunchtime deadline. Marilyn also stated that she needed more time to process lunch orders. The cutoff time for orders to be sent via the computer system was moved from 10:30 a.m. to 10:15 a.m. so that Marilyn could begin processing orders 15 minutes sooner. This new schedule meant that Marilyn had to move her breakfast break, which had been from 10:00–10:30 a.m., to 9:45–10:15 a.m.

In the area of trayline accuracy, Marilyn's performance went from 84 percent to 72 percent. This was attributed to the fact that lunch was a more complicated meal than was breakfast, with more choices and, therefore, more chances for errors. When one such error was significant enough to pose a safety concern for a patient (a confused patient on a pureed diet received beef stew, tried to eat it, and choked), the manager had no alternative but to initiate the disciplinary process for poor performance related to tray accuracy. A verbal warning was given on March 25.

points for discussion

1. Should the problems of late traylines and of tray accuracy be dealt with as one issue or as two distinct issues?
2. Has the manager made an error in not addressing these problems sooner?
3. What can be done to assist Marilyn in correcting the problems?
4. Is Marilyn's age an issue?

In response to the verbal warning about tray accuracy, Marilyn decided to concentrate on this problem. Her accuracy improved to 90 percent at breakfast and 83 percent overall. This was a very positive change. However, to achieve this level of improvement, the process of checking trayline became considerably slower. Breakfast trayline finished later than before, and now Marilyn could not begin her morning break until 10:00 a.m. Because this was an unpaid meal break, cutting the break short (to 15 minutes) resulted in the daily use of overtime. Once again, the manager spoke to Marilyn. Marilyn was praised for her increased accuracy with trays but was reminded of the cost of overtime and the need to keep it to a minimum. No disciplinary action *was taken when they discussed this on April 3.*

points for discussion

5. What is the problem now?
6. Has the accuracy problem been resolved?
7. What can Marilyn and the manager do to effect a solution to the problem(s)?

Marilyn perceived that there was nothing she could do to solve the overtime problem without compromising accuracy. Then an idea came to her. If she started work 15 minutes early (when nobody else was in the office), she could "punch in" at the regular time, get trayline started on time, and maintain the accuracy she wanted. Because no one knew she was starting work early, she would not report the overtime and the manager would be happy. Marilyn knew that she needed to hide this behavior, but she did not feel that it was wrong because she knew that Metro Hospital was in financial difficulty; she also knew that she needed to keep this job.

But someone did know about it. The night security guard noted the change when the Clinical Nutrition Department's lights went on in the morning. He reported it to the head of security, who reported it to Marilyn's manager. The manager asked security to provide the data generated by Marilyn's badge when she entered the parking lot over the past month. The data indicated that prior to April 10, Marilyn entered the garage at 5:45 a.m.; since that date, she entered the garage at 5:30 a.m. The manager rechecked the time cards and noted that the start times were always at 6:00 a.m. No change was noted after April 10. The manager then checked the trayline logs, which indicated that the breakfast trayline usually started late before April 10 but started on time after that date.

Now the manager was faced with a dilemma. Marilyn was falsifying an official document (her time card) in order to complete the assigned tasks on time and with the accuracy needed.

points for discussion

8. What should the manager do now?
9. How do you think that Marilyn will react?
10. Which of the problems that has been identified is the most serious?
11. What potential solution(s) do you think could be implemented at this time?

outcome. On April 22, the manager gave Marilyn a verbal warning related to the falsification of her time card. After that time, Marilyn never worked when she was not "punched in." However, her work deteriorated from that point onward. Both timeliness and accuracy suffered, and progressive discipline was begun on timeliness and continued on accuracy. When she was suspended for allowing a diabetic patient to be served a high-carbohydrate dessert that had not been ordered or authorized, Marilyn filed a grievance against Metro Hospital claiming age discrimination. The hospital admitted no wrong but agreed to count the suspension as a written warning and to pay her for the days that she was suspended. However, progressive discipline was still in process, and if Marilyn had continuing problems with accuracy on trayline, she would be suspended again, this time without pay. She was fully aware that continued errors could lead to her termination.

Problems with accuracy continued, and Marilyn was eventually terminated. The entire disciplinary process related to trayline accuracy that was initiated on March 25 was concluded when she was terminated for this same performance problem. The entire process took 2½ years.

activity 5

Write a verbal warning for the incident that was discussed on March 25 or for the incident that was discussed on April 22.

to study further

Additional information on the development of human resources policy and procedure manuals, employee discipline, termination, and employee assistance programs can be found in the following materials.

- Arthur, D. *Managing Human Resources in Small and Mid-Sized Companies.* 2nd ed. New York: AMACOM, 1995.
- Arthur, D. *The Complete Human Resources Writing Guide.* 5th ed. New York: AMACOM, 2005.
- Cascio, W. F. *Managing Human Resources: Productivity, Quality of Work Life, Profits.* 9th ed. New York: McGraw-Hill/Irwin, 2012.
- DuBrin, A. J. *Coaching and Mentoring Skills.* Upper Saddle River, NJ: Pearson/Prentice Hall, 2005.
- Eaton, A. E. and J. H. Keefe, eds. *Employment Dispute Resolution and Workers Rights in the Changing Workplace.* Champaign, IL: Industrial Relations Research Association, 1999.
- Falcone, P. *101 Sample Write-ups for Documenting Employee Performance Problems: A Guide to Progressive Discipline & Termination.* 2nd ed. New York: AMACOM, 2010.
- Mannion, L. P. *Employee Assistance Programs: What Works and What Doesn't.* Westport, CT: Praeger, 2004.
- Rusch, Patricia H. *Foodservice Policies and Procedures for Residential and Intermediate Care Facilities,* Chicago: American Dietetic Association, 1997.

scholarly journals

- *The Health Care Manager*
- *Employee Responsibilities and Rights Journal*

relevant websites

- Employee Assistance Programs for a New Generation of Employees: Defining the Next Generation. Washington, DC: US Department of Labor's Office of Disability Employment Policy.
  http://www.dol.gov/odep/documents/employeeassistance.pdf
- *Alcoholism in the Workplace: A Handbook for Supervisors.* Washington, DC: US Office of Personnel Management, Office of Workforce Relations.
  http://www.opm.gov/employment_and_benefits/worklife/officialdocuments/handbooksguides/alcohol/index.asp#Alcoholism

in practice

The following is a Policy and Procedure governing *corrective action (discipline)*. It is an example of a more-detailed policy than that described in Chapter 10. It is presented here to show the type of organizational policy dietetics managers may need to administer in the workplace.

corrective action (discipline)

All employees are expected to meet performance standards and behave appropriately in the workplace. Corrective action is a process of communicating with the employee to improve unacceptable behavior or performance after other methods such as coaching and performance appraisal have not been successful.

The goal is to guide the employee to correct performance or behavior by identifying the problems, causes and solutions, not to punish the employee. If there is no improvement or if there are repeat occurrences, correction action may be appropriate. In general, corrective action should be progressive, i.e., beginning with the lowest severity action before employing actions of more severity. Any formal corrective or disciplinary action must follow the principles of "Just Cause." After establishing that corrective or disciplinary action is warranted, use some or all of the following steps:

oral warning

The supervisor should:

- Set a time and place to ensure privacy.
- Make notes about what they want to say in advance.
- Remember that the employee has a right to choose representation. (Weingarten Rights)
- State clearly that they are issuing an oral warning.
- Be specific in describing the unacceptable performance or behavior.
- Remind the employee of the acceptable standards or rules. If they are available in writing, they should be provided to the employee.
- State the consequences of failure to demonstrate immediate and sustained improvement: Further disciplinary action may be the result.
- Note the oral warning on their calendar.

written warning

If the supervisor gave an oral warning and the problem performance or behavior persists, a written warning may be warranted. This action may be used more than once, however if the problem continues to persist repetitive letters may not be the solution. A template letter may be requested from an Employee Relations Consultant. A written warning should:

- State clearly at the outset of the letter that it is a written warning, and cite the appropriate personnel policy or contract provision.
- Describe the performance problem(s) or work rule violation(s) in very specific detail and attach documents which support the supervisor's conclusions.
- Outline previous steps taken to acquaint the employee with the issue and attach copies of the documents that are referred to.
- Describe the impact of the problem.
- Note the employee's explanation or that the employee declined to offer one. If it was unacceptable, the supervisor should explain why.
- Explain the expectations regarding behavior and/or performance.
- Clarify that if the employee doesn't demonstrate immediate and sustained improvement, the consequence may be further disciplinary action, up to and including dismissal.
- Note the appropriate policy or contract provision for the employee's appeal rights.
- The warning letter should be delivered to the employee using appropriate delivery procedures such as Proof of Service, and a copy forwarded to HR to be placed in the employee's personnel file.

suspension without pay

A suspension may be the next step in progressive corrective action after written warning(s) and typically prevents an employee to work and is without pay for one to ten working days, as specified in the letter. The letter should:

- State that the action is a suspension without pay.
- Inform the employee of the number of days they will be suspended with the beginning and ending dates.
- Describe the problem, the previous corrective measures, and the impact of the continued behavior or performance.
- State the supervisor's expectations and the consequences of failure to improve.
- Notify the employee of their appeal rights, if appropriate.

Depending upon the contract or personnel program the employee is covered by, a letter of intent to suspend may be required, which provides the employee with the right to appeal the intended action to the next higher management level before the action is implemented. Contact your Employee Relations Consultant as well as the appropriate policy or contract for more information. A template letter may be requested from your Employee Relations Consultant.

reduction of pay within a class

This alternative is normally used when a supervisor does not wish to remove the employee from the work site, but serious discipline is appropriate. Contact your Employee Relations Consultant for more information regarding this corrective action.

demotion to a lower classification

This action involves moving an employee to a lower level position, and may be temporary or permanent. Demotion may be appropriate in cases of inadequate performance of responsibilities at a particular level, rather than violation of work rules. It should be based upon a reasonable expectation that the employee will perform successfully in the lower classified position. Contact your Employee Relations Consultant for more information regarding this action.

dismissal

This action may be appropriate after performance counseling and progressive corrective action have failed to get the employee to correct the problem(s). Contact your Employee Relations Consultant for more information regarding this action.

Central HR: Human Resources Administration Building, University of California, Davis One Shields Avenue, Davis, CA 95616

references

1. Jesseph, Steven A. "Employee Termination: Some Do's and Don'ts." *Personnel* 66, February 1989: 36–39.
2. Bing, Stanley. "Stepping Up to the Firing Line. (Tips on how to fire employees)." *Fortune* 135, February 3, 1997: 51–52.
3. Haskins, Sharon A. and Brian H. Kleiner. "Employee Assistance Programs Take New Directions." (Brave New Workplace: Issues and Trends for Human Resource Management.) *HR Focus* 71, January 1994: 16.
4. Baron, Robert A. and Jerald Greenberg. *Behavior in Organizations.* Upper Saddle River, NJ: Prentice Hall, 1997, p. 241.
5. Bellison, Jerry. "Are EAPs the Answer?" *Personnel* 68, January 1991: 3–4.

part four

managing the work

Organizations exist because there is work to be done. That work needs to be managed to ensure that it is done efficiently, effectively, appropriately, and adequately. In addition to human resources, there must be adequate material resources and appropriate tools to create the product, processes for the actual production, and ways to measure the outcomes of work.

It is relatively simple to look at work and the management of work when the product is tangible. It is more difficult to look at the work when the product is intangible, like service, education, or an idea. Managing work includes managing the system that produces the product. This includes overseeing the inputs that are necessary for the accomplishment of work. Part IV deals with inputs such as material and time. Work processes and facilities are discussed as they relate to the jobs that must be done to create the product. Chapter 13 deals with the measurement of the work that has been completed.

In Chapter 2, the organization was described as a system in which inputs were transformed into outputs. It is not possible to control the productive work done during transformation if the inputs and outputs of work are not also controlled. Managing work includes the managing of all aspects of the system (inputs, transformation, and outputs), either directly or indirectly.

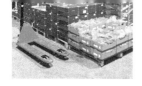

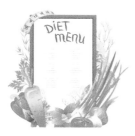

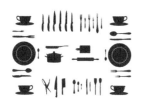

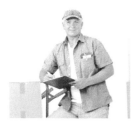

chapter eleven

material management

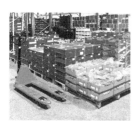

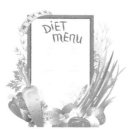

learning objectives

1. Define *purchasing authority*.
2. Describe the various ways in which purchasing is done.
3. Discuss how foodservice menus are written.
4. Discuss each of the five components of a specification.
5. Differentiate among supplies, groceries, perishables, and equipment and capital equipment.
6. Describe the difference between performance and technical specifications.
7. Write specifications for different types of products.
8. Describe the various ways of receiving goods and material.
9. List the equipment needed for receiving in foodservice and non-foodservice operations.
10. Determine the different ways material may be stored.
11. Describe the equipment needed for storage of perishable and nonperishable goods.
12. List the general principles that should be used for all types of storage.
13. Differentiate between perpetual and physical inventory methods.
14. Describe the various ways to distribute material from stock.
15. Determine how inventory is valued.
16. Discuss the use of Hazard Analysis and Critical Control Point (HACCP) in the procurement of food products.

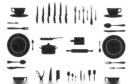

overview

One area of responsibility for many managers is the acquisition and distribution of the material and other inputs used in the production of goods, services, and ideas. **Material management** (sometimes called materials management) has a substantial effect on any operation where raw material is converted into tangible goods because of its impact on the bottom line. In foodservice, menus are the basis for procurement. Even in situations where the primary product is a service and little raw material is required, some purchases must be made. Though these items may not make up a large percentage of the budget (as compared with other items such as labor or benefits), making the right choices about purchases can still have a major effect on the organization's financial health and productivity. This chapter is about the procurement and management of material resources.

What and how much raw material is purchased is one aspect of material management. Other parts of material management include the handling, storage, distribution, valuation, and control of materials from the time they are received until production occurs and the material is transformed into products or used in the production process. Consideration will be given to perishable and nonperishable material as well as to items that are either reusable or disposable. There will also be a description of how to purchase capital goods. Costly items like computers, copiers, ovens, dishwashers, and automobiles are included under this heading.

Material Management.
The process of controlling the acquisition and distribution of material within an organization.

procurement parameters

The **procurement** of raw material is important to an operation for a number of reasons. First, there is the necessity of having the right material available at the right time in order for production to occur. It is also important to avoid having an excess of material on hand. Excessive amounts of material tie up financial resources and take up storage space, which is often limited and costly. Finally, there is the need to obtain the goods in a cost-effective way so that financial resources are not wasted.

Procurement.
Purchasing, or otherwise obtaining, material for use in an organization.

Hospitals and other large institutions frequently have a material management department that is responsible for doing the procurement for the organization. This department may take on the responsibility of obtaining all nonperishable goods for the entire organization. Despite this, it is typical that a foodservice within such an organization will do its own purchasing, or at least the procurement of perishable goods. When dietetics professionals manage in non-foodservice departments of large organizations, the bulk of the purchasing may be done through the material management department. In small institutions and organizations where there is no material management department, each manager will purchase goods as needed.

management practice in dietetics

Procurement includes writing specifications for the items to be purchased and establishing the terms and conditions related to the delivery of these goods. The quantity to be ordered must be determined, orders must be transmitted, and receipt of goods must be verified. Follow-up on incomplete orders is also part of the procurement process. In addition, arrangements must be made between suppliers and the organization regarding terms of payment. When there is no material management department or purchasing manager to take the responsibility for these functions, it becomes the responsibility of individual managers to assume or to delegate these tasks within their own departments or areas.

purchasing authority

Procurement is such a major part of management that **purchasing authority**, in dollar amounts, is one of the ways that a manager's level of authority is measured. Purchasing authority is the amount of the organization's money that an individual manager can spend on individual purchases without having to get the permission of superiors. The authorization to spend the specified amount of money is an inherent part of the management position. In general, as managers attain more responsibility, the dollar amount that they can spend on individual items increases. This means that the manager has a degree of financial control that is commensurate with the position held.

Some positions, by their very nature, require spending a lot of money and thus seem to have a greater purchasing authority than other positions. For example, purchasing managers in foodservice who must acquire lots of low-cost raw material on a daily basis would probably spend more money each week than a clinical nutrition manager whose product is more service-oriented and requires less raw material. This is independent of the organization chart, which may indicate that the clinical nutrition manager holds a position that is higher than that of the purchasing manager. In this example, the clinical nutrition manager would be allowed to purchase more-costly individual items, like office furniture or computers, than the purchasing manager would be authorized to buy. Though the purchasing manager spends a total number of dollars that is greater than the clinical nutrition manager spends, the overall purchasing authority of the clinical nutrition manager on an item-by-item basis is greater.

methods of purchasing

Hospitals, large organizations, and foodservices in institutions may purchase from a number of different sources or may have a **prime vendor** arrangement with a supplier from whom most of their purchasing is done. This prime vendor arrangement may be made between the provider of raw material and a single organization. Foodservice

Purchasing Authority.
A measure of a manager's control over the procurement of material; the amount a manager is allowed to spend without obtaining permission from his or her supervisor.

Prime Vendor.
The supplier that provides most of the material purchased by an organization.

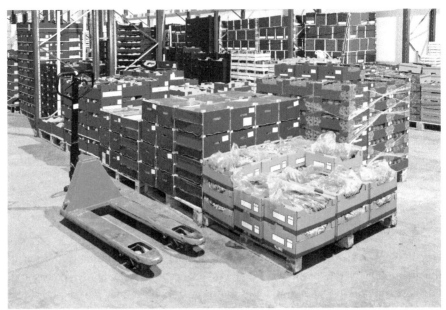

Produce is warehoused in a refrigerated storage area until it is shipped to the foodservice customer.

Purchasing Cooperative. *A group of buyers who join together for the purpose of negotiating better purchasing contracts with vendors.*

management companies generally use a single prime vendor for all of the operations they manage. Alternatively, a small, independent organization may join a **purchasing cooperative** that contracts with a prime vendor. In this case, all of the members of the purchasing cooperative use the same prime vendor. Because of the combined volume of business, each member of the co-op gets better prices and service than would be available to individual customers. An advantage of this type of purchasing arrangement is that it reduces the paperwork involved when buying from several vendors, and thus lowers costs. Individual products may cost less, as well. Another advantage is that all goods arrive in a single delivery, which allows the receiving personnel to work more efficiently. Using a prime vendor does not mean that other vendors are never used, but makes it less attractive to use multiple vendors. Prime vendors provide their customers with the ability to customize the ordering system to meet their own specific requirements and to process orders electronically. Typically, orders are placed through the Internet.

Multiple Vendor Purchasing. *Procurement of goods from several vendors; may be motivated by the desire to improve selection or the need to get the lowest price.*

Other methods of purchasing are also used (see Table 11.1). One such method, often used by small or specialty operations, is **multiple vendor purchasing**. In this situation, the operation has accounts established with several vendors and "shops" these vendors for the best prices on the needed items. The shopping takes place via phone or on the Internet. The advantages of this type of purchasing are the availability of more products and, at times, access to sale prices on raw material. In the past, most foodservices purchased this way. The disadvantages are that more vendors mean that more deliveries must be received, more invoices are generated, and more bills have

management practice in dietetics

| Prime vendor contracts |
| Multiple vendor agreements |
| Bid purchasing |
| Warehouse club buying |
| Retail purchasing |

Table 11.1 Commonly Used Purchasing Methods

to be processed. Orders may be placed by phone, fax, through a salesperson who visits the foodservice, or electronically. With the high cost of labor in today's marketplace, the multiple vendor approach is almost always more costly than using a prime vendor. This type of purchasing is usually driven by the need to purchase specialty items, like prime cuts of meats, out-of-season produce, and other gourmet items for which the buyer (typically a fine-dining establishment) is willing to pay premium prices. If, on the other hand, this type of purchasing is driven by the need to find the lowest price for each item to be purchased, it may follow that quality of goods and level of service provided by vendors decrease.

In foodservice, it is possible to have both a prime vendor agreement for bulk purchases of groceries and paper supplies as well as agreements with other small vendors for specific product lines. The prime vendor might be a nationwide provider, whose service is supplemented by local meat, dairy, bakery, and produce purveyors. The local vendors could provide daily deliveries for perishables while the larger supplier might provide weekly or biweekly deliveries of nonperishable material.

A more formal purchasing method is called **bid purchasing**. For this type of purchasing, the buyer specifies the item or items needed and asks for vendors to submit bids to provide the material. Several weeks' or months' worth of product may be requested. The lowest bidder who can meet all of the specifications for the product usually gets the contract for the goods. This type of purchasing is also used for capital equipment and contracted services such as pest control.

Bid purchasing is being used with decreasing frequency for raw material for foodservice operations, though some large, governmental institutions (hospitals, military operations, and prisons) still purchase this way. It is a cumbersome and time-consuming process. With improved technologies and reliable transportation systems, the cost of carrying extensive inventories outweighs the benefits of this type of purchasing for most operations. In today's marketplace, bid purchasing is most widely used when purchasing items like large, expensive equipment or service contracts. This method is no longer widely used for purchasing the provisions needed for foodservice production.

Bid Purchasing. *A type of purchasing that requires vendors to bid on the item or items an organization specifies in order to be eligible to get the business; used mostly for capital equipment and contracts. The business is generally awarded to the lowest bidder who meets the specifications.*

A variation of bid purchasing is the process used to select a prime vendor. A prime vendor may submit a "bid," which outlines the goods and services that will be provided for a specified period of time (perhaps a year, or a period of several years). Firm prices may be established for certain high-use products. Alternatively, the vendor may agree to provide goods on a **cost plus** (actual cost plus a set percentage to cover the vendor's handling and profit) basis. Once the prime vendor is selected and a contract negotiated, the purchasing method becomes the prime vendor method, which means that goods are ordered and delivered as needed; the purchaser does not need to receive large deliveries and store large quantities of material in inventory.

The least-formal type of purchasing is one in which the purchaser goes to the store and buys whatever material is needed. Warehouse clubs are available for a variety of supplies, such as food and groceries, office supplies, building supplies, and so on. Commercial customers may get special pricing levels or additional services (for example, delivery) that are not available to individuals who purchase smaller volumes of material for their own personal use. Small businesses and organizations find **warehouse club buying** convenient and cost-effective.

Purchases of individual items that are needed immediately might be made at a local **retail** establishment. Though the prices are often higher, it is a way to acquire small or unusual items in limited quantities. This method is also used for "emergency" purchases. Because retail sales are not usually covered by a purchasing agreement, payment is typically made with petty cash or a company credit card. It is desirable to limit this type of purchasing because it is generally more costly, both in time and money, to acquire goods in this way. Some organizations restrict the use of this type of purchasing to emergency situations.

menus as the basis for procurement in foodservice

Professionals who work in foodservice are involved in the procurement of food items. The items that are to be purchased are based on the menu that is used. Essentially, the menu is the basic plan for the foodservice, as it is closely related to every other aspect of the business. There is a critical relationship between the menu, the foods that are purchased, the production of that food, the type of service, the level of expertise the kitchen and service staff need, the cost of doing business, customer satisfaction, the physical facility, the equipment required, and so forth. Sometimes the menu is determined by the system, as it would be in healthcare or school foodservice. At other times, the system is designed for the menu, as it the case with quick service restaurants and with fine-dining establishments. In either situation, one is dependent on the other. Creating menus for foodservices is one of the most difficult, challenging, and creative jobs done by dietetics professionals. Prior to getting into the specifics of purchasing, it is necessary to take a look at how menus are developed.

types of menus

Basically, there are three kinds of menus. The first is a **single-use menu** designed for an event and not to be used again. An example of a single-use menu would be one planned for a wedding reception. Some fine-dining establishments pride themselves on presenting single-use menus, which change each day depending on the creativity of the chef and the seasonal foods available.

The second type of menu is the **static menu**—that is, one that remains the same from day to day. Typically, quick service restaurants and casual-dining restaurants use the static menu. Static menus frequently, though not always, offer many choices to the customer. Though the menu remains the same over a period of time, the length of time a menu is used has contracted in recent years. Restaurants are finding that they must create new products and new menus to keep their customers coming back.

Finally, there is the **cycle menu**. Cycle menus are used mostly in onsite foodservices where the same customers frequent the foodservice on a regular basis. A cycle menu is one that is different every day for a specified period of time—for example, three weeks—and then repeats. Cycle menus vary in length from several days (for hospital patient foodservice, where the patient stay is only a few days) to six weeks for campus and business dining facilities. However, cycle menus are also not permanent but need to be changed periodically in response to both the customer base and to the marketplace from which food is procured. Many onsite foodservices change the menu cycle with the season, in order to incorporate the use of locally produced fruits and vegetables.

Sometimes menus are a combination of these types. For example, a restaurant with a static menu might have daily specials printed on the menu, like spaghetti on Monday and crab cakes on Friday, or a soup du jour. This uses the principles of static and cycle menus. The use of a "monotony breaker" by a university foodservice, in which a single-use menu is implemented occasionally (for example, corned beef and cabbage on St. Patrick's Day), is another example of how different types of menus are used in combination.

Menus also vary in the amount of choice offered. Very limited choice (or no choice) is evident on airlines, in elderly nutrition programs, and in childcare feeding. Hospitals and skilled nursing facilities often offer more choices to their clients through the use of selective menus. Some healthcare facilities are developing new menus for use with room service. Others are making the transition to a cook-chill system, which requires a completely different set of menu parameters. Quick service restaurants generally often offer fewer choices than casual-dining restaurants.

Single-Use Menu. *A menu that is designed to be used only once.*

Static Menu. *A menu that is used from day to day; it usually has a wide range of items from which the customer can choose.*

Cycle Menu. *A menu that varies from day to day, but repeats itself when the cycle is complete. The menu cycle may be a few days or several weeks in length.*

Menus for onsite foodservices are designed to meet the needs of customers.

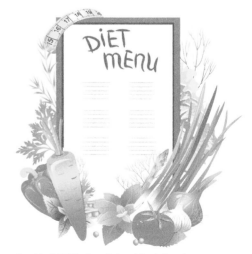

creating the menu

The first step in creating a menu is to determine what the needs of the particular foodservice and its customers are. The menu for a fine-dining operation may require only lunch and dinner selections, as well as Sunday brunch. Elementary schools need only weekday breakfasts and lunches. Full-service restaurants and healthcare facilities, which operate seven days a week, provide choices for breakfast, lunch, dinner, and perhaps between-meal selections, too.

The next step is to identify the constraints of the system for which the menu is being written. Possible system constraints are listed in Table 11.2. These include factors ranging from the availability of staff to the customer base to the space available for the foodservice operation.

Once the type of menu, the specific meal requirements, and the system constraints have been identified, the attributes of the meal itself must be determined. There are regional characteristics of meals (like grits for breakfast in the southern United States or the copious use of fresh vegetables in California), different nomenclature (for example, "dinner" or "supper"), and variation in the actual kind and type of items that make up a meal. In some places, a meal may include meat, starch, and a cooked vegetable, whereas in another area, it might include soup or salad in place of the cooked vegetable. In some regions, it is not necessary to include meat as part of a meal; in others, it is the norm.

The next step is to begin to create the menu. It is appropriate to start by planning the center-of-the-plate item for the main meal of the day (usually the evening meal), followed by the same item for the other non-breakfast meal. It should be noted that it

---

- Government regulations, including those for nutritional quality
- Size of facility
- Equipment available
- Skill level of staff
- Financial resources
- Numbers of customers to be served in a finite period of time
- Customer demographics, including age, religion, disposable income, and so forth
- Health of the clientele
- Preferences of the clientele
- Food availability

Table 11.2 Potential System Constraints on Menu Development

management practice in dietetics

is not necessary for the center-of-the-plate item to be a high-protein food. In fact, the use of meats or cheese as accompaniments, sauces, or garnishes instead of as entrées is gaining widespread acceptance.

Once the center-of-the-plate item has been established, the next step is to complete the main plate by adding accompaniments and garnishes. The accompaniments may include vegetables, starches, meats, fruits, or sauces to complement the main item. Care must be taken to ensure that all of the items on the plate are balanced in color, shape, size, texture, and flavor. Garnishes should be planned, not randomly selected as an afterthought.

After the main plate has been determined, the remainder of the meal is planned. There should be some pattern to how this is carried out. Typically, the items served before the meal are considered first. Starters include such items as juice, soup, salad, bread, and so forth. Finally, the after-meal items are established. These may include a salad (if not served before or with the main course) and the dessert. Beverage choices might also be included.

If breakfast is being served, it is usually planned after the other meals are completed. It may actually be planned independent of all other meals, because breakfast foods are different from those served at the other meals. The method of planning, however, remains the same. Start with the center-of-the-plate item and work outward from there.

Cycle menus require some additional considerations. The meals should be laid out on a spreadsheet so repetitious patterns can be identified and eliminated. The same vegetables, for example, should not be served at consecutive meals or on adjacent days. Center-of-the-plate items should not recur on the same day of consecutive weeks. The menus should be viewed as a cycle, so that the last week is evaluated in terms of the first week as well as the week that preceded it.

Once the menu is completed, it must be shared with others involved in its implementation. In health care, the clinical dietitians will consider the menu in terms of the patient needs, the chef will evaluate it for potential production problems, the purchasing manager for availability of product and for cost, and so on. Sometimes new items are pilot-tested to determine customer acceptance. Based on feedback from these other sources, the menu must be tweaked, adjusted, revised, and refined several times before it is actually implemented. In some onsite foodservice situations, the menu may have to comply with governmental regulations as well. For example, school lunches must include one third of the Daily Values (DV) of certain nutrients for its participants, and school breakfasts must provide 25% of the DVs. School meals must also meet the Dietary Guidelines for Americans. Dietetics professionals need to be aware of the regulations that apply to their own operations and be sure that their menus are in compliance with prescribed nutritional standards.

Finally, it should be noted that, at the moment, there is no computer program available to create foodservice menus. Computers are very effective at assisting with identifying market trends, aiding in the implementation of new menus, printing the actual menu, analyzing the menu for nutrient content, and other supportive functions. However, no one has yet found a way to incorporate the art of creating a menu into a computer program. Perhaps the variables are too numerous, perhaps food preferences are too individual, or perhaps it's just because computers do not know how to taste food. There have been and continue to be attempts to develop such programs, which may become available in the future. For the present, though, this is one job that is best done by people.

the specifics of purchasing

Once it has been determined that something needs to be purchased, whether it be food required to produce the menu, or stationery for the business office, the items need to be described accurately, so that the items that get ordered and delivered are those that are actually needed. Failure to establish precisely what is needed can result in waste of time, money, or both. As an example, if one needs legal-size envelopes and receives smaller personal-size envelopes, the order would either have to be returned (a waste of time, and perhaps money if the vendor has a restocking charge) or even discarded (if they were imprinted with the company logo). In either case, a new order would have to be made. To avoid such wasteful errors, purchasers must be able to state exactly what they need.

specifications

Specifications.
Written descriptions of the material to be purchased, including item name, form, quantity, quality, and pricing unit.

Specifications are descriptions of the item to be purchased. They need to be clear enough that both the purchaser and the supplier know exactly what is required. There are typically five parts of a **specification**, though six may be listed on a specification form. The usual components are the item name, form, quantity, quality, and pricing unit. Any additional information is included under the sixth category, miscellaneous. (See Table 11.3.) It may not be necessary to actually write complete specifications for each product, because some products are standardized. For example, if legal pads were needed, only the quantity, the price, and the pricing unit would be specified because the item name is descriptive of both the form (size and color) and the quality of the item.

Item Name.
The name of the product that is purchased; may be generic or brand specific.

item name. Under this heading, the name of the thing that will be purchased is listed. Often, the listing is generic, such as orange juice, 1 percent milk, file cabinet, copier, desk, letterhead, pens, napkins, chicken breasts, ground beef, and so on. When the **item name** is written in the generic form, it is necessary that the other parts of the

Component	Description of Component	Example
Item Name	Name of the product that is needed	Eggs
Form	Description of item (weight, size, whether it is fresh, frozen, or canned) and its packaging	Large, fresh whole eggs packaged 30 dozen per case
Quantity	How many are needed	60 dozen
Quality	Description of the minimum acceptable characteristics for this product	Grade A
Pricing Unit	Price per item, package, or other shipping unit	Price per case
Miscellaneous	Other information for the vendor from the purchaser	Delivery temperature between 38 and 41°F

Table 11.3 Specifications

specifications, particularly the quality descriptors, be detailed enough for the vendor to know what is needed. Sometimes brand specifications are used. For example, one may specify "Post-It" notes. In this case, there is no real need for quality descriptors in that section of the specification form because the brand name implies the quality that is desired.

When a prime vendor is being used, the brands of the product may be limited by the inventory that the prime vendor carries. There may be three brands of paper cups, for example, each of a different quality. When the purchasing agent chooses the brand, the quality is also chosen. In today's marketplace, the specifications are often determined by the availability of a product. When purchasing items that are usually mass-produced, custom-designed alternative goods are expensive and only the biggest purchasers have enough volume to influence large-scale manufacturing practices. For example, a national chain of quick service restaurants might have enough purchasing power to write their own specifications for the size and shape of their napkins and still command good prices on that product. An individually owned family restaurant will probably choose a napkin of a standard size and shape, perhaps customizing the standard napkin with a logo.

With large-ticket items, such as refrigeration units in a kitchen or a camper that has been outfitted to serve as a mobile WIC clinic, the specification will determine how the product is manufactured. The incremental costs of custom designs for such major purchases may not be as great as the cost of changing the design of a mass-produced item. For these items, the additional cost is often offset by increases in productivity.

form. The **form** indicates how the product is to be delivered to the buyer. Descriptors that fall into this category relate to the product itself, and to its packaging. If, for

Form. *A description of the product, which may include weight, size, packaging, and so on.*

Quantity.
*The amount of
a product to be
purchased, often
stated in multiples
that relate to how
the product is
typically packaged
(that is, each, case,
box, dozen, gallon,
pound, and so on).*

example, the item was hamburgers, the form might be specified as "four-ounce frozen patties, not to exceed 23 percent fat; packaged in cases of twenty pounds each containing four, five-pound plastic bags of patties with double layers of waxed paper between each patty." Using menus for patients as another example, the form could be written as "shrink-wrapped in quantities of 500 menus."

quantity. This states the amount that is to be purchased. In general, vendors prefer not to open packages and may charge a premium to do so. Therefore, the **quantity** of material ordered is usually in multiples that coincide with how the item is packaged. For example, canned peaches for foodservices are packed in cases of six No. 10 cans. Therefore, orders will usually be placed as cases or in six-can increments. If a buyer orders only two cans (an **odd lot**), the price may be higher. Unless there is a compelling reason to order goods in odd lots (for example, it would take three years to use an entire case of the item), orders should be placed in standard shipping units so that vendors do not have to break cases.

Odd Lot.
*An amount of a
product that is
different from
how a product is
typically packaged.
Orders in odd lots
require the vendor
to open packages
to deliver the
specified amount.*

For some heavily used items, like coffee and copy paper, quantities are determined by establishing a **par level** for the item. This is the minimum amount that is to be kept on hand at all times. A **reorder point** is set so that an order is generated when the amount of product on hand falls to near the par level. Items that are used less regularly are ordered by the production staff based on anticipated production needs. If a computerized system is in use, the computer generates the orders based on usage history, production estimates, and inventory. Even so, there is usually a safeguard built into the system that does not allow the order to be entered without authorization by a responsible person. The person is presumed to know facts that may not be "known" by the computer, such as shipping delays, upcoming holidays, special events, larger-than-usual production needs, new products to fabricate, and so on. That person should review and make appropriate adjustments to every order before executing it.

Par Level.
*The minimum
amount of a
specific item that
is to be kept on
hand at all times.
Sometimes the term
par stock is also
used.*

quality. **Quality** indicates those characteristics of the item that the purchaser feels represent the minimum acceptable standards for the item. Brand names (see "Item Name," above) or government grades can be used to specify quality. Alternately, a detailed written description of the product can be specified. With bid buying, brand names are usually not indicated because this limits the number of vendors who can bid on an item and diminishes competition, which may increase prices. For products for which grades are unavailable and brand names are disallowed in the bidding process, detailed written descriptions are used. If purchasing needs to be done using descriptive written quality parameters, it would be a good idea if the person writing the specifications did research into the process of writing specifications as well as into the product line being specified to determine what needs to be included in the specification. Some references to assist a manager with the development of written specifications are listed in the "To Study Further" section at the end of this chapter.

Reorder Point. *The
inventory level that
is set for an item
that triggers the
placement of an
order for more of
that item so that the
stock on hand does
not fall below the
par level.*

pricing unit. The **pricing unit** is the unit under which the item will be billed, not the actual cost of the product. Some items are listed by count. If the item to be purchased was a laser printer, it is likely that the pricing unit would be "each"—that is, a single machine. If an organization bought three identical printers at one time, the price for each printer would be listed along with the quantity (in this case, three) ordered. Other possible pricing units are weight (for example, 35 pounds of individual, quick-frozen chicken breasts), cases (for example, five cases of No. 10 cans of peaches), volume (for example, five gallons of liquid eggs), or the number (for example, one dozen dinner plates). It is essential that the pricing unit be agreed to by both the purchaser and the vendor before the price is negotiated.

miscellaneous. The **miscellaneous** section of the specification can cover any items that are not covered elsewhere. This might be a required delivery date, the frequency of deliveries, a service contract for a new piece of equipment, or the temperature at which goods should arrive. Other miscellaneous considerations could include how the goods are to be unloaded to facilitate receipt by the purchaser or an agent of the purchaser, how back orders will be handled, terms and conditions of payment, performance requirements, and so on. When a prime vendor is used, many of these items are covered in the contractual agreement between the purchaser and the vendor, so they do not have to be repeated for each item purchased. This may hold true for other vendors as well, but it is not universally true. If there is any doubt about terms and conditions, the purchaser can (and should) issue more detailed specifications.

The categories listed above are the usual parts of specifications for all material that is purchased. In practice, however, the specifications may not always be written down. When the individuals who are doing the purchasing and the vendors who supply the goods know what is required through experience, they may choose not to use a written description. For example, most people know that a case of cola consists of twenty-four 12-ounce cans of soda. There would be little need to specify anything but the number of cases needed and the brand name to get the desired product. However, if a purchaser wanted 6-ounce cans of the soda, the size of the container would need to be specified under "form." In another example, the purchasing agent may know that a specific type of flatware is needed for patient tray service, because the food-service department has a standardized tray setup. In this case, the flatware would be ordered by the manufacturer's item number, without detailed specifications, because the decision about what to purchase was made in the past, and what is being ordered now is classified as "replacements."

other considerations

Though written specifications for most material usually follow a standard format, there are some item-specific considerations that are helpful for the buyer to know. This section is an attempt to deal with some of the more universal aspects in purchasing.

Quality. *A description of the minimum acceptable characteristics of an item, which can be represented using brand names, government grades, or detailed descriptions.*

Pricing Unit. *The unit on which the price of the item is based.*

Miscellaneous. *Any additional information the purchaser includes for the vendor's information to ensure receiving the correct product under the right conditions.*

As the manager becomes more familiar with the vendors and the products available in the marketplace, this general information will be replaced with more detailed information based on experience.

supplies. The type of material that includes items with no finite shelf life is known as **supplies**. It includes office supplies, paper goods, disposable serviceware (paper plates, biodegradable utensils, placemats, napkins, and so on), cleaning supplies, and similar products. Though these items do not spoil when they get old and large amounts can be stored, it is usually inappropriate to tie up more money in supplies than necessary. In most cases, supplies are single-use items that are disposed of after being used. For bulky items like cleaning supplies and disposable serviceware, storage space is an issue. Small items like pens and paper clips, which take little space, are easily pilfered if they are too readily available. Depending on the usage of this material, deliveries may be scheduled on a daily, weekly, or monthly basis. Enough supply should be kept on hand to meet the anticipated need until the next scheduled delivery, with a small cushion added for safety. Overstocking of supplies should not be considered unless the storage space is readily available at no additional cost, the savings realized by large-scale purchasing is substantial, and the goods can be properly secured.

Some items are customized for use in an organization. These items might include pens, stationery, nutritional assessment forms, placemats, napkins, and menus. Customized products are often purchased in large quantities, because the printing or engraving cost decreases with increased volumes. The savings related to buying large quantities of these items may offset the cost of maintaining a larger-than-usual inventory. Sometimes an arrangement can be made with the supplier or printer of custom material to warehouse it and deliver the product on demand. The purchaser owns the goods and has paid or is paying for them. However, the cost of storage is minimized. When ordering supplies in this way, note that changes in the item cannot be made until the existing supply is nearly exhausted, unless one is willing to incur a loss. Customized supplies should be ordered with this in mind so that changes in information like phone numbers, e-mail addresses, or uniform resource locator (URL) do not make the supplies obsolete.

groceries. For purposes of this discussion, **groceries** are defined as those food products that are purchased in a form that is shelf-stable at room temperature. They can usually be stored at room temperature and include such items as canned goods, cereals, bread, spices, and so on. Though shelf-stable, groceries may have a defined **shelf life**, which is identified with a "use by" date on the package. When purchasing such products, one should be familiar with the typical shelf life of each product and purchase only amounts that can be used before the expiration date. The specifications for such products might indicate that the "use by" date be a minimum of a defined period of time (for example, 30 days) after the date of delivery, to ensure that all of the product can be used before that date. Vendors have different policies for dealing with returns of outdated food products. If the policy is not spelled out in a purchasing agreement, it should be detailed on an item-by-item basis in the specification.

Supplies. *Products characterized by having no finite shelf life.*

Groceries. *Food products that are shelf-stable at room temperature.*

Shelf Life. *The amount of time groceries can be used until they expire; indicated by a "use by" date.*

management practice in dietetics

Some grocery products have a shelf life of a week or less. For these products, quality deteriorates in a relatively short period of time. Therefore, the suppliers of products with a short shelf life, such as breads and other baked goods, may have a delivery routine whereby dated goods are removed at the time a delivery is made. Restaurants may have standing orders with bakeries to keep the stock at a predetermined par level. When such standing orders exist, there should be a requirement for stock rotation or the removal of old stock so that the product on hand is always fresh and usable.

perishables. **Perishables** are those foods with a limited shelf life and usually require cold-temperature storage, either refrigerated or frozen. These include meats, fish, poultry, fresh produce, dairy products, and eggs. When specifications are written for these items, the **HACCP** principles should be utilized. HACCP (Hazard Analysis and Critical Control Point) is described in the "In Practice" feature at the end of Chapter 12. Specifications should include such requirements as "internal temperature between 38 and 41 degrees Fahrenheit at the time of delivery" or "packed in ice covering the entire product."

small equipment. Two kinds of equipment are purchased. Some equipment is large, capitalized equipment, which will be described later. The other type of equipment is the reusable, small variety. **Small equipment** includes flatware and service utensils, dishes, linens, pots and pans, and similar items in foodservice, and skinfold calipers, thermometers, sphygmomanometers, and so on in clinical situations and community nutrition settings. Data storage devices, toner cartridges, and file folders may also

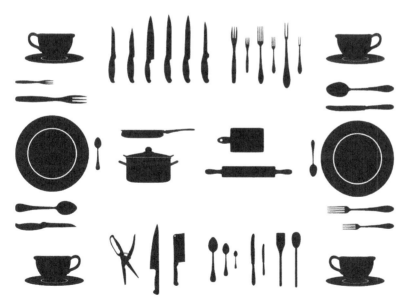

Copyright © 2010 by Depositphotos/Biljana Kordic.

In foodservice, small equipment includes tools and serviceware like the items shown here.

Perishables. *Food purchases characterized by a limited shelf life and usually requiring cold storage such as refrigeration or freezing.*

HACCP (Hazard Analysis and Critical Control Point). *Process that promotes food-safety protocols and outlines steps in the preparation of a food item starting from its point of delivery all the way to consumption.*

Small Equipment. *Reusable equipment that costs more than supplies and has a longer life expectancy.*

be categorized as reusable, as are smaller pieces of electronic equipment like video cameras, projectors, and telephones. In general, these items are costlier than supplies and have a longer life expectancy. They may be used for several months or years before they get used up, worn out, stolen, or broken.

Replacements.
Products that are purchased to replace items that have been lost, broken, stolen, or worn out with use.

For small equipment that gets used up in a normal operation, **replacements** must be purchased. Usually, the replacement is identical to the item that is being replaced. For example, the 24 dinner plates that are purchased to replace those that were broken last month are likely to be the same size, shape, pattern, and style as the plates that were broken. The original specifications can be reused for this type of replacement goods. When such items are ordered, the order will need to be placed with a vendor who can supply the dishes that are needed. (It should be noted that, when a prime vendor is changed, the new vendor might not be able to provide the replacements needed to match existing goods.) Other replacement items are toner cartridges, batteries, light bulbs, cutting boards, scoops and ladles, and so on.

Some small equipment is purchased less frequently, and because of technological advances, the new equipment is likely to be different than (and often better than) the item it replaces. Document cameras, laptop computers, and telephones are among the items that fall into this category. When these items are being purchased, the available options should be examined and the desired features specified. For example, one could specify a laptop computer with a larger memory and extended battery life as compared to the older model it replaced. Once the desired features are described, it becomes relatively easy to find the right piece of equipment to meet the specifications.

delivery options

Another integral part of the procurement process is the delivery requirements of the purchaser relative to the delivery capabilities of the vendor. The time and frequency of deliveries will have an impact on staffing and security and should not be left to chance. In general, a vendor's largest customers are likely to be able to specify conditions of delivery. A smaller customer often has to make accommodations to fit the vendor's routes and schedules. In this era of service management, however, prime vendors try to accommodate the customer's needs as much as possible. Another factor that will affect deliveries is the location of the purchaser. Facilities in rural areas may have access only to weekly or biweekly deliveries, whereas customers in urban areas may be able to get deliveries every day.

Frequency of Delivery.
The number of times deliveries are made by a vendor to a purchasing organization, which could be daily, weekly, or monthly.

Of the factors to be considered when negotiating terms of delivery, the first is the **frequency of delivery**. With daily deliveries, it is possible to order most goods to arrive when they are needed. This means that the material can go directly into the production area without having to be stored and distributed from storage. This reduces the need for manpower in the storage area and also reduces the cost of maintaining storage space. Loss from theft may also go down, because there is little inventory available to steal. A disadvantage of daily deliveries occurs when the delivery is late, because production may have to be delayed until the delivery arrives. Another possible concern is that if the delivery is missing items, there may not be adequate backup stock to support production. Daily deliveries that are taken directly to the production area may interfere with the systematic rotation of goods into and out of inventory. Care must be taken to ensure that the material in storage does not become outdated or obsolete.

Conversely, less-frequent deliveries mean that needs must be anticipated for a longer time span. Under these circumstances, and considering the possibility that deliveries may be delayed, care must be taken to maintain adequate stock on hand to cover contingencies. With less-frequent deliveries, each order is relatively large and needs to be put into storage quickly. This may affect staffing patterns on the day or days that deliveries are scheduled. In addition, large inventories increase the need for security. The value of inventory is inversely proportional to the frequency of delivery, and as value increases, so does the possibility of significant theft.

A second delivery factor to be considered is the **timing of the deliveries**. It is necessary to coordinate timing with both production needs and the schedule of the receiving personnel. If all deliveries were scheduled to arrive at nine in the morning, there could be a waiting period for trucks at the loading dock. In addition, the receiving personnel would be overwhelmed at that time of the day. That could lead to confusion and errors in the checking in of material. When perishables are included in the deliveries, delays involved in getting the goods into proper storage could create a problem with food safety. Finally, with too much product sitting on the loading dock, the potential for theft increases. If possible, deliveries should be staggered so that this type of backlog does not occur.

Timing of the Deliveries. *The time of day deliveries should arrive; should correspond with production needs and the receiving personnel's schedule to ensure a smooth delivery and proper storage of goods.*

In an operation that is open seven days a week, it is necessary to decide whether weekend deliveries are desirable or necessary. Some operations prefer to forgo weekend deliveries altogether, in order to decrease staffing on Saturdays and Sundays. Other operations choose to allow weekend deliveries of goods that will be transported directly to the production area by the delivery personnel. The delivery is checked in by the supervisor, rather than by storeroom personnel. If it needs to be stored, the supervisor assigns someone to put the material into storage. In operations that do full-scale production on a daily basis, daily deliveries may be required. In such cases, the delivery routine is the same on weekends as it is on weekdays, provided the vendor is willing and able to accommodate this schedule.

Finally, the responsibility for transporting the product from the loading dock to the storage area, or to another location in the operation, must be specified. Some deliveries are made to the loading dock, where they are received by the organization. The transport and storage of those products within the facility are the responsibility of the purchaser. This decreases risk by assuring that the storerooms are secure and that access to inventory by outsiders is limited. For other items, the delivery is actually made to the production area or to the point of service. Examples of foodservice products that may be stocked by the vendor are breads, chips, frozen confections, and specialty cold beverages. In other situations, service contracts for copying machines may include paper that is delivered to the location of the copier on a regular basis. In non-foodservice operations, coffee for leased machines, bottled water for water coolers, and items for stocking vending machines are among the goods usually stocked by the vendor.

capital goods and equipment

Capital Goods.
Large equipment, considered fixed assets, that is durable and can be depreciated over a period of time.

Large-ticket items, like cooking and refrigeration equipment in foodservice, large-volume copiers, computer systems, and furniture in all operations, may be among those items purchased by the dietitian or dietetic technician manager. **Capital goods** are those goods that are durable in nature and are depreciated over a discrete period of time. From an accounting perspective, capital goods are fixed assets. They differ from inventory, which is considered to be a current (or liquid) asset.

If large numbers of capital items are being purchased, as for the renovation of a kitchen or a cafeteria in a foodservice, the dietetics professional may work with a kitchen design engineer, an architect, or another consultant with expertise in institutional equipment. Experts are also generally consulted if one is making major systems changes in an office, such as upgrading a telephone system, installing a computer network, or coordinating furniture for a group of offices. The experts can provide design and implementation ideas that can greatly enhance the efficiency of an operation. The expert may be hired as an independent contractor or consultant, or the vendor who is providing the equipment may provide the design service.

There is almost always a cost for design services. The fee may be direct—for example, a fee for the design work done by an architect or interior designer—or indirect, wherein the fee is included in the commission that the vendor earns on the capital goods purchased. Though it is reasonable to expect to pay something for design services, it is prudent to note that individuals who work on commission increase their earnings as the cost of the goods purchased increases. Some of these individuals may try to sell premium items or more equipment than is needed in order to increase their own income. Knowing this, the purchaser should have a firm idea of what goods are needed before the consultation is undertaken.

Sometimes capital goods are bought as individual pieces; expert assistance may not be available for such purchases. This means that the dietetics manager will need to become familiar with the options available and make selections from those options. The necessary expertise can come from trade publications, meetings and exhibitions, networking, visiting other facilities, and shopping. Suppliers of capital equipment are often willing to tell potential customers where their product is installed and

management practice in dietetics

being used. By exploring the pros and cons of various products with individuals who actually use the equipment under different circumstances, a purchaser can greatly improve the chances of making a good purchasing decision. Information on foodservice equipment is available on the Internet.

Descriptions for capital equipment often include **performance specifications** that must be met by the product. For foodservice equipment, these might include things like preheat times for ovens or fryers, energy usage of the equipment, production capacity (for example, the amount of food that can be cooked each hour), and maintenance requirements. The In Practice feature at the end of this chapter deals with this concept in greater detail. With computers, speed, sound, networking, and graphics capabilities are among the performance standards that may be specified. For copiers, the machine's capacity per minute, its ability to produce colored or two-sided copies, the capability to scan documents, and whether or not it can collate and staple finished documents are performance variables. Performance specifications can be written to describe the precision of an instrument such as a thermometer, a scale, or a set of calipers. It is not always necessary to have the biggest, best, fanciest, or most accurate piece of equipment, as long as the piece meets the needs of the purchaser.

Technical specifications are also written for capital equipment. In general, technical specifications include things that can be determined by some objective test or measurement related to physical attributes rather than to performance. This includes the overall dimensions or the footprint of the piece, which is especially important for equipment that must fit into a defined space. It could also include such things as the thickness of the metal in stainless steel equipment, the capacity of the paper tray in a copier, the weight of a piece of mobile equipment, or the percentage of various fibers in carpeting.

It should be noted that technical and performance specifications could be written for any product, not just capital goods. Conversely, one can choose to purchase capital goods using brand (or brand and model numbers) specifications instead of written performance or technical specifications. The way that the specification is written will influence the number of competitive bids that can be solicited for a given product or group of products. If a limited number of bids is desirable, the specifications should be very precise; if many bids are being solicited, the specifications might need to be less rigid.

The most important part of writing specifications is not how the specification is written, but that the specification is written in such a way that the buyer gets the best possible product for the intended use at a fair price. It should also be noted that the lowest price is not always an indicator of which product to purchase because service, maintenance, and reliability are other variables that should have an impact on purchasing decisions.

Performance Specifications.
Written descriptions of how a piece of equipment is required to act, including factors that relate to speed, safety, production capacity, accuracy, and so on.

Technical Specifications.
Written descriptions for capital goods or other products that specify functions that can be determined by an objective test or measurement; includes such factors as type of material, dimensions, and weights.

receiving

After the purchasing decision has been made, the order is placed and the vendor ships the goods to the purchaser. The next step in material management is **receiving** the product or products and acknowledgment of its receipt. Large organizations usually assign an individual or several individuals to perform the receiving function and train them in the intricacies of the process. As with procurement, the process should be planned and deliberate. It should not be haphazard. The individual who does the receiving is also responsible for the rejection of products that do not meet specifications and for communicating with the rest of the organization about what has been received, what has been rejected, and what goods were missing from the delivery. Sometimes the receiving personnel are responsible for the storage and distribution of material as well.

methods

If the receiving is done at the loading dock or a specified receiving area, the designated individual from the purchasing organization should know when to expect the delivery. Upon arrival, it is usually accompanied by some sort of **invoice** or shipping document, which provides information regarding what was shipped. The amounts shipped may or may not be included on the shipping document. If the amounts are included, the process is called **invoice receiving**. With this method, the job of the receiving staff is to count the material received and sign the document as acknowledgment that the products listed on the document were actually delivered. If the document does not coincide with the shipment, notations should be made on all copies of the shipping/receiving document to indicate shortages, back orders, and so on before the document is signed to indicate that the material has been received. A copy of the document stays with the delivery person, and another copy goes to the accounting department of the purchasing organization. There should be an established method of notifying management of shortages and back orders so that appropriate changes in the production schedule can be made, if necessary.

If the amounts of product are not included on the receiving documents, the receiver should note the amount of each product that was delivered. This process is called **blind receiving**. The method was established to ensure the honesty of the delivery and receiving personnel, neither of whom is supposed to know what amounts were ordered, by placing the reconciliation of invoice and order in the hands of a clerk who did not handle the goods. The organization pays only for what was actually received, and the vendor covers all discrepancies. It is questionable whether the method has more positive or negative effects. Theoretically, it saves the organization from losses at the loading dock by dishonest employees, but the method itself shows a basic distrust of staff members who have been given positions of responsibility and may undermine the morale of the staff.

management practice in dietetics

Furthermore, blind receiving adds another step to the process and may delay the transmission of crucial information about missing items to the production area. In today's information-intensive environment, blind receiving may not be justified unless the function is automated with barcode readers or similar technologies. Another justification that has been used is a history of documented loss in the receiving area. In the latter event, other steps to decrease security risk can be implemented. These alternate methods could have a less-negative effect on the movement of information and on morale. One commonly used device is video surveillance of the delivery area. When blind receiving is automated and the transmission of information is instantaneous, this type of procedure may be an appropriate way to receive goods.

documentation

After goods are received, the documents that acknowledge the receipt of the product must be processed. The document may either be an invoice, which requires processing for payment, or a **packing slip**, which must later be reconciled with an invoice that is sent separately. In many cases, these documents are forwarded to the accounting department for processing. However, before forwarding the documents, there should be a procedure to identify missing items and back orders and to transmit that information to the production staff and the procurement staff.

Packing Slip.
A shipping document used to verify the receipt of a product, which is later compared to the invoice.

If the vendor is out of the item, it may be automatically back-ordered, meaning that it will be sent to the purchaser when it becomes available. This is fine if the purchaser has adequate stock to get through until the next delivery. However, if the purchasing organization procures the item from another source, the back order must be canceled to avoid stock duplication and excessive inventories. Sometimes a purchasing agent does not know that an item is back-ordered and orders the item a second or third time. When the item finally becomes available, all of the back orders could get delivered, resulting in an excess of that item. This is one of the reasons that communication is such an important part of the receiving process.

Tickler File.
A method of reminding oneself of "loose ends" that need follow-up. Often used for tracking procurement discrepancies such as back orders, cancellations, and shortages to ensure smooth production and proper payment, and to document vendor performance.

In an alternate scenario, it may be the vendor's policy to cancel orders for goods that are not available at the time of delivery or to cancel back orders after a predetermined period of time has passed. If this is the standing procedure, it is imperative that the procurement staff and the production staff be notified so that they do not run out of raw material for production. It is helpful if someone from procurement or receiving is assigned the task of maintaining a **tickler file** to follow up this type of procurement problem. In addition to communicating information about back orders, canceled orders, and shortages, information about products that were rejected at the receiving dock should be reported. This information is needed to replace the product, alter production schedules, and ensure that correct payment is made, as well as to document vendor performance. Past performance is one factor that is considered when a prime vendor is selected.

the receiving area

The equipment that is needed in the receiving area will be dependent on the type of product received. In an organization that provides a service product out of a small office suite, no specialized equipment is necessary. Most of what is received is in envelopes or small packages that can easily be moved by hand. In larger operations where items such as paper and janitorial supplies are purchased in bulk, it becomes necessary to have a cart or a hand truck for moving heavy boxes from place to place. In operations where large amounts of goods are received and produced, heavier equipment such as carts, dollies, and forklifts are needed.

The receiving area may be the reception desk at the entrance to an office where most deliveries come via the postal service or a delivery service such as UPS or Federal Express. In other situations, there may be a specially designed receiving area with loading docks designed to accommodate large vehicles such as trucks and semitrailers. The space requirements and the design of the receiving area will be based on the amount and type of material that is usually received by the business.

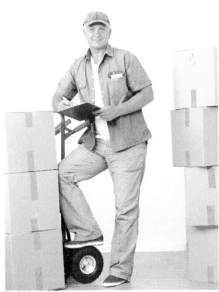

Copyright © 2011 by Depositphotos/CandyBoxImages.

Receiving personnel check in orders and transport goods to the storage area.

The receiving staff should have the knowledge and the authorization to reject shipments that do not meet specifications or that have been damaged in shipping. For some types of goods, this means that any damaged container is opened and the contents inspected. The delivery may then be accepted "as is," accepted with the damage noted for correction in the near future, or refused. Again, the variation between what was ordered and what was received intact should be noted and the information forwarded appropriately. For perishable products like food, the process is more complex and is described in detail below.

receiving food products

Because food products are often ordered by weight or count, and because much of what is received is perishable, the procedure for receiving food products differs from the procedure for receiving other types of products. If a foodservice is freestanding, like a restaurant, the foodservice will do all of its own receiving. If the foodservice is part of a larger organization like a hotel or a hospital, it may do all or a part of its own receiving. It is very rare to find a foodservice that delegates the entire task of receiving to another department. Supplies and replacements may be handled by a material management department, while perishables and other groceries are handled by the receiving personnel in the foodservice.

equipment/space requirements. The receiving area of a foodservice should be in an area where deliveries can be monitored and where there is a reasonable chance of excluding intruders from the area. If there are no employees stationed there, the area should be equipped with a system to secure the area and let the foodservice receiving personnel know when a delivery arrives so that it can be received properly. Ideally, the receiving area should be near both dry and refrigerated storage areas. If possible, freezers should also be located nearby.

Foodservice receiving areas need scales for weighing the product that comes in, thermometers for checking the temperature of perishables, and a sink if any pre-preparation is required. Also required are adequate equipment for moving the product into storage, a desk and writing supplies, and miscellaneous small equipment for opening containers, cutting boxes, and resealing packaging as needed. In automated systems, a computer terminal and a handheld barcode reader are essential.

HACCP. When perishables are received, attention must be paid to food safety using the HACCP system. (See In Practice feature at the end of Chapter 12.) The receiving personnel should be food safety–certified, using ServSafe or another similar certification system.

The first consideration is at the point of acceptance to ensure that the product is safe when it is delivered to the foodservice. It is appropriate to check the temperature and compare it to the standards set in the FDA's Food Code, which state recommendations related to food temperature and individual specifications for particular food items. For example, if it were specified that whole chickens be covered with ice and the ice had melted before the item was delivered, the item could be refused. Poor packaging can also lead to food contamination and might be a cause for concern. If the packing material for a perishable product like eggs was wet and soiled, the product probably should be rejected. Substandard perishable goods should never be used in foodservices because of the potential harm that can be caused to large groups of customers. If there appears to be a compromise in food safety, the product should be refused. It is better to be overly cautious than to take any health risks in foodservice.

The second safety concern at the receiving area is the time it takes to get perishable goods from the receiving area into temperature-controlled storage. This is always a concern, but more care needs to be taken when there are extremes in temperature, either hot or cold. Perishable products should be moved into temperature-controlled storage as soon as they are received. This does not mean that a product must be placed into its proper inventory control space right away, but it is imperative to get the product into the cooler or freezer. Often, perishable food is put into the cold storage area on a cart or similar piece of equipment while the rest of that day's deliveries are being received and secured. When time permits, the staff member returns to the refrigerator or freezer to redistribute these items onto shelves to ensure that they are properly stored. This immediate storage serves three purposes: to address food safety concerns, to secure the product from theft, and to save energy needed to cool a product that has been allowed to get too warm.

FDA's Food Code.
Food and Drug Administration guidelines that specify correct food-handling techniques.

FDA Food Code.
http://www.fda.gov/ Food/FoodSafety/ RetailFoodProtection/ FoodCode/ FoodCode2009/ default.htm

ServSafe.
http://www.servsafe. com/home

storage

All goods that come into an organization are either taken immediately to the point of use or stored until they are needed. Taking them to the point of use does not ensure that they will be used immediately, but it does allow the goods to be stored near where they are to be used so that they will be readily accessible when needed. This reduces the amount of handling needed. However, there may be limited space in the production area for large quantities of raw material. The organization has two options. It can choose to use **just-in-time** deliveries so that small quantities of goods arrive when they are needed and never have to be put into storage at all. Alternately, limited amounts of material can be stored in the production area and the remainder of the material held in a **storage area**.

When material is being stored, there is a need to monitor what is in storage and the age of that stock. **Stock rotation** is implemented so goods, especially perishables, do not go out of date. Older goods should be routinely used before newer goods. This is an issue in two situations. The first occurs when untrained personnel place newly received product in front of older goods, making it difficult to get to the older stock. The new product gets used before the older stock, which eventually becomes outdated and must be discarded. The second situation occurs when goods are delivered directly to the production area, bypassing storage. If a backup of product is kept in reserve, care must be taken to track this backup stock and replace it with fresh product often enough to allow all goods to be used before the expiration date. This is especially true of groceries, nutraceuticals, and other dated products. In this latter situation, there is some additional handling of product involved to ensure that no product is discarded because of expired **use-by dates**.

storerooms

Today, the space requirements for inventory are much less than they used to be. This is a result of advances in transportation and information technology, which enable most goods to be delivered within a day of being ordered. It is no longer necessary to keep large inventories in stock to cover for deficiencies in the procurement and delivery systems. This dramatically reduces the cost of inventory and thus the cost of doing business. It has also decreased the amount of storage space needed for inventory and improved the quality of products (reduced spoilage of perishables and less "freezer burn" for frozen products). It is rare for an operation that produces nonperishable goods to maintain an inventory of more than one week's raw material in stock. Some businesses (usually not foodservices) can operate exclusively on just-in-time deliveries. Well-run onsite foodservices maintain no more than 7 to 10 days' worth of inventory unless they are located in a place where deliveries are both infrequent and unreliable. Restaurants frequently have only 3–5 days' worth of food product on hand.

Store frequently used material near the entrance to the storage area.

Store material that is rarely used away from the entrance.

Store heavy items near the floor.

Place lightweight items on upper shelves.

If stacking items, put light items on top of heavy ones.

Assign and label space for each inventory item.

Keep each item in its assigned space.

If possible, secure shelving to the floor, the ceiling, or a wall.

Storage areas must be able to be secured, but with devices that ensure egress if someone is inadvertently locked inside.

Secure expensive or controlled substances (needles, alcohol, narcotics) at all times.

Table 11.4 General Storage Principles

Storage areas may range in size from a closet for copier supplies in a service-based operation, to multiple, temperature-controlled areas in a foodservice. Some storage principles are universal and should be used for any material. See Table 11.4.

In foodservices, there are additional requirements. The dry goods storage areas must have shelving that keeps all food products off the floor and, if possible, away from walls. The shelving should be easy to clean; newer shelving systems disassemble so that their components can be run through commercial dishwashers. If packaging is vulnerable to penetration from insects or rodents (for example, rice or flour packaged in paper bags), the product should be stored within bins or other sealed containers. The storeroom should be well lit, well ventilated, and humidity controlled if possible to prevent molds and mildew from forming. It is helpful to have temperature control as well. There should also be adequate space for all products to be viewed directly without having to move goods around to see what is behind them.

The Food Code requires that foods be stored in an area separate from nonfood chemicals. This includes cleaning supplies like soaps, bleaches and other sanitizers, pesticides, solvents, and so on. Such supplies must be stored in a locked storage area; they may not be stored in an open area of a foodservice.

refrigeration. Ideally, a foodservice will have walk-in types of refrigerators and freezers. Some small operations may have only one walk-in refrigerator and a small, reach-in freezer. Large operations will have separate walk-in refrigerators for meats, dairy, and produce (and perhaps one for leftovers, too). Each of these units will be set at the appropriate temperature and humidity for the product it holds. The freezer may be freestanding or may be located behind the refrigerator so that one must enter it through the refrigerator. This configuration conserves energy but limits the refrigerated storage available, because the refrigerator must accommodate two doors and more space-consuming traffic patterns.

Walk-in refrigerators and freezers are equipped with thermometers that can be read from the outside, without opening the doors. This feature was designed for energy conservation. Some have alarm systems that warn the foodservice personnel when the internal temperature reaches a predetermined threshold. Newer models may have automated systems that record the internal temperatures at predetermined intervals and send warning messages to management if these are exceeded. In any case, some monitoring system should be in place to meet HACCP guidelines.

Refrigerators should be maintained regularly and checked to be sure that their gaskets and seals are not worn, cracked, or dirty. Walk-ins should be equipped with strip curtains. Care should be taken to avoid frost buildup inside of the units, because this decreases efficiency. Shelving should keep all products off the floor and should be removable for cleaning. When there is only one walk-in in a facility, sections should be designated for each type of product kept there. That is, dairy should be separated from produce, which is separated from meats and opened containers of products like salad dressing or condiments. All products should be covered before being refrigerated to prevent the transfer of flavors or contamination from spills. Open packages should be dated when they are opened, and leftovers should be labeled and dated with the production date. If warm products are to be refrigerated, they should be placed in small, shallow containers to facilitate cooling. If there is a blast chiller available, all warm items should be chilled before being placed into the refrigerator. For additional details on food storage, consult the Food Code or the *ServSafe Manager Book*.

Smaller, **reach-in refrigerators** or **pass-through refrigerators** are often used in foodservice. These include point-of-use units such as a cook's refrigerator, or point-of-service units that may be found in cafeterias or on traylines. Sometimes these units are stocked from deliveries rather than from larger in-house storage units. As stated earlier, this method eliminates some of the double handling of a product but should be used with caution to guarantee that the product in storage is rotated in a timely manner.

inventory

The final part of the material management process is the managing of **inventory**, the raw material and goods kept for use in production. As discussed earlier, the quantity of goods kept on hand for production purposes has been decreasing in recent years. This has led to more efficiency in operations and to reduced costs. Despite these benefits, inventory management has become more difficult in that adequate production inputs must be available without any excess stock. It is no longer acceptable to keep large stockpiles of extra product on hand for emergencies.

Inventory control has three parts. The first of these is knowing exactly how much is on hand. The second is the distribution of material from the inventory, including how to account for these items. The final part of inventory control is establishing the value of these goods.

physical inventory

For accounting purposes, it is necessary for businesses to take a physical inventory of all of the material in storage once each year. This is probably sufficient for a small operation that has a perpetual inventory system in place, or for an operation with a service product, rather than goods. An operation with a large inflow of goods and outflow of product would do well to conduct a physical inventory each month. In foodservices, many managers prefer to conduct weekly inventories to better track the product on hand.

The physical inventory consists of counting the material that is on hand at a specific time (for example, every Thursday, or the first Monday of every month). When retail stores conduct a physical inventory, they may precede the count with a sale to reduce the inventory on hand so they have fewer items to count. When foodservices perform weekly or monthly inventories, they are frequently done before a large order is delivered so that fewer goods are on hand to count.

It is standard practice for two individuals to do inventory, one who actually counts the products in storage and the other who records the data. Often, one of these individuals is a manager—for example, the purchasing manager or the production manager. Though the two-person inventory team may not be essential with the use of barcodes and scanners, it is still the method of choice because it builds verification into the physical inventory process. With the scanners, the barcode of an inventoried product is read and the amount of that product is entered into a handheld device. This device then downloads data into a computer that processes the actual inventory records.

Procedures for physical inventory should be spelled out for individual operations. Some foodservices, for example, exclude just-in-time items like milk and bread from the inventory because unused or outdated product is removed from the operation by the vendor without cost to the foodservice. Other operations count only those items in storage; some count every item that is on the premises, regardless of its location.

Physical Inventory. *The process of counting each item that is in storage at a specific time to determine what product is on hand.*

Taking inventory is facilitated by the use of barcode readers.

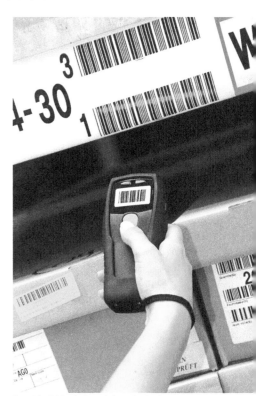

Copyright © 2011 by Depositphotos/Benjamin Haas.

perpetual inventory

A **perpetual inventory** system is one in which goods on hand are determined by using an initial physical inventory, adding goods that have been purchased, and subtracting goods that have been distributed or used in production. Because it is ongoing, it is theoretically possible to know exact amounts of what is on hand at any given time. This system can be **real time** thanks to computerized inventory management systems. The perpetual inventory system precludes the need to perform frequent physical inventories, though accounting standards require that a physical inventory be done at least once a year.

When there are good controls related to the issuing of material from a storeroom, and documentation that the physical inventory and the perpetual inventory are in agreement at the 90 to 95 percent level, foodservice operations may reduce the frequency of physical inventory from weekly to monthly. Material management departments and warehouse operations often choose to do quarterly physical inventories on a rotating basis. That is, they may verify on a quarterly basis the data that come from the perpetual inventory for each item they stock. Each item is counted quarterly, with about 8 percent of items counted during any given week. This saves the warehouse personnel from doing a massive physical inventory once a year, verifies that product is rotated and does not become outdated, and validates (and corrects as necessary) the data generated by the perpetual inventory.

distribution from storage

The control of items leaving storage is crucial if a perpetual inventory method is to function properly. Methods must be in place to assure that every item leaving the storage area is accounted for and recorded. Though this sounds like a relatively simple procedure, it is very difficult to achieve in the context of day-to-day operations.

Sometimes crisis situations arise that cause employees to enter the storeroom and obtain needed material without recording what was taken. This causes a discrepancy in the perpetual inventory. If multiple individuals have access to the storeroom, or if the storeroom is not secured, a perpetual inventory system cannot work.

open storeroom

Many small operations run with an **open storeroom** system. In this situation, any staff member can retrieve items from the storeroom at any time. When this system is used, weekly physical inventories are essential to ensure that raw material is available when needed.

ingredient room

In large, onsite foodservices, the perpetual inventory system works best in conjunction with an **ingredient room**. This may be an actual room or a designated area of the food production facility where ingredients are measured and assembled for each recipe that is to be prepared. Sometimes pre-preparation, such as peeling, chopping, or dicing, is also done in the ingredient room. With this method, the only individuals who have access to the storage areas are designated people who place the delivered goods into storage and those who assemble ingredients to distribute to the production staff. Because one of the primary functions of the ingredient room staff is inventory control, accountability is greater and the perpetual inventory system works well. Sometimes the ingredient assembly worker is the same individual who receives and stores the deliveries, which puts all of the accountability into the hands of one person. Similar systems are used in non-foodservice operations, though the term *ingredient room* is not used outside of foodservice.

Ingredient Room.
A designated area of a food production facility in which the items needed to prepare a certain recipe are measured and assembled; some pre-preparation may also be done here.

point-of-sale systems

Point-of-sale inventory systems are those that link the cash register to the inventory control system. It works well in retail operations, like grocery stores, where barcodes are located on each product and individual items are rung up using barcode readers. It also works well in restaurants with limited menus, where products are uniform and there are not large numbers of items made from "scratch" using complex recipes. As items are sold and "rung up," each item is subtracted from inventory. To work properly, this inventory control system must be able to identify each item separately. If barcodes are not used, then the item must be represented by an individual cash register key—for example, 8 oz. low-fat milk, large fries, cheeseburger, and so on. When one key is used for multiple items of the same price (for example, 12 oz. soft drink) the effectiveness of the point-of-sale system is compromised.

Point of Sale.
An inventory system in which the cash register is linked to inventory control, automatically subtracting an item as it is used or sold.

inventory control methods

Inventory is controlled using a number of different strategies. Items are arranged to minimize handling and injuries to workers (for example, light items overhead, heavy items on lower shelves). Once the storage area is arranged, the computerized inventory program can be sequenced in the same order, so items can be counted in sequence. A sort function can then be used to rearrange the inventory into product categories for ordering. Thus, the arrangement of the storeroom for efficiency is the driving factor behind inventory management.

A second factor to consider is stock rotation, in which old product should always be used before newer product. To meet this goal, there must be adequate space in the storeroom to stock product without having to move the goods that are already in stock. In older facilities, there is usually excess storage space, because these facilities were designed when organizations needed to keep high inventory levels on hand. In newer facilities with less square footage devoted to storage, shelving that can be approached from either side assists storeroom personnel with this process. **High-density shelving** that can be moved on tracks (much like the movable stacks in some libraries) is effective in saving space while fostering efficiency.

Keeping the storage area secure, by staffing it continually, locking it, or otherwise limiting access, is crucial to managing inventory. It is necessary to prevent theft and to promote accountability. Unsecured storage areas are invitations for dishonest people to help themselves to whatever is available.

valuation of inventory

Finally, it is necessary to place a value on the inventory that is in stock. Acceptable accounting practices allow for three possible ways to value inventory. The first method values the stock at the actual price that was paid for each item. The second assigns a value at the current price, which is the cost of replacing each item. The third establishes a weighted average value for each item. The second method (replacement value) actually places a higher value on inventory than the other methods, because the cost of items usually goes up over time.

If the value of inventory is small, it appears that the organization has fewer assets. This means that the cost of raw material seems larger, and profits appear to be less. From the perspective of tax liability, it is desirable to have lower profits. Conversely, if the inventory value is larger, profits appear larger, too. From the perspective of attracting investors, it is desirable to appear more profitable.

Despite the temptation to use different methods of valuing inventory for different purposes, it is illegal to do so. The organization must make a decision about how it wishes to value inventory and stick to that method over time. Once the method of valuing inventory has been determined, it is unlikely to be changed.

A more useful management tool is the value of the inventory relative to time. In some onsite foodservices, for example, it is desirable to keep a maximum of 7 to 10 days' worth of inventory in stock. Other foodservice operations may want between 4 and 7 days' worth of inventory on hand. To calculate the value of inventory as it relates to time, start by determining the cost of all products used in a given period. The difference in value between the beginning and ending inventories plus the cost of purchases during the period equals the total cost of material used. That number is then divided by the number of days in the period to determine the daily cost of raw material.

management practice in dietetics

Next, divide the value of the current inventory by the daily cost of raw material to determine the number of days' worth of product on hand. Small foodservices in rural areas may need to keep more on hand because of infrequent deliveries; large operations in urban areas might get by with fewer days' supplies on hand. Usually there is a standard amount of inventory that should be kept on hand for different types of businesses. This is one of the items that may be benchmarked for accountability purposes (see Chapter 13).

conclusion

This chapter has described the process of material management. This includes the procurement, the receiving and storage of goods and material, the distribution of that material from storage, and the determination of inventory. The following are the main concepts discussed in this chapter.

1. One measure of the scope of management of an individual is the manager's purchasing authority.
2. A variety of purchasing methods are available, ranging from the most formal—bid purchasing—to the least formal—retail purchasing. In today's marketplace, prime vendor contracts are becoming the norm for most large operations.
3. In foodservices, the menu serves as the basis for purchasing.
4. Specifications include the name and form of the product needed, as well as the quantity, quality, and pricing unit; miscellaneous data can be added as necessary.
5. Both technical and performance specifications can be written for material.
6. Material purchases include, but are not limited to, the major categories of supplies, groceries, perishables, small equipment, and capital equipment.
7. Good receiving practices include accountability for and the safe handling of all material received.
8. Goods should be properly and securely stored as soon as possible after delivery.
9. A method must be in place to account for inventory on a regular basis. This includes knowing what is received and what is distributed from stock, as well as the total amount (and value) of stock on hand at any given time.
10. HACCP principles must be used throughout the procurement process.

activities

activity 1

Write specifications for products assigned by your instructor. If your instructor does not assign specific products, choose one product from each of the following categories.

- Supplies
- Small equipment
- Perishables
- Groceries
- Large (capital) foodservice equipment
- Large (capital) office equipment

activity 2

Visit a foodservice operation or a grocery store when a delivery is scheduled to arrive. Observe how receiving is done in that facility. Analyze what you observed in light of HACCP guidelines and security. Write a brief report on what you observed.

activity 3

Determine how many days' worth of inventory is on hand for a foodservice with an opening inventory valued at $26,000, a closing inventory (one week later) of $28,000, and purchases of $18,000 for the week. How does this value compare with the 7- to 10-day standard for foodservices?

to study further

Additional information on material management, writing specifications, foodservice equipment, and HACCP can be found in the following books and on the websites noted below.

- Birchfield, J. C. and Birchfield J. *Design and Layout of Foodservice Facilities.* 3rd ed. Hoboken, NJ: John Wiley and Sons, Inc., 2008.
- Katsigris, C. and C. Thomas. *Design and Equipment for Restaurants and Foodservice: A Management View.* 3rd ed. Hoboken, NJ: John Wiley and Sons, Inc., 2009.
- Kotschevar, L. H. and R. Donnelly. *Quantity Food Purchasing.* 5th ed. Upper Saddle River, NJ: Prentice Hall, 1999.
- Lynch, F. T. *The Book of Yields: Accuracy in Food Costing and Purchasing.* 8th ed. Hoboken, NJ: John Wiley and Sons, 2012.
- McVety, P., B. J. Ware, and C. L. Ware. *Fundamentals of Menu Planning.* 3rd ed. Hoboken, NJ: John Wiley and Sons, Inc. 2009.
- National Restaurant Association. *ServSafe Manager.* 6th ed. Chicago, IL: Pearson College Division, 2012.
- Payne-Palacio, J. and M. Theis. *Introduction to Foodservice.* 11th ed. Upper Saddle River, NJ: Pearson Prentice Hall, 2009.
- Gregoire, M. B. *Foodservice Systems: A Managerial and Systems Approach.* 8th ed. Boston: Pearson, 2013.
- Spears, M. C. *Foodservice Procurement: Purchasing for Profit.* Upper Saddle River, NJ: Prentice Hall, 1999.

scholarly journal

- *Journal of Foodservice Business Research*

other relevant periodicals

- *Food Management*
- *Foodservice Director*
- *Foodservice Equipment and Supplies*
- *Foodservice Equipment Reports*
- *Nation's Restaurant News*

relevant websites

- FDA's Food Code http://www.fda.gov/Food/FoodSafety/RetailFoodProtection/FoodCode/FoodCode2009/default.htm
- Food Safety home page www.foodsafety.gov
- Energy Star http://www.energystar.gov/

in practice

specifying performance in foodservice equipment

Foodservices, especially onsite foodservices and those small restaurants that are individually owned, often have to make do with less-than-optimal foodservice equipment. For budgetary reasons, the "mom and pop" operations may purchase low-cost, low-efficiency equipment in the first place. Institutions and large facilities might have had state-of-the-art equipment when it was purchased and installed, but often the workhorse pieces like dishwashers and ovens wear out and are held together with proverbial "baling wire."

Dietetics professionals do not often have the opportunity to build new facilities from the ground up, and when this does occur, architects and kitchen designers are usually contracted to assist with facilities design and equipment specification. Though this is a real help to the RD or the DTR in charge of a foodservice, it must be remembered that the architect and designer will move on after the project is completed and it is the manager who must live with the kitchen and its equipment on a daily basis.

Whether designing a whole new facility or merely replacing one or two old pieces of equipment, it is important for the manager to know what equipment is available and how to write specifications that consider energy usage, water usage, and performance. A new efficient piece of equipment, be it oven, dishwasher, or blast chiller, can contribute to increased productivity, decreased energy and water consumption, conservation of resources, and to the bottom line, as well.

For years the Environmental Protection Agency (EPA) has mandated that cars sold in the United States specify fuel efficiencies. The Energy Star logo has been attached to household appliances like dishwashers, clothes dryers, and computers, so that consumers have guidance about which appliances have the highest energy efficiency. Generally, the technology in Energy Star appliances is the most advanced available. In 2001, the EPA began to designate some categories of foodservice equipment as Energy Star. At this writing, qualified dishwashers, fryers, griddles, hot food holding cabinets, commercial ice machines, commercial ovens, refrigerators, freezers, and steam cookers can be labeled with this Energy Star. It is anticipated that other classes of foodservice equipment will have Energy Star standards set in the near future. In many states, the purchase of an Energy Star appliance qualifies the purchaser for a rebate.

If a foodservice operation is paying for its own utilities, it is relatively easy to justify the higher costs for appliances that conserve fuel and water. Even though these items tend to cost more, the savings are measurable and a payback period can be calculated. That means that one can determine how long it will take to recover the additional cost of the equipment with savings in utility costs. Unfortunately, for the small operator, the initial cost of the more efficient piece of equipment may be prohibitive. In institutions where the manager may not have to pay for utilities, there is little motivation to search for the most energy-efficient unit. However, from an environmental perspective, the foodservice manager needs to consider the cost of resources to the community at large, not just the economic impact of the purchase on the facility's capital budget.

The type of fuel that an appliance uses may be an issue. Though electric appliances are usually more efficient than those that use natural gas or propane, many chefs prefer to cook with gas, since it is easier to control, especially in surface cooking units like ranges and woks. However, the cost of these fuels varies from location to location. For example, electricity costs more in California than it does in the Tennessee; the opposite is true of natural gas.[1]

Both gas and electric foodservice equipment should be UL approved, which indicates minimum standards have been met for construction and safety, and certified by the NSF International, which focuses on the equipment's contribution to food safety, not the least part of which is how easily it can be cleaned/sanitized. Until recently, however, the foodservice operator has had few objective measures for evaluating the performance of foodservice equipment. By and large, manufacturers have been able to make outrageous claims about the performance and energy efficiency of their products, with no way to support or disprove their claims. Operators needed to network with colleagues who owned the equipment to validate the claims, and though this type of information is better than no information, it is highly subjective and not reproducible.

Large users of equipment, such as restaurant chains, identified that not all fryers were created equal. There was a large-scale saving potential if the most energy efficient equipment was purchased for all of their operating units. Enter some new players who identified the gap in credibility of information given to foodservice operators by some manufacturers. These include the ASTM, the North American Association of Food Equipment Manufacturers (NAFEM), the Food Service Technology Center (FSTC), and two trade publications dealing exclusively with foodservice equipment *Foodservice Equipment Reports* and *Food Service Equipment and Supplies*. Working together, these organizations have developed and publicized standard test methods for many different types of foodservice equipment.

There were also food safety concerns related to some equipment. At least one instance of death from *E. coli* 0157:H7 was associated with both contaminated hamburger meat and uneven heat on a grill. The grill cooked at a higher temperature in the center of the cooking surface than on the perimeters, and the items cooked at the edge of the grill did not reach a high enough temperature to kill the bacteria. The development of standards for grills not only provided information on the safety of existing equipment and the evenness of the heat on the cooking surface, but also led to the development of newer technologies, better-functioning equipment, and improved energy efficiencies.

---

[1] U.S. Energy Information Administration http://www.eia.gov/. Accessed August 27, 2012.

Advances in the technology of foodservice equipment started slowly, but have moved forward at lightning speed during the last decade. At the present time, it is possible to measure hourly energy use for fryers, broilers, grills, griddles, refrigeration units, holding cabinets, warming drawers, booster heaters for dishwashers, various types of ovens, and even toasters and coffee pots. In addition, data are available on the number of French fries that a fryer can produce per hour, the number of burgers that a specific grill can cook to a safe level of doneness per hour, the amount of ice that an ice maker can produce, and the time, water, and energy it takes to wash and sanitize a rack of dishes. Mostly, all that one has to do is ask, and then make sure that the data are comparable to similar data from other manufacturers—in other words, that the standard test methods of the ASTM are being used. "Life Cycle and Energy Cost Calculators" to help managers compare different pieces of foodservice equipment are available at http://www.fishnick.com/saveenergy/tools/calculators/.

Electronic monitoring of foodservice equipment has been or is being developed; sophisticated systems will soon be commonplace. Managers will be able to monitor equipment performance such as temperature of refrigeration units and blast chillers, obtain real-time sales and inventory data, and determine productivity from local or remote computer terminals. Equipment such as ovens or grills will be able to sense when food is being cooked and automatically adjust energy usage to the production needed. Induction units including woks, stockpots, and ranges are already available; these use no energy until a pan is placed onto the cooking surface. Rapid-cook ovens that combine microwave with convection technology reduce cook times and energy usage without having negative effects on product quality.

It is no longer sufficient to look only at the footprint of a piece of equipment, or to specify the thickness of the stainless steel from which it is made. Though these characteristics are still important, it is now possible to measure and specify energy use and productivity as well, and to insist that manufacturers provide you with reproducible data obtained from an independent testing facility. Managers should never again have to rely on unsubstantiated claims or hearsay regarding performance of foodservice equipment. Further information is available at the following websites:

UL http://www.ul.com/global/eng/pages/
NSF International http://www.nsf.org/
ASTM International http://www.astm.org
North American Association of Food Equipment Manufacturers http://www.nafem.org
Foodservice Equipment Reports http://www.fermag.com
Foodservice Equipment and Supplies http://www.fesmag.com/
Food Service Technology Center http://www.fishnick.com

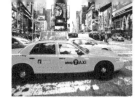

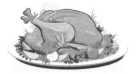

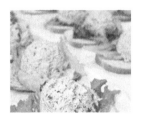

chapter twelve

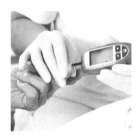

workflow and production

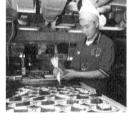

learning objectives

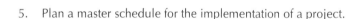

1. Describe how work should move through the workplace.

2. Discuss how to design work processes.

3. State the interrelationship between facilities design and process design.

4. List factors to be considered when planning a master schedule.

5. Plan a master schedule for the implementation of a project.

6. Define *task analysis, work simplification, job rotation, job enlargement,* and *job enrichment.*

7. List factors to be considered when writing a work schedule for employees.

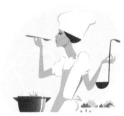

8. Prepare an employee schedule.

9. Define *production.*

10. Describe each of the steps in production planning.

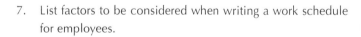

11. Discuss what types of tools are used to control production.

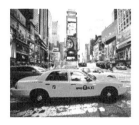

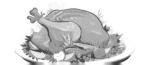

overview

Work does not just happen. In order for work to occur, there must be something that needs to be done, and someone who takes on the task of getting that "something" done. The work may be the transformation of raw materials into a tangible product. It may also be providing a service or the creating and implementing of an idea. Work may occur in a random manner, or may be planned and done in an organized way.

Usually there is a degree of trial and error involved when the work to be done is new to the worker. As the worker acquires experience with the task to be done, efficiency increases and the work is done in less time with fewer errors. Along the way, the worker acquires the tools to do the tasks more efficiently. Productivity increases as does the satisfaction that is gained from doing a job well.

It is not necessary for everything to be learned through trial and error. We use personal, institutional, or global history to learn how to do much of what we do. We read directions to learn how to prepare foods or how to assemble toys for our children. We study mathematics in order to learn how to balance the checkbook, and we use "help menus" to operate new computer software. Sometimes we get instruction from a teacher or another expert in order to learn. There is still some trial and error, but it is less than what was needed by those who first performed the task.

Consider the personal computer, which started to appear with regularity in American homes in the early 1980s. The few people who owned them spent hours installing and figuring out how to operate software that would allow them to do the task now known as "word processing." Because systems have been refined, sophisticated word processing programs are now available to anyone who has access to a computer. Today's students learn to use this tool in days rather than in the months that it took for their predecessors to learn the same task. For those introduced to word processing in the twenty-first century, the use of this software is mostly intuitive. The difference is partly due to advances in technology, but it is also due to the fact that word processing is now considered to be a tool rather than a novelty. As more people use word processing, it becomes easier for everyone to use. Soon, keyboarding will be completely optional, as voice recognition software continues to mature. Similar analogies can be made with the introduction of other technologies, from the mass-produced automobile at the beginning of the 20th century to (presumably) space travel in the near future.

This chapter will deal with the process of work and how to organize it so that there is the least amount of trial and error. There will be a discussion of how work moves through space and time. Consideration will be given to designing the flow of work to minimize duplication, backtracking, and cross-traffic. There will also be a discussion of how individual tasks within a job can be designed to increase efficiency while, at the same time, decreasing risk to the worker. The process of writing good work schedules for employees will be described, as will production planning and control.

management practice in dietetics

the flow of work

The shortest distance between two points is a straight line. It is a simple fact of geometry that most of us learned early in life. It is logical to expect that work will be done most efficiently if it is carried out in a linear fashion, moving forward along a plane until it is complete. Though this is a sound concept, the nature of work is such that there are variations that make simple linear movement impractical, if not impossible. Still, the principle remains that work should move forward, even if the movement is not strictly linear.

In this section, **workflow** will be discussed. This includes factors that facilitate the flow of people and product through a workplace, with emphasis on the design of the facility. Next there will be a discussion of the processes involved in moving work through a facility. Finally, there will be a description of the movement of work through time, which focuses on the development of a master schedule.

Workflow. *The way in which people and products move through a workplace.*

facilities design

It is easy to think about **facilities design** and the movement of people through the workplace by examining traffic patterns on the roads that we use every day. Consider a location where perpendicular roads intersect. Usually some sort of traffic control (stop signs or a traffic light) is in place to make sure that two vehicles do not meet

Facilities Design. *The layout of a workplace (including traffic patterns), which affects the flow of people, goods, and services within a designated space.*

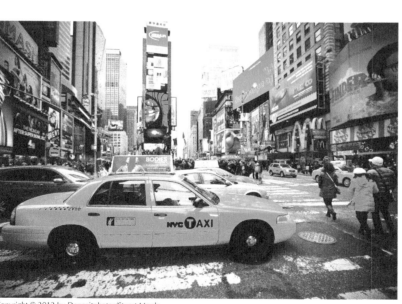

Just like on roads, traffic patterns through facilities should be planned and controlled.

(collide) in the intersection. The traffic control prevents accidents but also slows the rate of progression through the intersection.

Employees in a kitchen, an office, or a clinic should not have to compete at "intersections." Nor should customers in a cafeteria or in a clinic have to deal with traffic congestion in order to get the desired product or service. Because it is not practical to install mechanical traffic controls, it is useful to construct the "roads" through a facility with as few intersections as possible.

This can be accomplished with a straight-line design, but such designs are often impractical because the distance between one end of the operation and the other would be too great; the employees or the customers would have to walk great distances. The workplace should be designed in a way that work can flow forward over a limited amount of space. This might mean that there are turns and parallel workstations, but there should be as few intersections as possible.

Figure 12.1 shows the design of a kitchen that is conceptualized in a linear fashion. Note that the kitchen layout is planned so that raw materials (food) enter the facility on the left and the finished products (meals) leave on the right. There is little cross-traffic among workers because the employee who receives and stores the food does not have to enter the pre-preparation area and the pre-preparation worker does not have to enter the production area. The food moves in one direction, from left to right. However, the hot and cold food production workers have to go around each other to get to the service area or preproduction area, respectively. Figure 12.2 improves on the linear design by eliminating cross-traffic. Both of these configurations have the disadvantage of compartmentalizing workers, which interferes with their ability to work as a team. In fact, a strictly linear design is seldom used in foodservice.

Even if linear designs worked for foodservice, the space that is allocated is not likely to lend itself to linear design. However, the facility can be designed so that traffic patterns are considered and the need for multiple intersections can be avoided.

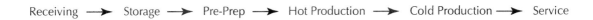

Receiving → Storage → Pre-Prep → Hot Production → Cold Production → Service

Figure 12.1 Kitchen with a "Straight Line" Traffic Flow

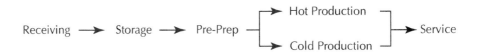

Figure 12.2 Kitchen with a Modified "Straight Line" Traffic Pattern

management practice in dietetics

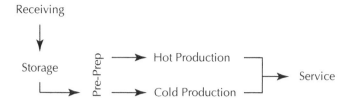

Figure 12.3 Kitchen with a "No-Intersection" Traffic Flow

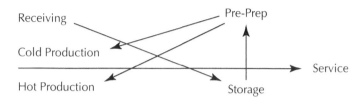

Figure 12.4 Kitchen with Multiple Intersections

Figures 12.3 and 12.4 show two kitchen designs using the same space. It is easy to see how traffic patterns between work areas in Figure 12.3 minimize the potential for workers to get in each other's way while the product moves forward continuously. In contrast, the layout in Figure 12.4 has so many intersections that it looks like "an accident waiting to happen."

It is not quite as easy to conceptualize traffic patterns when the product is purely a service. If the service is nutrition counseling, whether group or individual, the traffic pattern can be considered to be the client entering the room, attending a session with the dietitian, then exiting. That is an oversimplification. In fact, there are many other factors that must be considered. The client may have to park a vehicle (Is there parking available?) or take public transportation (How far is the bus stop from the building?). After the client enters the building, what must be done to locate the meeting room? Is the way to this room straightforward or as circuitous as a maze? If it is circuitous, is the client provided with clear directions for getting there? Is there a waiting room? Who else uses the waiting room? Where are the restrooms in relation to the waiting room and the meeting room? Is there a back way out to ensure privacy, if needed? Is the meeting place private so that the session will be undisturbed, or will the client be seen in a room that other practitioners also use? Will the counseling be done in a hallway, a hospital's emergency room, or (perhaps the worst possible option) in a hospital cafeteria? All of these facilities design issues must be addressed if counseling services are to be delivered in an appropriate and effective way.

Dietetics professionals sometimes plan meetings for local, state, and national dietetic associations. The facilities design concepts are a necessary consideration for event planners. Additional considerations for traffic flow for large meetings include transportation to and from airports, hotel accommodations, conveyance between hotels and meeting and exhibit sites, and optional activities for guests, families, and participants. At the meeting site itself, there should be maps or posted directions to the registration area, various meeting rooms, exhibits, professional services, restrooms, food vendors, and so on.

From this brief discussion, it can be seen that the arrangement of the physical facility is crucial to the movement of people and of product. The ease with which the movement takes place has a major impact on the actual process of work. The internal design of the facility, or changes to an existing design, are usually the responsibility of the manager. In addition, it has been noted that the location of the workplace relative to the community at large is also of importance, though this is not usually the responsibility of dietetics managers.

process design

Process Design.
The methods and procedures used to facilitate the movement of people, work, and materials through space and time.

Sometimes it is necessary to move all of the people involved through a single area—for example, the waiting room in a clinic or the reception area at a meeting site. In such situations, it is impossible to eliminate cross-traffic and congestion. Still, there should be a plan to facilitate the movement of people through the space. If it is not possible to eliminate the source of congestion, the problem can be addressed through **process design**. This can be likened to traffic lights and stop signs used to control traffic on roadways. It might be appropriate to adjust staffing so that more staff is available to assist clients at peak times. Staggering appointments at a clinic can flatten peaks so that not all clients arrive at the same time; meeting participants can preregister. These are issues of process rather than issues of facilities design, and are of equal importance to the movement of work.

Process design is even more dramatic when the movement of goods through a workplace is considered. In the kitchen illustrated in Figure 12.3, the materials proceed in a single direction, from raw materials to finished goods. There is no backtracking. But that is not the entire story about product movement. As materials move through a production area, effort should be made to keep handling to a minimum and to avoid redundancy whenever possible. For example, in a hospital kitchen, milk could go from receiving to refrigerated storage and subsequently could be redistributed to the patient trayline, to the cafeteria, and to the food production area. However, it would increase efficiency to take the milk directly from receiving to the areas where it will be used (point of service). This reduces the number of times that the milk has to be handled, and could impact the number of labor hours needed.

One of the factors related to having a product delivered directly to the point of service (rather than to storage) is the amount of space needed to store the product there. In order to overcome this problem, one can either increase the amount of point-of-service storage (a facilities design issue), or one can decrease the size and increase the frequency of deliveries (a process design issue). Increasing storage may not be a viable option because of limited space and the cost of equipment. The trend is toward increased numbers of smaller deliveries. In fact, it is common in most businesses to reduce inventories, which also reduces the cost of storage by using just-in-time delivery.

Another consideration for process design is the form in which the raw materials arrive. If it is possible, specifications (see Chapter 11) should be based on how the product is to be used so that there is a minimum waste of labor and packaging material. Again, using milk as the example, the milk for the production area should come in large containers so that the cook is not required to open, empty, and dispose of 16 eight-ounce cartons to get a gallon of milk. Conversely, the milk for the trayline needs to be delivered in eight-ounce portion-controlled (PCs) containers so that no labor is required to pour the milk into eight-ounce containers for service.

Process design also takes advantage of a factor known as **economy of scale**. This implies that it is more efficient to do a task once on a large scale than it is to do the same task multiple times on a smaller scale. An example of this can be seen in a bakery. If production for a day is 20 sheet cakes, it is appropriate to mix the batter for 20 cakes in a large mixer, then divide it into 20 pans so that the cakes can all be baked at once. This is much more efficient than mixing 20 individual batches of cake batter and baking the 20 cakes sequentially. Economies of scale can easily be achieved by forecasting and planning production rather than responding to each request individually. It might even be possible to bake twice as many cakes every other day and bake pies on the alternate days to further increase efficiency.

Economy of Scale.
A concept that it is more efficient to complete a task once on a large scale versus repeating the same task on a smaller scale to reach the same output level.

These and similar process design techniques to increase the ease of work and decrease the amount of redundancy in the workplace apply to all types of work, though the examples are not as obvious in service settings. Three examples follow. First, computer-generated diet orders could be processed as they arrive in the diet office (one at a time), or they could be held until just prior to a meal and processed all at once. This allows the diet clerk or DTR to complete other tasks (for example, heading menus or completing the production forecast) without interruption until just prior to meal service, and then process all of the diet changes. Efficiency is increased when one task is completed before another is started.

Another example is the assignment of clients to nutritionists working in a home healthcare agency based on geography, to lower the travel time and expenses associated with that travel. This might mean that one nutrition support dietitian is assigned the western part of a city and a second is assigned the eastern part. Alternately, it could mean that a single dietitian sees patients in the north on Monday, in the east on Tuesday, in the south on Wednesday, and in the west on Thursday, leaving Friday as an office day for completing paperwork and other tasks.

Finally, a laundry service could be contracted to make deliveries of clean linens each day instead of twice weekly. This would decrease the number of linens that needed to be stored and decrease the amount of the investment needed to own the larger inventory. All three of these examples address the process of work rather than the physical setting in which work occurs.

Though facilities design and process design have been separated for purposes of this discussion, the two are seldom that clearly separated. The relationship between facilities design and process design is complementary, and each must be viewed in light of the other. It might be necessary to adapt a process to accommodate the constraints of the physical site, or it might become necessary to renovate the site in order to accommodate an updated process. In foodservice, both the process and the facilities design will depend on the type of foodservice offered, cook-serve or cook-chill. Dietetics managers must consider all of these factors when setting up a new unit or when redesigning an existing one.

the movement of work through time

Just as managers design workspace and work processes, they must also plan time schedules for completion of work. Whether the work to be done is the implementation of a new computer system, the revision of a menu, or the processing of diet orders for trayline, it will be done better if it has been planned and implemented according to a **master schedule**.

Master Schedule. A time-based written outline, usually for complex or non-routine jobs, that plans the movement of work across time and is used to follow progress and keep work on time.

For routine tasks, such as the processing of diet orders or the preparation of a meal, the schedule will be familiar to employees. In fact, routine tasks are seldom supported by a written schedule. It is more likely that the schedule for such tasks is passed on from one employee to another through on-the-job training. If it is written at all, it will be found in the job analysis for whatever position is responsible for doing the task. However, non-routine tasks need some planning, which makes the master schedule a valuable resource. Master schedules may be devised for single use, such as the implementation of a new computer system, or for cyclical use. An example of a the latter is a schedule for heavy cleaning in a foodservice operation, which assures that major equipment like refrigeration units, ventilation hoods, and so forth are cleaned routinely, though not necessarily on a on a daily, weekly, or even a monthly basis.

Even the most experienced person will prepare a master schedule when doing tasks that are complex or non-routine. The schedule starts with the expected end point and works back from that time. As an example, consider the master schedule for the preparation of Thanksgiving dinner. To prepare the production schedule, the manager relies on personal experience as well as information (such as recipes, yield data, and portion sizes) about the foods to be prepared, and knowledge about the equipment and staff available for food preparation. The production schedule might look like the one shown in Table 12.1.

The principles of writing a master schedule are the same, whether it is for a small task or for the implementation of a major project. The only real differences are the

management practice in dietetics

Thursday	2:00	Serve dinner
	1:30	Carve turkeys/bake dinner rolls/steam vegetables
	1:15	Make gravy
	1:00	Place dressing (stuffing) in ovens
	12:00	Prepare dressing (stuffing)
	11:30	Proof frozen dinner rolls
	10:30	Put turkeys in the oven
	10:00	Prepare turkeys for roasting
Wednesday		Determine amount of food to be prepared; adjust recipe quantities as needed
		Confirm final meal count
		Make pies
		Pre-prep all vegetables
Tuesday		Order perishable foods
Monday		Place turkeys in refrigerator to thaw
		Order groceries needed for food production
Friday		Estimate meal count; determine quantity of food to be purchased
		Order frozen turkeys for Monday delivery
Thursday		Finalize menu
		Write specifications for foods to be purchased

Table 12.1 Master Production Schedule for Thanksgiving Dinner

complexity of the project to be scheduled and the amount of time available. The plan for the movement of work through time is often represented on a **Gantt Chart**,[1] a two-dimensional representation of a project schedule. In this graphic, activities are listed on the left side of the figure and times are represented across the top. The Gantt chart attempts to represent, graphically, the answers to the questions outlined in Table 12.2.

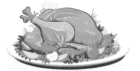

Gantt Chart. *A two-dimensional diagram of a master schedule on which activities are listed on the left side of the figure and times are represented across the top. It depicts the movement of work through time.*

When must the work be completed?

When can the work start?

How long will the work take to complete?

What work cannot be started until other work has begun?

What work must be completed before other work can begin?

What types of work can go on simultaneously?

Table 12.2 Questions Considered in the Gantt Chart[2]

A Gantt chart for the production of Thanksgiving dinner is shown in Figure 12.5.

Note that all of the tasks related to the preparation of the turkey are related to one another in that one must be completed before the next task can begin. The pies, rolls, dressing, and turkeys all require the use of ovens. In the example shown here, the production manager is aware that there is not enough oven space to cook all of these items at one time, so the cook times are staggered. The pies are baked a day in advance, and the turkeys are finished before the rolls are baked. Implicit in the design of the master schedule is a consideration of the physical environment, as illustrated by the limited oven space just described. The availability and skill level of personnel are also taken into account. If only one cook had been available to prepare the entire meal, more of the work, like baking the rolls or prepping the dressing, would have been done the day before.

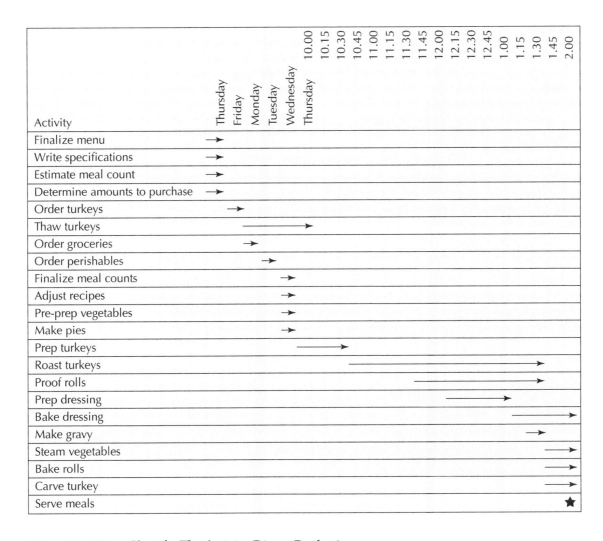

Figure 12.5 Gantt Chart for Thanksgiving Dinner Production

management practice in dietetics

In long-term or very complex projects, the sequencing of events will be related to the number of staff, to physical constraints, or to both of these factors. For example, if it takes 1,000 hours to complete a data entry project, one could assign one person to enter the data over a period of 25 weeks, or 25 people could be assigned to complete the job in one week, given enough data entry terminals. Physical constraints would interfere if there were only a few data entry terminals. It would not be possible to enter all of the data in one week if only five terminals were available, because the maximum capacity of the system is limited. Even if staff worked around the clock for seven days, only 840 hours would be available (5 terminals × 24 hours per day × 7 days per week = 840 hours).

Master schedules are used to plan and to monitor the movement of work across time. They are often expressed in the form of a Gantt chart. Once written, this schedule should be used to follow the progress of the work and to make adjustments as necessary to keep the work on schedule. Adjustments frequently involve altering the number of people available or modifying physical factors that impact the schedule.

job design

There has been much talk in recent years about **job reengineering**. The concept is not a new one. In fact, job design has been an issue since the industrial revolution. The principles of job design have expanded over the years, and the definitions are broader than before. In many cases, what is happening today is more appropriately called *job redesign* than *job design* because jobs are changing rapidly in response to the environment, information and other technologies, and the needs of society.

Job Reengineering. *The process of restructuring jobs to fit the needs of employees and to respond to the continuously changing environment, technology, and needs of society.*

If an organization believes that human resources are a valuable asset and that a competitive advantage can best be achieved by allowing worker participation in the workplace, it follows that the workers must take an active part in job design. In fact, individual workers know more than anyone else about the jobs that they perform. Efforts at job redesign should be employee-centered and should focus on empowering employees.

Job design is important for a number of reasons. How a job is performed is one of the factors that determine whether the job is rewarding and satisfying for the employee. Job satisfaction (or lack of it) ultimately affects productivity. Some of the issues dealt with under the heading of *job design* are task analysis, work simplification, job rotation, job enlargement, and job enrichment. Task analysis and work simplification were used extensively in the early part of the twentieth century to streamline production in the workplace. Job rotation, job enlargement, and job enrichment are more recent developments.[3]

task analysis

Task analysis is just what the name implies. It involves looking at each task within a job and analyzing it to determine just how the job is carried out. The ultimate goal of task analysis is to find better ways to get the tasks done (_better_, for purposes of this discussion, can be defined as more efficiently, more safely, or both). In task analysis, the job is broken down into its component parts. This is done through direct observation of one or more workers doing the job. One might analyze a single worker sorting mail to see where the inefficiencies in the process are, or one could study an entire patient trayline to determine how efficient each position is relative to the others. In the classical situation, observation is done through the use of video recordings, which can be studied after the task is completed. Videos have the advantage of being available to more than one observer and can be replayed as needed to facilitate accurate analysis of the data.

Task analysis is done for two reasons. The first is to identify inefficiencies that can be minimized or eliminated. An example of this might be the placement of dishes in the hot foodservice area of a cafeteria. If they are located to the right of a right-handed server, the plate would be picked up in the right hand, then transferred to the left so food items could be served with the right hand. Moving the plates to the left of the server would eliminate the step of transferring the plate from one hand to another by allowing the worker's initial motion to be picking up the plate with the left hand. The second reason to do task analysis is to identify and eliminate those activities that could lead to worker injury. For example, plates stored on a shelf behind the grill would force the worker to reach over a hot cooking surface, thus increasing the chance for burn injury. If the plates were moved to a cart beside the worker, this risk would be eliminated. The information gathered when doing a task analysis is used in the process called work simplification.

work simplification

Individual tasks within a job can be designed or redesigned in a manner that will increase efficiency while at the same time reducing the potential for injury. Originally, the emphasis in **work simplification** was to reduce the number of motions involved in doing a task. It was thought that work simplification decreased the energy expenditure and thereby increased the output of a worker. However, with advances in technology, work simplification is less critical today than it was during the industrial age. This is because much of today's work is being done with equipment designed to lighten the physical burden of work. Much of what was learned from earlier task analysis and work simplification projects has been incorporated into facilities and equipment design. In addition, it is now known that repeating the same few motions for long periods of time leads to **repetitive stress injury**. This is not acceptable in today's workplace.

Consider the way that deliveries are made today. Trucks back into a loading dock that is the same height as the floor of the vehicle. Next, the palletized, shrink-wrapped delivery is off-loaded with a motor-driven forklift and moved into (or at least near) the storage area. Then the items on the pallet are unwrapped and moved, individually, to the proper inventory space in the storeroom. Only the final step in this process is done using manual labor. Historically, each individual item would have to be manually off-loaded from the truck to the ground, then moved (often up stairs) into the building, and carried into the storeroom (sometimes with the help of a dolly or a cart). The differences between how it was done and how it is done today are based on innovations developed from the task analysis and work simplification that took place in the past.

Even though work simplification does not seem to be as important as it used to be, there are still some tasks that are done manually for which efficiencies can be gained by using work simplification techniques. For example, a foodservice worker could portion rice by weighing each serving to be sure it was the exact weight desired and then transferring the serving to the customer's plate. Another option would be to choose a serving utensil that consistently delivers the desired amount of rice. The latter technique simplifies the work by eliminating the step of "weighing." Table 12.3

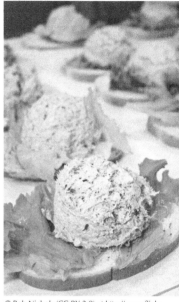

Tuna salad sandwiches being assembled for a school lunch program.

Original Method of Making 36 Tuna Salad Sandwiches	Take one slice of bread from a package.
	Put spread on one slice of bread.
	Scoop a portion of the tuna salad onto the bread.
	Spread the tuna salad.
	Add three slices of tomato.
	Add a piece of lettuce.
	Put another piece of bread on the top.
	Cut the sandwich in half.
	Wrap the sandwich.
	Label each sandwich.
	Repeat the entire process 36 times.
"Simplified" Method of Making 36 Tuna Salad Sandwiches	Lay out 36 pieces of bread.
	Put spread on all pieces of bread.
	Put a scoop of tuna salad on every piece.
	Spread each portion of tuna salad.
	Put three slices of tomato on each sandwich.
	Put lettuce on all sandwiches.
	Put the second slice of bread on each sandwich.
	Cut each sandwich in half.
	Wrap and label each sandwich.

Table 12.3 Work Simplification Technique

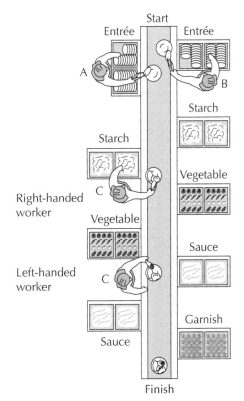

Start
Entrée | Entrée
A | B
Starch
Starch
Right-handed worker | Vegetable
C
Vegetable | Sauce
Left-handed worker
C | Garnish
Sauce
Finish

Figure 12.6 Plate Assembly Line

Ergonomics. *The physical aspects of work and movement; how movement relates to the performance of a task.*

represents a work simplification technique used in sandwich making. Note that the latter technique is more efficient, in both the time and the effort expended to make the sandwiches. The design of the workstation and the relative location of each of the ingredients and utensils are also important to efficient work design.

Of equal or greater importance than gaining efficiency when performing task analysis and redesigning jobs is consideration of the ergonomics of the job. It is desirable to reduce the potential for work-related injury, including repetitive stress injury. This is illustrated in Figure 12.6, which depicts an assembly line for the plating of meals in the staging area of a hotel's banquet facility. In this example, plates are placed directly on a mechanized belt, and each worker puts only one item on the plate (for example, entrée, starch, vegetable, sauce, and garnish). To speed the process, there may be two workers for every food item, so that each worker puts food on every second plate. It is possible to plate 50 or more meals per minute using this system.

If the hot foods are placed in warmers that are parallel to the moving belt (A), workers are required to reach and bend over the hot food to place items on the plate. This increases the risk for both burn injury from the hot food and for lower back injury because of the need for repeated reaching and bending. Alternately, the warmers could be placed perpendicular to the belt (B) so that there is less reaching and the worker does not have to reach over heated serving tables. This worker can remain erect at all times. Because workers should always be able to see what is coming down the belt, they should face either the beginning of the assembly line or the line itself. Thus, the position of the worker varies based on which is the dominant arm for that worker (C). Asking a left-handed worker to work from a right-handed position will cause increased turning movements that could lead to injury.

These principles can be used in clinical and office settings as well. Something as simple as correlating the sequence of the information obtained on a diet history form with how the information is entered into a computerized nutrient analysis program enhances the efficiency of the data entry process. The diet clerk or dietetic technician can enter the data in the same order that they are recorded on the history form, without the need to search for the information as the computer program requests it. This enables the data entry process to proceed in an orderly, sequential, and efficient manner. Data entry can also be enhanced by using ergonomically designed computer workstations, chairs, keyboards, mouses, and other related equipment to decrease repetitive stress injuries in office workers. For more information on ergonomics, see the ergonomics page of the Occupational Safety and Health Administration.

management practice in dietetics

job rotation

Job rotation is a method that is used to enhance job satisfaction and to decrease the risk of repetitive stress injury. It involves the **cross-training** of individuals (often within a specific job classification) to be able to perform more than one job. For example, a foodservice worker may be able to work as a porter, a trayline server, a cafeteria runner, or a tray server in the patient care area. A clinical dietitian may be cross-trained to function as the foodservice manager in the manager's absence. With job rotation, each job remains essentially the same, but people can move between jobs to decrease boredom and enhance job satisfaction.

Job rotation benefits the organization because workers who are cross-trained allow for greater flexibility in scheduling. For the worker, job rotation reduces the potential for repetitive stress injury and increases job security. In addition, workers who know how to perform a variety of jobs may have an increased chance for promotion within an organization.

job enlargement

Another job design technique that is used to improve job satisfaction is **job enlargement**. This involves teaching employees some additional skills that are needed to perform jobs other than their own. It is sometimes called **multi-skilling**. Job enlargement gives employees the chance to learn more about the overall operation and to see the larger picture, rather than having a narrow perspective based on their individual job tasks. Job satisfaction is enhanced by this broadened perception, as is the individual's sense of accomplishment in being able to participate in a greater part of the total work process. Job security for the employee may increase as well, because having additional skills makes the employee more valuable to the organization.

It would be of great value, for instance, for foodservice management dietitians to learn some of the skills that cooks and chefs have. This would allow them to "pitch in" during crisis situations, to be sensitive to the factors that have an impact on the chefs' jobs, and to be better supervisors of cooks and chefs. For dietetic technicians, job enlargement could include knowing how to measure heights and weights correctly so that they can perform these tasks when nurses are not available to do them. Likewise, it is useful for clinical dietitians to be able to take blood pressures, identify bowel sounds using a stethoscope, give injections, use glucose monitoring devices, and so on.

Even when multi-skilling is not appropriate (for example, it would not be desirable to teach a hospital's cooks to screen clients for nutritional risk), there is value in introducing information about other jobs in the organization. Experiences that allow cooks to go to the clinical areas with clinical dietitians to visit patients increase the cooks' knowledge of the customer and enhance their perception of the importance

Job Rotation.
The practice of having workers do different jobs at different times to improve job satisfaction and minimize the potential for repetitive stress injury.

Cross-Training.
Preparing employees to perform various jobs within a work setting.

Job Enlargement.
The practice of increasing the tasks done within a specific job; increasing the number and types of skills workers use in their jobs.

Multi-Skilling. *The process whereby workers learn to perform new tasks and to develop techniques that, in turn, enlarge their jobs.*

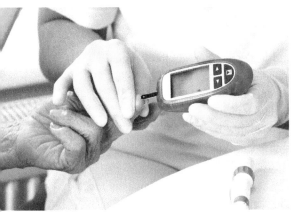

Multiskilling for a clinical dietitian may include learning to use glucose monitors.

Job Enrichment.
The practice of adding variety and, simultaneously, increasing the knowledge required to do a job. Job enrichment activities should be designed to respond to each employee's unique characteristics.

of their own jobs. It also makes requests for "special" food items seem a little more reasonable. Conversely, the clinical dietitian or diet technician who spends time working with food production staff will have a better understanding of just how the cooks' jobs are done and how special requests impact the "back of the house." This may serve as an incentive to limit special requests to those that are essential. In general, expanding employees' knowledge of the total workplace increases respect for personnel performing other functions within the organization, and improves job satisfaction, which could lead to increased productivity.

job enrichment

Job enrichment increases job satisfaction by supporting the employee to do something extra that will enhance the job for that particular employee. It increases the variety of work within a job and the skill and knowledge required for that job. A greater level of responsibility and autonomy for the employee may result from job enrichment programs.

Job enrichment is a viable way to foster loyalty in employees when budgets are tight and it is not possible to give substantial financial rewards, either as salary increases or as bonuses. The clinical nutrition manager who knows the clinical staff well might offer different job enrichment opportunities to each of three dietitians. For example, one of them may be offered the opportunity to develop management skills by learning to write work schedules for employees. The second dietitian might be given work time to write a paper for publication, while the third is provided with tuition support to attend computer classes. The options would be determined by the available resources along with recognition of the needs and interests of each member of the clinical staff. Each of these dietitians would learn new skills, and their resumes would be enhanced by the additional activities.

Job enrichment activities need not be costly, but they must be tailored to the needs of both the organization and the individuals involved. If a clinical dietitian has no aspirations for becoming a manager, it may be perceived as an additional burden to learn management tasks. Job enrichment for this staff member would be better if it was directly related to the job she was doing, which might include writing a needed clinical protocol or developing standards of care for a specific medical/nutrition problem. Even routine tasks, such as revising a menu or updating a diet manual, can be job-enriching experiences if managed in the correct way. Such projects are necessary, are cost-effective, and enhance the jobs of individual staff members.

Jobs can be designed or redesigned to increase job satisfaction and to improve productivity. These factors benefit both the organization and the employee.

management practice in dietetics

Techniques that are available for reengineering jobs include task analysis, work simplification, job rotation, job enlargement, and job enrichment. Because employees know more about their jobs than anyone else does, it is best to include them in the process of job design or redesign. The process works best when it is employee-centered and its implementation is based on empowerment of staff rather than on managerial control.

labor schedules

The **labor schedule** for employees is another tool that is used by managers to facilitate getting the work done. The schedule is, first and foremost, a management tool, and because it is the employer who is paying the worker, management's needs are the primary needs that must be met through the work schedule. If a business needs to be open seven days a week, it would be unwise for management to guarantee weekends off to all permanent workers. That being said, it is also appropriate to plan labor schedules with fairness, consistency, and consideration for the needs of employees.

Schedules should be written in such a way that employee preferences are considered whenever it is possible to do so. Schedules should follow a pattern so employees can anticipate days off and be able to plan their lives. In addition, if an employee wishes to take some time off for personal reasons (for example, to attend an event, such as a graduation or a wedding), the manager should make an effort to adjust the work schedule to meet the employee's need.

Because the schedule is a management tool, there is always room for adjustment. Even when computers are used to write work schedules, following a standard procedure for schedule-writing, the process is either implemented or reviewed by a manager to be sure that it is fine-tuned for the specific circumstances reflected in a particular schedule covering a discrete period of time.

Consider the allocation of paid time off for holidays. Sometimes employees want to work on holidays. One reason for this is the need for extra income, because premium wages are usually paid to workers who agree to work. Another reason may be that the employee has no activities planned for the holiday and would prefer to be at work rather than be alone. Conversely, some employees have social commitments that make it undesirable for them to work on holidays. A manager should acknowledge these different needs and preferences when writing a schedule. Even if each employee's preferences cannot be granted on each occasion, adjusting the schedule when possible demonstrates the manager's desire to be flexible and to treat the employees as individuals. Computers cannot know these individual needs unless the schedule-writer inputs the appropriate data.

Labor Schedule. *A management tool used to designate the hours and days each employee is to work.*

Some managers use the work schedule as a means to reward or to punish employees. In the case of holidays, a manager could disregard the preferences noted above in order to punish a troublesome employee by scheduling the employee with outside commitments to work on the holiday, while denying an employee who wishes to work the opportunity to earn additional pay. Conversely, the manager could preferentially give one employee more opportunities to earn overtime pay than other employees have. Such use of work schedules to punish or show favoritism is a potentially dangerous practice because the entire workforce will recognize it. This lack of fairness will undermine the credibility of the manager. In a unionized workplace, such inequitable treatment of individuals will lead to the initiation of the grievance process.

Schedules can greatly enhance or diminish an individual worker's quality of work life and job satisfaction. It is difficult to cope with a schedule with every other day off, with long numbers of consecutive days at work, or with shifts that vary on a daily basis. In general, employees need to know what their regular work hours will be. Employees need to be informed of work schedules as far in advance as is practical, so that they can have control over the rest of their lives. If there need to be changes in usual work hours, it is common courtesy to consult with the employee before the schedule is posted to explain the need and to seek that employee's cooperation. It is quite a shock for an employee to expect to have a set schedule and then see a different schedule posted.

Weekends are another area that demand some consideration. If employees know in advance that there is a work requirement on the weekend, and that the schedule will require them to work every second or every third weekend, then they can plan to engage in leisure activities on scheduled (week) days off. Managers should not rearrange these usual days off without checking with the employees to see if they are willing to adjust personal schedules to meet the organization's needs. Employees should be able to plan for leisure activities whether or not their jobs require that they work weekends.

Though writing a work schedule is never an easy task, the process can be organized in a way that will make the task easier. The most important part is to know the needs of both management and employees so that one can attempt to balance these needs when writing the schedule. This takes time and is the reason that it becomes easier for a manager to write a schedule as that manager's tenure in a position increases. Managers should know how many workers are needed each day, and what positions need to be covered. It is also necessary for the manager to know who is able to work each position, and who has been cross-trained to work in other positions. New managers might find it useful to work from lists that include this information. Seasoned managers internalize this information and do not need to rely on lists.

When writing the actual schedule, the manager should use a grid that shows the employees on one axis and dates on the other axis, with boxes where rows and

	Sun	Mon	Tue	Wed	Thur	Fri	Sat
Aaron Noe	1	1	1	1	Off	Off	1
Wei Huang	Off	Off	3	3	1	1	3
Agnes Schulz	3	3	Off	Off	3	3	2
Latifa Brown	Off	2	2	2	2	2	Off
Tony Arch	2						

Positions 1 = Porter   6–2:30
           2 = Dishwasher 8–4:30
           3 = Potwasher   7–3:30

Figure 12.7 Sample Employee Schedule

columns meet (see Figure 12.7). This provides space for position numbers or work hours to be entered in the boxes. Any type of notation is acceptable, as long as it provides employees with enough information to know what job each of them will be doing on a given day. Positions may be designated by job number, job title (for example, porter, dishwasher, potwasher, and so on), work hours, or any other coding system that is easily interpreted by all.

To begin writing a schedule, enter the days off for all employees. This includes regularly scheduled days off, holidays, vacations, and special requests. The next step is to write in hours for all full-time employees to ensure that they are scheduled for their guaranteed number of hours (or get holiday or vacation time instead). In the event that an employee has an extended illness, sick time may be scheduled as well. The next step is to schedule the guaranteed hours for part-time and short-hour employees. Finally, casual employees are scheduled to fill in positions as needed. When the schedule is completed, it should be cross-checked to ensure that all positions are filled and that all employees have been scheduled for their guaranteed hours, but none is scheduled to work more than full-time. (An employee who works more than 40 hours per week gets overtime compensation for those hours, usually at the rate of time-and-a-half. To avoid these additional costs, increase scheduled hours for part-time, short-hour, and casual employees as needed.) Overtime hours may be authorized on a day-to-day basis to respond to changing needs but should not be scheduled in advance, except in unusual circumstances.

Another factor to consider is the cost-effectiveness of the schedule. For example, if a diet clerk and a dietetic technician are cross-trained and can each perform both jobs, one could theoretically schedule either employee in either position.

workflow and production   395

But if the dietetic technician position is one that commands a higher salary, the options for managers change. Because the technician would maintain the higher salary while working as a clerk, it would be wasteful to schedule the dietetic technician to do the clerk position except in an emergency. On the other hand, it is acceptable to schedule the clerk to work as a dietetic technician, because the clerk will receive the higher salary only when scheduled to work in the higher-paying position.

When possible, days off should be scheduled consecutively. This should be balanced by a limit on the number of consecutive days the employee is scheduled to work. People get too tired if required to work long stretches without a day off. It is probably better to split days off than to require an employee to work eight days in a row, because fatigue can lead to on-the-job injuries. Individuals should be scheduled to work hours that are as consistent as possible, working day shifts, evening shifts, or afternoon shifts rather than alternating work hours to a large degree within the space of a few days. Employees should not be scheduled to work an evening shift followed by an early-morning shift without adequate time for rest. Work schedules that are employee-friendly and try to meet the workers' needs contribute to job satisfaction, while those that consider only management's needs may result in employee fatigue, drops in productivity, and increased job-related injuries.

In some cases, it may be possible to delegate the preparation of schedules to the employees themselves. For example, if there were five clinical dietitians employed in a healthcare facility, requirements could be established that allowed the staff to determine their own schedules. Such requirements might include:

- Four dietitians must be on duty on weekdays.
- One dietitian must be on duty on Saturdays, Sundays, and holidays.
- Weekday coverage must extend from 6 a.m. until 7 p.m.
- Weekend coverage must extend from 8:30 a.m. until 5 p.m.

With these parameters established, the clinical dietitians should be able to prepare their own work schedules, consulting management only when the scheduling requirements cannot be met.

Employee schedules are a management tool that can be used or misused. When managers abuse their power or neglect their responsibilities when scheduling employees, the results include fatigue, injury, resentment, and loss of productivity. If the schedules reflect fairness and management's flexibility in meeting employee needs, there will be increased job satisfaction and trust in management. It is in the best interest of the manager to consider employee issues when planning work schedules.

production and productivity

The actual process of converting inputs into products, whether these products are goods, services, or ideas, is known as **production**. Production adds value to the inputs or raw material while creating products to be sold. Production is planned, controlled, and measured using a variety of management tools and techniques. Some of those tools have already been described in this chapter. Others include forecasting, production schedules, production meetings, production controls, and productivity measurements. The remainder of this chapter will focus on these tools that are used to plan and control production.

Production.
The process of converting inputs into products such as goods, services, or ideas.

planning production

There are three basic steps in production planning. The first is the determination of what is to be produced in what amounts. Accurate forecasts are needed to bring in raw materials, schedule labor, and plan how the work will get done. The second step in production planning is the production schedule, which outlines what needs to be done by each worker at a given time. The production schedule also takes into consideration physical factors such as the equipment available. The final step is to communicate with the workforce, either in writing or verbally. Production meetings are especially useful in that workers can help to identify potential problems, which can then be avoided or minimized. Two-way communication between a group of workers and management at production meetings can help determine what the variables in workload are, and how these can be evened out in order to distribute work equitably.

forecasting. The determination of how much of which products to make is called **forecasting**. The range of products to be made is usually known for ongoing operations. (Research and development efforts and marketing programs are used in new product development that may broaden the range of what is produced.) Once products have been identified, the amount of product needed must be determined so that inputs are available for the production level required.

Forecasting. *A tool used to predict the quantities of product needed.*

Accurate forecasting is necessary because both underproduction and overproduction are costly to an organization. Too little product can result in lost business because customer demand cannot be met. Overproduction leads to wasted resources. If the product is perishable, it will spoil. If the product is not perishable, the loss is due to the cost of storing the product until it is needed.

Thus, it is imperative that some sort of forecasting method be used to determine what will be produced during a given period. This discussion will center on short-term forecasting, which is used in day-to-day or week-to-week operations. Long-term forecasting is used more in strategic planning than in daily operations planning.

**Subjective
Forecasting.**
*A forecasting
method that uses
information, experi-
ence, and intuition
to determine the
amount of product
needed.*

The amount of each product to be produced is determined by using one of a number of forecasting methods. The simplest of these models is **subjective forecasting**. This involves someone (perhaps a manager or a technical expert) deciding how much of each product to make based on a combination of information, experience, and intuition. This type of forecasting (sometimes called *visionary*) works for small, entrepreneurial operations and for situations in which reliable historical data are not available. However, it is not a very sophisticated model and is only as reliable as the person doing the forecasting. In general, the use of subjective forecasting should be discouraged.

Manual Tally.
*The physical
counting of
orders received to
determine produc-
tion needs.*

Another simple method is the actual counting of orders. Production is based entirely on the **manual tally**. Technically, this is not "forecasting" because actual orders are used to set production levels. It is appropriate to use this method in some situations such as preparing food in fine-dining establishments where the meals are prepared "to order." The tally method is also appropriate when the product is a big-ticket item with limited production, such as customized computer systems or commercial aircraft.

Manual tallies are often used in hospitals to determine how much food to prepare for patients. This is not a good use of the tally method because patients are admitted, are discharged, and have their diet orders changed from meal to meal; the tallies are seldom accurate. Manual tallies are labor-intensive, are costly to produce, and yield very poor results. In hospital foodservices, where much of the preparation is done in advance of customer selection, the use of more sophisticated methods of forecasting is required. If manually produced tallies are used at all, they should be used exclusively for items that are not on the standard menu. The only other reason to hand-tally orders is to provide baseline data for a more sophisticated forecasting system. Theoretically, this will be limited to periods of time immediately following the introduction of a new menu.

**Percentage
Forecasting.**
*Determining how
much of a specific
item is needed as a
percentage of the
total number of
items needed.*

A forecasting method that does not require the use of computers and works well in small operations is the use of percentages to determine the proportion of specific products needed relative to total production. In **percentage forecasting**, it is necessary to know the usual proportions of product used and the total amount to be produced. The next step is to multiply the total by the various percentages to compute the specific production levels for each product. As an example, consider a lunch menu that offers hamburgers, a cold plate, and a pasta dish. If historical data show that 50 percent of the orders are for burgers, 20 percent for cold plates, and 30 percent for pasta, one could estimate the total meals needed for a given day and multiply by these percentages. In a school, the total might be based on attendance; in a patient foodservice, the total is the number of patients in the facility. If 200 customers are expected, then 100 burgers, 40 cold plates, and 60 servings of the pasta entrée need to be produced. With this method, some **padding** needs to be added to avoid short-

Padding. *The
practice of ordering
and producing
more product than
is actually needed
in order to avoid
shortages.*

ages of each product. A designated individual should do this. Padding is not a random task done by multiple individuals, because that leads to overproduction and loss.

With the increased use of computers for information management, **computer fore-casting** models are now commonplace for anticipating production requirements. These can be used in all areas of dietetics, from predicting caseloads at WIC sites to projecting participation in school lunch programs. Computer systems are widely used to forecast food production. A variety of mathematical models may be applied, including the time-series model, the moving average model, exponential smoothing, and multiple regression analysis. The specific model, and thus the accuracy of the forecast, will be dependent on the software being used. Once a computerized fore-casting system is in place, it is very easy to use.

Computer Forecasting. *Using computer-generated forecasts to determine production needs. Accuracy is dependent on reliable historical data.*

Managers should select software that meets the needs of the operation. Software specifications can be written to require a specific mathematical forecasting model if the manager is willing to pay for enhancements to a generic program. In general, the more kinds of data that can be entered into the computer system, the more accurate the forecast will be. In foodservice, data might include the amount ordered, amount produced, overproduction, underproduction, substitutions (including amounts used), date, day, meal, competing items, weather, customer demographics, and special circumstances. It should be noted, however, that a high degree of accuracy is not always necessary.

The most critical part of computer forecasting is ensuring the accuracy of the (historic) data entered into the system. The program can produce good forecasts only if the data in the system are reliable. Some people claim that subjective forecasts are as good as computer models. This is untrue. When computerized forecasting models are inaccurate, it is due to the lack of accurate data input. Common reasons for this phenomenon are outlined in Table 12.4.

Forecasting is the initial step in production planning. It allows the manager to deter-mine the volume of goods, services, or ideas that will be needed and to provide for adequate inputs to meet that production need. Accuracy in forecasting is necessary, though the same degree of precision is not necessary in all situations.

Incomplete recording of information

Failure to record amounts that are padded, if padding is done manually

Neglecting to record foods as they are "batch cooked" (prepared as needed)

Discarding leftovers without recording the amounts

Neglecting to document substitutions and numbers of portions of these that were used

Intentional or unconscious attempts to undermine the computer system

---

Table 12.4 Reasons for Inaccuracies with Computer Forecasting Models

Forecasts are used in all areas of dietetics. It is a typical pattern, for example, that elective surgery is not usually scheduled during the winter holidays in late November and in December. Therefore, it may be appropriate to allow hospital clinical dietetics staff to schedule time off during these periods without having to replace the workers. On the other hand, the volume of catered events may increase during the holidays, so additional foodservice staff may be needed. Schools and colleges can decrease production during times when school is not in session. There may be greater attendance at group weight-reduction classes in the spring (just prior to the bathing suit season) than in the fall. Making use of this kind of data allows staffing and budgets to be adjusted to be in line with the expected customer volumes.

production scheduling. Once forecasting has been done, the next step in production planning is to prepare a **production schedule**. The production schedule is like the master schedule, except that it covers a shorter period of time—for example, a shift, a day, or a week. Because the workers who are doing the production are familiar with the tasks involved, production schedules do not typically use a Gantt chart. In most cases, the time needed to construct such a chart is too great in relationship to its overall contribution to output. The production schedule is usually a less formal document that specifies what is to be produced, in what quantities, at what time, and by whom. Written production schedules also have the flexibility to provide for the addition of special tasks, activities to be completed during downtime and idle periods, and comments or special instructions.

Production Schedule. *A document that specifies what is produced, how much, at what time, and by whom.*

Consider the DTR whose job includes screening patients for nutritional risk. If this DTR can perform one screening every 10 minutes and is given a total of two hours to complete screenings each day, it is assumed that 12 patients can be screened each day. This DTR's production schedule would include the screening of 12 patients for nutritional risk between 1 p.m. and 3 p.m. each day. If the dietetic technician was asked by a supervisor to give a diet instruction during this time (assuming the instruction will take 30 minutes), the number of screenings will be reduced to nine. Conversely, if only six patients needed to be screened, the DTR might be asked to distribute and collect 12 patient satisfaction surveys (taking 5 minutes each) in lieu of completing six of the screenings. The production schedule for the specific time period will vary from day to day, depending on the forecast of production needs. In the case of this particular dietetic technician, the production schedule might be prepared by a clinical dietitian or a clinical nutrition manager, or be a self-designed schedule. It may even be in the form of a verbal directive, rather than a written schedule.

Production schedules are particularly useful when prepared for groups of workers rather than for a single individual. In a foodservice where several cooks work at the same time, one may be scheduled to produce a specific number of entrées, another may prepare vegetables and soups in the forecast amounts, and others may do cold production, desserts, grilled-to-order items, and so on. Depending on the size of the operation and management staffing, the production scheduling for cooks will be prepared by a food production manager, a chef, or a lead cook. The production schedule for cooks includes both production for today's needs and some pre-preparation for future needs. For example, if the vegetable/soup cook has free time as the meal service reaches completion, that cook might begin to gather and prepare ingredients that are required for tomorrow's soup. The schedule also takes into account what equipment is available so that its use is also scheduled.

production meetings. Though a written production schedule may be enough to communicate what needs to be done, **production meetings** are a more valuable tool in that they allow for two-way communication. Production meetings may be scheduled daily, weekly, or monthly, as needed in the individual work setting. They may be one-on-one consultations between a manager and a staff member or may be a meeting that includes all members of the work group or team. Though the underlying purpose of these meetings is production, other topics may be included on the meeting agenda. In fact, the meeting may not be called a production meeting but may be called a staff meeting, team meeting, or department meeting instead.

The major benefit of using the meeting format is to facilitate communication that goes in both directions, to the staff and from the staff. Managers who use this technique provide their staff with opportunities to participate in the management process by soliciting their input and considering their ideas. Potential problems may be identified and dealt with during these sessions.

For example, a production meeting between a chef and several cooks may have to deal with the fact that the president of the organization has called an emergency board meeting on the same evening that three other special events were planned. The menus for the scheduled events require the use of all of the available oven space. To accommodate the extra event, a menu would have to be planned that does not require the use of any oven space; however, the president is insistent on serving roasted Cornish game hens. Alternatives include cooking some items in advance and holding them until serving time, changing the recipes or menus to include items that don't require the use of ovens, rescheduling one of the events for a different day, or leasing/purchasing the additional oven capacity needed. It is likely that the group will come up with more alternatives than would one individual. In addition, the group has the ability to make a good decision about how to solve the problem, and the solution is likely to work because everyone had input in the decision.

Production meetings may include such agenda items as tasks to be done, productivity goals and deadlines, work and job schedules, other input requirements, and so on. The meeting may also be used as a time to review safety protocols, topics related to policies and procedures, or issues related to the overall functioning of the operation. In fact, probably the only items that should not be discussed at these meetings are confidential personnel issues. As these meetings are part of paid work time, an effort should be made to keep the meeting directed toward work, even though some purely

Production Meetings. *Planned or scheduled times when employees and managers gather to discuss production issues. Often used for information dissemination and for problem solving.*

social interaction is both necessary and inevitable. It is important that managers participate in and expect the participation of their staff in these meetings so that the value of the interaction is acknowledged by all involved. The arbitrary cancellation or postponement of production meetings undermines their importance in the minds of all participants. "Not enough time" is an overused and often invalid excuse for meeting cancellation. If the manager sees the meeting as important, time will be made available. The meetings do not have to be lengthy. In fact, these meetings should be long enough for adequate communication but brief enough that they do not interfere with the other work that needs to be done.

Production meetings, like production schedules, are useful in all areas of dietetics, not just in foodservice. However, in non-foodservice areas of practice, the meeting is more likely to be called a staff meeting. They are as important to a WIC director or a clinical nutrition manager as they are to a hospital foodservice director. For example, a WIC director may schedule staff meetings to assure that the service being given in various clinic sites meets the needs of the clients, the staff, and the funding agency. Such meetings may include agenda items such as how to best balance individual and group interactions with clients, the computerization of data collection and reporting, client and staff scheduling, nutrition education content and materials, issuing of vouchers/EBT cards, and so on. These meetings also serve to enhance communication that allows staff working at different sites to produce similar outputs.

The three components of production planning (forecasting, production schedules, and production meetings) are integral to the smooth operation of an organization. Though these tools are traditionally utilized in situations where the product is a tangible one—that is, goods—they are equally useful when the products are either services or ideas. Production planning, in essence, is the blueprint for where production is going and who will do what along the way. It also includes provisions for various contingencies so that outputs can be maintained when things do not go as planned.

production control

Production control involves monitoring production during and after it has occurred to determine if plans are being met. The controls used during production include the various protocols and procedures that are in place in a setting. In clinical nutrition, these would include timelines for doing screenings and assessments, guidelines for determining desirable body weight, formulas used to estimate nutrient and energy needs, and clinical pathways for the treatment of various nutrition-related disorders, decision trees, and so on. In a well-baby clinic, it would include procedures for the measurement and recording of anthropometric data and developmental milestones. In a WIC setting, it could include lesson plans for the classes attended by new mothers.

Production Control.
The process of monitoring production during and after it has occurred to determine if plans are being met and to make adjustments as required.

The "Virtual" Nutrition Center.
http://www. martindalecenter. com/Nutrition.html

When it is determined that the production plans are not being met, one of two things must be done. If the plan is unreasonable, it must be changed so that goals are realistic and achievable. If the plan is determined to be a good one, adjustments must be made in the facility, the process, or the various schedules so that the production goals can be achieved. In order to control production, it is necessary to monitor and measure what is being produced and to make adjustments as necessary.

production controls in foodservice. There are some production control tools that are unique to the area of food production that cannot be universally applied to other areas of dietetics management. These include the use of recipes, yields, portion control, temperature, and taste tests. All of these items have a major impact on the quality or the quantity of the food that is produced in a foodservice operation. Extensive information related to food production is available at the "Virtual" Nutrition Center.

First, consider the use of recipes. Though some chefs feel that it is their prerogative to be creative with the food they prepare, in most large-scale operations it is more appropriate to use **standardized recipes**[4] to control the quality of the product and to ensure that it is consistent each time it is produced. A standardized recipe is one that has been adapted for use in a specific foodservice operation so that a high-quality product can be reproduced time after time. It has been tested under real conditions using the equipment available in that facility, the personnel working there, the available ingredients, and so on.

Standardized Recipe. *A production control that gives a known quantity of known quality ingredients to establish amounts needed to continuously reproduce the same high-quality product.*[4]

Preferences of the customer base are also considered in preparing a standardized recipe. For example, in California, which has a large Asian population, it would be appropriate to use short-grain "sticky" rice with a stir-fried vegetable entrée. In the Midwest, the customers may prefer "converted" long grain rice. Tacos served in southern Texas might have shredded beef as an ingredient, whereas the same dish in New England might be better accepted if made with ground beef.

Recipes are usually standardized by repeatedly testing an existing quantity recipe (or enlarging a home-size recipe) until a product that is acceptable to a taste panel is achieved. Adjustments are made in the recipe each time it is produced, and all changes are recorded, so the finalized recipe is accurate and reproducible. The recipe is then entered into the computer database or into a traditional recipe file. The number of tests needed to achieve a good recipe is dependent on a number of variables, including the experience of the chef or cook, the need to use substitute ingredients, the degree of enlargement needed, the specificity of the procedures described in the original recipe, and so on.

Standardized recipes used in an institution should follow a consistent format, should be written in language that allows no room for interpretation, and the font should be large enough to be read from a distance of several feet. In addition, the actual written recipe should be either single use (computer generated for use on a specific date) or

Item name and ID number

List of ingredients in order of use

Amount of each ingredient to be used

Procedures for production (including HACCP information)

Cooking time and temperatures, as needed

Expected yield

Portioning information, including portion size, number of portions, serving guide-lines, and serving utensil to be used

(Optional) Miscellaneous information, such as photo or sketch of the plated product, garnishing ideas, suggestions for accompaniments, and so on

Table 12.5 Parts of a Recipe[5]

laminated to prevent damage to the recipe. The parts of a recipe are shown in Table 12.5. A sample recipe is shown in Figure 12.8.

Yield is the amount of product that can be expected after all of the waste associated with the production process has been factored into the equation. Factors affecting yield include trimming and slicing losses, cooking losses, and the inevitable handling losses of product, which include scraps such as the food that remains attached to equipment during production and service. The method of cooking and the time and temperatures used may also influence the yield of the product. Usually the amount of product is less than the amount of the ingredients purchased. The relationship between the ingredients **as purchased** (AP) and the **edible portion** (EP) is known as the yield. Quantity food purchasing and food production texts are available with tables to assist the foodservice manager to project yields. Managers may have to conduct their own yield studies when dealing with a product that is new to the foodservice market.

Portion control is another foodservice production control. Portion control is achieved in several ways. Commonly used methods include pre-portioning, scoring an item to indicate the correct portion size to the server, weighing each portion, displaying a weighed portion for the server to use as a guide, or specifying a standard serving utensil. An alternative to portion control is self-serve, where customers determine their own portions and pay for the product by weight.

Pre-portioning the food to be served entails placing a specified amount of the finished product on a serving dish or a disposable unit. An example of this type of portion control is the sandwiches that are made up in advance of a meal peak at a typical quick service restaurant. Pre-plating of items like cakes and pies is fairly labor inten-sive, and the portioned products require a great deal of space. This technique is still used in full-service restaurants and by caterers who do table service, but is losing

Yield. *The amount of a product available for consumption from a specified quantity of ingredients after adjusting for losses that occur during production and service.*

As Purchased (AP). *The amount of a product (food item) acquired before any production loss has occurred.*

Edible Portion (EP). *The amount of food that can be consumed after accounting for preparation and/or cooking losses.*[6]

Portion Control. *A form of produc-tion control to regulate serving size.*

Portion Size Used: 4 oz   (use #8 scoop)   Recipe: 151044, Casserole Sweet Potato

Portion Count Used: 200

Yield Amount: 800 oz

Ingredient Name	A.P. Amount Required	E.P. Amount Required
yams, cut canned	8 10 CN 3 lb 1 oz	37 lb 8 oz
sugar, brown		5 lb 7 oz
cornstarch		5 3/4 oz
SP cinnamon, ground		11/2 tsp
nectar, apricot (NBL) 46 oz	2 46 oz 1 cup	3 quarts 1/2 cup
water		1 quart 2 1/4 cups
margarine, solid		12 oz

Method of Preparation

1. Drain potatoes and place 14 lbs in each 2 inch full line pan.

2. Combine brown sugar, cornstarch, and cinnamon.

3. Stir in apricot nectar and hot water.

4. Bring to boil, stirring constantly for 2 minutes.

5. Remove from heat and stir in margarine.

6. Pour 21/2 quarts sauce over the potatoes.

7. Bake uncovered at 350 F for 20–25 minutes.

HACCP Notes

1. Maintain above 135 F.

2. Check and record temperature every 2 hours.

3. Cover, date, and label.

4. Chill to 45 F within 2 hours.

5. Reheat to 165 F within 30 minutes.

Figure 12.8 Sample Recipe

Portion control is sometimes achieved by pre-plating the food for the customer.

ground in facilities where labor is expensive and cafeteria and buffet style service are the norm.

Scoring an item for service by a foodservice employee means making marks or cuts on the product, but not putting the item onto a plate or container until the customer requests it. Examples include a pie that is marked in eighths on the crust, or a lasagna in a rectangular casserole where the portion size is "3 × 8." See Figure 12.9.

Weighing each portion is time-consuming, so it is used only in situations where exact portions are absolutely necessary. Variations include weighing a sample portion that is available throughout the meal period for the server to use as a visual comparison, or weighing specific (for example, every tenth portion) or random portions. This latter technique is frequently used in ice cream or frozen yogurt shops to determine the accuracy of the food server.

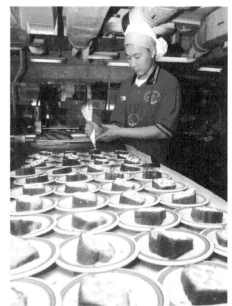

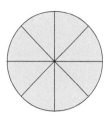
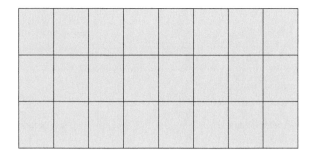

Figure 12.9 Scoring for Portion Control

Finally, portion control can be obtained through the use of a standard serving utensil or service piece. For example, a #8 scoop should deliver four ounces (by volume) of a product. (The ounces in a scoop are equal to the ounces in a quart—that is, 32 divided by the number of that scoop.) However, this implies that the scoop is a level one, not heaping. A four-ounce portion size might be achieved by using either a level #8 scoop or a heaping #10 scoop. Ladles, spoons, and slotted spoons are also used to deliver standard-size portions. The cups, bowls, and glasses used to deliver the product to the customer might also be used to achieve portion control.

Quality control in foodservice always includes tasting the food before serving it.

Taking and recording the temperature of food is essential in storage, preparation, and service, as is checking and recording the temperature of the equipment being used. The issue here is safety, because food products have the potential to carry a variety of microorganisms that can lead to illness, or even death. (See the "In Practice" feature at the end of this chapter.)

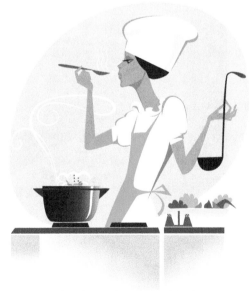

The last production control for foodservice is, perhaps, the most important. It is the actual tasting of the product before it is served to customers. This is an essential step in ensuring the quality of a product, but one that is often bypassed. Several individuals should do tasting from a sample plate that has been assembled from the foods to be served at that meal. Each taster should use a clean, reusable utensil for each item tasted, or a new disposable utensil for each item. The purpose of the taste test is to determine that the recipe has been followed as prescribed, that no ingredients have been omitted or added, and that the product is fit for customers to eat. If you ever tasted scrambled eggs in which sugar was inadvertently added in place of salt, or been served breakfast pancakes with garlic butter instead of butter, you will understand the importance of this step. Some production errors can be identified only by actually tasting the food.

management practice in dietetics

It is unlikely that one food product will satisfy all potential customers. Each customer has individual preferences and tastes that are dependent on cultural, physical, and environmental variables. However, production controls like those described in this section increase the likelihood that food products will be reproducible and served in a safe and uniform way.

conclusion

This chapter has dealt with how work moves through space and time, considering variables such as facilities, process, and job design. Time management was described from two perspectives—project management and management of labor hours. Production was discussed with emphasis on the planning and control of work. The major concepts that were presented in this chapter are summarized below.

1. How work moves through the workplace is dependent on both the physical layout of the workplace and on the processes delineating how the work is done. Facilities and process design are interdependent—that is, alterations in one will inevitably lead to changes in the other.
2. For major projects, a master schedule is used for time management to assure that the work is proceeding according to plan.
3. Individual jobs are designed using task analysis, work simplification, job rotation, job enlargement, and job enrichment techniques, all of which may make a positive contribution to the employees' level of satisfaction with their jobs.
4. Employee work schedules are a management tool that should be used to meet both the needs of management and those of employees.
5. Production planning tools include a forecasting method, production schedules, and production meetings.
6. Production controls are used to direct the conversions of inputs into products that are uniform and reproducible.

activities

activity 1

Design a trayline for a hospital's foodservice. Consider both the physical layout and the work processes involved. Students should work in groups of five or six to complete this project. Information on the types of equipment used in patient traylines can be obtained from your instructor, from a local restaurant supply company, or on the Internet.

Variations for this project include:

1. Three-person trayline that produces 40 trays in 50 minutes.
2. Five-person trayline that produces 100 trays in 60 minutes.
3. Eight-person trayline that produces 150 trays in 60 minutes.
4. Nine-person trayline that produces 200 trays in 90 minutes.
5. Eleven-person trayline that produces 275 trays in 90 minutes.

Make the assumption that the total number of positions includes all trayline workers, a checker, and a runner. (A runner is an individual who replenishes food as supplies dwindle, or who locates and delivers missing items for trays.) Supervisors are not included in the number given. If you make other assumptions, please enumerate them in the assignment.

activity 2

Design a master schedule for the implementation of a computer system in a campus dining facility. Construct the skeleton of a Gantt chart using the following information.

1. It is now August 15, and you have just learned that the university has budgeted enough money to capitalize a computer system for dining services. You must have the new system operational by the beginning of the next fiscal year, which will occur on July 1. There are 10.5 months to purchase, install, and test the new system.
2. The specifications for the new system were made during the previous budget cycle; the decision regarding what hardware and software to buy has already been made. The package will be purchased immediately, with a delivery date of August 31.
3. Final testing of the system will take a month, so the system should be up and running in its entirety by June 1.

management practice in dietetics

The other activities to be included on the master schedule are

1. installation of equipment
2. rewriting recipes for compatibility with the new system
3. compiling a list of all ingredients needed
4. establishing inventory levels and prices for each ingredient
5. entering data for items 2 through 4 into the new computer system
6. designing procedures for using the system
7. training the staff on the new system

The additional information you will need follows.

1. Existing management staff will provide the information needed for data entry, but they must also continue to perform their regular jobs.
2. Two thousand hours will be needed to enter the data.
3. Each of eight work-study students can work 15 hours each week doing data entry.
4. Five computer terminals are available for the students to use.
5. A consultant will be hired for 20 hours per week for three months to write procedures and train the staff.

activity 3

Please read the all of the instructions for Activity 3. Once you have read this in its entirety, you will have the information that you need to complete a work schedule for all foodservice workers in a department, or for a specific group of workers within that department. This schedule does not include cooks, management staff, or diet office personnel.

1. Pay rates are

    SK—Storekeeper   = $12.35 per hour
    DR—Dishroom Staff = $11.95 per hour
    KH—Kitchen Helper = $11.27 per hour

2. All employees can work any position except SK; this position requires additional training that has been completed only by SK1, KH3, and KH4. No one else can do this job.
3. DR1, DR2, DR3, DR4, and DR5 get paid $11.95 no matter what job they are doing; SK1 gets paid $12.35 no matter what job he does. All other employees get paid $11.27, unless they work as a DR or an SK, in which case they get paid the wage for the position they work.
4. Shifts listed as 6:00–2:30, 7:30–4:00, and so on are considered to be eight-hour shifts with a 30-minute (unpaid) meal break.

5. The SK position works Monday through Friday and is unfilled on weekends (a weekend is designated as Saturday and Sunday, together). SK1 is guaranteed a 40-hour week and is scheduled off every weekend.

6. There are four DR positions scheduled each day; 3 DRs work 7:00–3:30, and one DR works 8:00–4:30. DR1 and DR2 have seniority and, therefore, get every other weekend off. DR3, DR4, and DR5 get every third weekend off. All five DR employees are guaranteed 40 hours each week.

7. KH1, KH2, KH3, KH4, KH5, KH6, KH7, KH8, and KH9 are all full-time employees, are guaranteed 40 hours each week, and get every third weekend off.

8. There are eight 8-hour shifts for KHs scheduled Monday through Friday. These are

5:00–1:30	1 shift
7:00–3:30	3 shifts
7:30–4:00	1 shift
10:00–6:30	1 shift
11:00–7:30	1 shift
12:00–8:30	1 shift

On weekends, one of the 7:00–3:30 shifts and the 12:00–8:30 shift are eliminated.

9. KH10, KH11, KH12, KH13, and KH14 are all part-time employees. Each is guaranteed 20 hours per week and at least every third weekend off.

10. KH15 is a short-hour employee who is guaranteed 16 hours each week and every third weekend off.

11. There are five 4-hour shifts on weekdays. They are all 3:30–7:30, and three of the positions work in the dishroom, so they get DR pay. On weekends, there are four 4-hour shifts; three are 3:30–7:30 in the dishroom, and the fourth is 4:30–8:30.

12. KH16, KH17, KH18, KH19, and KH20 are casual employees with no guaranteed hours. KH20 is a college student and can work only on weekends.

13. Short-hour and casual employees receive no benefits but are paid 12.5 percent differential in lieu of benefits.

14. Overtime pay (150 percent of base pay) is earned by any employee who works:
    a. more than 8 hours in a day
    b. more than 40 hours in a week (week begins Sunday and ends Saturday)
    c. any shifts that are not separated by 12 hours (the second-shift work is paid overtime)
    d. any days after the seven consecutive days have been worked

15. A shift differential of $.50 per hour is paid for:
    a. any shift that begins before 6 a.m. or after 12 noon
    b. any hours worked after 6 p.m.

16. Employees should be scheduled to work the same shifts, whenever possible.

17. Consecutive days off should be given when possible.

18. The following vacations have been approved:

    a.   SK1   3/28–4/1 inclusive
    b.   KH6   3/21–3/26 inclusive
    c.   DR4   3/26–4/3 inclusive

activity 3a

Write the schedule on a form like that shown on the next page for the SK and all of the required dishroom shifts. In order to do this, some KH positions will be needed to work in the dishroom. The schedule should run from Sunday, March 20, through Saturday, April 9. Make every effort to keep labor costs to a minimum by avoiding overtime. When you have completed the schedule, calculate the number of FTEs who worked in the SK position each week and the number who worked in the dishroom each week. Calculate the gross labor costs for each week; do not include the cost of benefits and vacation pay.

activity 3b

For extra credit, you may want to try to fill in the remainder of the schedule, filling all of the shifts, and meeting all of the scheduling requirements for employees noted in items 1 through 18 above.

Time Schedule

	S 3/20	M 3/21	T 3/22	W 3/23	T 3/24	F 3/25	S 3/26	S 3/27	M 3/28	T 3/29	W 3/30	T 3/31	F 4/1	S 4/2	S 4/3	M 4/4	T 4/5	W 4/6	T 4/7	F 4/8	S 4/9
SK1																					
DR1																					
DR2																					
DR3																					
DR4																					
DR5																					
KH1																					
KH2																					
KH3																					
KH4																					
KH5																					
KH6																					
KH7																					
KH8																					
KH9																					
KH10																					
KH11																					
KH12																					
KH13																					
KH14																					
KH15																					
KH16																					
KH17																					
KH18																					
KH19																					
KH20																					

to study further

Materials to supplement this chapter can be found in the following sources.

- Blecher, L. "Using Forecasting Techniques to Predict Meal Demand in Title IIIc Congregate Lunch Programs." *Journal of the American Dietetic Association.* 104:1281–1283, 2004.
- Brown, D. M. "Process Analysis Improves Quality and Volume of Nutrition Screenings." *Journal of the American Dietetic Association.* 96:381–383, 1996.
- Buchanan, P. *Quantity Food Preparation: Standardizing Recipes and Controlling Ingredients.* 3rd ed.
- Chicago: American Dietetic Association, 1993.
- Dittmer, P. and J. D. Keefe. *Principles of Food Beverage and Labor Cost Controls.* 9th ed. Hoboken, NJ: John Wiley and Sons, 2009.
- Dutta, S. and J. F. Manzoni. *Process Reengineering, Organizational Change and Performance Improvement.* New York: McGraw-Hill, 1999.
- Gregoire, M. B. *Foodservice Organizations: A Managerial and Systems Approach.* 8th ed. Boston: Pearson 2013.
- Gregoire, M. B. and M. F. Nettles. "Is It Time for Computer-Assisted Decision Making to Improve the Quality of Food and Nutrition Services?" *Journal of the American Dietetic Association.* 94:843–845, 1994.
- Katsigris, C. and C. Thomas. *Design and Equipment for Restaurants and Foodservice: A Management View.* 3rd ed. Hoboken, NJ: John Wiley and Sons, Inc. 2009.
- Knight, J. B. and L. H. Kotschevar. *Quantity Food Production, Planning and Management.* 3rd ed. New York: Wiley, 2000.
- Kotschevar, L. H. and R. Donnelly, *Quantity Food Purchasing.* 5th ed. Upper Saddle River, NJ: Prentice Hall, 1999.
- Lientz, B. P. and K. P. Rea. *Project Management for the 21st Century.* 3rd ed. New York: Routledge, 2011.
- Lynch, F. T. *The Book of Yields: Accuracy in Food Costing and Purchasing.* 8th ed. Hoboken, NJ: John Wiley and Sons, 2012.
- Payne-Palacio, J. and M. Theis. *Introduction to Foodservice.* 11th ed. Upper Saddle River, NJ: Pearson Prentice Hall, 2009.
- Sharp, A. and P. McDermott. *Workflow Modeling: Tools for Process Improvement and Application Development.* 2nd ed. Boston: Artech House, 2009.
- van der Aalst, W. and Kees, M. van Hee. *Workflow Management: Models, Methods, and Systems.* Cambridge, MA: MIT Press, 2004.

scholarly journals

- *Applied Ergonomics*
- *Human Factors: The Journal of the Human Factors and Ergonomics Society*

other relevant periodicals

- *Food Management*
- *Foodservice Director*
- *Foodservice Equipment and Supplies*
- *Foodservice Equipment Reports*
- *Nation's Restaurant News*

HACCP

Richard Lawley—September 2008

what is HACCP?

HACCP is an acronym for Hazard Analysis Critical Control Point, a science-based food safety management system that has become the preferred method of ensuring safe food all over the world. The HACCP approach to food safety is based on a detailed examination of every stage in the production process for an individual food product. The objective is to identify where and when hazards could occur and to design effective controls for each hazard. In other words, HACCP anticipates food safety hazards in a process and builds in safeguards to prevent them occurring.

HACCP has its origins in the US manned space flight programme of the 1960s and '70s. It was vital that the food provided for astronauts was completely free from foodborne pathogens and other hazards, since any illness in flight would have serious consequences. NASA, in collaboration with the Pillsbury Company, therefore adapted analytical techniques used to anticipate failures in the engineering industry to develop the first HACCP system.

This early version of HACCP has since been further developed by the food industry and over the last 20 years it has been widely adopted by many food manufacturers. More recently, HACCP has increasingly become a basic requirement of complying with food safety regulations in many countries.

HACCP basics

The HACCP system is based on, and defined by, seven underlying principles. However, these principles use some important terminology that needs to be defined first.

definitions

Control measure—An action or an activity that can be used to prevent, eliminate, or reduce a food safety hazard to an acceptable level.

Corrective action—An action to be taken when loss of control at a CCP is indicated by monitoring.

Critical Control Point (CCP)—A step in the production process at which control can be applied and is essential to prevent, eliminate, or reduce a food safety hazard to an acceptable level.

Critical limit—A predetermined value for a control measure marking the division between acceptability and unacceptability.

Hazard—A biological, chemical, or physical agent in, or property of, food that has the potential to cause an adverse effect on consumer health.

Hazard analysis—The process of collecting and assessing information on the hazards and the conditions leading to their presence to determine which are significant for food safety and should therefore be addressed in the HACCP plan.

Monitoring—Conducting a planned sequence of observations or measurements of control parameters to assess whether a CCP is under control.

Step—A raw material, location, procedure, operation or stage in the food production process from primary production to final consumption.

Validation—Obtaining evidence that the elements of the HACCP plan are effective.

Verification—The application of supplementary information, including methods, tests and other evaluations, in addition to monitoring to determine the effectiveness of the HACCP plan.

the seven HACCP principles

1. Conduct a hazard analysis (identify hazards and control measures)
2. Identify the critical control points (CCPs)
3. Establish the critical limit(s) for each CCP
4. Establish a system to monitor control of the CCPs
5. Establish the corrective action to be taken when monitoring indicates that a CCP is not under control.
6. Establish verification procedures to confirm that the HACCP system is working effectively.
7. Establish documentation concerning all procedures and records appropriate to these principles and their application.

the application of HACCP

Although HACCP has been shown to be an effective means of managing food safety, there are a number of prerequisites for the successful application of the HACCP principles.

It is essential that any food business is already aware of appropriate food safety requirements and good hygiene practice before developing a HACCP plan. HACCP is not a substitute for basic hygiene and good manufacturing practice. Adequate staff training procedures should also be established in advance of applying HACCP principles.

A high degree of management commitment is also necessary for the successful application of HACCP. A food safety management system that does not have the full backing of the managers implementing it is unlikely to be effective. Clear definition of individual responsibilities with regard to the HACCP system is also essential.

Finally it is essential that managers and staff have appropriate knowledge and skills to undertake a HACCP study and some training is likely to be required. Smaller businesses may lack the technical and scientific expertise needed to identify and evaluate hazards and controls. It may therefore be necessary to seek expert advice and support from trade associations, independent consultants, or enforcement officers. A great deal of information about HACCP and its application is freely available and some web-based resources are listed below.

stages of the HACCP process

1. Assemble the HACCP team

The development of an effective HACCP plan normally requires a multidisciplinary team to ensure that appropriate product-specific expertise and knowledge is available. The team should comprise individuals familiar with all aspects of the production process, plus specialists with expertise in specific areas, such as engineering or microbiology. It may be necessary to use external sources of expertise in some cases.

The scope of the HACCP study should be determined by defining the extent of the production process being considered and identifying the classes of hazard being addressed (e.g. biological, chemical, and/or physical hazards).

2. Describe the product

It is important to have a complete understanding of the product, which should be described in detail. The description should include all relevant safety information and should cover factors such as composition, physical and chemical structure (including A_w, pH etc), processing conditions (e.g. heat-treatment, freezing, fermentation, curing, smoking etc), packaging, shelf life, storage and distribution conditions and use instructions. Where a range of similar products are being considered, these can be grouped together if their characteristics and processing steps are similar.

3. *Identify intended use*

The intended use should be based on the expected uses of the product by the end-user or consumer (e.g. is a cooking or reheating process required?). It is also important to identify the consumer target groups. Vulnerable groups, such as children or the elderly, may need to be considered specifically.

4. *Construct flow diagram*

The HACCP team should construct an accurate and detailed flow diagram of the manufacturing process being considered covering every individual step and providing sufficient technical data for the study to progress. It should provide an accurate representation of each step from raw materials to end product and may include details of the factory and equipment layout, ingredient specifications, features of equipment design, time/temperature data, cleaning and hygiene procedures and storage conditions. The same flow diagram can be used where a range of similar products are being produced on the same line.

5. *On site confirmation of the flow diagram*

The HACCP team should confirm that the flow diagram it has drawn up matches the process that is actually carried out in practice. The operation should be observed at each stage and any discrepancies between the diagram and normal practice should be recorded. The diagram should then be amended to take these discrepancies into account. The production process should also be observed outside normal working hours, such as during night shifts, as practice may vary between shifts. It is essential that the flow diagram is accurate, since the hazard analysis and identification of CCPs relies on the data it contains.

6. *List all potential hazards associated with each step, conduct a hazard analysis and identify control measures for each hazard*

The HACCP team should list all hazards that may reasonably be expected to occur at each step in the production process.

The team should then conduct a hazard analysis to identify those hazards that are of such a nature that their elimination, or reduction to acceptable levels is essential to the production of safe food.

Wherever possible, the hazard analysis should include consideration of:

- the likely occurrence of hazards and the severity of their adverse health effects;
- the qualitative and/or quantitative evaluation of the presence of the hazards;
- survival or multiplication of pathogenic microorganisms;

- production or persistence in foods of toxins, chemicals or physical agents;
- conditions leading to the above.

The HACCP team should then consider what control measures exist that can be applied to each hazard identified. Some hazards may require more than one control measure for adequate control and a single control measure may act to control more than one hazard.

Note: it is important that no attempt is made to identify CCPs at this stage as this may disrupt the analysis.

7. Determine critical control points

The determination of the CCPs is the key stage in a HACCP study, since the final HACCP plan will focus on the control and monitoring of the process at these points. It is vital that the HACCP team has sufficient technical data to determine the CCPs effectively and it is also important to be aware that more than one CCP may exist for a single hazard.

The determination of a CCP can be facilitated by the use of a decision tree (diagram 2.) to provide a logical, structured approach to the decision making. However, the decision tree is for guidance only and its application should be flexible. Its use may not always be appropriate. Training in the effective use of the decision tree is recommended.

If a realistic hazard has been identified at a step where control is necessary for safety, and no control exists at that step, or any other, then the production process should be modified to include a control measure.

8. Establish critical limits for each CCP

Critical limits must be specified and validated for each CCP. More than one critical limit may be defined for a single step. For example, it is usually necessary to specify both time and temperature for a thermal process. Criteria used to set critical limits must be measurable and often include measurements of temperature, time, moisture level, pH, A_w, available chlorine, and sensory parameters, such as visual appearance and texture.

9. Establish a monitoring system for each CCP

Monitoring is the planned and scheduled measurement or observation of a CCP relative to its critical limits. The monitoring procedures must be able to detect loss of control at the CCP and should provide this information in time to make appropriate adjustments so that control of the process is regained before the critical limits are violated. Where possible, process adjustments should be made when monitoring results indicate a trend towards a loss of control at a CCP.

Monitoring should either be continuous, or carried out sufficiently frequently to ensure control at the CCP. Monitoring procedures for CCPs must be rapid so that results are available quickly enough to maintain control at the CCP. Therefore, physical and chemical on-line measurements are usually preferred to lengthy microbiological testing.

The information derived from monitoring must be evaluated by a designated individual who has the knowledge, training and authority needed to act effectively on the basis of the data. The data must also be properly documented and recorded by that person.

10. *Establish corrective actions*

For each CCP in the HACCP plan, specific corrective actions must be developed that can be applied when the CCP is not under control. If monitoring indicates a deviation from the critical limits for a CCP, action must be taken that will bring it back under control. Actions taken should include proper isolation and disposition of any affected product and all corrective actions taken should be recorded and documented.

11. *Establish verification procedures*

Verification and auditing methods, procedures and tests, including product sampling and analysis, should be used frequently to determine whether the HACCP system is working correctly.

Responsibility for verification activities should be given to someone other than the individual responsible for monitoring and corrective actions. In some cases, this may mean that verification activities are performed by external experts.

Verification procedures should include detailed reviews of all aspects of the HACCP system and its records. The documentation should confirm that CCPs are under control and should also indicate the nature and extent of any deviations from the critical limits and the corrective actions taken in each case. Information such as customer complaints and returns may also be useful for verification.

12. *Establish documentation and record keeping*

Efficient and accurate record keeping is an essential element of the application of a HACCP system. All HACCP procedures should be documented. However, documentation and record keeping should be appropriate to the nature and size of the operation, but sufficient to ensure that the business is able to verify that controls are in place and are being properly maintained.

Examples of appropriate documentation include:

- Hazard analysis
- CCP determination
- Critical limit determination

Examples of appropriate recorded data are:

- CCP monitoring activities and results
- Deviations from critical limits and corrective actions taken
- Verification procedures performed
- Modifications to the HACCP plan

A record keeping system should be clear and simple so that it can be easily maintained and communicated. It may be helpful to integrate HACCP records with other documentation. For example, product temperatures can be recorded on delivery invoices.

review of the HACCP plan

It is important to remember that a HACCP plan is a dynamic system and must be kept up to date at all times.

The plan must be reviewed following any changes to the production process, including changes to raw materials, processing conditions or equipment, packaging, cleaning procedures and any other factor that may have an effect on product safety. Even small modifications to the product or process can invalidate the HACCP plan and introduce potential hazards. The implications of any such changes to the overall HACCP system must be fully considered and documented and adjustments made to procedures as necessary.

sources of further information

published

Taylor, E. and Taylor, J.
HACCP: 12 Steps to Success (second edition)
Manchester, Practical HACCP Publishing, 2006.

Mayes, A. and Mortimore, S.
Making the Most of HACCP: Learning from Others' Experience
Cambridge, Woodhead Publishing, 2001.

Mortimore, S., Wallace, C., and Cassianos, C.
HACCP (Food Industry Briefing)
Oxford, Blackwell Science, 2001.

Mortimore, S. and Wallace, C.
HACCP: A Practical Approach (second edition)
Gaithersburg, Maryland, Aspen Publishers Inc., 1998.

on the web

Codex Alimentarius Commission—Recommended International Code of Practice: General Principles of Food Hygiene CAC/RCP 1-1969, Rev. 4-2003 (Includes Annex on HACCP, pages 31–43)
http://www.codexalimentarius.org/

Canadian Food Inspection Agency—Food Safety Enhancement Program HACCP Generic Models http://www.inspection.gc.ca/

Generic HACCP models from USDA/FSIS
http://haccpalliance.org/alliance/haccpmodels.html

The Seafood Network Information Center—Generic HACCP plans
http://seafood.ucdavis.edu/HACCP/Plans.htm

UK Food Standards Agency—HACCP in Meat Plants
http://www.food.gov.uk/foodindustry/meat/haccpmeatplants/

Source: http://www.foodsafetywatch.com/public/745.cfm

references

1. Leintz, Bennet P. and Kathryn P. Rea. *Project Management for the 21st Century.* San Diego: Academic Press, 1995.
2. Sears, Woodrow H. Jr. *Back in Working Order.* Glenville, IL: Scott, Foresman, 1984.
3. Champagne, Paul J. and R. Bruce McAfee. *Motivating Strategies for Performance and Productivity.* Westport, CT: Quorum Books, 1989.
4. Donnelly, Richard and Kotschevar, Lendal H. *Quantity Food Purchasing.* 5th ed. Upper Saddle River, NJ: Prentice Hall, 1999, p. 105.
5. Spears, Marian C. and Mary B. Gregoire. *Foodservice Organizations: A Managerial and Systems Approach.* 5th ed. Upper Saddle River, NJ: Pearson Prentice Hall, 2003, p. 207.
6. Ibid. p. 236.

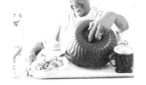

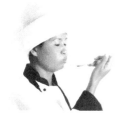

chapter thirteen

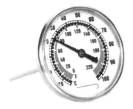

productivity and accountability

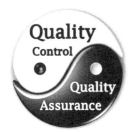

learning objectives

1. List the various groups to which an organization may be accountable.

2. Describe why accrediting agencies are interested in the accountability of the organizations and programs that they evaluate.

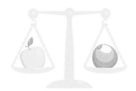

3. State reasons for measuring productivity.

4. Differentiate among quantitative, qualitative, and outcome productivity measures.

5. Describe how to measure productivity for various types of workers.

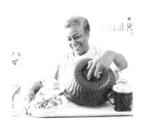

6. State why fiscal accountability is necessary.

7. Determine why it is necessary for an organization to be accountable to its employees.

8. List various ways organizations measure accountability to their employees.

9. Distinguish between quality control and quality assurance.

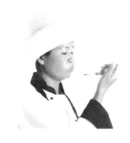

10. Discuss the standard systems used for quality management, including quality assurance, continuous quality improvement, and total quality management.

11. Define *benchmarking*.

12. Differentiate between internal and external benchmarking.

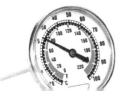

overview

Accountability is a part of business just as it is a part of life. Without accountability, individuals and organizations could act with absolute autonomy, without any responsibility to other individuals, groups, or society as a whole. Although autonomy may be a good thing in the hands of responsible people, it has the potential for creating chaos when exercised by unscrupulous people. Thus, there is a system of checks and balances, called accountability, built into today's business environment. It provides a framework within which individuals and organizations achieve and maintain individual and social responsibility.

There are many constituencies to which one may be accountable as a manager. These include the organization itself, the financial backers (owner, bank, or stockholders), the customers, the general public, the employees, the accrediting body, one's profession, and oneself. Each of these constituencies may be harmed when management behaves irresponsibly, and each benefits from systems that are put into place to guarantee accountability.

Accountability includes a variety of performance measurements that look at the quantity and quality of production as well as the outcomes related to what is produced. These are called *productivity measures*. Other measurements are those that relate to financial performance that, though related to productivity, are best measured in terms of dollars. Additional measures are related to human resources, such as job safety issues, amount of sick leave or overtime used, and job satisfaction. All of these and any other indicators of accountability that an organization measures can be used to compare that organization with its own past performance, with similar organizations, or with industry standards. This process of comparison is known as *benchmarking*. Both internal and external benchmarks are used to determine how an organization is measuring and improving its performance. Good management requires that managers know how they are doing in comparison to benchmark data, even if their constituencies do not require that they report this type of data.

Over the years, accountability systems have been refined and streamlined. What was originally known as quality control developed into quality assurance, then into quality improvement systems such as TQM (total quality management) or CQI (continuous quality improvement). These systems continue to develop. This chapter will describe some of the more universal aspects of measuring productivity, benchmarking, and quality management.

constituencies

Businesses and organizations are often viewed from a systems perspective in which resources, known as inputs, undergo transformation and are changed into products, called outputs. At every point in the system, individuals and groups are involved, and the organization becomes accountable to all of those people who are directly or indirectly related to the organizational system. These include those who provide the various resources from which the product is made. The organization is also accountable to the employees who actually produce the product. Finally, the organization is accountable to its customers to deliver a safe, useful product that will perform as advertised and not cause harm.

vendors

When raw material is used in production, the supplier is entitled to payment for that material. Usually there is some sort of agreement that identifies the terms and conditions for payment by the organization to the vendor. There are a number of possible arrangements—for example, paying bills a certain number of days after delivery, or the first day of the month after the delivery date, and so on. Whatever the agreement, the vendor has the right to expect payment by the date agreed upon, and the purchasing organization is accountable to the vendor to pay the bills by the expected date. When an organization is late with its payments, it is not being accountable to its vendors. Over time, this practice could result in less-favorable terms, increased prices, decreased service, and so on. If the purchasing organization does not pay its bills on time, it will eventually lose its credit rating, which could have a negative effect on the organization by increasing both the cost of goods and the cost of borrowed money. This decreases the organization's potential for earning a profit.

People who supply other services to the organization or business—such as consultants, contractors, management advisors, and others—are entitled to the same fair treatment as those who supply material inputs. The services and ideas that are utilized as inputs in a business are as important a part of the system as the more-tangible material inputs.

financial backers

Along with the vendors who must be satisfied, the financial backers of a business have a right to expect a reasonable return on their investment. If the backers are owners, stockholders, or banks, they will expect to make money from their investment. This means that the organization must earn a profit that can be returned to the investors or paid to lenders in the form of interest.

If the financial backers are taxpayers, and the organization is a public one, these taxpayers have a right to expect a certain level of quality or service in return for their tax dollar. For example, the taxpayers have a right to quality education from a public college or university; if a hospital is supported by taxes, efficient, effective, appropriate, and adequate health care should be provided by that hospital.

U.S. Department of Agriculture.
http://www.usda.gov/wps/portal/usda/usdahome

Food and Drug Administration.
http://www.fda.gov/

Health Canada.
http://www.hc-sc.gc.ca/index-eng.php

The public, as taxpayers, has a right to accountability from the government and its agencies. It is not unreasonable for the public to expect that the government will assure the safety of the food supply. In this case, agencies such as the U.S. Department of Agriculture (USDA), the Food and Drug Administration (FDA), and Health Canada are accountable to the public at large, because taxes support these agencies that oversee the safety of the food supply. If an outbreak of food-borne illness occurs (for example, *E. coli* in burgers or *Listeria* in cheese), the public has the right to know why the problem occurred and what steps are being taken to prevent future outbreaks.

employees

It has been a major focus of this book to demonstrate the importance of the worker to the organization. It is the job of the management to provide a safe, harassment-free work environment and a fair wage to all of those who work in the organization. It is also important to provide for open communication, empowerment, and fairness to all employees. Management is accountable to the organization's employees.

The labor movement grew out of an era when managers considered employees to be mere "inputs" that could be used without regard to such issues as safety, security, and employee rights. Employees needed only to be paid for the number of hours worked. This is no longer the case. The labor movement has made business accountable to its employees in many other ways. Although this evolution might have occurred spontaneously, it would never have happened as fast as it did without the influence of organized labor. The horrors that were evident in the factories and mines of the early industrial period are, for the most part, over. In economically developed countries, the workers are considered to be valuable resources who will produce more and better products if they are treated and respected as individuals who have rights and expectations beyond that of merely earning a paycheck.

customers

In today's world, it is no longer acceptable for a business or an institution to make a product and sell it to any customer who can afford to purchase it. It is also necessary that the product perform, that it meet the need of the customer, and that it not harm the customer, either individually or as a group. In recent years, there has been a differentiation between types of customers. Both internal and external customers have been identified as being important to the success of an organization.

External Customer.
The end user of the product made by an organization.

An **external customer** is the end user of the product. In a college or university, for example, there are two major external customers. The first is the student, who is entitled to a good education in exchange for the money spent on that student's behalf. The second is the person or group who pays the university to educate the student.

This may be a parent or a guardian, the student herself, or a government agency that provides the student with funding. Both of these customers need some assurance that the students are, indeed, getting a quality of education that will be recognized in the future and that will give the students the skills and tools to succeed in their chosen fields. In a healthcare system, an external customer is the patient.

Internal customers are those individuals within an organization who provide direct service to the external customers. Again using the educational institution as an example, the internal customer might be the faculty (who teach the students), the librarians (who provide students with learning resources), or the campus police (who ensure safety and security for the students). All of these groups are internal customers of one or more other groups within the institution.

For example, the three groups listed here are the internal customers of the payroll department that provides them with their paychecks on a regular basis. Without a smoothly operating payroll department, the internal customers might not get paid regularly. As a result, they could become angry and stop providing quality service to the external customers, the students. In healthcare systems, internal customers include the physician, physician's assistant, or nurse practitioner who brings the patient into the system and the nursing personnel who give direct care to the patients.

Hospital foodservices have inpatients, outpatients, and their families as external customers, and hospital employees as their internal customers. As with the educational institutions and healthcare systems, the hospital foodservice must satisfy all of its customers if it wants to have repeat business and achieve growth. In today's mobile society, having a **captive clientele** is rare because customers have choices about where to purchase goods and services. It is necessary to be accountable to the entire customer base, both internal and external.

professional/accrediting agencies

In some situations, the public, either as a financial backer of an organization or as a customer, does not have enough information to know if the goods and services that they are getting are appropriate. This does not mean that they are at fault for not being well informed, but more that they lack the training and education to sort through the complex data available. For example, many consumers of health care do not have enough information about medicine to judge the quality of service that they get from healthcare systems. Thus, it is important that some group be given oversight to protect the public. In health care in the United States, the oversight organization is the Joint Commission for the Accreditation of Healthcare Organizations (JCAHO). The Accreditation Council for Education in Nutrition and Dietetics (ACEND) oversees dietetics education. These and other oversight organizations—such as state and local health departments, the FDA, the USDA, and similar agencies—make sure that

Internal Customers. *Those individuals within an organization who provide direct service to the external customers.*

Captive Clientele. *Customers who must use a product or a service because they have no other options.*

Joint Commission on Accreditation of Healthcare Organizations. *http://www. jointcommission.org/*

Accreditation Council for Education in Nutrition and Dietetics. *http://www. eatright.org/ ACEND/*

businesses and organizations are accountable to the public. Because these groups are composed of professionals in the specific area of expertise that is needed, they often assure accountability to the profession as well. (Recall from Chapter 7 that a professional is a member of a group that is self-regulating.) For example, JCAHO ensures that healthcare systems meet minimum standards for the provision of health care; ACEND assures quality in dietetics education. The FDA and the USDA oversee food safety in the United States.

Finally, professionals are accountable, on a very real and personal level, to abide by the ethical code of the profession (See "In Practice" feature, Chapter 1) to which they belong. For example, it is assumed that pilots will not fly commercial aircraft after consuming alcohol, that physicians will not prescribe treatments that will harm patients, and that nutritional professionals will not dispense nutritional supplements whose sole purpose is to decrease the weight of the consumer's wallet.

productivity

Productivity.
Measurement of the relationship between outputs or products and inputs such as time, money, labor, and raw material. Productivity may be measured quantitatively, qualitatively, or in terms of outcomes.

Once one has determined the constituencies to whom organizations are accountable, it is necessary to develop measurements of accountability. The most commonly used are measures of productivity that can be adapted to any system that produces a product, including goods, services, and ideas. The simplest definition of productivity is the comparative relationship of inputs to outputs. Productivity is measured to determine how product (output) is associated with the time, money, labor, raw material, and other resources used (inputs) to create the product. As with other management tools, productivity measurements have become more sophisticated over time. It is no longer enough to measure how much is produced. It is also necessary to measure productivity in terms of quality and outcomes as well.

measuring productivity

Two illustrations will be used to describe how productivity is measured at the three levels. Again, productivity measurements may focus on the quantity of what is produced, the quality of the product, or the outcomes that occur as a result of the production.

Quantitative Measure. *A type of productivity measure that focuses on the quantity of product produced.*

First, consider the patient trayline in a hospital. The **quantitative measure** of trays produced can be reported as trays per minute (total trays produced divided by the number of minutes needed to produce the trays). It can also be reported as person-minutes per tray (number of minutes needed to produce the trays multiplied by the number of people working on the trayline divided by the number of trays produced). See Table 13.1.

management practice in dietetics

Trays per Minute	Person-Minutes per Tray
Data needed:	**Data needed:**
Duration of trayline in minutes = 60	Duration of trayline in minutes = 60
Number of trays served = 165	Number of trays served = 165
	Number of trayline workers = 8
Calculation:	**Calculation:**
165 trays / 60 minutes = 2.75 trays per minute	60 minutes × 8 people = 480 person-minutes
	480 person-minutes / 165 trays = 2.9 person-minutes per tray
Use:	**Use:**
Internal comparison; comparison of traylines with the same number of workers	External comparison; comparison with traylines with different numbers of workers

Table 13.1 Trayline Productivity (Quantitative)

Trays per minute is a measurement used for internal comparison with past performance or for comparing two similar traylines at different facilities; person-minutes per tray is used for purposes of external comparison with traylines that are staffed with different numbers of workers. Another quantitative measurement related to tray service could be the time that it takes to get the tray from the assembly point to the point of service—that is, the patient's bedside.

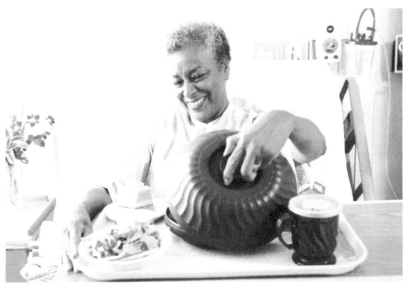

Quantitative, qualitative, and outcome measures are used to measure productivity related to patient trays in healthcare organizations.

Qualitative Measurement.

A type of productivity measure that is concerned with the accuracy and quality of what is produced.

Outcome Measurement.

A type of productivity measure that determines whether or not the product did what it was supposed to do.

Occupied Beds.

A measure hospitals use to quantify the work that they do; the number of patients who occupy a bed in the facility on a specific day for a 24-hour period. These data are often obtained by determining the number of patients who are physically present at a specific hour during the night (for example, 2 a.m.).

The **qualitative measurement** goes a step further and looks at whether or not the patient trays that were produced were complete and correct. This might measure accuracy—that is, if each tray has all the required items in the correct amounts with no extraneous items. Other possible qualitative measurements could include food temperatures at the point of service, sensory quality of the food, or the neatness of the tray when it is served (for example, proper arrangement of tray items, no spills, and so on).

The **outcome measurement** looks at additional information to determine if the purpose of the production was fulfilled. In the case of the patient trays, one could determine whether or not the food was consumed by doing plate-waste studies when the trays are returned for dishwashing. Alternately, one could evaluate whether the patient consumed the food as intended, or whether a visitor or a staff member consumed it. Another way to measure quality and/or outcomes is by conducting regular surveys to determine patient satisfaction with the meal service. Queries can be structured to evaluate both quality and outcomes.

In the clinical setting, it is possible to look at the productivity of the clinical dietitian related to nutritional assessments. Quantitative measurements might be either the number of assessments the dietitian completes in a prescribed amount of time, or the amount of time needed for the dietitian to complete each assessment. A qualitative measurement would relate to the correctness of the assessment—that is, if the prescribed protocols were followed, the calculations were done accurately, and the resulting chart note met procedural guidelines. The outcome measurements would include whether or not the recommendations made were followed by the primary care practitioner (physician, physician's assistant, or nurse practitioner) and the related questions, "If not, why not?" or "If followed, did the recommendations result in the improved nutritional status of the client?" The actual outcome measured—for example, weight gain, weight loss, improved protein stores, decreased cholesterol levels, better diabetes control, and so on—would be dependent on the characteristics of the client population.

Even though the trend is toward measuring outcomes, quantitative and qualitative measurements are still very valuable management tools. Such measures are important for comparative purposes (benchmarking) and for quality management. The measurements chosen need to be product specific, and need to include adjustments for peculiarities within the setting. Standardized measurement devices and tools are used for external comparative purposes to make the data from one facility more readily transferable to a different, but similar, setting. In addition to person-minutes per tray, described earlier, two other tools for external comparison are described in the following paragraphs. These are cited as examples of many such tools that can be used or designed to meet the needs for measuring productivity in an organization.

Hospitals used to use the number of **occupied beds** to compare their staffing levels to those of other healthcare facilities. In today's healthcare environment, the number of patients who occupy a bed for 24 hours (historically, the definition of *occupied* *bed*) has decreased, though the number of procedures performed, such as births and surgical procedures, has remained the same or increased. Hospitals can use a measure known as **adjusted occupied beds** to compare staffing levels with those of similar, but different, hospitals. This number corrects the number of occupied beds to include the care given to patients who are not officially admitted as inpatients for an entire 24-hour period of time. The adjustment is based on a number of variables, including outpatient volumes, utilization of surgical facilities, patient acuity, and so on. It allows hospitals to compare their staffing levels to those of other hospitals that have different occupancy levels and different volumes of outpatient work. This measurement recognizes the uniqueness of each facility while still allowing for comparisons among diverse healthcare organizations.

In foodservice, the productivity of cooks might be measured in terms of the number of **meals** served, because cooks actually produce meals (often defined as starter, entrée, starch, side dish, and dessert). However, some restaurants and cafeterias do a large volume of sales of between-meal snacks, such as pastries, desserts, beverages, and so on. In foodservices where many of the sales are not actual meals, comparing this year's sales in dollars to last year's sales is a viable tool for doing internal comparisons. However, it does not allow for comparison with other facilities where the food costs and/or the pricing of food products is different. In order to compare the productivity of such different foodservice operations, **meal equivalents** may be used. This number is obtained by determining the total sales for a facility and dividing it by the average cost of a typical meal within that facility. Meal equivalents allow the production of different facilities in different geographic regions to be compared. Both adjusted occupied beds and meal equivalents are quantitative measurements of productivity.

Qualitative measurements look at those factors that deal with the correctness or the accuracy of production, and are integrally related to quantitative measures. The volumes that are produced are important only if what is produced is correct. If a DTR screens 15 clients for nutritional risk, instead of the 12 required, the quantitative productivity increases. However, if that same technician neglected to record heights and weights for those clients, the work is incomplete and must be redone. Thus, the qualitative measure considers the precision of the work that is done, recognizing that only work that is complete and correctly done is truly done. Quantitative measurements are meaningful only if the quality consistently meets the standards that have been set for the product.

In foodservice, one of the qualitative measurements is the sensory characteristics of the food—that is, does it look, taste, and smell good? If a foodservice produced a batch of scrambled eggs to which sugar had been inadvertently added instead of salt, the product would fail the sensory evaluation test. The food would not be edible and, though it was actually produced, the production had no value because the product was not of acceptable quality. This is one of the reasons that food should always be evaluated before it is sent to the customer. It is prudent to check the quality of what

Adjusted Occupied Beds. *A measure generated through the use of a mathematical formula to adjust the actual number of occupied beds to reflect the work that is done in the hospital for patients who are not actually admitted for 24 hours or are not in residence at the time when the occupied bed census is taken. The formula is based on the hospital's usual activity patterns, volumes of outpatient visits, day surgeries, patient acuity, and so on.*

Meals. *A group of foods that are usually eaten together; typically, a meal includes an entrée, a starch, a side dish, and a dessert (it may also include an appetizer and/ or a salad). The number of meals prepared is often used to quantify the productivity of cooks.*

is produced to correct errors before they reach the customer. Poor-quality food can quickly ruin the reputation of the organization. Nevertheless, tasting food for quality is a step that many foodservices, both commercial and onsite, often fail to take. That is one of the reasons that it is not uncommon to get cold food or inappropriately seasoned food from commercial and onsite foodservices.

Another qualitative measure in foodservice revolves around the issue of food safety. Though it is easy to quantify the number of instances of food-borne illness that occur in a foodservice, it is obviously not enough to note that these situations occurred. It is necessary to take steps to prevent those instances from occurring. Food safety certification for staff and a HACCP system should be in place to assure accountability in the area of food safety. HACCP is described in more detail in the "In Practice" feature following Chapter 12.

Food should be checked for appearance, taste, and temperature before it is served to the customer.

Outcomes are more difficult to measure because they are out of the control of the person or group doing the production. Outcomes may not become apparent until a long time after the production has taken place. This is especially true in clinical dietetics. If a dietitian does a series of classes on cardiac risk reduction, the outcome is best measured by a decrease in the number of heart attacks among those who attended the class. However, it may take years to determine the effectiveness of the intervention. Clinical dietitians are learning to identify outcomes that can be measured in the short term—like decreases in total and saturated fat consumption, weight loss, and lowering of LDL cholesterol levels—to measure interim outcomes. Positive results in these measurements are extrapolated to predict that a decreased number of heart attacks will occur in the future.

Outcome measurements in restaurants and other dining facilities can be determined by looking at plate waste, by customer satisfaction surveys, and by repeat or increased business. One very perceptive foodservice manager stated it well by saying that his goal was not only having the customers like the food but having them come back to eat at his restaurant on a repeated basis. In addition to the food, this manager identified and measured productivity in terms of ambience, value, and service.

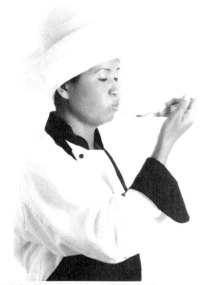

Copyright © 2012 by Depositphotos/Christophe Kajzar.

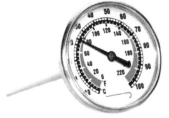

Copyright © 2011 by Depositphotos/ Valentyna Antonenko.

use of productivity records

Monitoring productivity has little value unless the resulting data are used. Managers should make a habit of monitoring productivity on an ongoing basis and using the resulting data as a management tool, whether or not the various constituencies require that the data be reported. The gathering and recording of the data on a daily or weekly basis take just moments, and the records can be used immediately to reward good work or to identify and correct problems. If the data are allowed to accumulate before being processed and analyzed, it becomes an overwhelming project to compile the data. If one chooses to look at the data on a quarterly or an annual basis, the data are so old by the time they are compiled that they are of limited value as a management tool. Old data are useful for writing reports but cannot be used to identify and respond to trends as they occur.

Computerized spreadsheet programs make it easy to record the data as they are generated. Trends are then easy to identify, and reaction time is shortened. Consider, for example, the clinical nutrition manager who has been monitoring the labor hours of DTRs and diet clerks in relation to the patient census by entering the number of hours worked each day and the number of occupied beds for that day into a spreadsheet program. Data show that it took 40 hours of labor per day to do screenings and menu processing for an average census of 200 occupied beds. Thus, the total diet office labor was 12 minutes per patient day (40 hours × 60 minutes = 2,400 minutes / 200 occupied beds = 12 minutes per patient). If the patient census suddenly drops to 150, then the diet office should be able to complete the work with 30 hours of labor. Conversely, if patient days increase to 250, then an additional 10 hours of labor per day can probably be justified. Without the productivity data, gathered on an ongoing basis, the staffing reduction or increase would be no more than an educated guess on the part of the manager.

In a different scenario, consider that this same manager had been keeping productivity records over time and had evidence that the staff had reduced the amount of time spent in diet office activities from 20 minutes per patient day to 12 minutes per patient day. This was accomplished by changing the jobs and job processes (an example might be the use of a computer forecasting system rather than a manual tally) to eliminate overtime, which was a daily occurrence prior to the implementation of the changes. If across-the-board layoffs were pending in the facility, this manager could use the quantitative productivity data on hand to show that a 40 percent reduction in time had already been achieved *in advance of the proposed layoffs*. This might be enough to insulate the diet office staff from layoffs and protect their jobs.

Another use of this same datum could be to monitor the staff during change. If the diet office staff is asked to work with a new patient menu, time will be needed to adjust to the new format, food items, nutrient composition of the items, and so on. All of the diet office functions will slow during the implementation of this new menu. To cope with the change, DTRs may do fewer nutritional screenings, and diet clerks may have to prepare manual tallies instead of forecasting food production needs. The manager will be able to monitor the labor minutes per patient day to determine the progress of the transition. This will provide data that can be used to provide additional support, encouragement, or congratulations for a job well done. When productivity levels return to normal, the manager will know that the transition to the new menu is complete.

Thus far, this discussion has been confined to the use of quantitative productivity data. The use of the qualitative and outcome productivity data is of equal or greater value as a management tool. These types of data, however, are best used in the context of quality management. Data on quality are used for benchmarking and for comparing an organization's products against those of similar organizations. Data on outcomes are often used to determine cost effectiveness and to justify the appropriateness of nutritional interventions.

quality management

As mentioned earlier, accountability within organizations has been evolving over the years. First, the problems of making a product had to be solved. Then, the focus changed from production itself, to the amounts of product made, then to the quality of the product. Initially, quality management focused on measuring quality. Over time, the process evolved to one of improving quality. Recently, quality management has begun to look at the quality of the production of the organization as a whole, rather than the quality of what each of its parts produces.

quality assurance

Quality Control (QC). *A method to determine if the products being made meet minimum standards of acceptability.*

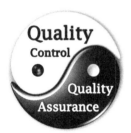

Copyright © 2011 by Depositphotos/Dtjs.

Quality control and quality assurance are complementary processes.

Quality Assurance (QA). *The process of identifying and solving problems within a department or area of an organization.*

At one point in the evolution of accountability in health care, **quality control** (QC) was the focus. Each department in an organization measured the quality of the product that it produced. Unfortunately, it is human nature for managers to want to "look good" to accrediting bodies and oversight committees, so they often chose to measure quality in those areas where they were already performing well, or chose measurement tools that would make them look good. For example, if a foodservice had a state-of-the-art food transporting system, it might measure food temperatures at the point of service to demonstrate excellent performance. A foodservice with poorer-quality equipment might use the same measurement (temperature) at the point of assembly, so that the temperatures appeared to be good, even though temperatures at the point of service were less than desirable. In the latter case, the measurements looked good on paper but may not have been a true indicator of quality.

The next step in the evolution of quality management was **quality assurance** (QA). It is the process that identifies a "problem" area, takes action to correct the problem, and then monitors the results over time to see that the problem is solved and remains solved. In the case of poor temperatures at the point of service, perhaps new equipment could be purchased to hold better food temperatures, or new processes could be developed to transport the trays to the point of service more rapidly. In either case, the changes need to be developed and implemented, with the results monitored over time. Once it is documented that a problem was solved, a new problem needs to be identified and addressed.

management practice in dietetics

In clinical nutrition, typical problems include the timeliness of screening to identify high-risk patients, variation among clinical dietitians in determining the kilocaloric requirements of obese patients, or inconsistent methods for determining desirable body weight for individuals with developmental disabilities. Quality assurance monitors and corrective actions led to the development of policies and procedures and patient care protocols to ensure consistency from practitioner to practitioner (and therefore from patient to patient) within an organization.

continuous quality improvement

As QA became more sophisticated, it became apparent that problems could be and were being solved. Indeed, over time, some of the more universal problems related to food and nutrition services in healthcare organizations were managed successfully and eliminated. As the quality of services improved, it became obvious that improvements could be made in areas that were not being identified as problems. For example, it is probably acceptable to screen every patient in a hospital for nutritional risk within 72 hours of admission, but in some cases (perhaps for patients who have specific diagnoses—for example, cystic fibrosis) it might be better if screenings were completed within 24 hours of admission. Thus, quality management evolved into the process called continuous quality improvement (CQI).

CQI is the process that looks at what things within an organization can be improved, and what can be done to achieve that improvement. Using hospital foodservice as an example, the results of patient satisfaction surveys may indicate that the majority of clients are satisfied with the quality of food served in a hospital. However, the surveys may also identify that there is a subgroup of the population that is not satisfied with the quality of the food because it does not contain items that are culturally suited to them because of their ethnicity. Even though the overall food quality is good, an alternate menu could be developed to meet the needs of the subgroup, which may be Asian American, Moslem, Hasidic Jewish, African American, or Latino. By establishing alternate menus, the facility can improve the quality of service to some clients, even though no major "problem" was ever identified.

total quality management

In the search for ways in which to improve services that were already good, or at least acceptable, it became apparent that problems still existed that had not been solved. When these problems were studied, a common thread that defined them was that they were all issues that involved more than one department in a facility. Thus, CQI must be complemented with the concept of total quality management (TQM), which is designed to look at problems and improvements that could be made across departmental boundaries. In essence, TQM is a strategic concept that is supported by QC, QA, and CQI.[1]

Continuous Quality Improvement (CQI). *The processes of identifying areas in a department that can be strengthened and working to make those areas better.*

Total Quality Management (TQM). *The application of quality management processes throughout the organization. This includes working on problems and strengthening areas that cross departmental lines.*

Some problems that commonly exist in healthcare operations that involve dietetics professionals are tray delivery, late tray service, adequacy and use of floor stock, data accumulation for kilocaloric counts, recording of actual (rather than reported) heights and weights, billing for enteral feedings, and so on. These problems have often developed over time and may have political implications. For example, it may be that each of the departments or units involved in the problem blames it on another department and takes no responsibility for either the problem or the solution. It may seem easier to blame someone else than it is to make the changes necessary to correct the problem. The larger and stronger departments usually have more personnel and thus more ability to control how things get done. They may look at what is convenient for them, rather than what is good for the organization or for the customer.

TQM puts the focus on the problem (or the product to be improved). The process is interdepartmental and is assigned to a committee that is established with representation from all departments that might be able to contribute to a positive outcome. Often, the committee is a self-managed team that is drawn together for the TQM project and then disbanded. Sometimes the group is assigned a group leader or facilitator who is neutral and has no vested interest in any specific outcome, only that a satisfactory outcome is reached. TQM teams work best when a consensus is reached by all group members regarding the proposed solution, which is then implemented, refined, and, if it works, monitored over time to see if the solution is sustainable.

Dietetics professionals are involved in all of the variations of quality management that have been described. In addition, there are other systems that have been or are being tested and refined. The process of quality management is still evolving and is at different stages in different settings. Some organizations are still working on solving existing problems within individual departments; others have sophisticated systems in place for institution-wide TQM. However, it must be remembered that though these processes appear to be evolving from one to the other, the implementation of the more sophisticated types of systems does not replace the need for the basic systems for measuring quality. Rather, TQM and CQI build on QC and QA. One cannot be successful at dealing with institution-wide problems if individual departments are not functioning well as independent units.

use of outcome data

The measurement of outcomes is also in an evolutionary phase. The profession of dietetics is still in the process of determining how to best measure outcomes and how to use these data in a way that is both meaningful and quantifiable. To date, outcome data have been widely used in public health to measure the impact of such programs as the National School Lunch Program, the Supplemental Nutrition Assistance Program, WIC, and other public health nutrition programs. The data obtained from public health interventions are both quantifiable and useful for such things as showing the effectiveness of the programs and justifying continued funding for them.

Clinical outcomes data have documented the effectiveness of nutritional interventions for patients with diabetes and renal disease.[2, 3] These studies have served as the impetus for the coverage of Medical Nutrition Therapy as a reimbursable treatment for these diseases by Medicare. It is anticipated that the data generated by ongoing work will provide validation of the cost-effectiveness of clinical nutrition services to treat other diseases such as cardiovascular disease and obesity. Nevertheless, the dietetics profession is just beginning to make significant progress in this area. It is anticipated that the use of standardized *International Nutrition and Dietetics Terminology*[4] in electronic medical/health records will facilitate the data-gathering process. It will allow for the electronic search of keywords to measure outcomes as a matter of course, so that the data are routinely available to management personnel as well as to the profession.

The outcome data related to the foodservice side of dietetics practice have been in use for longer periods of time. Studies that measure over- and underproduction of food are used to refine production forecasts so that enough food is produced with a minimum of waste. This information, when accurate, can be used in conjunction with sophisticated computer programs to decrease waste and save money. Plate-waste studies look at what is discarded relative to what is served so that menus can be altered to better respond to the needs of the foodservice customer. Satisfaction surveys are somewhat more meaningful in foodservice than in clinical or community nutrition in gathering outcome data, because customers are more familiar with food and foodservice than they are with other types of nutrition services. That is, they know how to measure the quality of the food that they eat more accurately than they know how to measure the quality of a diet instruction they receive or a supplement that is prescribed.

Remember that there are different constituencies to which an organization is accountable. Though most of what has been discussed in this section has been related to the types of productivity measurements that relate directly to products and outcomes related to customers and clients, dietetics professionals are also accountable to vendors and employees. For vendors, one might look at what proportion of bills are paid on time, how frequently delivery people are made to wait at the loading dock before goods can be off-loaded, how often they are required to make "emergency" deliveries due to poor ordering procedures, and so on. Financial backers have a right to know information like the size of the inventory, the profit and loss statements, the balance statements, the length of time that accounts receivable remain outstanding, and so on. Accountability to employees might relate to the numbers and types of on-the-job injuries or to the health and safety programs available to workers. It can also be measured by the percentage of workers participating in each of these programs, the organization's history of promoting employees to more-responsible positions, information on the standards used to evaluate employee performance, and so forth.

benchmarking

Benchmarking means using the data that have been gathered for comparative purposes. Generally, there are two kinds of benchmarking that an organization uses. The first is **internal benchmarking**, which compares current data to records of past performance within an organization to determine if its own standards are being met or surpassed. The second is **external benchmarking**, in which the organization compares itself with data derived from other organizations.

internal benchmarking

Internal benchmarking has been mentioned before. The illustration of the clinical nutrition manager using data gathered on DTR and diet clerk time per patient day is an example of this. In the examples given, the clinical nutrition manager had the option of using the internal data to avoid layoffs in one case and to monitor adaptation to change in the other case. The data set the standard for how the DTRs and diet clerks usually performed from the perspective of time, which could be used as a benchmark against which current performance is measured. Those were fairly dramatic examples of how the data could have been used. More often, the data are used to monitor what is happening in an organization on a routine, day-to-day basis.

When variations from the benchmark or standard occur, the variation should alert the manager that something has changed. The manager should be able to review the situation and identify why the variance occurred. Often, the reason is obvious and justifiable. Considering diet office labor time, one reason that could justify an increase from 12 minutes per patient day to 15 minutes per patient day is a breakdown in the computer system. Others include the training of a new employee, a drop in patient census, or the need for several staff members to attend in-service training. Individual variations from set standards that can be justified are a normal part of how an organization operates.

Sometimes patterns and trends can be identified when looking at internal benchmarking data. A perceptive manager will recognize these patterns and use the information to adjust staffing or work processes accordingly. For example, it might consistently take 12 minutes per patient day to process diet orders on Monday, traditionally a high admission day, but productivity may decline to 15 minutes per patient day on weekends, because the census is usually lower on weekends. The manager could decide to decrease staffing on the weekends so that fewer hours are scheduled when fewer patient days are anticipated. Alternately, if the clerks and DTRs are required to be present to deal with phone calls and trayline activities, and it is known that weekends have light workloads, additional tasks could be assigned to the staff on weekends. Activities such as filing patient records, restocking supplies, or compiling the data gathered from patient satisfaction surveys could be assigned to the clerks and DTRs as weekend activities to compensate for the lighter workload.

management practice in dietetics

Sometimes the trends that are seen are not easily explained. In these situations, the manager needs to look beyond the obvious reasons for an explanation. Decreases in productivity might be due to worker illness or be a reaction to some job-related stress. Increases in productivity might be due to a change in the employee benefits package, an improvement in the work environment, or other factors. Changes in productivity could also be due to alterations in work processes, or changes in equipment. Something as simple as a new, more comfortable computer mouse might have a positive impact on one worker's productivity.

Whenever variations occur from the quantitative, qualitative, or outcome benchmarks that an organization has established, the reason for the change should be identified. If the change is a positive one, effort should be made to capitalize on the newly discovered advantage. If the changes are negative, the underlying problem needs to be identified and corrected as soon as possible.

It has been stated that data should be monitored on an ongoing basis to note day-to-day variation in productivity. It is equally important to look at the bigger picture—that is, the changes that occur over longer periods of time. The total number of meals produced by a foodservice may look stable when viewed on a daily or weekly basis. For example, the average number of meals served in January might be 1,050 per day, compared with 1,045 average meals per day in February. The drop in meals produced was equivalent to about one half of one percent and is probably not significant. However, if over a year the trend continues so that the meals served dropped by 5 per day each month, the total number of meals served in December might average 990 per day. The total drop, about 9.5 percent, is significant. Therefore, it is important to look at the data both in the short and in the long term.

Internal benchmarking is a management tool that is used to monitor short- and long-term performance within an organization. It provides managers with information on trends that might not become obvious if the information were not monitored. Once productivity measurements have been established, they can be used to set benchmarks for performance within an organization, which are tracked over time. As with productivity, benchmarks can be set for quantity, quality, and outcomes.

external benchmarking

Though it is nice to know how an organization is performing in comparison with its own past performance, sometimes it becomes necessary to determine how an organization's performance compares with the performance of other organizations. External benchmarking is somewhat more complex than internal benchmarking because of the competitive nature of business and because organizations are different enough that comparing them is much like comparing apples to oranges (though both are fruit, they vary extensively in color, texture, flavor, and so on).

External Benchmarking. *The process of an organization comparing its performance and productivity with those of other comparable organizations to determine whether it is performing at, above, or below the industry standard.*

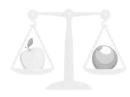

*If not done correctly,
external benchmark-
ing can be like
comparing apples
to oranges.*

The first obstacle to external benchmarking is locating organizations that are similar enough for the comparisons to be meaningful. A small community hospital with 50 beds is not comparable to a 700-bed teaching medical center. Nor is a pediatric tertiary care center comparable to a Veteran's Administration Medical Center. Public facilities are different from private ones. To be able to draw valid conclusions from benchmarking data, the organizations being used to set the standards must be similar to one another. For hospitals, this means that pediatric facilities are compared with other pediatric facilities, community hospitals with other community hospitals, and teaching medical centers with other teaching medical centers. The facilities must also be similar in size.

The other major obstacle in comparing one organization with another is the competitive nature of business. When an organization identifies another that is comparable and can provide meaningful benchmarking data, it is not uncommon that the organization is a competitor. In such situations, it is unlikely that benchmarking data will be freely shared, because such data sharing may lead to one organization gaining a competitive advantage over another.

When faced with the situation of not being able to obtain benchmarking data from comparable sources, some businesses have found it useful to benchmark themselves with businesses that, though not comparable, are similar enough to be able to make some meaningful comparisons. A hospital cafeteria, for example, may compare itself with a business dining operation or with a school foodservice; a weight-control clinic might find it useful to benchmark itself against a cardiac rehabilitation program or an outpatient hemodialysis center.

Press Ganey.
*http://www.
pressganey.com/
index.aspx*

Hospitals are in the unique position of being part of a large industry with wide geographic distribution. There are professional organizations, purchasing coopera-tives, and healthcare consortiums that have banded together to gather benchmarking data for various segments of the industry. Most hospitals have the ability to utilize one or more of these services. In this situation, the hospital reports its data to a central clearinghouse (for example, Press Ganey) that pools data from the industry as a whole, as well as from comparable facilities. It then generates reports that show the individual hospital how it compares with both the industry and with its peers. Because the data are not reported on an institutional basis, but rather as a pool of data, the security of competitive information is assured. Benchmarking for the hospital industry is in widespread use because of the availability of this type of data.

When data are gathered industry wide, no matter what the industry, there must be some consistency in what is reported. Hospitals that participate in benchmarking programs usually take advantage of uniform reporting methods and use standard-ized survey forms. The benchmarking data are reported in generic terms. This means that data are reported in units like adjusted occupied beds, meal equivalents, and person-minutes per tray, rather than as occupied beds, meals served, and trays per

management practice in dietetics

minute. Adjusting the data for relative labor costs and cost-of-living indices in each geographic region minimizes differences inherent in the data.

conclusion

This chapter has provided an overview of how organizations are accountable to their constituencies. Accountability systems that are used include the measurement of productivity and the comparison of these data against standards known as benchmarks. This process falls under the general heading of quality management, a system that is continuously evolving. The major concepts in this chapter are the following.

1. Organizations are accountable to a variety of constituencies, including those who contribute resources, both human and material, and the end users of the product.
2. When the customer is identified as the public, the organization is often accountable to an oversight group, representing the public.
3. Productivity is measured in relation to quantity, quality, and outcome.
4. The measurement of productivity is a management tool. It is most effective when productivity is monitored in both the short term and in the long range.
5. Discrete measures, other than productivity, are used to demonstrate fiscal accountability and accountability to staff.
6. Quality management programs include quality control, quality assurance, Continuous Quality Improvement and Total Quality Management.
7. Benchmarking is one of the processes used to measure an organization's performance against internal and external standards.

activities

activity 1

Activity 1 in Chapter 12 described traylines for hospital foodservice. For each of these, calculate the trays per minute and the person-minutes per tray.

activity 2

Establish a quantitative, a qualitative, and an outcome measurement of productivity for one of the following workers:

- dishwasher
- waitress
- secretary
- meeting planner
- office manager
- nutrition aide in an elementary school
- National Nutrition Month coordinator for a local dietetic association
- professional recruiter for dietetics professionals

activity 3

Explore the website for the American Hospital Association (www.aha.org). Write a brief report about what you find there about benchmarking. Do a similar study of the National Restaurant Association's website (www.restaurant.org). Compare the differences of the types of data that appear on each of these sites.

to study further

Additional information on productivity measurement, quality management, and benchmarking can be found in the following material.

- Barnard, C. *Benchmarking Basics: A Resource Guide for Healthcare Managers.* Marblehead, MA: HCPro, Inc., 2006.
- Goetsch, D. L. and S. Davis. *Quality Management of Organizational Excellence: Introduction to Total Quality.* 7th ed. Upper Saddle River, NJ: Prentice Hall. 2012.
- Johnson, B. C. and J. Chambers. "Expert Panel Identifies Activities and Performance Measures for Foodservice Benchmarking." *Journal of the American Dietetic Association.* 100:692–695, 2000.
- Johnson, B. C. and J. Chambers. "Foodservice Benchmarking: Practices Attitudes and Beliefs of Foodservice Directors." *Journal of the American Dietetic Association.* 100:175–180, 2000.
- Kelly, D. L. *Applying Quality Management in Healthcare: A Systems Approach.* 3rd ed. Chicago: Health Administration Press, 2011.
- Larsen, Eric. "Quality Management and the Dietetics Professional." *Journal of the American Dietetic Association.* 104:1070–1072, 2004.
- Lighter, Donald E. and Douglas C. Fair. *Quality Management in Healthcare: Principles and Methods.* 2nd ed. Sudbury, MA: Jones and Bartlett, 2004.
- McLaughlin, C. P., J. K. Johnson, and W. A. Sollecito. *Implementing Continuous Quality Improvement in Healthcare.* Sudbury, MA: Jones & Bartlett Learning, 2012.
- Stapenhurst, T. *The Benchmarking Book: A How-To Guide to Best Practices for Managers and Practitioners.* Oxford: Butterworth-Heinemann, 2009.

scholarly journals

- *American Journal of Medical Quality*
- *Benchmarking: An International Journal*
- *Health Care Management Review*
- *International Journal of Productivity and Quality Management*
- *Journal for Healthcare Quality*

relevant websites

- The National Restaurant Association http://www.restaurant.org/
- American Society for Quality http://asq.org/index.aspx

in practice

evidence-based practice

From the early days of the profession, dietetics practitioners have tried to find effective means of carrying out their jobs, based on the best information that was available to them at the time. Back then, there was much less information to process, and the knowledge required to be a dietitian was significantly less than it is today. Dietetics in the early 20th century consisted mostly of managing the preparation and delivery of healthy foods to groups of individuals. Dietitians often worked in the military or in healthcare facilities. The only way to nourish individuals was with whole foods because very few processed foods existed. Many hospitals had their own gardens, bakeries, and butcher shops. Little was known about food safety.

Fast-forward to the 21st century. Dietitians still work in foodservices. In that setting advances in science and technology have been relatively definitive. Science has provided evidence of the conditions that are conducive to the growth of microorganisms. (Remember FATTOM—Food, Acid, Time, Temperature, Oxygen, and Moisture?[1]) Based on this evidence, principles of food safety have developed. These include such concepts as the temperature danger zone, prevention of cross-contamination, potentially hazardous foods, and HACCP, which have been guiding dietetics practitioners in foodservice for years. The information related to the growth of pathogens also provided the impetus for technologic innovations in foodservice equipment to complement other food-safety activities. The widespread availability of blast chillers, for example, has drastically reduced the length of time that foods stay in the temperature danger zone. It should be noted, then, that dietetic practitioners working in foodservice settings have been using the concept of "evidence-based practice" for years.

Today, we know a lot more about food than our predecessors knew. Processed foods outnumber whole foods in supermarkets. We can accurately measure the macro- and micronutrients in a food or food product and can alter an individual's diet to modify the amount of nutrients and phytochemicals. It is also possible to nourish individuals without using any of the items that early dietitians identified as "food." In fact, it is commonplace to bypass the mouth and feed patients directly into the gastrointestinal (GI) tract, or even to bypass the GI tract entirely and deliver nutrients directly into the circulatory system. Such advances in the sciences that support innovation in clinical nutrition are far more complex than those that have driven the advances in foodservice. Clinicians need to deal with individuals with many different diseases and disorders, and have a myriad of tools to use in treatment. Because of the complexity of each condition, it has taken much longer for evidence-based guidelines to be established for clinical practice than it did for foodservice.

---

[1]University of Iowa Extension. http://www.extension.iastate.edu/foodsafety/Lesson/L4/L4p1.html. Accessed September 7, 2012.

One of the most difficult parts of being a clinical dietitian is making sure that the care you provide for clients is based on the most up-to-date scientific information. This is very difficult to do in the information age where so much new information is being published each month. It is nearly impossible for an individual to work full-time and still remain current in all aspects of clinical nutrition. This is part of the reason that many dietetic professionals tend to specialize in one or two areas of practice, like diabetes, or maternal nutrition, where they are able to keep up with changes impacting their practice area. However, sometimes practitioners are required to step out of their comfort zone, and when they do so, they must base their care on the best available evidence.

The first publication to address the issue of evidence-based practice for clinical practitioners appeared in the *Journal of the American Dietetic Association* in September of 2001.[2] By 2006, the organization has established an evidence-analysis library (EAL) to gather, evaluate, and summarize current research on important questions related to clinical nutrition practice.[3] The EAL provides the practitioner with a bibliography of articles included in a review of major research papers on defined topics. Conclusions, based on the literature review are then published, along with a grade based on the quality, consistency, quantity, and potential clinical impact of the evidence.[4] The following grades are assigned to the conclusion statements:

- Grade I if the evidence is Good
- Grade II if the evidence is Fair
- Grade III if the evidence is Limited
- Grade IV if the evidence is Expert Opinion Only
- Grade V if a grade is not assignable[5]

By 2012, evidence analysis had been completed on 39 topics including more than 20 diseases and conditions, several nutrients, foods, life-cycle issues, and the nutrition-care process.[6] This process of evidence analysis helps the practitioner review materials related to one or more of these topics. It saves both time and effort, in that the actual research papers have already been reviewed by colleagues who are experts

[2]Myers, Esther F., Ellen Pritchett, and Elvira Q. Johnson. "Evidence-Based Practice Guidelines vs. Protocols: What's the Difference?" *Journal of the American Dietetic Association.* 101:1085–1090, 2001.

[3]Blumberg-Kason, Susan and Ryan Lipscomb. "Evidence-Based Nutrition Practice Guidelines: A Valuable Resource in the Evidence Analysis Library." *Journal of the American Dietetic Association.* 106:1935–1936, 2006.

[4]Research and Strategic Business Development. Academy of Nutrition and Dietetics. *Evidence Analysis Manual: Steps in the Academy Evidence Analysis Process.* Chicago: Academy of Nutrition and Dietetics, 2012.

[5]Ibid.

[6]Academy of Nutrition and Dietetics Evidence Analysis Library. http://www.ada evidencelibrary.com. Accessed September 7, 2012.

on the topic. Practitioners can access both the bibliography and the conclusions that have been drawn from the evaluation of these papers.

Based on these reviews, the first clinical practice guideline was released in September 2006. The guideline was entitled "Evidence-Based Nutrition Practice Guideline on Critical Illness."[7] Since the release of that document, additional guidelines have been established for nearly 20 other diseases or conditions, including diabetes, hypertension, and chronic kidney disease.[8] The guidelines are updated as new information becomes available (e.g., the Critical Illness Guidelines were updated in 2012). All guidelines are designed in part to assist clinical practitioners provide consistent nutritional care to their patients.

Evidence-based practice guidelines provide recommendations that are rated using two complementary assessments. The first is based on the strength of the evidence used in developing the guideline. Recommendation may be rated as strong, fair, weak, consensus, or insufficient evidence. The second rating is related to whether or not the recommendation statement is conditional or imperative. If a recommendation is rated as Strong/Imperative, it means that this should be a part of routine care for patients with this condition.

For example, one of the recommendations for Adult Weight Management is "Individualized goals of weight loss therapy should be to reduce body weight at an optimal rate of 1–2 lbs per week for the first 6 months and to achieve an initial weight loss goal of up to 10% from baseline. These goals are realistic, achievable, and sustainable."[9] Since it is rated as Strong/Imperative, it should be a standard strategy for dietitians working with overweight adults to use in their practice.

On the other hand, in the guidelines for celiac disease, one of the recommendations is "The registered dietitian (RD) should advise individuals with celiac disease who enjoy and can tolerate gluten-free oats to gradually include them in their gluten-free dietary pattern. Research on individuals with celiac disease reports that incorporating oats uncontaminated with wheat, barley or rye at intake levels of approximately 50g dry oats per day is generally safe and improves compliance with the gluten-free dietary pattern."[10] The rating for this recommendation is Fair/Conditional, which indicates that it may not be appropriate for all clients.

The EAL represents a significant step forward for the profession. It increases the accountability of clinical practitioners by providing standards against which they can judge their own performance. As the library continues to grow, and guidelines are

---

[7]Blumberg-Kason, op.cit
[8]Academy of Nutrition and Dietetics Evidence Analysis Library. http://www.ada evidencelibrary.com. Accessed September 7, 2012.
[9]Ibid.
[10]Ibid.

management practice in dietetics

developed for more conditions, the value of this tool will continue to grow. Dietetic practitioners can access the EAL either online or using the smartphone app called NutriGuides.

references

1. Kelly, Diane L. *Applying Quality Management in Healthcare: A Process for Improvement.* Chicago: Health Administration Press, 2003, p. 9.
2. Franz, Marion J. "The Lenna Francis Cooper Memorial Lecture—The Future of Clinical Dietetics: Evidence, Outcomes, and Reimbursement." *Journal of the American Dietetic Association* 103:977–981, 2003.
3. Academy of Nutrition and Dietetics. *Which Nutrition Services Are Covered?* http://www.eatright.org/HealthProfessionals/content.aspx?id=8175&terms=medicare+reimbursement#.UEe1d43a2VF. Accessed September 5, 2012.
4. Academy of Nutrition and Dietetics. *International Dietetics and Nutrition Terminology (IDNT) Reference Manual: Standardized Language for the Nutrition Care Process.* 4th ed. Chicago: 2013.

part five

managing financial resources

Money management is a very broad topic, which ranges from managing personal funds using cash, a checkbook, credit cards, and Internet banking, to managing the funds in the work setting. Sometimes it is easier to handle money that belongs to an organization than it is to handle your own. The risks involved are not as personal, and therefore require less justification. Organizations know this, and compensate by exerting more control in the area of financial management than in other areas. Budgets are required. Managers must explain when they do not adhere to budgets. Multiple financial reports are generated and studied on a regular basis. Top management requires this degree of accountability because it knows that the work of the organization cannot be accomplished unless there is financial stability.

Part V deals with fiscal management for the new manager by providing the information and terminology necessary for the initial confrontation with financial management. It will provide enough familiarity with financial management for the manager to know what additional information is needed. It should allow the person facing the budgeting process for the first time to do so with a moderate level of comfort. Beyond this, the best teacher of all will be experience in the realm of finance.

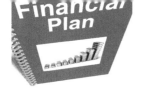

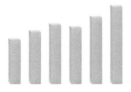

chapter fourteen

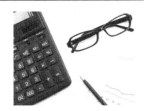

the budgeting process

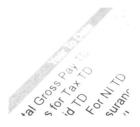

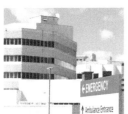

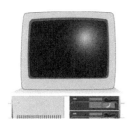

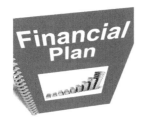

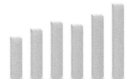

learning objectives

1. State why organizations develop budgets.

2. Differentiate between the master budget, the operating budget, and the capital budget.

3. List the four possible kinds of operating budgets.

4. Describe the advantages and disadvantages of the incremental budget.

5. Describe the advantages and disadvantages of the zero-based budget.

6. Describe the advantages and disadvantages of fixed budgets.

7. Describe the advantages and disadvantages of variable budgets.

8. State the differences between a cost center, a revenue center, and a profit center.

9. Describe how an operating budget is prepared.

10. Define each sub-budget that can be included under operating expenses.

11. Discuss each of the steps involved in preparing a capital budget.

overview

Writing a budget is like preparing an income tax return. Few managers have any formal training in how to do it, but they must do it anyhow. Most have some intuitive knowledge that budgeting would be a part of their management responsibility, but choose to suppress that knowledge for as long as possible. The task seems intimidating but is really fairly simple. And yet, just as individuals avoid preparing income tax returns until the last possible minute, procrastination is elevated to an art form for many managers working on their departmental budgets. It is the job that managers love to hate.

This chapter is designed to take some of the mystery away from budgeting. The goal is to familiarize readers with the reasons that budgets are needed and to introduce them to the basic terminology related to budgets. In addition, an outline of the budgeting process will be presented with consideration of both operating and capital budgets.

Budget. *An estimate of the income and expenditures during a given period of time based on the mission, goals, and objectives of an organization. In other words, an organization's business plan expressed in financial terms.*

the purpose of budgeting

Believe it or not, organizations do not establish budgets for the sole purpose of making work for their managers. A **budget** is the organization's business plan expressed in financial terms.[1] As such, it should be based on the mission, goals, and objectives of the organization and should be consistent with these. A good budget does much more than quantify the allocation of resources. It makes sure that those resources are being used to accomplish the overall purpose of the organization, rather than to support the agendas of individual managers.

There are a number of reasons for preparing budgets. The first is that the budget helps to set the parameters for activities to be done during the budget period. That is, it gives the managers guidance about what financial resources are available to carry out their work. It makes managers plan ahead and think about the certainties and relative risks of their decisions. Budgets also act as a control device for regulating spending in the organization. Large variances from the budgeted amounts should alert managers and their superiors to potential problems that can be identified and addressed. Finally, budgets provide an objective set of criteria against which a manager's performance can be measured. Though a manager's overall accomplishments should not be judged solely on financial performance, it is usually one of the major considerations for evaluating a manager.

Often, the word *forecast* is used in conjunction with the budgeting process. Indeed, much of budgeting involves forecasting what revenues and expenses are to be expected in the immediate future. Budget forecasting is not unlike the forecasting that is done in foodservice to determine how much food should be prepared on a specific day. However, because annual organizational budgets involve far more resources than do daily food production forecasts, the margin for error (as a percentage of the

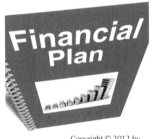

The budget is the financial plan for an organization.

total) is smaller. Because the numbers are so large and because many managers have little formal training in preparing budgets, it is wise to use information management systems to support the budgeting process.

When dealing with budgets, it should be noted that budgetary terms are not uniformly defined. In general, a **master budget** consists of an operating budget, a capital budget, a cash budget, and a budgeted balance sheet. The **cash budget** deals with such concepts as cash on hand, accounts payable, accounts receivable, the cost of credit, and cash flow. Cash budgets project when funds will become available and when they can be spent. Dietetics professionals do not often deal with this type of budget unless they have moved into upper-level positions or operate their own businesses. Likewise, the **budgeted balance sheet** is an organizational document that is not usually considered by the dietetics manager, except from an observational perspective. In situations in which it is necessary for dietetics professionals to prepare cash budgets or budgeted balance sheets, there are accounting personnel, consultants, or bankers to help with the task. Neither of these will be included in the following discussion. The remainder of this chapter will concentrate on the operating budget and the capital budget.

operating budgets

Operating budgets are those that project the income of the organization and allocate the funds for the accomplishment of work. They are prepared for the entire organization and for each individual operating unit. There are two major categories of operating budgets—incremental and zero-based. Each of these categories can be further characterized as fixed or variable. Thus, it is possible to use any of the four distinct types of budgets listed in Table 14.1.

Budget Type	Characteristics
Incremental/Fixed	The budget is based on the previous budget cycle; once the percent change has been established, the budget is set at that level for the next budget cycle.
Incremental/Variable	The budget is based on the previous budget cycle; the actual dollars allocated will vary in proportion to the amount of work done.
Zero-Based/Fixed	The budget is written "from scratch" for each budget cycle; once the numbers have been established, the budget is set at that level for the budget cycle.
Zero-Based/Variable	The budget is written "from scratch" for each budget cycle; the actual dollars allocated will vary in proportion to the amount of work done.

Table 14.1 Types of Operating Budgets

Master Budget. *Consists of an operating budget, a capital budget, a cash budget, and a budgeted balance sheet.*

Cash Budget. *An estimate of the anticipated cash flow (that is, cash on hand, accounts payable, accounts receivable, and the cost of credit) that can be used to project the availability of funds.*

Budgeted Balance Sheet. *A statement of the assets and liabilities of an organization based on budget estimates.*

Operating Budget. *Budget that takes into account the revenue, expense, direct labor, direct material, and overhead budgets as well as other operating expenses. It is used in projecting the income of an organization and in allocating funds within an organization.*

Because operating budgets are normally planned for an entire year, the discussion that follows will apply to that time frame. However, budgets may be planned for shorter or longer periods of time, as required by the organization. Another basic piece of information that cannot be ignored is the differentiation between **fiscal year** and **calendar year**. The calendar year begins January 1 and ends December 31. A fiscal year can begin on any date and end 365 days later (366 in leap years). Organizations often choose to begin and end their fiscal years on dates that are different from the calendar year. One reason for this is that many additional accounting activities must be done at the end of a fiscal year, and it is sometimes better if these can be done at a time of year when staff is not involved in holiday activities and personal travel.

Another common variable is the way an operating budget is divided for purposes of reporting. Some organizations use the calendar month as the **accounting period**. This means that there are 12 reporting periods in each year, which vary in length from 28 to 31 days. Other organizations use four-week blocks that end on Saturdays and begin on Sundays (or any other consecutive days). With this configuration, there are 13 accounting periods each year instead of 12. A third option is to have periods that vary in length but end and start on the same consecutive days (for example, end on Friday and start on Saturday). This keeps the number of accounting periods consistent with the calendar, which has 12 periods; it is accomplished by having two 4-week accounting periods followed by one 5-week period each quarter. Though these three plans are commonly used, an organization may choose to use other accounting periods to monitor their financial performance.

An interesting characteristic of operating budgets is that they do not carry over from year to year. If a manager saves money this year, it cannot be spent next year. This explains why some managers frantically seek ways to spend money in the last days of the fiscal year. They know that money that is not spent will be lost to them. Though it is prudent to hold some money in reserve for the last part of the fiscal year, frenzied spending often leads to unwise purchasing decisions. If a manager chooses to hold some funds in reserve until the end of the year, this cache should be identified as such and a contingency spending plan should be implemented in a planned and orderly fashion as the year-end approaches.

incremental budgets

An **incremental budget** is one that is based on the previous year's budget. The standard way to manage this type of budget is to determine what was allocated in the previous year and adjust the amounts based on a predetermined increment. There are a number of factors involved in setting what the increment will be. One is to look at the inflation rate and tie the increment to it. Other considerations are related to labor contracts, profitability, operating losses, restructuring, reengineering, and so on. The common factor is that the previous budget is used as a base for setting the proposed budget.

management practice in dietetics

For example, if the budget is increased by 3 percent, the entire budget is increased by that amount. Therefore, if the total budget for a clinical nutrition department was $500,000 last year, the new budget will be $515,000. Once the departmental allocation has been set, three options exist. The first is that every item is automatically increased by the predetermined increment. This means that each line item is increased by 3 percent. In this situation, salaries will go up by 3 percent, as will travel allotments, funds for overhead, those for supplies, and so on. Under these circumstances, managers have little say in establishing their budgets. They are given a plan and told to manage within its parameters. This type of budget is being used with less frequency than it was in the past.

Another way to handle the incremental budget is to allocate the entire budget to the manager, who must project how the money will be spent and disburse funds as necessary. The only restriction is that the total stays within the $515,000 limit. It is up to the manager to decide how the money will be used. The manager may choose to use it for travel, for salaries, for supplies, for overhead, or for any combination of these items. There is no requirement that the allocation for any specific item increases. This means that the manager can decrease the money spent on supplies and overhead and increase travel allowances for staff. This type of budgeting empowers the manager to assume both responsibility and accountability.

The third way to handle incremental budgets is to give the manager the same funds allocation as in the previous year and then accept requests for increases for the coming year. In this case, each request for additional funds must be justified. Upper management reviews only the requests for increased allocations. Whatever was allocated in earlier years is untouchable and is not subject to review.

Though it is normal for incremental budgets to increase from year to year, this may not always be the case. In economic downturns or after an organization has been downsized, it is possible that budget allocations will be decreased by a certain percentage. Thus, a manager may be faced with having fewer funds to allocate than in previous years. This type of belt-tightening activity is a difficult, but necessary, part of being a manager. It is much easier to live with increased budgets than with decreased ones.

Incremental budgets usually increase from year to year, but this is not always true.

There are several advantages to the incremental budget. It is relatively easy to prepare. Often, the allocations are programmed so that little actual decision making is required. It is based on accurate records of an organization's financial history, so the budget is likely to be fairly precise. There are few surprises and little reason to expect major change as a result of budget activities.

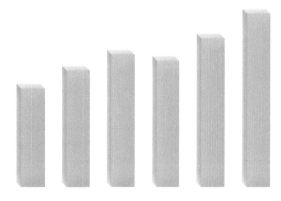

Disadvantages include the fact that the incremental budget is not responsive to change; it maintains the same relative funding levels for different work groups. It does not differentiate between departmental workloads, changes in technology, and other factors that contribute value to the organization. In fact, incremental budgets support the status quo and discourage innovation. By not reviewing what went before, incremental budgets tend to hide inefficiencies in an organization, perpetuating activities long after they are no longer needed.

zero-based budgets

To avoid the pitfalls of using incremental budgets, **zero-based budgets** have gained widespread acceptance in recent years. A zero-based budget assumes that no budgeted item is sacred and that every item is subject to scrutiny. In essence, the manager is asked to justify every dollar of proposed spending for the coming year.

It is often thought that the zero-based budget ignores history and requires managers to compute all values from scratch. This is not true. Historical data are acceptable and useful if they can be justified. For example, the manager is free to use existing data on salaries and typical salary increases to determine what the cost of labor will be. However, it is incumbent on the manager to justify the number of employees who are needed to perform the work, and to prove that the work is essential to the organization.

Consider, for instance, the situation in which a full-time employee is assigned to prepare and distribute enteral nutrition products in a skilled nursing facility. The position was justifiable in the past when many of these products were prepared onsite from complicated recipes and others were mixed just prior to their delivery to the bedside. Today, most of these products are standardized and come to the facility pre-packaged and labeled. They can be delivered to the nursing units for storage and distributed directly to the bedside as needed. The need for a full-time employee to prepare and distribute enteral products has been eliminated. However, with incremental budgeting, a facility might retain this position and use the employee to distribute the standardized products. This means that the product is handled twice, once getting into the formula preparation area, and again getting to the point of use. There are usually more efficient ways to handle the distribution of enteral products than having a full-time person dedicated to this task. The justification process required in the zero-based budget method would show that this position is expendable.

Though the zero-based budget is not always used as described in theory, the goal is for managers to separate out each function that happens within their span of control. If that is done, then an annual cost can be assigned to every function that occurs in an organization. In hospital foodservices, for example, costs would be assigned to such functions as cafeteria operations, patient services, clinical nutrition services, quality management, procurement, and so on. In a public health clinic, funds might be allocated to nutrition screening, nutrition education, social marketing, and grant-writing activities. Then the organization would rank these functions in term of their value to the organization and fund those that are most important.

Zero-based budgets make organizations responsive to their environments. They work well when used in situations involving restructuring of an organization, where transformation is happening rapidly. They also work well in start-up companies and in high-tech industries where the products and production methods change dramatically in the short term. The use of a zero-based budget forces organizations to examine their structures and processes in order to eliminate waste and redundancy.

Nevertheless, zero-based budgets are not well suited to all situations. They are difficult to prepare, consuming a lot of management time and energy. This alone makes the project costly for any size organization. For large bureaucracies, the costs are enormous (though these are the very organizations that would probably benefit the most from using this technique). The politics inherent in the large organization may undermine the purpose of zero-based budgeting. Then, too, managers bias the process by overselling the projects that they want to have funded.

Proponents of the zero-based method argue effectively for the process, whereas detractors find the process unwieldy. Though there are some obvious benefits, they probably do not justify the additional costs in all situations. Perhaps some sort of combination of these two methods will evolve, in which zero-based budgeting is used one year and incremental budgeting the following year. Another alternative is using the zero-based format for 25 to 50 percent of an organization's units each year (on a rotating basis), and incremental budgeting for the other departments.

fixed budgets

The term **fixed budget** refers to a variation in budgeting that can be applied to either the zero-based budget or to the incremental budget. It is characterized by firm projections that are set for the entire budget cycle. For example, if an organization has a fiscal year that started July 1, 2014, and ended on June 30, 2015, the budget that was implemented in July would have projected income and expenditures for 12 months. Fixed budgets (also called *static budgets*) assume that business will be stable during the entire budget cycle. This means that if salaries are estimated to be *X* dollars in December, then the manager is meeting the goal if *X* dollars are spent.

Historically, most budgets were fixed. This model was developed before information technology was widely available, when budget calculations were done manually. In fact, the earliest budgets allocated funds for the entire year, then divided the total into the number of accounting periods per year. Thus, the budget for each accounting

Fixed Budget.
Budget plan for which funds are allocated for the entire fiscal year. It is also known as static budget and can be applied to either the zero-based budget or to the incremental budget.

period was identical to that for every other accounting period during the budget cycle. Because fixed budgets are used to compare actual financial performance with expected performance, there were serious limitations because seasonal variation was not built into the budgets.

Refinement to the fixed budget came with the application of information technology to the budgeting process. It became relatively easy for managers to project the use of funds during each individual accounting period. Fluctuations in expenses can be predicted. For example, one might project that fewer dollars will be spent on energy in the spring and the fall, when outside temperatures are moderate, than in the summer and winter, when buildings need to be cooled or heated. Campus dining services can anticipate lower food costs in March, when many students leave campus for a week during spring break. With this improvement in how budgets are written, it is easier to monitor performance during the budget cycle because the projections, adjusted for seasonal variation, are more accurate.

Fixed budgets are good in that they provide managers with goals for financial performance that can be measured each accounting period. However, they do have one serious limitation. Fixed budgets, by virtue of the fact that they are fixed, do not have enough flexibility to be responsive to changes in the volume of work that needs to be done. In fact, they are based on the premise that the volume of work was predicted accurately when the budget was prepared. If the volume of work changes (for example, if a natural disaster caused an influx of patients admitted to a county hospital), there is no budgetary mechanism to deal with the change in volume. Under these circumstances, there is no way that the budget can be accurate, nor is it likely that a manager can stay within the prescribed budget.

variable budgets

Variable Budget.
Budget plan for which expenses will vary in response to actual production, volume, or revenues. It is also referred to as flexible budget *and can be used in conjunction with either the zero-based budget or the incremental budget.*

Another budgeting concept that can be applied to either the incremental or zero-based budget is called the **variable budget**. This type of budget projects expenses based on production, volume, or revenues. It is designed to address the shortcomings of the fixed budget. When income increases, more money can be spent to accomplish the work; when income decreases, fewer dollars should be spent. In other words, the expense portion of the operating budget is dependent on the revenue portion of that budget.

Variable budgets take into account the fact that some costs do vary with volume. Costs such as labor and materials will vary, even though items like rent will not. Variable budgets are designed to be flexible so that organizations are poised to react to change as it occurs. They work best when information technology permits the rapid turnaround of data. If data on August performance figures do not become available until September 30, there is little value to using flexible budgeting. It works best in situations where production data is available on a daily, or at least weekly, basis.

There are drawbacks to variable budgeting. First, this type of budgeting is more reactive than predictive. In essence, it tells the organization how it should have performed rather than setting goals for future performance. Second, many organizations are not able to respond quickly to decreases in volume. For example, employees are often scheduled to work two to three weeks in advance. When the volume of work increases, it is relatively easy to add additional labor, either by calling in casual workers or by authorizing overtime. However, once the schedules are posted, labor hours are not likely to decrease, especially if the scheduling process is regulated by a union contract. At best, it takes nearly three weeks to respond to a spontaneous, unpredicted decrease in workload. Often it takes longer.

preparing the operating budget

Now that the different types of budgets have been identified, the actual preparation of an operating budget can be described. It is a stepwise process that is generally directed by the financial department of the organization. In its simplest form, individual managers are told what their budgets are for the coming year. Then managers must decide how to produce the anticipated revenue and operate within the expense allocations. More often, though, in keeping with newer management theory that stresses participative management and empowerment, the managers will take an active role in setting their own operating budgets.

Typically, managers will deal with one part of the budget at a time. One way to do this is to project revenues first. This includes the volume of work to be done, the price of the product, anticipated price increases, and income from other sources like grants or subsidies. Next, the managers can estimate their labor needs and anticipate the cost for that labor. Then, non-labor expenses will be computed. Finally, the various pieces of the budget will be combined to project profit or loss. The parts of an operating budget are described in Table 14.2.

Though businesses generally expect to make a profit, nonprofit organizations are required only to break even. This is not true for every department in an organization. Within any establishment (either for-profit or nonprofit), there are some departments that operate solely as **cost centers**. These are not expected to generate a profit or to break even. Often support departments like payroll, human resources, and material management are considered to be cost centers.

If a department also generates some income, it is both a **revenue center** and a cost center. A revenue center may or may not produce enough income to offset its cost of operation.

Cost Center. *Any unit within an organization that has expenses. Some cost centers, like foodservices and pharmacy, also generate revenues. Others, like payroll, human resources, and materials management, are not expected to generate a profit or to break even.*

Revenue Center. *Any department within an organization that generates an income.*

Planning a departmental budget is hard work for the manager.

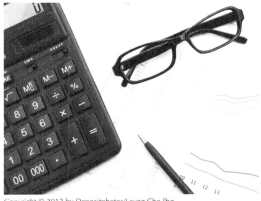

Revenue Budget	Projects income from sale of products, based on volume and price, as well as income from other sources
Expense Budget	May be a single budget plan for all anticipated costs or be divided into two or more of several sub-budgets, including labor, material, overhead, and other expenses
Direct Labor Budget	Predicts labor costs needed to perform the work; does not include cost of benefits
Direct Material Budget	Projects the cost of raw materials to be used in the production of goods
Overhead Budget	The cost of facilities, including rent or mortgage, utilities, repairs, and maintenance
Other Operating Expenses	All other operating costs that can be anticipated for the budget cycle

Table 14.2 Parts of an Operating Budget

An example of a revenue center is the clinical nutrition service in a hospital, if it charges for services like nutritional assessments, kilocaloric counts, diet instructions, and so on. Foodservice is another example of a revenue center, as is the pharmacy or the laboratory.

Profit Center. *Any department within an organization with an income that exceeds operating costs.*

When income exceeds cost by a substantial amount, the revenue center is also considered to be a **profit center**. Clinical nutrition services do not usually operate as profit centers, because their revenues seldom exceed the cost of providing services. Foodservices, on the other hand, can and do earn a profit. The profits from foodservice are often used to subsidize the clinical nutrition services in a healthcare facility. If an organization is to be viable over time, profit centers must produce enough excess income to compensate for those support departments that do not earn substantial revenues.

revenues

Revenue Budget. *The projection of the income of an organization or a department based on the sale of products. It is a part of the operating budget.*

A **revenue budget** is a projection of the income of an organization. It is a part of the operating budget. Like every other part of the operating budget, it is projected for the entire year and then divided into projections for each accounting period. Revenue budgets are written only for revenue centers. They are not prepared for departments that are solely cost centers.

Some organizations project their revenues for the coming budget cycle as the first step in the budgeting process. For these organizations, it is felt that once income levels are known, it is possible to prepare a realistic expense budget that is in balance with income. Alternatively, it is possible to prepare expense budgets first and then project revenues to cover operating costs and the amount of profit needed, if any. In either case, there are two steps to computing anticipated revenues. One is to project the volume of goods or services to be produced and the other is to set the price of those products.

Often, there is an inverse relationship between price and volume. For example, if a weight-loss program charges $250 per session, there will probably be fewer people enrolled in it than in a program that charges $25 per session. This relationship is even more obvious in foodservice. Quick service restaurants rely on large numbers of customers who eat relatively inexpensive meals. At the other end of the spectrum, fine-dining restaurants focus on providing high-cost meals to a few select customers.

Managers need to estimate both the price and the volume of products. Any price adjustment has the potential for impacting volume. Historically, health care has been exempt from this effect because the service providers were few. However, in recent years, competition has intensified the inverse relationship between price and volume in healthcare settings. Insurance companies and other third-party payers now have the ability to direct their clients away from facilities and services that they feel are overpriced. Also, contracts between facilities and payers discount the fees that an insurer will pay for a service. Pricing is critical, because overpricing will drive away potential and existing consumers, while underpricing will cut into profits. When setting prices, it is useful to have access to reliable market research data.

Two other considerations might be included in revenue budgets. One is revenue from sources other than the sales of a product. Money from grants, matching funds, charities, and subsidies are all income and need to be included in revenue projections. (Sometimes grant-funding sources require that a separate budget be prepared for any grant awarded to an organization.) The other consideration is that there is no guarantee that all of the money that is billed will be collected. Some people do not (or cannot) pay their bills. Bad debt and discounts to major accounts will erode the actual income. Insofar as this type of data is available, it should be included in revenue projections. For example, if the fee for a nutritional assessment is $200, but there are data that say that for the past five years, the collections were 80 percent of billings, then the anticipated revenue should be 80 percent of anticipated billings. Unfortunately, this information is not always available to the manager who is preparing the budget.

expenses

The operating budget also includes an **expense budget**. This is prepared for every department in an organization, including those departments that are exclusively cost centers. On a department-by-department basis, there is no mandate to cover expenses with revenues, but on an organizational basis, there is a clear need to do so. For-profit organizations need an excess of revenue over operating costs; nonprofit organizations need to break even.

Expense Budget.
Component of the operating budget that deals with all anticipated costs, which can further be divided into a number of sub-budgets (for example, labor, material, overhead, and other expenses).

Labor Budget. *A prediction of the labor costs needed to get work done; does not always include the cost of benefits. It can be written as part of the expense budget or as a separate part of the operating budget.*

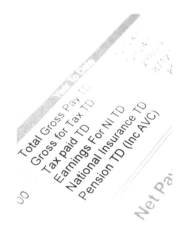

Copyright © 2012 by Depositphotos/Katie Nesling.

Direct Labor Costs. *Labor costs that are related to the actual performance of work (for example, base pay, overtime, pay in lieu of benefits, and so on). These are the projections that get written into the labor budget.*

Indirect Labor Costs. *Labor costs over which managers have little control. These include benefits like insurance, taxes, and paid time off, which are not always included in the labor budget.*

There may be one overall expense budget for a department that includes all anticipated costs, or there may be several sub-budgets. For example, the expense budget is frequently divided into two parts—labor and other expenses. Alternately, the expense budget may be divided into a greater number of sub-budgets, including labor, material, overhead, and other expenses. The number and names of the sub-budgets are dependent on how the organization chooses to manage financial information. A description of some kinds of sub-budgets follows.

labor. The **labor budget** may be prepared as a separate document or may be written as part of the larger expense budget. Except during restructuring, this particular part of the budget is fairly easy to project. Managers know how much labor they use, who their employees are, how much each earns, how much vacation time they have accumulated, and when pay raises are due. In addition, managers can often predict what the pay raises will be. Experienced managers usually also know approximately when turnover in staff will occur, what it will cost to hire and train a replacement worker, what type of vacation relief is required, and so forth.

Direct labor costs are those labor costs that are related to actually doing work. Direct labor costs include straight-time pay, overtime, pay in lieu of benefits, and so on. These are the labor costs that managers have a degree of control over, and this is the part that is projected in the budget. **Indirect labor costs** are those over which the manager has little control. These include benefits like insurance, taxes, and paid time off. In many cases, indirect labor costs are not included in the labor budget.

material. Frequently, a **direct material budget** is computed for those departments that produce a tangible product. It is common for foodservices to have a direct material budget in order to plan and monitor the outlays for the ingredients that are used to produce meals. In this case, the budget for foods and related goods would be separate from the budget for other items that are used in the department, like computer paper, pens, books, dishwashing chemicals, and so on, which are included in the **indirect material budget**. In departments or units where the primary product is service, like an outpatient nutrition clinic, there is little need for a direct material budget.

overhead. Overhead is another item that may or may not be included in a departmental operating expense budget. In a very large physical plant, like a hospital, it is not particularly useful to measure the costs of lighting, heat and air-conditioning, gas, steam, housekeeping, and so forth on a department-by-department basis. Therefore, the cost of overhead items is charged to one department (perhaps engineering or

management practice in dietetics

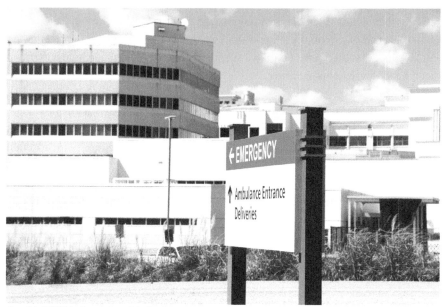

Copyright © 2010 by Depositphotos/John Panella.

In hospitals, overhead costs (heating, cooling, water, and electricity) may be included in the budget of the engineering or the building department rather than charged to individual departments such as foodservice or pharmacy.

buildings and grounds) as part of its overall budget. In this situation, other departments are not charged for overhead. If, however, the department is at a remote site, like a satellite clinic in a suburban office complex, the overhead costs are finite and would be charged to the individual department. If a department is responsible for paying its own overhead, this item must be included under operating expenses.

other operating expenses. The category that is listed as **other operating expenses** includes everything else that a department plans to spend for operations. The type of items that fall under this heading are telephone bills, copying charges, printing, office supplies, books, travel, journals, postage, fees and licenses, and so on.

When preparing an operating budget, it is in each manager's best interest to be as accurate as possible. This is especially true when determining when the funds will be spent. Even though it is usually acceptable to divide the money equally across all accounting periods, it is easier to use the budget to monitor actual performance if the funds are allocated to the period in which they will be spent. It is definitely worth the added effort to fine-tune these forecasts as much as possible.

For example, if it is anticipated that direct labor costs will decrease in December because individuals will take time off and not be replaced (because the workload is historically lower during that month), then the labor budget for December should

Other Operating Expenses.
Subdivision of the operating budget that encompasses all other anticipated costs of operation. Items usually included are telephone bills, copying charges, printing, office supplies, books, travel, journals, postage, fees and licenses, and so on. Organizations that do not use sub-budgets would also include the costs of labor, overhead, and material under this heading.

be lower than that for October. In a school foodservice, if inventories are depleted in June at the end of a school year, and stockpiled in August for the coming semester, then the budget should reflect minimal spending on direct material in June and heavy spending for these items in August.

Because the budget is used to monitor a manager's performance, making the budget as accurate as possible means that there will be less variance between what is budgeted and what is spent during each accounting period. In the long term, accurate budget forecasting saves the manager the time and effort needed to justify variances to administration after the fact. Accurate budgets also help the parent organization to manage cash flow and reduce the cost of borrowing funds from an outside source. Though managers dread the budgeting process, they often find the completed operating budget to be a very useful tool to monitor their own performance and that of their departments.

capital budgets

Capital Budget.
Projects spending on items that are costly and durable such as land, buildings, and major pieces of equipment.

The other part of the master budget that requires consideration is the **capital budget**. Large investments in land, buildings, and major pieces of equipment are considered to be capital expenditures. These items are both costly and durable. They are expected to last for a long time, and their value can be depreciated over time. Many organizations set a dollar value for capital goods; any item that costs more than the designated amount is defined as a capital expenditure. Ovens, dishwashers, computer systems, and automobiles are other examples of items that would be included in a capital budget.

Because of the relatively high cost of capital expenditures, there is usually an organization-wide system for the allocation of these funds. Department managers are not allocated capital dollars and allowed to spend them as they see fit. Rather, managers write a proposal for the capital goods that they need and submit the proposal to a budget committee of some sort. Membership on this committee varies, but generally includes representatives of the financial department and representatives from upper levels of management.

Managers who request more than one capital expenditure are asked to prioritize these items. At the organizational level, all the capital requests are evaluated and resources are allocated based on, among other factors, the urgency of the request, the worthiness of the proposal, the cost of goods, and the availability of funds for capital expenditures. Sometimes capital budgets are projected for more than a year at a time to allow an organization to accumulate funds for major undertakings.

preparing the capital budget

For the individual manager, the preparation of the capital budget is a five-step process. Essentially the process allows the manager to determine the unit's needs and attempt to justify the expenditures necessary to satisfy those needs. After the capital budget is proposed and submitted, the manager must wait to see which, if any, of the requests are approved. If the response is positive, an implementation plan must be developed and put into effect. Sometimes an outline of this plan is included as part of the justification for the capital outlay.

Determine what capital goods are needed

Prioritize the items on the list of needs

Estimate the cost for each proposed capital expenditure

Prepare the capital budget request/s including justification and cost data

Submit the proper paperwork to formalize the request/s

Table 14.3 Steps for Preparing a Capital Budget

the five-step process

The first step in preparing a capital budget is to determine what types of capital goods are needed for the budget period. There may be years when no capital items are needed. For example, if a Meals-on-Wheels program moved into a new (and newly furnished) facility one year ago, it is unlikely that capital purchases will be required during the next few years. On the other hand, a foodservice that has occupied the same space for 20 years and is still using original equipment might need to make several capital purchases within one year.

Once the list of items needed is generated, the manager should prioritize the items on that list. This is done early in the process so that the manager can decide how much time should be spent on each individual request. Obviously, the item that is needed the most should get the most attention in order to document sufficient need and provide adequate justification. Items that do not have very high priorities can be left until later in the process so that, if time runs out, it is those items that have less-compelling justifications. In any case, the prioritization will have to occur before the requests are submitted, so it is a good idea to complete this step as soon as possible.

The third step is to estimate the cost for each item. Note that the operative word is "estimate." It is not necessary to come up with an exact cost for three reasons. First, the cost is likely to change between the time that the budget is prepared and the time that the project is funded. The second reason is that it is probably too early to select a specific product to meet the need. Again, time is the important variable. Technological advances may mean that something that is specified may become obsolete in a matter of months. Rather than request a specific item, therefore, it is usually considered to be prudent to make the request in generic terms and estimate the cost based on a range of prices at which that product is available. It is common for managers to estimate cost for capital goods on the high side, so that they are not limited in their choices if the item is funded. The final consideration is the time a manager has for preparing the capital budget. Often that time is extremely limited. The manager would not have time to make a good decision about what, specifically, to purchase. This is even more of a problem if more than one item is being requested. If the funds were not allocated for an item, then the manager's time would have been wasted. It is best not to invest the time in making a firm decision until it is known if money will be available for the purchase.

When the cost estimates are completed, the actual budget request is written. The format for the request is organization-specific. Usually there is a distinct form that needs to be completed and submitted. The form includes such information as department, person making the request, item requested, cost data, priority, urgency, justification, proposed implementation schedule, and so on. The amount of information requested varies from organization to organization. The documents submitted should be concise, so that the reader is able to evaluate it quickly.

Sometimes it is easy to justify the replacement of an outdated piece of equipment.

Though all of the information in a capital budget request is important, the justification is probably the most critical part of the document. This is especially true if the budgets are tight and the request is for something that is not absolutely essential. For example, a manager may want a bigger, faster copier even though the existing copier still works well. In most cases, critical items will be funded first, with little regard for the way the justification is written. After that, the items that get funded will be those that have the best justifications to support their purchase.

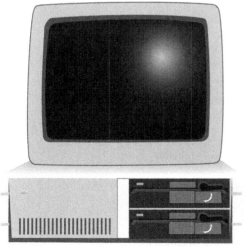

The final step in preparing the capital budget is to submit the required paperwork. This should be done on time and in the approved format. Sometimes a manager will be asked to defend the request verbally in a formal budget session, but this type of situation usually occurs only in large bureaucracies, not in smaller organizations. Dietetics professionals who work for governmental agencies may be asked to participate in such budget sessions.

The only thing left to do after the capital budget is submitted is to wait to hear the outcome. If the item is funded, then the decision-making process related to its purchase, installation, and implementation begins. If it is not funded, the document can be used as the basis for resubmission during the next budget cycle.

management practice in dietetics

conclusion

This chapter has explored the mysteries of budget preparation, which includes defining terms, and outlining how the process is carried out. The key ideas that were covered in this chapter include those listed below.

1. Budgets are an important management tool that should be based on the mission, goals, and plan of the organization.
2. The master budget has four distinct parts—the cash budget, the budgeted balance sheet, the operating budget, and the capital budget.
3. Budgets can be either incremental or zero-based. Either of these budget types can be further characterized as fixed or flexible.
4. Operating budgets include revenue and expense budgets. Revenue budgets project both production volume and cost. Expense budgets may be simply one budget listing all expenses or may be a compilation of two or more sub-budgets.
5. Operating budgets are more useful over the life of the budget if they are as detailed as possible.
6. Capital budgets are for large, costly items. The process for developing a capital budget is outlined in the five steps of determining need, prioritizing, estimating cost, writing the request and justification, and submitting the request.

activities

activity 1

Prepare an operating budget for yourself for one month. For revenue, you should include allowances, earned income, and/or money that you have saved to live on for the following month. List all of the operating expenses that you anticipate on a weekly basis, including housing, food, transportation, phone, clothing, and incidentals.

Please keep this budget. You may want to use it for the exercise at the end of the next chapter.

activity 2

The purpose of this assignment is to familiarize you with the process of writing a justification for a piece of equipment that needs to be proposed as part of a capital budget. The piece of equipment is a convection oven. Noting the assigned piece of equipment below, you should compare models available, determine which piece of equipment you want to purchase, and write a justification showing why you need the oven and why you chose a particular piece of equipment.

step 1:

Your assignments are as follows:

- Please choose one gas and one electric convection oven from the list at http://www.fishnick.com/publications/appliancereports/convectionovens/. Make sure that the two ovens that you choose are "full size." Also, make sure that the oven you choose is **not** Energy Star–rated as listed at http://www.energystar.gov/ia/products/prod_lists/comm_ovens_prod_list.xls.
- Review the summary report for each of the ovens that you have chosen and determine the preheat energy, the idle energy rate, the heavy-load energy efficiency, and the production capacity.
- Note that the initial cost of each of the ovens is as follows:

	Gas	Electric
Base Efficiency Oven	$3725.00	$2309.00
Your Oven	$4891.00	$3185.00
Energy Star Oven	$6328.00	$5428.00

- The annual maintenance cost for each oven is as follows:

	Gas	Electric
Base Efficiency Oven	$168.00	$127.00
Your Oven	$124.00	$115.00
Energy Star Oven	$96.00	$84.00

- Using the life cycle cost calculator at http://www.fishnick.com/saveenergy/tools/calculators/, input the preheat energy, idle rate energy, heavy load energy efficiency, and production capacity for your ovens. Use the default numbers for "Oven Usage" and "Utility Cost and Lifespan." Next input the initial cost and the maintenance costs for your oven, the base efficiency ovens, and the Energy Star oven.
- Calculate the results and print these for the gas and electric convection ovens, making sure that the page you print shows the results for all three levels of ovens. (If you use the "Click to Print Results" button at the bottom of the page, you will print the results only for your oven.)
- Write a report about the six ovens that you have evaluated and make a recommendation about which of the six you would like to buy. Since your manager is making the final decision, you need to justify the recommendation that you make.

to study further

- Finkler, S. A. *Financial Management for Non-Financial Managers*. 4th ed. Chicago: CCH, 2011.
- Finkler, S. A., T. Calabrese, R. Purtell, and D. L. Smith. *Financial Management for Public, Health, and Not-for-Profit Organizations*. 4th ed. Upper Saddle River, NJ: Prentice Hall, 2012.
- Lalli, W. R., ed. *Handbook of Budgeting*. 5th ed. Hoboken, NJ: John Wiley and Sons, Inc., 2012.
- McMillan, E. J. *Not-for-Profit Budgeting and Financial Management*. 4th ed. Hoboken, NJ: John Wiley and Sons, Inc., 2010.
- Peterson, P. P. and F. J. Fabozzi. *Capital Budgeting: Theory and Practice*. New York: Wiley, 2002.
- Person, Mathew M. III. *The Zero-Base Hospital: Survival and Success in America's Evolving Healthcare System*. Chicago: Health Administration Press, 1997.
- Seitz, Neil and Mitch Ellison. *Capital Budgeting and Long-Term Financing Decisions*. 4th ed. Mason, OH: Thomson/South-Western, 2005.

scholarly journals

- *Management Accounting Research*
- *The Health Care Manager*
- *Management Accounting Quarterly*

other relevant periodical

- *Healthcare Financial Management*

in practice

the clinical nutrition manager meets the budget

In healthcare nutrition, as in other patient care settings, the professionals who do patient care seldom need to be knowledgeable about budgetary issues, since they are not responsible for financial management of a department in an organization. However, these individuals might be responsible for certain aspects of the financial plan, like keeping records of productivity, billing for services, ordering patient education materials, or submitting expense accounts for business travel.

It is nearly impossible for a practitioner to completely avoid the repercussions of belt-tightening when the regional economy is in a downturn, even if one has no direct responsibility for financial management. If nothing else, limited pay raises or loss of the ability to replace old computer systems in a timely manner will have an impact on the way that work is perceived and on what can be accomplished within the fiscal constraints imposed on a service area. Therefore, clinicians should be concerned with the budget, the budgeting process, and the overall financial position of the parent organization, whether or not they want to be involved with financial matters.

Unfortunately, the clinical RD and DTR often become so wrapped up in the science of nutrition and the details of patient care, that they do not put a high value on learning about financial planning and management. They tend to be on the receiving end of the process, rather than the controlling end. In the long term, this dissociation can have a negative impact on patient care since, if needs are not well articulated in a language that can be understood in financial circles, the needs may not be translated into a line item on the master budget for an organization.

Clinical nutrition managers, promoted into their positions largely from the ranks of clinical staff, are often unfamiliar with financial management when they are new in their positions. If the clinical services are integrated into a larger food and nutrition services department, there may not be a separate budget for the clinical services. Thus the clinical manager may become accountable for the financial performance of part of the larger department without being responsible for financial planning. This is not a good situation for a number of reasons, not the least of which is the lack of ability to set priorities for clinical services.

Given modern accounting procedures and the use of technology to separate various parts of budgets electronically, it is possible for the clinical manager to take on the management of finances for all the clinical services. This should occur to assure that responsibility and accountability rest with the same person, and to allow that person to exercise a degree of control over the services being provided. It is no longer acceptable for a clinical manager to rely on the foodservice director to take on all the responsibility for preparing the budgets. By doing so, the clinical manager is not managing the service area completely, and is delegating part of the management position's responsibility to another manager. Though it may be easier to avoid budgeting than to learn how to do it, it is a mistake to do so.

Budget-phobia can limit your upward mobility. Usually one progresses up the management ladder by taking on additional responsibility relative to total span of control as measured by the number of employees reporting to the manager and his or her subordinates, and by becoming responsible for progressively larger total operating budgets. If you do not take the first step to learn about the budgeting process, you effectively limit your upward progress through various levels of management. This is an example of how to create your own "glass ceiling."

Budgeting is as much a matter of logic and common sense as it is of mathematical prowess. Probably the best way to learn the process is to do it, but there are a number of things that a beginner can do to facilitate the process. The first is to review general accounting terminology as well as the specific terminology that is used by the facility's accounting department. Terms like FTE, direct labor costs, indirect labor costs, supplies, overhead, utilities, accounting periods, fiscal year, and so forth are essential to the budgeting process. Second, knowledge about an organization's rules and guidelines related to labor, pay scales, and benefits is necessary for preparing a labor budget. It is also helpful to have some budget history to determine how funds have been spent in the past. This information can be obtained from past operating reports. Finally, a mentor who has done budgetary work in the past within the organization can be a useful ally. This mentor need not be your boss or administrator; a colleague with a like-size budget and a bit more budgeting experience than you have will serve as a good resource.

The Chief Financial Officer and his or her staff may make an outline of the organization's specific budgeting process available to managers and perhaps even offer classes or discussion groups for managers as they go through the budget process. Take advantage of these resources until you develop a level of competence and confidence that satisfies you and your direct manager.

Networking is another very useful tool for learning new skills. Contacting colleagues in the Clinical Nutrition Management Practice Group with questions about budgets will give you a feel for how peers handle similar challenges. Even if the information obtained is not directly transferable to your setting, the ideas generated may help you formulate a plan that can be used in your specific situation. For example, a colleague in California may have developed a fee schedule based on an hourly rate of $100.00 per hour for clinical services because the average RD salary there is approximately $50.00 per hour. If your staff earns only an average of $40.00 per hour in Louisiana, you may not be able to charge the same $100.00 per hour for service, but may be able to justify a charge of $80.00 per hour by using a factor of two times salary to establish a fee schedule.

The first budget that you prepare will be the most difficult. This is largely due to the fear of the unknown coupled with the knowledge that you will have to live within the constraints of that budget for the next fiscal year. A prudent manager will build in some degree of cushion, if a way can be found to justify that cushion. However, in order to make subsequent budgets easier to design and manage, it is useful to prepare variance reports on a monthly basis during the year. (See Chapter 15.) This will enable you to understand the actual accounting from both the figures and the underlying facts that supported those figures. Thus, if labor costs rise in the summer when regular staff is on vacation and more casual labor needs to be added to cover the caseload, then you can incorporate this information into the budget for the coming year, increasing the labor budget for those specific months.

In reality, preparing the budget for a clinical service is a great jumping-off point for learning financial management. Clinical budgets are much less complex than budgets needed for foodservices. The clinical revenue budget is relatively small, and contains only a few line items. It is accompanied by an expense budget that is mostly labor, with other operating expenses being minimal. In contrast, foodservices budgets involve larger revenues generated from cafeteria meals sold, catering, patient meals, floor stock, and vending. Labor expenses are higher than they are for clinical services since there are more employees. There are large expenditures for food products on a daily basis. Clinical Nutrition Managers may even learn that they like having the increased clout that comes from managing a budgetary unit, and find that their career takes on a new direction after these challenges are met.

reference

1.   Bryan, Robert M. "The Basics of Budgeting." *Association Management,* January 1998, pp. 65–67.

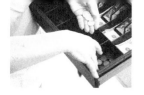

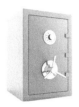

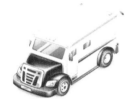

chapter fifteen

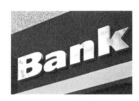

financial management

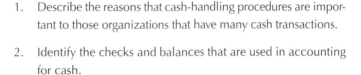

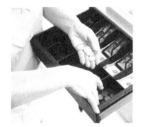

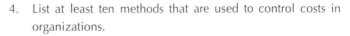

learning objectives

1. Describe the reasons that cash-handling procedures are important to those organizations that have many cash transactions.

2. Identify the checks and balances that are used in accounting for cash.

3. State the precautions that need to be taken to secure cash in a retail operation.

4. List at least ten methods that are used to control costs in organizations.

5. Describe the operating statement.

6. Discuss how a variance report is prepared, using the operating statement as its basis.

7. Describe the characteristics of a profit and loss statement.

8. State the uses for the profit and loss statement and the consolidated profit and loss statement.

9. Describe the characteristics of a balance sheet.

10. Differentiate between assets and liabilities.

11. Define *owner's equity* and *stockholders' equity*.

12. Discuss the uses of the balance sheet and the consolidated balance sheet.

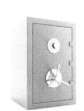

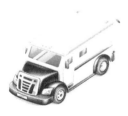

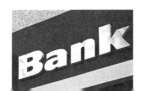

overview

Many managers, including dietetics professionals, would like to believe that managing human and material resources is enough and the money will take care of itself. This is just not so. In today's economy, money is the common denominator for trade. Not that money is always defined in terms of currency ... credit and debit cards, checks, electronic transfers and payment systems, and other mediums of exchange all are used as substitutes for money. Without money, workers would not work for long, no matter how motivated and dedicated they are. Without money, there would be no raw materials to use in production. Without money, no one would consume the products made. Without money, the workplace we know would cease to exist.

Therefore, managers have fiscal responsibility and must manage money, either by default or by choice. Financial management, like budgeting, is an essential part of the job of every manager. Whether it is more or less important than managing people is a philosophical question that the readers are free to answer for themselves. There will be no attempt here to establish the relative importance of this management function.

With financial management, as with budgeting, there are many more intricacies than can possibly be discussed in one chapter. Financial management, like information management and marketing, is a discipline in its own right. Just as everyone must know a little about nutrition in order to live a healthy life, everyone must know something about money management to survive in today's world. This chapter is an attempt to describe some basic financial concepts to the dietetics practitioner. The content that is covered here includes only those topics that dietetics professionals deal with routinely. Those who have moved into upper-level management and those who are self-employed will need to know much more about financial management than is described here.

This chapter will begin with a discussion of how to handle situations in which the revenue comes in the form of cash, rather than as credit cards or checks. This will be followed by a review of various ways costs are controlled in organizations. The chapter will conclude with a description of some of the financial reports that dietetics professionals in management positions may encounter.

cash handling

It is a fact that cash is being used less and less for transactions in the twenty-first century. It has been predicted that cash will eventually cease to exist, at least as a medium for exchange.[1, 2] However, for those businesses that use cash today, the manner in which it is handled is an area of vulnerability. Just the presence of cash increases the potential for theft. There are multiple factors to consider when handling currency, including the amount of cash that is on hand, the way that it is handled, the types of cash registers used, and the amount of data they generate. The procedures for reconciling cash at the end of the day, how the cash gets to the bank, and security for both the cash and for the personnel who handle it are also necessary considerations.

Cash is used in most retail businesses. In those organizations that employ dietetics professionals, foodservice is the only one that is likely to involve large numbers of cash transactions and handle large amounts of cash. Most other non-foodservice transactions use other forms of payment such as credit cards, bank transfers, and occasionally checks. Foodservices sometimes use alternatives to cash payments like credit cards and debit cards, meal passes, digital wallets, and so on. However, whenever large amounts of cash are present, controls need to be in place to safeguard it.

Cash handling has several components and needs to be standardized within each setting in a way that meets the requirements of the setting and the information needs of the manager. The standards are in place to protect both the management and the employees who handle cash. Some of the key components to cash handling are described in this section.

Cash Handling.
The management of cash transactions (includes the receiving, storing, counting, recording, withdrawing, and depositing of cash).

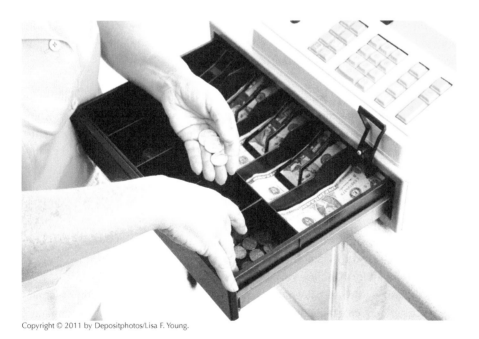

Cashiers need to verify the amount of cash in their banks at the beginning and the end of their shifts.

checks and balances

The checks and balances that are required for the handling of cash involve the routine reconciliation of cash with transaction records. At the beginning of a shift, the cashier should verify the amount of money that is in the cash register drawer. This is called the **bank**. At the end of the cashier's shift, the money is counted once more. The money in the drawer at the end of the day less the starting bank is the day's **cash receipts**. The amount is recorded and verified by another person (a supervisor, a manager, or someone with accounting responsibilities). After the money has been counted and verified, the cash receipts from all cash registers are pooled and prepared for deposit in a commercial bank. Cash receipts should be transferred to a **commercial bank** each day, if possible. In the meantime, the money should be secured. The cash register drawer's bank is left intact, to be used as the next day's starting bank.

The **cash register**, itself, is a computer that is capable of providing much useful information. Some of the information is related to inventory; some is related to cash. In general, the managers should know the features of their cash registers, how to operate them, how to program them, and how to use the information that is generated. More sophisticated cash registers include **point-of-sale (POS) systems**, which are capable of tracking individual items sold and deducting those items from inventory, giving a real-time dimension to the perpetual inventory system. This type of system, coupled with barcode technology, is used in supermarkets and other large retail operations. It provides managers a wealth of data that can be used for reconciling sales, cash, and items sold. In addition the POS registers aid in the forecasting of production, in procurement, and in inventory control.

Periodically (sometimes daily, sometimes at the end of each cashier's shift), cash receipts must be reconciled with the data generated by the cash register. Typically, only a manager or supervisor can clear the accumulated data off the register at the end of the day. (This requires the use of a different key or password than the cashier has.) There are usually a variety of ways to clear a cash register, each of which yields different kinds of information on a printed tape that is used to verify cash sales at the end of the day.

The **cash register tapes** are used to determine the cash sales for the day. This number is compared to cash receipts. The numbers should coincide. An individual who has no responsibility for handling cash should carry out the comparison, if it is at all possible. Cash registers also keep duplicate records, sometimes as electronic files and sometimes as duplicate tapes that are stored in the machine. These act as a permanent record of transactions. These tapes are among the financial records that need to be saved for several years. Managers who work in cash sales operations should be well versed in cash-handling procedures. They should carry out frequent spot checks to make sure that the process is working as it should. It is relatively easy for an astute

---

Bank. *The amount of money that the cash register drawer contains at the start of a shift.*

Cash Receipts. *The amount of money that is present in the cash register drawer at the end of the day minus the starting bank.*

Commercial Bank. *A banking institution that handles the everyday financial transactions of businesses.*

Cash Register. *A machine that records and displays the details of a sales transaction (such as the quantity and price of items purchased), as well as acting as a storage unit for the cash involved in these transactions.*

Point-of-Sale (POS) Systems. *Cash register computer systems that are capable of tracking individual items sold and deducting those items from inventory.*

management practice in dietetics

thief to manipulate cash register tapes to cover theft. If random checks of the entire cash-handling process are not being done, the theft could go on for years and the losses could be staggering.

Another set of checks and balances occurs when the money arrives at the bank. The bank's staff validates that the deposits and withdrawals coincide with what is written on the supporting documents. Whatever cash comes back to the organization (usually coins and small bills to be used to make change) is double-checked by a supervisor or manager before being secured on site.

security

Security related to cash handling is quite complex and has to be adapted to each different situation. It is pretty obvious that a quick service restaurant in an impoverished inner-city neighborhood will need a different type of security than the pub on the rural campus of a small private college. Nevertheless, there are some precautions that are universal.

First, a limited number of people should have access to the money, and those people need proper authorization. In some large organizations, individuals who are designated to handle cash may need to be **bonded**. Small operations tend to operate more on trust and instinct. People who handle cash need to be trained on the organization's cash-handling procedures and the reasons for following them. They should be taught the basics about cash control so that they do not leave themselves vulnerable, either as potential victims of theft or as suspects when a loss occurs.

Second, the money should be secured whenever it is not being handled. Cash should never be left unattended. This means that cash register drawers are closed between transactions, and are locked when no one is around. Some cash registers have keys that allow access to the cash drawer; others use codes or passwords. If keys are used, they should stay in the possession of authorized personnel during work hours. Keys should not be left in an unattended cash register. The keys themselves should be secured at the end of the day. These should not go home with staff members. If passwords or codes are used, they should be handled like other computer passwords and should never be shared between employees.

When money is being counted for any purpose, it should be done in a secure area. Those who are doing the task should be free from distraction and interruption. If interruptions occur, the cash should be secured, if at all possible. As soon as the money is counted, it should be stored in closed containers, in as safe a place as possible. This may be a safe or a locked closet, cabinet, or desk. The room should also be locked as an additional precaution. When large amounts of cash are involved, even these redundancies may not be sufficient to secure it.

Cash Register Tapes. *A record of cash transactions made and stored by the cash register that contains information about daily cash sales.*

Bonded. *To bind by an agreement to pay a certain amount of money upon failure to complete a job properly; insuring an organization against financial loss incurred by such.*

Safe. *A place or container used to secure valuables from theft.*

If a **safe** is available, it should be used routinely. The combination for the safe should be known to a limited number of management-level staff. If any of those people terminates affiliation with the organization, either voluntarily or involuntarily, the combination on the safe should be changed immediately. If a person who knows the combination takes a new position within the organization, but no longer requires access to the safe, the combination should also be changed, but the reprogramming can be done with somewhat less urgency. Those with access to the safe and its contents should commit the combination to memory; combinations that are written on a piece of paper are vulnerable.

Armored Transport. *Transport of money between retail facilities and commercial banks by licensed and bonded companies.*

If large amounts of cash are handled each day, its movement between the facility and the commercial bank should be contracted out to a licensed and bonded **armored transport** service. These companies routinely carry money between retail facilities and banks while taking the responsibility for its safety. For transport, the money is placed in locked containers to protect the armored guards from suspicion if shortages occur. If there is minimal cash and the management chooses not to use an armored transport service, appropriate measures should be taken to ensure the safety of whoever makes the bank deposit.

Note that cash moves in both directions between the foodservices and the bank. Bank deposits are not the only cash transactions that take place. Coins and small-denomination bills are obtained from commercial banks for the purpose of making change. Money is also needed for petty cash funds. Any money that is delivered to an organization needs to be stored in a protected place immediately after the delivery is verified. If verification cannot be done immediately, the money should be secured until the verification can be done.

Petty Cash. *Money that is kept on hand for making emergency purchases or for minor expenditures that cannot be made through regular vendors in a timely manner.*

petty cash

Petty cash is money that is kept on hand to use for emergency purchases. For example, if a healthcare foodservice needs to purchase soy bread for a newly admitted patient

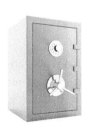 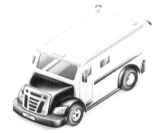 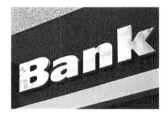

Cash must be secured on site and during transport until it is delivered to the commercial bank.

management practice in dietetics

who is allergic to wheat, the soy bread may be obtained from a retail store. Petty cash funds should be used only for emergency purchases and for items that cannot be obtained from regular vendors. Sometimes managers overuse this fund to avoid paperwork, or to compensate for poor planning. This is not a good idea. Nearly always, items purchased using petty cash cost more than they would otherwise.

Petty cash funds are necessary for all types of businesses and organizations, whether or not they routinely handle cash sales. However, some businesses that have significant cash revenue choose not to have a petty cash fund. Instead, they pay for emergency purchases out of the cash receipts for the day. This should not be done. From an accounting perspective, it creates headaches because it is very easy to lose track of cash that is spent this way. Receipts tend to get lost or disappear. It is better to keep petty cash as a separate fund and to require a receipt for any money withdrawn from it. This way, revenues are always revenues, and all expenses are clearly identified as expenses.

A petty cash fund should contain enough money for about a month's worth of transactions. When the cash in the account is running low, all of the receipts are totaled and submitted, much like an invoice would be, to accounts payable. When the monies for this "invoice" are available, they are used to replenish the petty cash fund.

It is also possible to set up a procedure that uses a credit card instead of petty cash. Though this type of procedure is gaining acceptance, it is not used in all situations because it limits the number of people who are able to purchase items needed for emergencies. Nevertheless, in an organization with only a few individuals who purchase retail items, a Visa, MasterCard, or similar credit card could replace cash for petty cash transactions.

controlling costs

It is important to manage expenditures and to control the amount that is paid for goods and services. Many of the principles of cost control were discussed in detail earlier in this text. The major aspects of cost control will be reviewed here in order to give perspective on how these relate to overall financial management. Cost containment has been considered in purchasing, receiving and storage, inventory control, production, and labor management. Other considerations in cost control that have not been mentioned previously include maintenance, energy management, and risk management.

material management

Cost control includes negotiating good prices for items that are purchased, but it does not always mean accepting the lowest price. Low prices do not guarantee high-quality goods. Thus, specifications are the part of cost control that assures recourse if the products bought do not meet standards. Cost control may also mean using a prime vendor, whose price for some items may be higher than the competition's, but savings are realized from reduced labor in the receiving area and decreased paperwork to process. Group purchasing may also help to reduce costs.

Other cost-control measures can be implemented in the receiving, storage, inventory, and distribution functions. A balance must be struck between keeping enough material on hand to meet an operation's needs while not tying up excess dollars in inventory. Just-in-time delivery is one method that is used to manage inventory. Another is accurate recordkeeping that allows the manager to know what is available at any time so that orders can be adequate without being excessive. POS cash register systems assist with cost-effective inventory management.

Finally, security is an essential part of cost containment in material management. Open storerooms and unlocked refrigeration units, especially those not monitored with security cameras, are an invitation for thieves. Receiving and storage areas near street exits to the facility are often accessible to outsiders, but sometimes the theft is done from within the organization. Both types of vulnerabilities must be guarded against by implementing appropriate security precautions.

workflow

Another area for cost control is in the movement of work across space and time and the processes used to carry out the work. If work moves in a forward motion, with smooth flow, minimal backtracking, and the elimination of redundancy, both labor and material are conserved. Often, economies of scale will be realized as well. Production cost controls in foodservice include using planned menus and standardized recipes, measuring yield, and establishing portion control. In all dietetics specialties, cost control involves monitoring output and making sure that both the quantity and the quality of work done are meeting standards. Decreases in the amount of output lessen the revenue needed to offset expenses, and poor quality increases costs because the errors need to be remedied.

the workforce

Measuring and improving productivity is also used to manage the cost of labor. Other labor controls include monitoring actual work hours, limiting the use of overtime, and using workers in the appropriate jobs for their skill sets. For example, a cook should not be routinely assigned to wash dishes, and a dietitian should not routinely perform clerical tasks. Scheduling employees in a humane manner so that they are not required to work long hours or erratic schedules will provide them with the time needed to get adequate rest, which also can lead to productivity improvement and reduction of errors.

facilities maintenance

Preventive maintenance is another way to control costs and manage expenditures. When a piece of equipment is not working, there are usually associated losses. If a computer is down, the loss often takes the form of the overtime it takes for employees to do the work manually. If a large refrigerator is not working, there could be deterioration of large quantities of food. Worse yet, there could be an outbreak of food-borne illness due to inadequate refrigeration. A broken dishwasher will increase the use of disposable serviceware. A broken air conditioner or heating system can lead to poor productivity among workers who are either too hot or too cold to work efficiently. Even burned-out light bulbs cause headaches and poor productivity associated with eyestrain. All of these losses can be converted to dollars. Keeping the equipment in good working order is one way to reduce this type of non-budgeted expense.

management of utilities

It is also necessary to manage utilities, including energy (gas and electricity), water, and waste disposal. Though these costs are typically less than the cost of labor and materials and make a smaller difference in the monthly operating expenses, they can have a significant financial impact over the course of a year. The environmental costs of poor resource management are significant, too. Although it is not always possible for older facilities to become certified as "green" businesses, becoming "greener" by managing utilities well should be a goal of all businesses.

With some simple precautions it is possible to control energy usage and associated costs. In general, gas cooking equipment is cheaper to operate than electric cooking equipment. This is especially true where gas is less expensive than electricity, offsetting the fact that gas equipment is less efficient than electric equipment. In addition, there are ways to reduce energy use regardless of the type of the fuel being used. One way is to idle equipment when it is not in use, rather than leaving it run at peak capacity all day long. Another is to maintain gaskets on refrigerators and ovens; clean, unworn gaskets decrease heat transfer, thus limiting energy consumption. Heating and warming equipment like hot holding cabinets, warming drawers, and proofing ovens need to be well insulated. This not only makes the piece of equipment more energy efficient, but also reduces the need for tempering the room air.

The use of double-paned glass and insulated window coverings in offices and dining facilities can help to control energy loss while maintaining a comfortable ambient temperature. Energy-efficient lighting systems are available with sensors that extinguish lights when a room is vacant. These and other similar interventions can significantly reduce energy costs with little capital outlay.

Controlling the use of water is an area where technology is advancing rapidly. Water-conserving fixtures for restrooms have been available for years. Low-flow spray nozzles for pre-rinsing dishes are widely available and so inexpensive that they pay for themselves in a matter of weeks or months. Dishwashers that recycle some of the water from rinse cycles to be used in subsequent wash cycles are more widely available than in than they were in the past. Garbage disposals, which consume large amounts of water and create excess amounts of sewage, are being replaced with systems that have a less-negative impact on resources. Recycling, composting, and similar strategies are being implemented to reduce costs, both from the environmental and the financial perspectives. For more information on this topic, refer to Chapter 17.

risk management

Finally, a form of cost control that is more indirect is known as **risk management**. Risk management covers a broad spectrum of issues related to liability for what an organization does or does not do. Risk management principles can be applied to a wide variety of situations, from product liability for goods that do not perform as promised to injuries that occur to the public as a result of the organization's negligence.

In healthcare settings, risk management includes making sure that the nutritional status of the clients does not deteriorate while they are in residence. Children in pediatric hospitals must continue to get enough nutrients to maintain their growth, hospitalized patients need adequate nutrients to recover from the procedures that are done, and residents of skilled nursing facilities must not develop malnutrition because of poor food quality. And the food must be safe for our clients to eat. The safety of customers should always be primary.

Of particular concern is the issue of workplace illness and injury to workers. When employees are hurt or disabled on the job, it is not just the employee who is affected. The whole organization pays. A replacement worker must be hired and trained, which is costly. Though workers' compensation pays the worker during any absence from work, the cost of this coverage is paid either directly by the organization (if it is self-insured) or by an insurance company. Too many claims on workers' compensation policies will result in higher insurance premiums. If the workplace is found to be unsafe by the **Occupational Safety and Health Administration (OSHA)**, substantial fines are levied against the organization. Also, there is the potential for lawsuits filed by workers who believe that their injuries were preventable. Again, the organization must pay for defending itself or for settlement (or both), either directly or through higher insurance premiums in the future. Keeping the workplace safe for everyone who works there is, undoubtedly, one of the biggest cost-control mechanisms of all.

Risk management is less easy to quantify as a cost control than the other examples presented in this section. For example, it is easier to measure the reduction in electricity used when ovens are idled between peak production periods than it is to determine how many hand injuries are prevented by providing "cut resistant" gloves to foodservice workers in the production area. It is difficult to quantify the number of repetitive stress injuries that are prevented by replacing an old computer mouse with one that has a more ergonomic design. Still, it is in the organization's best interest to invest in equipment and programs that will reduce its risk of liability because of job-related injury or stress.

financial reports

Attempting to control costs is one thing. Actually measuring and reporting those expenses is another. It is, unfortunately, common for a manager to do things correctly but not track them adequately. This is especially true in times when the overall economy is good and there are adequate resources for operations to run well. When no one is hovering over a manager asking for justification of every penny that is being spent, it is pretty easy to avoid looking at the overall financial picture, and its details, as well. After all, if the organization is performing efficiently, the manager must be doing everything right. During economic downturns, tighter fiscal controls are necessary, but this does not mean that fiscal controls should be ignored at other times.

In this section, several financial reports will be considered. These include the operating statement, variance analysis, the profit and loss statement, and the balance sheet. Except for the variance analysis, which is prepared by individual managers for their areas of responsibility, these financial statements are prepared by the accounting function in the organization. Of these reports, the operating statement and variance analysis are internal departmental documents that are used primarily as management tools. The profit and loss statement and the balance sheet are most often prepared for the entire organization, rather than for segments of it. Internally, they are used as a tool for upper management, but these documents are also used to report on the organization's financial performance to employees, bankers, stockholders, investors, and others to whom the organization is accountable.

operating statement

The **operating statement** (sometimes called a *performance report*) is a document that compares actual fiscal performance to the budget. The information on the operating statement includes the budget for the accounting period and the amount budgeted from the beginning of the fiscal year. It also provides data on what the actual revenue and expenses were for both the accounting period and for the year to date. These numbers are provided for each line item on each section of the operating budget. An example of that portion of an operating statement for the expense item described as "telephone" is shown in Figure 15.1.

Operating statements are generated by the accounting function of an organization as soon as possible after the accounting period ends. Because of the speed with which information flows through today's information systems, it is possible to generate these

Operating Statement.
A document prepared by the accounting department of an organization at the end of an accounting period that compares actual fiscal performance to the budget (also called a perfor-mance report).

Line Item	May Budget	May Actual	% Variance	Y-T-D Budget	Y-T-D Actual	% Variance
Telephone	$300	$700	+133%	1500	1650	+10%

Figure 15.1 Excerpt from an Operating Statement

statements in a matter of days. The sooner the report is issued, the more value it has as a management tool because more timely information about trends can allow the organization to make midcourse adjustments more quickly. For example, if a health club earned more money from new memberships in the past month, it may be necessary to increase hours of operation or add some new equipment to meet the needs of the growing membership. The increased membership dollars should alert the club's manager to monitor usage trends to see what corrective action is required, if any. If the manager learns of the increase one week after the end of the accounting period, corrective action can be taken more quickly than if the information does not become available for 45 days. By then, it may be too late to react quickly enough to keep those new customers happy.

variance analysis

The earlier discussion of budgeting alluded to the fact that budgets could be used to monitor the performance of managers. This is certainly true. In some organizations, managers are required to submit a **variance analysis** each accounting period to explain and justify any deviation from the budget. In other cases, this type of report is required quarterly or annually. Even if it is not required and no formal analysis is generated, good managers will look at their departments' actual financial performance in relation to the budget and attempt to explain why the variance happened. It is part of the job of management to know where the money is coming from and where it is going.

A **budget variance** is any deviation from budget. If the budget projected costs of $300 for the telephone bill in May, and only $299 was spent, there is a variance. However, this variance of $1.00 represents a deviation of only 0.33 percent of the budgeted amount, which is insignificant. There is no need to explain this discrepancy, because it is so small. Conversely, if the actual May phone bill was $700, the $400 variance is 133 percent of the budgeted amount and does require an explanation. Often, there is a specific level at which an explanation is required by upper management. For example, any item that is off (either over or under budget) by 5 percent or more may need explanation or justification.

In order to prepare a variance report, the manager must have the information from the operating statement. Despite the natural inclination of some practitioners to bury the financial paperwork at the bottom of their inbox, operating statements should be dealt with as soon as possible. The sooner the manager knows about a variance, the sooner something can be done to identify and correct any problems that emerge.

Managers who are not required to submit written variance analyses are not exempt from doing them. The manager is still responsible for what is spent in the department and for noting budget overruns and under-spending. The department and manager should be encouraged to take credit for any significant savings that are evident on the operating statement. At the very least, the manager should know when there is extra money to carry out additional work, or when belt-tightening is required. In addition, the manager may be required to verbally defend budget variances at any time. It is wise to make notes on budget variances when they are identified in order to be prepared for this eventuality.

Any one of a number of possible scenarios could have resulted in the $400 variation that was seen in the May phone bill example cited earlier. Perhaps the phone company bills were not processed the previous month and the $700 represents two months' charges. (This would have been reflected in April's operating statement and variance analysis, too.) Maybe the department's phones were used by volunteers for a phone-a-thon (an unplanned and unbudgeted event) to raise money for the organization. Maybe the phone system failed during the month and had to be replaced with updated equipment. In each of these situations, the manager would be aware of the situation and could explain the variance. Nevertheless, it will be necessary to continue to monitor phone expenses for the next few months until the year-to-date numbers are back on target.

When the manager cannot explain the variance, there is a cause for concern. Thus, the manager should seek to find the reason for all unexplainable variances. In the case of the $700 phone bill, it could be that an employee is making personal calls to friends who live out of town. It could be that whoever cleans the office at night is calling relatives who live overseas. It could be that someone is using the number to charge collect calls that are made from a pay phone. Whatever the cause of the unexplained variance, it needs to be identified and, if necessary, stopped.

For managers who analyze operating statements when they arrive and address discrepancies promptly, the exercise of doing budget variance analysis has the potential to stop problems before they get out of hand. Variance analysis is one of the tools that managers use to control finances in their departments and organizations. It should be used as a supplement to other cost-control efforts.

profit and loss statements

The **profit and loss statement (P&L)** is another document that is generated by the accounting department. It is similar to the operating statement in that it lists all the actual

Profit and Loss Statement (P&L). *A document generated by the accounting department of an organization that lists all the actual data accumulated for the accounting period, including controllable as well as uncontrollable revenues and expenses. It also shows a business's net profits or losses.*

data accumulated for the accounting period. P&L statements may also be produced as a year-to-date document, or on an annual basis. The frequency with which these documents are produced is based on organizational needs and priorities. It should also be noted that this document is usually produced for the entire organization and may not be produced for individual departments or operating units. Thus, a stand-alone restaurant is likely to have a P&L statement, but the foodservice in a private college may not.

The P&L statement lists all the revenues and expenses that were posted in the operating statement. However, these values are not compared with the budgeted amounts. An organization's ability to perform to budget standards is a separate issue from its ability to earn a profit. In addition, the P&L statement must include all of the revenues and expenses that are accrued to a department, an operating unit, or an organization, not just those that are controllable. For example, indirect labor costs like paid time off and employer-paid benefits appear on this document. In addition, assets and the depreciation of equipment are often included. Some examples of items that appear on the P&L statement that might not be included on an operating statement follow. The exact items that appear on a P&L statement are dependent on the individual characteristics of each organization. See the sample P&L statement, Figure 15.2.

inventory. In an earlier section of this text, there was a discussion of how inventory is valued. It was noted that inventory can be valued at its current value, at the value of the oldest item in stock, or at the actual purchase price of each item. In general, valuing the inventory at the replacement value means that the inventory is, at least on paper, worth more than it would be if other methods of valuing inventory were used. Also, it was stated that the higher the value of the inventory, the more apparent profit the business made. This is illustrated in Figure 15.2, where the value of the inventory is shown on the P&L statement. Had the closing inventory had a lower value, the expenses would have appeared higher, and the bottom line (net profits) would be less.

indirect labor costs. Many budgets and operating statements include only salaries for employees. These are items that the manager can control. However, employees accrue paid time off, have benefits like health and life insurance, and are covered by Social Security, unemployment, and workers' compensation insurance, and so on. These benefits may be determined on an individual basis or may be calculated for the entire organization and reported as a percentage of gross earnings. Whatever these costs, they must be included in a P&L statement, even though they may not be on an expense budget.

Social Security.
http://www.ssa.gov/

overhead. Overhead, including rent, was an item that may not have appeared on the operating budget. Recall that not all organizations separate out this expense and charge it off to individual departments. However, if one is to compute profit or loss accurately, these costs must be included in the P&L analysis. If it is not possible to ascertain the actual amount spent on these items, then a value that is based on a percentage of the larger organization's expenses for these items might be included.

```
                        Driftwood Diner
                   Profit and Loss Statement
                         October 20__

    Gross Income
              (less sales tax)                  $100,000.00

    Direct Material
              Beginning inventory       10,000.00
              Cost of goods           + 40,000.00
              Ending inventory         - 7,500.00
                                                42,500.00
    Gross Profit                                             57,500.00

    Labor
              Salaries                 28,000.00
              Taxes and benefits        8,400.00
                                                36,400.00

    Operating Expenses
              Rent                      3,000.00
              Utilities                   800.00
              Maintenance                 375.00
              Supplies                    525.00
              Cleaning services         1,200.00
              Interest on credit line     935.00
              Depreciation              3,000.00
                                                 9,835.00
    Total Expenses                                         46,235.00
    Operating Profit                                       11,265.00
    Income Tax                                              3,154.00
    Net Profit                                              8,111.00
```

Figure 15.2 Sample Profit and Loss Statement

depreciation. When an organization invests in capital equipment or buildings, it is assumed that the value will decrease over time. This is called **depreciation**. Eventually the items will wear out and need replacement. Rather than count the entire cost of the item as a loss when it finally wears out, the item is depreciated to spread the loss over the life of the item. If a copier system was purchased at a cost of $8,000 and is expected to last for five years, the copier will be depreciated at the rate of $1,600 per year. (This is merely an example; other methods for calculating depreciation may be used.)

taxes. This item includes the income tax that is paid on the profits that the organization earns. Sales taxes, if charged, are not included on the profit and loss statement because they are collected and paid to the government directly without ever being transferred into the organization's books either as an asset or as revenue. Taxes that the employer pays on employees' wages are reported under indirect labor costs.

Depreciation.
An accounting technique that spreads the expense of capital equipment or buildings over their life spans, because value decreases gradually with time. It is calculated by dividing the purchase price of an item by its expected lifetime.

Consolidated Profit and Loss Statement. *A report that merges all the data from the profit and loss statements of an organization from multiple years into one report. It can be used for identifying trends over time.*

Balance Sheet. *A financial report that summarizes an organization's assets, liabilities, and owners' equity. It provides the user with a snapshot of the organization's financial status at a specific point in time.*

Assets. *Items of value owned by a person or business (for example, checking and savings accounts, real estate, inventories, equipment, and so on).*

Liabilities. *Debts or other financial obligations of a business (for example, payroll, rent, invoices owed for goods and services recently purchased, loan or interest payments, and so on).*

consolidated profit and loss statements

Profit and loss statements are useful for businesses that are seeking financing from outside sources. They are also necessary for publicly held companies because the dividends that are paid to stockholders are based on the amount of net profits earned. Sometimes, for reporting purposes, an organization will merge the P&L statements from several years onto one report called a **consolidated profit and loss statement**. This allows interested parties who are reviewing the report to identify trends over time. The outline for a consolidated P&L statement is shown in Figure 15.3. None of the data are new for a report like this one, but are gleaned from earlier reports. It would be equally effective to review the individual report for three consecutive years, though not as efficient to do so.

balance sheet

The **balance sheet** is a financial report that provides the user with a snapshot of the organization's financial status at a specific point in time. It is usually prepared at the end of the fiscal year, but may be prepared at any time during the year that current information on an organization's financial condition is needed. Balance sheets are used for such purposes as obtaining loans, participating in mergers, reporting to stockholders, and for various other legal matters. The basic format of this tool is the listing of all of the **assets** and **liabilities** of an organization. As the name implies, the numbers in this report need to be in balance. This means that assets must equal liabilities.

Like operating statements and P&L statements, the balance sheet is prepared by the accounting department. In smaller organizations that do not have accounting departments, a firm of consulting Certified Public Accountants or an electronic business accounting program may be used to generate it. It is individualized to meet the needs of the organization and the type of business it does. The following section will explain some of the items that are found on balance sheets. The list is not all-inclusive, but illustrative of the kinds of information that are found on this document.

current assets. **Current assets** are those items that are readily available and can be converted into cash as needed. It includes such items as cash on hand and the money in checking and savings accounts. Other current assets include the value of the organization's inventory, both those goods to be used in production and those finished goods that are available to be sold. **Accounts receivable**—the money that is owed to an organization for products that have been delivered and billed—are included in this category. **Prepaid expenses** are also current assets. This includes any item that has been paid in advance, like insurance premiums that are paid once a year for the following year.

fixed assets. This category known as **fixed assets** represents tangible goods that have been capitalized and are being depreciated over time. The value that remains in these

management practice in dietetics

Driftwood Diner Consolidated Profit and Loss Statement			
	2013	**2014**	**2015**
Gross income			
(less sales tax)			
Direct Material			
Beginning inventory			
Cost of goods			
Ending Inventory			
Gross Profit			
Labor			
Salaries			
Taxes and benefits			
Operating Expenses			
Rent			
Utilities			
Maintenance			
Supplies			
Cleaning services			
Interest on credit line			
Depreciation			
Total Expenses			
Operating Profits			
Income Tax			
Net Profit			

Figure 15.3 Format for Consolidated Profit and Loss Statement

items is an asset that is not considered to be a **liquid asset**. This means that it cannot be easily converted into cash. In addition to property and equipment, any improvements that the business has made to rented space, like carpeting, paint, and security systems, fall under this heading. Such leasehold improvements are the property of the building owner at the end of the lease.

other assets. Any other item of value that is held by an organization is listed under other assets. These may include long-term holdings such as bonds, other securities,

Current Assets.
Cash and all assets that are readily available and can be converted to cash within a short period of time (usually one year).

Accounts Receivable. *Money that is owed to a business for products that have been delivered and invoiced.*

Prepaid Expenses.
Expenses that are paid for in advance, such as insurance.

Fixed Assets.
Nonliquid, tangible goods that have been capitalized and are being depreciated over time. Includes land, buildings, equipment, and any improvements like new carpeting, paint jobs, and the installation of security systems.

Liquid Assets.
Items, like inventory, that can easily be converted to cash. See current assets.

Current Liabilities.
Short-term debt that is due to be paid in the near future.

Accounts Payable.
Money that is owed by a business to a creditor for the purchase of products, rent, mortgage payments, and other outstanding loans.

Payroll Liability.
Any salaries and wages that are owed to employees on the day that the balance sheet is prepared.

Accrued Liability.
Expenses for which payment will be made in a future period, such as paid time off and income taxes.

Unearned Revenue.
Liability incurred from the advanced payments for products that have not yet been delivered.

or surplus real estate that cannot be converted into cash at the current time. It can also include funds that have been invested in product development for a product that is not yet ready to be marketed and sold. Finally, it includes the value of intangible assets like name recognition and reputation.

current liabilities. Current liabilities represent the short-term debt of the organization. This includes invoices that are owed for goods and services that have recently been purchased, which are called **accounts payable**. It also includes items such as rent and payments due on mortgages and other outstanding loans. Only the current portion of the mortgage is included here. The balance of the mortgage is considered to be long-term debt.

Any salaries that are owed to employees on the day that the balance sheet is prepared are known as **payroll liability**. It is very unusual for employees to be paid as soon as the work is done. Most are paid on a payroll cycle that is a few days behind the actual work period. For example, if a pay period ends on Friday, the employee may get paid for that week on Wednesday of the following week. Thus, on any given day, the organization has some payroll liability for the workdays that have passed but are not yet paid.

Another type of current liability is called **accrued liability**, which is money owed that will be paid at some time in the future. For example, employees earn and accumulate paid time off during the entire year. However, they are not paid for that time until they actually take a vacation, a holiday, or a sick day. This is an accrued liability because the organization "owes" the pay to the employee but defers paying it until the time off is taken. Income taxes are usually paid at the end of each quarter for the previous quarter. That portion of the tax bill that is owed on the date when the balance sheet is prepared may also be treated as an accrued liability.

The last type of current liability is called **unearned revenue**. It is used for items that have been prepaid but not yet delivered. An example of this is a vending card or a debit card that is used in dining halls on college campuses. Students purchase and pay for a meal plan in advance but consume those meals over time. Until the meals are actually delivered, the value of those transactions is considered to be unearned revenue.

long-term debt. Any debt that will become payable after a year is considered to be **long-term debt**. Such items as mortgages, long-term leases, and warranties on goods sold are included here.

other liabilities. If other liabilities exist and can be reasonably predicted, they would be included here. Items listed here might include post-retirement benefits for employees who used to work for the company or potential liability from pending lawsuits.

ownership equity. It was stated earlier that the balance sheet must be in balance; assets must equal liabilities. However, if the values for the above items were entered into a balance sheet, it is very unlikely that they would be in balance. This is due to the fact that the organization is usually owned by some person, people, or entity whose **ownership equity** also represents a liability to the organization. If there is one owner, the liability is called **owner's equity**. If there is more than one owner, the appropriate term is **stockholders' equity**.

Ownership equity represents the difference between assets and liabilities. It is a number that reflects the risk of ownership. If the organization performs well and the assets are much greater than the liabilities, then the ownership equity is high and the investment of the owner(s) is maximized. If, however, the assets and liabilities are not significantly different, then the ownership equity is low and is of little value to the owner(s).

The owners are the people who assume the majority of the risk. It is their personal investment that will fluctuate, because their claims are subordinate to those of any other creditors in the event of liquidation. This means that when a business goes out of business, everyone else will get paid first. The owner(s) gets whatever is left, which may or may not cover the initial investment that was made. It also means that, when a business is highly successful, the owner(s) has the most to gain.

There are other items that can appear on balance sheets. Most of these refer to publicly held corporations with large numbers of stockholders. These items are beyond the scope of this discussion. A sample balance sheet appears in Figure 15.4.

consolidated balance sheets

For purposes of clarity, it is often useful to prepare a **consolidated balance sheet**, so that this year's data can be compared with that from last year. These documents resemble the consolidated P&L statement, where the information from multiple years is entered on the same report. Consolidated balance sheets are used to document financial conditions over time. They are useful for both internal and external reporting purposes.

All the information contained on these financial reports is useful in managing an organization and can be analyzed to determine the value of the organization, its creditworthiness, whether or not it is a good investment, how it is performing relative to standards, and so on. As managers work with this type of data over time, they become more familiar with different ways of using the information in the reports and with making judgments based on the data found in them. As with other accountability measures, it is useful to have benchmarks against which to measure financial performance, just as it is useful to have benchmark data on productivity and quality.

Long-Term Debt. *Any debt that becomes payable after a year. Includes such items as mortgages, long-term leases, and warranties on goods sold.*

Ownership Equity. *An owner's net investment in a business after providing for full payment of all creditors; the difference between assets and liabilities. When assets are in excess of liabilities by a considerable amount, equity is said to be high. When assets and liabilities are not significantly different, equity is said to be low.*

Owner's Equity. *The term used to describe the ownership equity of a business with only one owner.*

Stockholders' Equity. *The term used to describe the ownership equity of a corporation for which there is more than one owner.*

The Fitness Center
March 31, 20__

ASSETS
Current assets

Checking	$ 12,300	
Savings	32,000	
Accounts receivable	6,250	
Inventory	1,200	
Prepaid expenses	5,875	
		$ 57,625

Fixed assets

Leasehold improvements	4,500	
Equipment	175,000	
		179,500

TOTAL ASSETS — $237,125

LIABILITIES
Current liabilities

Accounts payable	$ 1,700	
Payroll liabilities	8,783	
Accrued liability	11,947	
Unearned revenue	26,790	
		$ 49,220

Long-term debt

Loan (for equipment)	90,200	
		90,200

OWNERSHIP EQUITY 97,705

TOTAL LIABILITY AND EQUITY $237,125

Figure 15.4. Sample Balance Sheet

Finally, it should be noted that dietetics professionals are not expected to come into management positions as expert financial managers. There is a learning curve that comes with experience. Reading books or taking courses in those aspects of financial management that are used in the work setting can enhance knowledge of these concepts. It is also helpful to utilize the services of accountants and financial managers to help with the learning process. These individuals have much information to share and can help the beginning manager to see things from a different perspective. They can also help the manager to avoid some very costly mistakes.

conclusion

This chapter has introduced several aspects of financial management for dietetics professionals with management responsibilities. The topics that have been presented include the concepts listed below.

1. Money is vulnerable in any cash-based retail operation. A system of checks and balances must be put into place to account for and secure this asset and the personnel who handle it.
2. Cost control is a part of every manager's responsibility and can be implemented in many areas, including procurement, production, facilities and maintenance, labor management, and so on.
3. Operating statements and variance analysis are the tools that individual managers use to measure their performance in financial terms.
4. Profit and loss statements are tools that are used to show how an organization is performing financially.
5. Balance sheets provide a snapshot of an organization's financial standing. They balance the assets and liabilities of an organization with ownership equity.

activities

activity 1

You are the head cashier for the foodservice for homecoming weekend at your college or university. Your job includes the following:

- Arrange to have $3,575.00 in change prior to the event. This is to include:

50 rolls of nickels	$ 100.00
15 rolls of dimes	$ 75.00
40 rolls of quarters	$ 400.00
1,000 $1 bills	$1,000.00
200 $5 bills	$1,000.00
100 $10 bills	$1,000.00

- Arrange to have a two-part carbonless cash receipt book.
- Issue nine cashier bags (banks) of $300.00 each.
- Pick up keys to the safe from your manager at the beginning of the day.
- Check in at each of the two indoor and five outdoor cash registers every 30 minutes to ensure that each of the 7 cashiers has adequate change.
- Pull cash from each register when it exceeds $500.00; a minimum of $200.00 should be taken at each "pull."
- Whenever you pull cash, provide the cashier with a receipt indicating the amount of the pull, the name of the cashier, the time, and today's date. Both you and the cashier must sign the receipt. The original receipt stays in the receipt book; the duplicate goes to the cashier.
- Both parts of the voided receipts stay in the receipt book.
- At the end of the event, conduct a normal closing and place the money and the cashier balance sheets in the safe. Deposit the safe keys in the lock box for your manager to pick up in the morning.

Please answer the following questions.

1. Why are there nine banks when there are only seven cash registers?
2. How many of each type of coin and currency should go in each bank?
3. Why are there no pennies?
4. If the total needed for the banks is $2,700.00, why is the total cash on hand $3,575.00?
5. Identify two reasons the head cashier must visit each register every 30 minutes.
6. What is the purpose of having the receipts sighed by both you and the cashier?
7. Why are duplicate receipts kept?
8. Describe what you think the process of "normal closing" should be.

activity 2

Using the budget that you wrote for the previous chapter, prepare an operating statement that compares actual spending to budgeted spending for the past month. Write a variance analysis for any item that was over or under budget by 5 percent or more, explaining why the variance occurred.

activity 3

Create a profit and loss statement for yourself or your family for a month. Consider that your earnings, allowances, money from loans, and so on all represent revenues. All costs that you incurred should be listed as expenses, whether you actually paid for them or charged them to a credit card. Compute your profit (excess of revenues over expenses) or loss (excess of expenses over revenues) for the month.

activity 4

Looking at the operating statement and P&L statement you have made for the preceding two exercises, state five ways you could control your expenditures in the coming month.

activity 5

Prepare a balance sheet on yourself or your family, including all assets (such as cars, clothing, books, furniture, and so on) that you own and all liabilities that you have incurred (like loans, debts, and outstanding bills). Do your assets exceed your liabilities? When doing a personal balance sheet, note that ownership equity is known as net worth.

to study further

- Dittmer, P. R. and J. D. Keefe. *Principles of Food Beverage, and Labor Cost Controls.* 9th ed. Hoboken, NJ: John Wiley & Sons, Inc., 2009.
- Dopson, L. R. and D. K. Hayes. *Food and Beverage Cost Control.* 5th ed. Hoboken, NJ: John Wiley and Sons, Inc., 2011.
- Fields, E. *The Essentials of Finance and Accounting for Nonfinancial Managers.* 2nd ed. New York: AMACOM, 2011.
- Hopkin, P. *Fundamentals of Risk Management: Understanding, Evaluating and Implementing Effective Risk Management.* 2nd ed. Philadelphia: Kogan Page, 2012.
- Ormiston, A. and L. M. Fraser. *Understanding Financial Statements.* 10th ed. New York: Pearson Education, 2013.
- Schoenebeck, K. P. and M. P. Holtzman. *Interpreting and Analyzing Financial Statements: A Project-Based Approach.* 6th ed. Upper Saddle River, NJ: Prentice Hall, 2012.
- Stickney, C. P., P. R. Brown, and J. H. Wahlen. *Financial Reporting and Statement Analysis: A Strategic Perspective.* 6th ed. Mason, OH: Thomson South-Western, 2007.
- Vaughan, E. J. and T. M. Vaughan. *Fundamentals of Risk and Insurance.* 10th ed. New York: John Wiley & Sons, Inc., 2008.

scholarly journal

- *Journal of Healthcare Risk Management*

other relevant periodical

- *Healthcare Risk Management*

relevant websites

- Links to business journals and management magazines http://www.brint.com/magazine.htm#ISJbus
- Business Owner's Toolkit: Finance http://www.bizfilings.com/toolkit/sbg/finance.aspx
- Practical Risk Management http://www.pracrisk.com/

in practice

risk management on a personal level

One of the topics that was included in this chapter was risk management. It was described as minimizing the liability of an organization in areas such as work-related illness, job-induced injury or stress, and products whose performance fails to meet set standards. But dietetics professionals also need to be concerned about risk management on a more personal level. Specifically, what are the financial risks to an individual practicing in the profession and what, if anything, can be done to minimize those risks?

The first line of defense is to ensure that you are performing responsibly, in accordance with current best practices for the profession. In other words, you need to be accountable for your own performance and for remaining current in the field of nutrition, clinical nutrition, foodservice, or any other area of practice in which you work. (See the Code of Ethics for the Profession of Dietetics at the end of Chapter 1.) Maintaining competence is probably the best way to avoid being sued for malpractice.

Nevertheless, there is no guarantee that you will never be sued during your professional career, even if you are competent and ethical. In the litigious environment in North America, lawsuits (sometimes frivolous, sometimes not) are commonplace. Therefore, it is essential that professionals have adequate insurance coverage to protect themselves from financial loss in the event of such a lawsuit.

Frequently, dietetic education programs require their students to purchase liability insurance. This protects both the students and the program from risk if the student is named in a lawsuit. The cost of such student insurance is nominal. If your accredited dietetics program requires you to purchase this type of insurance, the requirement is disclosed as part of the information provided to prospective and to current students.

Often employers like healthcare facilities carry a blanket malpractice insurance policy that covers the institution and the employees who work there. Sometimes this is enough to protect you in your role as dietitian or dietetic technician. It is, however, your responsibility to determine if you are covered by your employer and what the limits of liability are. It is also up to you to evaluate the coverage and decide whether or not you feel it is sufficient protection for you. For example, if your employer covers you for $10,000 and you routinely deal with high-risk neonates in an intensive-care nursery, the coverage may not be enough. Similarly, this is probably not enough coverage for a professional who runs a major foodservice operation where there is always some risk of an outbreak of foodborne illness.

Even when your employer provides adequate coverage for you, it probably protects only you when you are performing your job. It is unlikely that it will protect you if you are moonlighting, making a presentation to a community group, or consulting. Theoretically, you could even be sued by a seat mate on an airplane or a casual acquaintance at a party if you promote yourself as a nutrition professional and then offer advice about food and/or nutrition. If you engage in such activities, it is prudent to consider purchasing malpractice insurance as a way to protect yourself from the financial risk associated with this type of activity.

The cost of malpractice insurance for dietetics professionals is not prohibitive. This is due to the fact that the relative risk for the profession is not high, especially as it compares to medical malpractice insurance for physicians. Nutrition professionals are not sued as frequently as physicians are, which helps keeps the costs moderate. Also, nutrition professionals can purchase different types of policies, depending on the number of hours they work and the type of work that they do. Malpractice insurance is not a "one size fits all" kind of coverage; you have the latitude to determine the extent of the coverage you need.

One particular practice setting where it is always prudent to carry professional liability insurance is in skilled nursing facilities. With the passage of laws relative to elder abuse, the aging of the population, and the prevalence of facility-acquired bedsores in some settings, litigation is on the rise. Nutrition professionals are particularly vulnerable because of the relationship between nutrition and decubitus ulcers. They are also vulnerable because some skilled nursing facilities fund only minimum consultant dietitian hours, which may not be sufficient to cover the work that needs to be done. If this is the case, the dietitian may be doubly liable because she agreed to work for the facility knowing that the hours were inadequate.

In conclusion, note that your responsibility as a dietetic professional is to ensure that you are covered by adequate liability insurance. If this is not the case, it is your responsibility to determine what additional insurance is needed and purchase it for yourself. It is even more important for independent contractors and consultants to maintain their own personal coverage, since they have no employer coverage at all. Hopefully, you will never need to use the benefits such insurance provides, but if you do, the cost benefit of having the coverage will become evident both in financial and in human terms.

references

1. Reich, Robert. "Why Cash Is Losing Its Currency." *CBS Sunday Morning*. March 25th, 2012. http://www.cbsnews.com/8301-3445_162-57404086/why-cash-is-losing-its-currency/. Accessed September 11, 2012.
2. Wolman, David. *The End of Money: Counterfeiters, Preachers, Techies, Dreamers—and the Coming Cashless Society*. Boston: Da Capo Press, 2012.

part six

new directions in management

The final part of this text deals with emerging management issues. These include the management of information, the application of the principles of sustainability, and the management of change. Though these topics are not new, conceptually, there is an emerging sense of urgency in dealing with these issues. Information is available in exponentially larger amounts than it has ever been, and needs to be handled effectively, so as to be useful without being overwhelming. Sustainability efforts must be implemented now in order for the planet to continue to support the population. Change is occurring at a faster pace than was anticipated. All of these developments are due, largely, to advances in science and in technology.

As technology improves, managers are faced with both too much and too little information. They must manage information as they manage time, material, money, or other resources, using the available technology to ensure that the flow of information is an asset rather than a burden. Managers must understand that, though they cannot control all of the information that is available, they can choose to direct or to limit the kind and amount of information that they access in order to support them in their roles as managers.

Sustainability impacts all aspects of life, from the conservation of energy and water resources to the use of land, from animal welfare to the diversion of waste from landfills. Science and technology have joined forces to enable us to move forward with efforts to recycle and reuse materials that were discarded only a few years ago. We can and must reduce our carbon footprint while ensuring social justice for workers, here and abroad.

Because of the increasing availability of information and the extraordinary progress being made in the sciences, organizations have to change more rapidly than ever before. Change has become a constant that must also be managed and controlled.

Part VI provides the reader with some insight into what is now happening and what is projected to occur in management in the near future. Since change is not wholly predictable, perhaps the best way to deal with the uncertainty of the future is to view it as an opportunity rather than as a barrier.

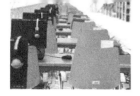

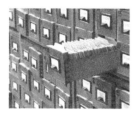

chapter sixteen

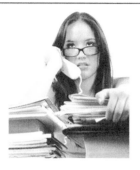

information management

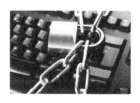

learning objectives

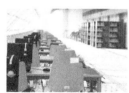

1. State why it is necessary for organizations to manage information.

2. Define *information management* and *informatics*.

3. Differentiate between information management and informatics.

4. State the difference between intrinsic and extrinsic information.

5. Discuss the different ways dietetics professionals and managers use information.

6. Describe how information overload and information shortage can coexist.

7. State why information systems need standardization.

8. Differentiate between internal and external information.

9. Discuss security issues related to information systems.

10. List the types of information processing systems designed specifically for dietetics professionals.

11. Describe how to determine what kind of information system an organization needs.

12. Discuss the process of bringing a new computer system on-line.

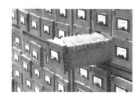

overview

Until the beginning of the twentieth century, the main way that information got exchanged was either through word of mouth or through print. There were books (first handwritten, then printed), newspapers, and magazines to record information and opinion and to transmit it from the writer to the reader. The typewriter sped the process along but had significant limitations in that it could make only a few copies at a time. This was followed by the broadcast media, which revolutionized word-of-mouth dissemination of information. The print media was enhanced by copiers, followed by word processors, desktop computers, and networked computers so that information generated in one place can be transmitted instantaneously around the world. Data are available digitally, so they can be accessed, read, manipulated, stored, transmitted, and received without ever being printed. Information technology has created an explosion in the amount of data and information that are available today, both to organizations and to individuals.

The information superhighway is here to stay, and the amount of information available will grow exponentially as the space required to generate, store, and transmit this information gets smaller and smaller. There is already more information available than any person can hope to sort through in a lifetime. Some of it is cataloged and accessible to those who want it. Other information is more obscure, so that finding it requires the assistance of a trained specialist, like a librarian. Then there is the rest of the information—it exists, but it either is not generally accessible or it cannot be used in the form that is available. The proliferation of information has effectively hidden a lot of meaningful data in a growing volume of irrelevancy.

Information management is an area of management that includes "the planning, budgeting, control and exploiting of the information resources of an organization."[1] It is a relatively new discipline, a specialty within management, just as is marketing or finance. Information management is not to be confused with **informatics**, which is the science of information, which "studies the representation, processing, and communication in natural and artificial systems."[2] In 2007, the American Dietetic Association's Nutrition Informatics Work Group defined **nutrition informatics** as "The effective retrieval, organization, storage and optimum use of information, data, and knowledge for food and nutrition related problem solving and decision making. Informatics is supported by the use of information standards, information processes and information technology."[3] An in-depth study of nutrition informatics is beyond the scope of this management text for dietetics professionals. However, some aspects of information management are necessary for any manager to know. This chapter will provide an overview of information management that can be applied in dietetics practice and dietetics management.

The basic topics to be covered include the types of information that are processed, uses for that information, information overload, and information shortages. This will

---

Information Management (IM). *An area of management that includes "the planning, budgeting, control and exploiting of the information resources of an organisation."*

Informatics. *The science of information, which "studies the representation, processing, and communication in natural and artificial systems."*

Nutrition Informatics. *"The effective retrieval, organization, storage and optimum use of information, data, and knowledge for food and nutrition related problem solving and decision making. Informatics is supported by the use of information standards, information processes and information technology."*

---

be followed by a discussion of techniques for managing information, including standardization, data storage, and movement of data from place to place. The issues of access to information and security of data within an organization are also addressed, with consideration given to the Internet. Finally, there will be a discussion of the types of systems that are designed for nutrition professionals, and some considerations for implementing these systems.

availability of information

To begin to make some sense of the many information resources that are available to dietetics professionals, it is first necessary to establish a basic understanding of some of the terminology used when discussing information technology (IT). It is necessary to differentiate between the types of information and how it is used by information processing systems. Though it is not possible to enumerate all of the uses for the information generated by these systems, some common uses are listed. The potential for and consequences of information overload and information shortages are also identified.

types of information

In general, two types of information are handled by information technology systems. The first is called **intrinsic information**.[4] It is the actual information that is processed. Intrinsic information includes the data that enter the system (input) and the data that are produced by the system (output). In general, intrinsic information does not require the use of high-tech systems to be processed. People can process it manually and have done so for years. There are several reasons that these tasks have been transferred to automated systems, though. The compelling reasons are that transactions can be processed more rapidly, there is a greater degree of control, and the chance for error is minimized.

Among the more sophisticated information handling systems in use today are those in libraries, where a student or other user can enter a subject, an author, or a title (input) and retrieve a list of references (output) within seconds. Though this type of transaction can still be done manually, it is no longer necessary to do so. In fact, the manual process is so cumbersome that traditional "card catalogues" have disappeared from many libraries. Print versions of book titles or journal articles have been replaced with searchable electronic files.

Search engines on the Internet perform a similar function. They allow the user to enter a topic of interest and quickly retrieve links to related websites. Unfortunately, not all of the searches lead to reputable Internet sites, so it becomes the searcher's responsibility to determine the reliability of the site, which may or may not be trustworthy. As an

Intrinsic Information. *Information that is processed; it includes the data that are entered into the system (input) as well as the data that are produced by the system (output).*

Search Engines. *An Internet tool that allows you to do keyword searches for information. Examples include Google, Yahoo!, Lycos, Ask, Metacrawler, and others.*

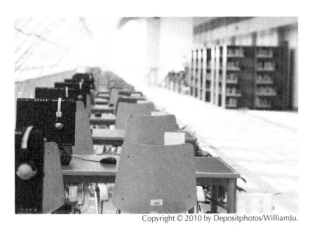

Copyright © 2010 by Depositphotos/WilliamJu.

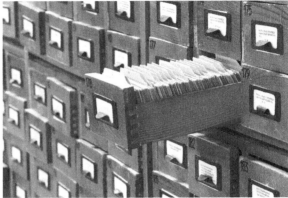

Copyright © 2011 by Depositphotos/Andrey Kuzmin.

Online catalogs have replaced card catalogs in libraries.

Extrinsic Information. *Information that is stored in a computer system for the purpose of processing intrinsic information. It includes the database and the program that contains necessary information for carrying out the actual processing.*

Database. *A set of related information that is organized and stored in a computer for access and is usually associated with software applications.*

Program. *The set of instructions that a computer follows when processing information. A program utilizes information from a database to transform input into output.*

example, questionable information is rampant on sites that provide information on botanicals and other nutritional supplements. In this case, valid information is likely to be housed on websites from educational (.edu) and governmental (.gov) sites. Sites that are in the business of selling products often offer less-objective information. Many college and university libraries offer guidance for judging the quality of Internet sources.

In dietetics practice, there are many transactions that rely on information technology. A few of many possible examples follow. Diet clerks enter a diet order, food allergies, and other patient information into a departmental computer system that produces a meal ticket for that patient. A dietitian inputs records from a food diary into a nutrient-analysis program at a health fair and produces a profile of the nutrients consumed relative to recommended values. Client information entered into a computer at a WIC clinic determines eligibility and enrolls families in the program. In foodservice, data about delivery, cost, and usage of goods are entered to generate perpetual inventory reports, production sheets, recipes, purchase orders, and so on.

Extrinsic information[5] is information that is stored in the system for the purpose of processing the intrinsic information. Extrinsic information includes both the **database** and the information needed to do the actual processing—that is, the **program**. The food list and nutrient database in a nutrient analysis program are examples of extrinsic information. They are there so that a nutrient analysis can be calculated from a list of foods consumed. In essence, the program utilizes the information in the database to transform the input into output. This system is used much the same way as raw ingredients (input) are processed by a cook (program) who uses recipes (database) to produce a meal (output).

It is necessary to differentiate between intrinsic and extrinsic information because, when information systems fail to produce the desired results, it is generally a result of faulty intrinsic data. For example, when foodservice computers fail to forecast

management practice in dietetics

food production needs accurately, it is frequently because data on previous usage were not entered or were not accurate. Inaccurate nutrient analyses can almost always be traced back to **input errors**. During the initial installation of a new information handling system, there may be problems with the hardware, the software, or other extrinsic information. However, once the bugs have been eliminated, it is the intrinsic data that determine the quality and reliability of the output, relative to system constraints.

use of information

Information, as a stand-alone entity, has very little value. The real value in information comes from using it.[6] It is people who access and use the information who determine its worth. For example, an article in a medical journal that describes a new method for performing liver transplant surgery is of no value to the teenager who is choosing an outfit to wear to a dance, but is of great importance to a surgeon who performs the procedure regularly. For the information to be of value, someone must choose to obtain and use the information.

An ever-increasing amount of information is available for people to use. It is generated automatically by today's information management systems. This means that the potential uses for information have also grown. All that is needed is someone who chooses to use the available information. In addition to completing transactions with accuracy and speed, information systems can produce reports that are used for quality management and benchmarking purposes. The information can also be used to manage finances, monitor productivity, control inventory levels, trigger orders for raw materials, issue invoices, pay bills, monitor safety in the workplace, track paid time off, issue paychecks, and many other tasks. Programs are available to support the decision-making process. The potential uses for information are limited only by the ingenuity of human beings.

When a new information processing system is introduced, it takes time for users to become familiar with both the functionality of the software and the format of the reports that are generated. Typically, individuals seek to use the functions that they have used in the past, and look for the kinds of information that they are familiar with. In many cases, new functions are ignored and additional data are overlooked for a period of time. It is advisable to review, periodically, the types of information that a system is able to generate. Such a review will help identify new ways for the program to generate additional data. For example, a detailed analysis of overtime may not have been necessary in the past, when there were plenty of resources to cover the costs. However, in an economic downturn, when every dollar spent must be justified, the analysis and control of overtime are imperative. The analysis will be easier if information can be retrieved (for example, from the payroll department's existing records) rather than having to be collected in the future.

Input Errors. *Errors that occur while entering data (intrinsic information) into a system that often account for the failure of information systems to produce the desired results.*

information overload

Information overload is the condition of having too much data available. This can actually slow down processes and interfere with getting things done. Information overload, for example, can give market researchers more information than they need to know about all segments of a population, when all they really need to know are the characteristics of a target market. Too much information about the alternatives available will slow the decision-making process on items of critical importance. Considering both internal sources like organization-wide computer systems, and external sources like the Internet, managers can easily get buried in too much data.

At some point, a manager must determine just what information is actually needed to complete a job. From then on, the extraneous information must be considered an added benefit that can be accessed and used if time permits. People learn their physical limits and are able to say no when asked to do something beyond their capacities (like being in two places at one time). Likewise, managers need to be able to set limits on the amount and kind of information they will utilize. The limits need to be set with knowledge of the value of the information in the current situation.

The operative words are *current situation*. Information needs must be reassessed and reconfigured in reaction to (or in anticipation of) a changing environment. It is a mistake for any manager to choose a set of data or an information source and rely solely on that information for extended periods of time. Requirements in both the kind of information and the amount needed change over time.

information shortage

Information Shortages. *The condition that exists when data are deficient or when not enough information is available to get a job completed.*

Sometimes, despite the availability of massive amounts of information, there are **information shortages**. This may occur, for example, when a manager wants to extend a clinic's operation beyond 9:00 a.m. to 5:00 p.m., Monday through Friday. The manager feels that there are adequate clients to warrant increased service hours, because the waiting list for clinic appointments is long. Evening hours are judged to be good because many clients are employed, as determined by insurance data. However, there are no data available on what hours clients actually work, and whether or not they will be too tired in the evening to go to a clinic. In addition, it is not known if clients would prefer weekend hours or evening hours. Despite all the data that are available, there are no data to answer the question at hand. The datum either does not exist or exists in an inaccessible form, so new data are needed before a decision can be made.

It is relatively easy to use information technology to gather data that are needed now or anticipated to be needed in the future. However, this should not happen without some thought and effort put into selecting the data that are needed, and how they are

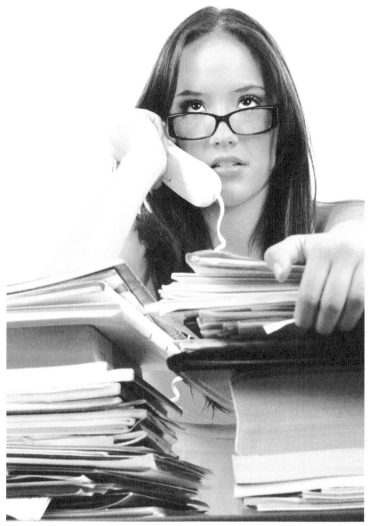

Copyright © 2011 by Depositphotos/David Castillo Dominici.

Sometimes a critical piece of information gets lost in the piles of data generated by today's information systems.

to be gathered. Clients can be given a questionnaire or asked some questions when they visit the clinic. **Online survey tools** can be used to contact clients at home and these make data collection very easy. In the clinic example mentioned, a detailed series of questions about each client's job, physical exertion level at work, working hours, days of the week worked, and distance between work and the clinic, could be asked to determine what additional hours the clinic should be open. On the other hand, it might be best to ask only a few close-ended questions like, "If necessary, could you come to the clinic between 6 and 8 p.m. on Mondays and Wednesdays?" and "If necessary, could you come to the clinic on Saturdays?" Since surveys that are clear and concise generate more useful responses than those that are too long or

Online Survey Tool. *An Internet tool that allows for the administration of online surveys. Examples include SurveyMonkey, SurveyGizmo, Kwiksurveys, and others.*

too complicated, care should be taken in writing the surveys. In this case, the latter example is probably the better choice.

Future information needs must be anticipated so that the system can capture information before it is needed without being burdensome to the respondent. However, it should be noted that the use of surveys generates even more data, which can contribute to the ongoing cycle of information overload.

information in an organization

Information systems in organizations evolved in a fairly haphazard manner and are continually changing as new information technology becomes available. Initially, there were data processing systems established to handle various individual functions in an organization—for example, word processing, accounts receivable, medical records, or payroll. Usually, individuals with knowledge in a particular specialty area managed these systems. Information systems were overseen by clerical, accounting, medical records, or payroll staff, independent of one another. Each may have had a system that worked in a given department, but these early data processing systems seldom communicated with each other.

As time passed and the complexity of information technology expanded, it became obvious that large organizations needed to consolidate the management of these functions in one place. During the 1970s and 1980s information management (IM) as a management discipline began to emerge, and the demand for IM managers far exceeded the supply. Therefore, people with any computer experience, either hardware- or software-related, were recruited to manage the new departments. Often these individuals had little or no management training or skills. For some organizations, the internal systems grew randomly, in a reactive fashion, rather than as a planned series of events. Frequently, the organization selected systems based on availability, without ever considering the organization's long-term goals. This was not due to poor management. Much of the problem centered on the rapid expansion of technology and the reality that products sometimes were eclipsed by newer versions before they were fully implemented.

Today, IM departments are likely to be directed by managers in staff positions. They report directly to the upper management of an organization. IM departments are charged with maintaining the various systems that exist in an organization, and with coordinating, standardizing, and controlling those systems throughout the organization. This includes training staff from all areas of the organization and providing support materials to users. Anything that other departmental managers choose to do with the information technology in their respective departments must be coordinated through the IM department, because it is ultimately IM's job to manage information flow within and between departments. In some situations, the IM department is required to deal with making older systems communicate with newer ones.

standardization

Organizations need to consider some degree of **standardization** concerning how they handle their information. In the past, this meant that the computers all had to be of the same basic type and the software written in the same programming language. This is no longer true because many of today's technologies allow for data transfer between systems. The critical factor is that computers and workstations are compatible enough to communicate with one another, through a **local area network (LAN)**, an organizational **intranet**, a server, or over the Internet.

One result of the indiscriminate addition of data processing programs over the years was that the various computer systems and software packages did not communicate with one another. Several classic examples exist in healthcare foodservices. Some sophisticated programs became available to manage onsite foodservices in the late 1980s. (Forerunners of these systems have been in use since the 1960s.) Unfortunately, they were self-contained packages that did not "talk to" the other systems that existed in the facility. For example, diet orders that came from nursing on the patient information system had to be retrieved by a diet clerk and reentered into the departmental system in order to generate menus, meal tickets, and nutrition-screening profiles. Perpetual inventory programs generated lists of products to be purchased, but those data had to be manually entered into the order-entry system for the prime vendor. The accounting department could not pay invoices until someone entered the data from the purchasing program into the organization's accounting system. Clinical dietitians had to input data twice, once to the accounts receivable system to generate a bill, and a second time to the departmental system to generate productivity figures.

Now technology exists to facilitate communication between systems that were once considered to be incompatible. In some cases, it is relatively simple to accomplish the task; in others, it is prohibitively expensive. It is likely that the incompatibility problem will eventually cease to exist. However, for the time being, some institutions still have some mismatched information handling systems and have to use manual approaches to solve the problems that the inconsistency creates. Most organizations cannot afford to revamp entire systems at once, so that an integrated plan often takes a long time to implement. Some organizations will find it necessary to live with what they have, at least for a while longer. (Please see the "In Practice" feature at the end of this chapter to read about how a fully integrated system might work.)

Other than the ability of computers to communicate with each other, there are several additional standardization issues to consider. One is that the word processing,

Standardization. *To make common or compatible.*

Local Area Network (LAN). *A type of data communications network in which a group of computers are interconnected in a small geographic area such as adjacent buildings.*

Intranet. *An organization's internal communications system, available for sharing information within the organization, but not accessible to the public.*

Spreadsheet. *A tool that allows input of numerical data into rows and columns for computation and analysis.*

spreadsheet, graphics, and presentation software should be institutionalized wherever possible. This means that departments should use the same programs for similar functions. Word processing, for example, might be standardized on WordPerfect or Microsoft Word. Lotus 1-2-3 and Excel are commonly used **spreadsheet** programs. The use of universal software within an organization simplifies the transfer of information between computers and among individuals. It also means that workers can transfer from one job to another within an organization without having to learn new software programs.

Another area that requires standardization is how files are named and stored. Items that are kept in the form of data files (rather than as hard copy) need to be retrievable, just as are medical records, cash register tapes, X-rays, and invoices. Organizations should have a systematic method for identifying data files so that the information can be stored and retrieved by many individuals, not just one or two. The standard method used should be enforced for anything that is put into an **archive**. Some organizations require that all employees use the standard system for items stored in personal computers, too. This allows others to access data in the event of one employee's absence. The business forms that are used within an organization can easily be transmitted electronically to the desktop units of staff members. To simplify this, the format should be consistent from form to form. All personnel forms, accounting forms, billing forms, payroll reports, and so on should be similar in format to facilitate an employee's use of each. They should be created on the same software, and all staff should receive training on how to use the software efficiently and effectively. When forms (or other documents, for that matter) require that they not be substantially altered, they should be converted to portable document format (.pdf) so that the person who downloads the document is unable to alter it, except for filling in requisite fields, as necessary.

Archive. *Stored information.*

As the profession of dietetics evolved, one thing that did not happen was the development of a standardized language for the profession. Clinical dietitians tended to think in medical terms, rather than in terms that were germane to the field of nutrition and dietetics. This all changed with the implementation of the nutrition care process[7] and the development of International Dietetics and Nutrition Terminology.[8] As these come into widespread use, it becomes possible to search for specific terms and measure outcomes for particular nutrition diagnoses and interventions.

All of these standardization practices should be institutionalized in the form of policies and procedures. Standards for compliance need to be established and routine audits conducted to determine if the standards are being met.

The IM department is accountable for the flow of information within an organization, just as any other department is accountable for its work. Quality, quantity, and outcomes are needed to measure and compare IM's performance to internal and external benchmarks.

information flow

Within organizations, information flows in many different directions. It always has, even though most official communication used to flow vertically. In recent years, the traditional flow of information upward and downward through an organization has eroded significantly. Even without information processing technology, the flattening of organizations and the empowerment of lower-level employees have increased information sharing. There is much less hoarding of information at the top of the hierarchy than there was in the past. Most managers have learned the value of sharing information, though some still cling to the notion that information is power, so they tend to share only that information that they are required to share.

Greater changes are on the horizon now that information can move in all directions very quickly. Layers of management can be bypassed through the use of e-mail and wide-reaching distribution lists. Frontline workers are able to e-mail the CEO and vice versa. Computer systems in one department are communicating with those in other departments and breaking down barriers that used to exist, both vertically and horizontally, within organizations. It is appropriate to take advantage of this increased information flow to improve performance, but it is also necessary to ensure that direct person-to-person communication does not get lost.

internal information. Some of the information that organizations generate is for internal use only. This information is found on the organization's intranet, which is protected by a **firewall** so that it cannot be penetrated from the outside. In business organizations, this includes information related to personnel, strategic plans, financial performance, product development, and so on.

In health care, **patient information systems** have been used for quite some time to process patient information such as height, weight, diagnosis, orders, and test results. A relatively recent development is the **electronic health record (EHR)**, which centralizes most of the health/medical data on individual patients in electronic documents that can be accessed by authorized personnel. At the moment, this information is usually available within a single institution or in a group of associated facilities, like Kaiser Permanente. The development of the EHR is paralleling the dietetic profession's implementation of the nutrition-care process and standardized language. When both are fully operational, the profession will have the information needed to establish the effectiveness of nutritional care.

It is anticipated that, in the future, this information will be available to most facilities in North America, once systems are in place to guarantee the security of personal information. Patient information is protected by law under the **Health Insurance Portability and Accountability Act (HIPPA)**, which was passed in the United States in 1996. Similar legislation has been enacted in Canada. Access to EHRs must be tightly controlled to maintain client confidentiality.

Firewall. *Software that protects a private network or organizational intranet from outside penetration.*

Patient Information Systems. *The management information system that is used for the processing of some patient information (patient records, orders, laboratory tests, and billing and financial information) in health care facilities.*

Electronic Health Record (EHR). *Computer-based electronic data processing and storage of complete client/patient records that eliminates the need for hard copies of these documents.*

Healthcare Insurance Portability and Accountability Act. *http://www.hhs.gov/ocr/privacy/*

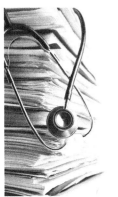

*Soon paper medical
records will be replaced
entirely by EHRs.*

external information. Organizations need to exchange information with the outside, too. The Internet is a major marketing tool for many organizations. Even the smallest mom-and-pop shops and restaurants now have their own websites. Consumers seek information about governmental programs, professional organizations, health care, schools, and other services by accessing the web using computers, netbooks, tablets, and smartphones. Not only is it essential to have a website, but that website also needs to be comprehensive and easy to navigate, so that consumers can find the information that they seek with relative ease.

Use of the Internet in the workplace is an area that can be either useful or detrimental to an organization. Many organizations need to give employees access to the Internet. For example, information on evidence-based practice guidelines is available from the Academy's Evidence Analysis Library. The Food Code is available on the FDA website. These and other professional resources are not generally available on a hospital's intranet, so it is essential for some individuals to have access to this information. On the other hand, Internet access has so many possible applications that giving free access to employees may be the equivalent of giving them license to use the system for personal purposes. It is not uncommon for an employee to perform such tasks as banking, shopping, and following social media from business computers.

If there is concern that employees are abusing the privilege or "surfing the net" when they should be working, some organizations put constraints into place to monitor Internet usage or to disallow access to specific websites. Other organizations prefer to measure productivity, instead of imposing restrictions. Essentially, this latter approach takes the perspective that, as long as the work gets done, the organization does not need to serve as police. It is an approach that is likely to gain more universal acceptance with the growth of telecommuting. As more and more employees work out of their homes, the trend will be toward measuring the work that has been accomplished rather than measuring the time spent doing that work.

A note of caution … information that is posted in the Internet can take on a life of its own, and once posted, it is difficult to retract. Though social media sites and blogs are useful and fun, they can also be a source of embarrassment if questionable posts or uncomplimentary photos are posted. Dietetics professionals need to be concerned about what is posted about them, since colleagues, clients/patients, and employers all use these sites, too.

security

When both internal and external information systems exist within an organization, some care must be taken to limit the flow of information between the two. It would be embarrassing (or disastrous), for example, if internal memos, balance sheets, or patient records were inadvertently available to the public through the Internet because of unlimited communication between systems. The IM department is responsible for the security of information, as well as its movement. This is accomplished by using a variety of tools available to IM engineers. The technology related to security for information systems is changing rapidly.

A system that is widely used for maintaining the security of information systems is a password, or the combination of a **log-on** identification and a password or passphrase. These methods are used to identify the user to the computer system. The system then "knows" what information the

Copyright © 2011 by Depositphotos/Vladimir Yudin.

individual is permitted to access and allows that individual only into those particular files. The system also controls who is able to enter or manipulate data. For example, a diet clerk in a health care facility should be able to retrieve diet orders, but not to enter them, because this is a responsibility of nursing personnel.

Though IM is responsible for the security system, overall, individual managers are responsible for seeing that the security guidelines are followed. It is imperative that employees understand the reason for having passwords, and the risks involved when the information system is not protected. Staff should not share passwords. Instead, individual passwords should be issued to new employees as soon as they are trained on the system.

Individual employees should log on to the system as required, and be sure to log off when they leave their workstations, so that the system remains protected. That minimizes the risk of unauthorized use. When security problems occur, IM needs to be able to identify who was on-line at the time in order to troubleshoot and take corrective action. If employees fail to identify themselves as a user, then this datum cannot be tracked. The sharing of information about passwords and entry codes can lead to breaches in security. As a result, it may be necessary for every user of the system to set up a new entry routine. This is a costly and time-consuming process that leads to inefficiency and frustration on the part of all those concerned. It is usually preventable by a little education and training.

Telecommuting is based on accessing the organization's information system from outside the organization. It is necessary for individuals who work from home or while traveling. This requires a different and more sophisticated type of security system to protect data. Redundancies are necessary for persons who need access to the organization's intranet from the Internet, since this type of access is particularly vulnerable to security breaches.

Systems must be in place to ensure the security of proprietary or personal information.

Log-on. *To start a session with a system by giving a user name and password as a means of user identification and authentication.*

Telecommuting. *To access the intranet of an organization from a remote computer.*

manuals

From the user's perspective, one of the most important functions of IM is training personnel on the use of the systems. Initial hands-on training is done organization-wide before a new system becomes operational. Sometimes formalized training on the computer systems is part of the new employee's orientation program. At other times, an experienced user teaches the new user how to operate the computer terminal to get the desired results. Though the training is important, it usually provides only the basic knowledge to the new user. As that individual gets more and more experience with the equipment and the program, more options become available.

User Manuals.
Online publications made available to employees in an organization for the purpose of communicating to them such information about how to operate and use equipment, programs, and information systems.

User manuals are one of the best ways to get the information out of the IM department and into the hands of staff. A well-written manual will be consulted frequently and will save many calls to the IM department. This, in turn, increases IM's efficiency and allows IM staff to concentrate on their work without unnecessary interruption. IM manuals should be available online, and should be written in simple language that can be understood by most readers. The directions on how to carry out a function should assume that the user has little knowledge of computers. Steps should be specified in detail and accompanied by screen shots so that nearly everyone will be able to follow them. Most importantly, user manuals should have a comprehensive, searchable index for locating information.

For internal systems, user manuals are normally customized for the facility or organization. The programs that organizations install control how specific tasks are to be done in that organization. For example, the types of passwords that are acceptable, the way an order is entered, the commands for printing, and so on are tailored to the setting. The manuals need to reflect any customization that was done to the software. This is relatively easy to accomplish by using a generic manual for the system and adapting it to meet the organization's needs.

Downtime. *The time during which a facility cannot function as usual, due to such disturbances as power outages and system failures.*

One part of the manual that must be written specifically for the organization is the section on **downtime** procedures. Many businesses are virtually paralyzed when the power goes out or the computer system fails. A common remedy is to close early for the day, send everyone home, and bring staff back when the system is again functioning. Hospitals are unable to do this. Step-by-step procedures need to be available in hard copy and followed in the event of downtime, because patients still need to be fed and to be given their medications and treatments, even when the computer is not working.

System disturbances seem to occur more frequently when a system is new. In a way, this is good, because personnel are able to recall the manual processes that preceded the system's installation and can revert to them in a crisis. However, after a system has been in place for a several years, the backup systems are forgotten. Therefore, it is necessary to review these procedures periodically and to revise them to meet

management practice in dietetics

current needs. Downtime procedures are an integral part of the IM manual and should be a topic for in-service training on a periodic basis.

access to information

Though IM staff are able to control an individual's access to information for security purposes, it is unlikely that they are knowledgeable enough about individual job responsibilities to determine what data an employee needs to be able to access. It is up to individual managers to specify what types of clearance should be given to their subordinates in different jobs. For example, diet clerks in a hospital need access to information about patients' diet orders, but probably do not need information about the results of patients' lab tests. Dietitians and dietetic technicians need access to lab data in order to carry out nutritional screening and assessment. Therefore, the dietitians and technicians would have access to a different **computer menu** than would the diet clerks. In most facilities, cooks do not need access to any of the data in the EHR system. Financial information should be available only to employees with management responsibility or those who work in the financial or accounting departments.

Managers are the people who know what information their subordinates require. They may make this determination with or without consulting the employees. When determining what information a specific individual or job classification needs, some care must be taken to be both realistic and cautious. Where issues of patient confidentiality are concerned, the fewer individuals who have access to data, the better. With organizational information unrelated to patient confidentiality, the manager needs to make sure that clearances are in line with usual organizational practice. If the organization is one that shares information freely across all levels, then each employee should have the maximum amount of access possible. On the other hand, if the organizational culture is one that restricts information, the manager should limit access to information that is essential for the employee to do the job.

Computer Menu. *A list of the available commands and operations performed by a computer from which a user may select.*

data storage

Today's desktop and laptop computers have significant amounts of storage built into them. If a user chooses to keep sensitive information on these devices, then the device should have a security program, as well. It is also prudent to back up the data onto a storage device periodically. These devices currently include external hard drives, CD-ROMS, memory cards, or USB flash drives. However, as technology moves forward, other types of storage devices may emerge and replace these, just as these have replaced floppy diskettes and magnetic tapes as storage devices. Some data that were stored less than a decade ago are irretrievable because of "data rot," which is essentially the degradation of the storage media, or the obsolescence of the technology or software used to retrieve the data. If the stored information is going to be needed far into the future, it is judicious to transfer it to newer storage media as it becomes available.

Many individuals and businesses choose to store their backup data on hosted storage sites on the Internet. In essence, they rent space at an external storage site (sometimes called a Cloud) on which to store their electronic documents, photos, presentations, and so forth. It is widely anticipated that EHRs will eventually be stored in this way, once security concerns are addressed.

information systems for dietetics professionals

Dietetics professionals have a variety of information systems available to help them do their work. Programs and systems exist for inventory control, menu processing, nutrient analysis, order processing, cost analysis, food/medication interactions, nutritional screening and assessment, and so on. The detailed analysis of each of these programs is beyond the scope of this text. Even if a comprehensive list of available programs were presented here, the list would be outdated in a matter of months. Managers must determine their own criteria and evaluate available programs before deciding which particular program or system to use. This section will attempt to provide an overview of the kinds of systems and programs that are available, along with the constraints that may limit each system's usefulness. There will also be a brief discussion of the process involved in implementing a new system.

what's available

hardware. Dietetics professionals deal with many different types of computers and computer applications in their work. The hardware is evolving along with the available software. Some of the hardware used in healthcare dietetics are terminals that are connected to the main patient information systems or EHRs, and are designed exclusively for internal communication. There are also the usual iterations of desktop workstations that are freestanding computers or docked laptops that may or may not be networked and may or may not be connected to the Internet. In addition, many dietetics professionals use netbooks, tablets, or other devices for such tasks as completing nutritional screenings and assessments, placing patient food orders in room service applications, and taking inventories in foodservice. Many of these devices have either wireless connectivity with the Internet or are capable of transmitting data to other computers using Bluetooth technology.

It should be noted that handheld devices and wireless systems are enabling clinical dietitians and dietetic technicians to do more and more of their work at the patient's bedside rather than at a remote computer terminal. This is a positive outcome of advancing technology, since quality patient care requires interacting with the patient, not with the computer terminal. Systems that enhance this interaction increase overall patient satisfaction and quality of care.

software. Some software applications in dietetics are generic programs that are adapted by dietitians and dietetic technicians to meet specific needs. An example would be a basic spreadsheet, which could be used as a grade book for a dietitian who is teaching a nutrition course at a community college, a form for measuring the productivity of clinical staff, or as the basis for an inventory control system. Generic materials include word processing programs, accounting programs, presentation software, and so on.

Other types of applications that dietetics professionals use are organization-based systems. These systems may process patient information or they may be dedicated to management of information that is unrelated to patient care. Generally, these systems are purchased and installed by IM personnel, with collaboration from others like dietitians, pharmacists, medical records staff, finance personnel, and so on. There are also systems designed strictly for the dietetics profession. These are the software systems that will be considered in this section.

One type of program that is available is the **nutrient analysis program**. This program contains extrinsic information like a list of foods and data related to the nutrients that each of those foods contains. These programs vary in many ways. The first is the size of the food list. Some programs contain as few as several hundred foods; others, like USDA's database, include a nearly comprehensive list of the foods available in North America. A second characteristic of these programs is the number of nutrients contained in the database. These range from those that list only the macronutrients (carbohydrate, protein, fat, and kilocalories) to those that list all known nutrients, including the amino acids and fatty acids. Obviously, the more foods and the more nutrients in the database, the more comprehensive the program is said to be. However, it should be noted that even the most comprehensive nutrient analysis program is incomplete, because all possible nutrients have not been identified and measured in every food.

Nutrient Analysis Program. *A program that consists of a database listing of food items and nutrients. It can be used to determine the nutrient composition of foods, recipes, or diets of individuals and groups.*

More is not necessarily better. The dietitian who is running a metabolic research unit may actually need the information about dozens of nutrients including individual amino acids or fatty acids. The dietitian who is operating a university dining program does not. If the dining program used a program designed for research it would provide too much information related to individual nutrients. On the other hand, the campus dining operation requires the ability to generate Nutrition Facts Labels, which are necessary for foods at both student dining sites and in campus retail operations. The software package for this application must have a list of foods that is large enough to meet the dining service's needs and the capacity to produce the required labels..

Some other considerations in choosing a nutrient analysis program include the source of the data used. Are the data from a reliable source, and are they the most recent

System Constraints.
Limitations that are innate in a system, in light of the particular application in which the system is being used. Examples include speed, size of database, user-friendliness, reliability, format of output reports, and so on.

Patient Services Program. *An information processing system used by dietetics professionals to process information related to patient meals and meal service.*

Interface.
Connection that allows communication and interaction between two software systems.

Foodservice Programs. *An information processing system for foodservices used to manage purchasing and inventory data, produce food production forecasts, generate quantity recipes, compute costs, analyze use, calculate waste, and so on.*

data available? There is also a question about missing data. If there are some pieces of information that are not in the database, like the selenium content of kiwi, is that datum simply not reported in the totals, or is there a note that states that the data are incomplete? Is there an ability to add new foods to the food list? For example, if a dining program in Hawaii uses papayas regularly, can nutrient information about papayas be added to the program database if it is not already there?

These types of issues are considered to be **system constraints**. They are the limitations that are innate in a system, in light of the particular application in which the system is being used. These limitations may be speed, size of database, user-friendliness, reliability, format of output reports, and so on. When choosing a system for a specific application, it is necessary to look at both what a computer program can do well and what it is unable to do. In many situations, a perfect fit for a unique application will not be available, and some compromise will be necessary.

Another type of information processing system that dietetics professionals use is the **patient services program**. These programs process information related to patient meals and meal service. The systems process information related to diet orders, food preferences, menu selections, and snacks. They are used to order patient foods, print meal tickets, produce labels for menus and for snacks, calculate the numbers of meals and snacks served, determine the percentages of patients served by diet type, and so on. In addition, these systems can be used to generate lists of patients who need to be screened or who require nutritional assessment or follow-up. A common constraint in this type of system is that it does not communicate well with the facility's patient information system, so that information about admissions, diet orders, and discharges may have to be entered manually. These systems can **interface** with compatible nutrient analysis programs so that the nutrients in foods ordered (or consumed) can be calculated with relative ease. They may also interface with other foodservice programs like food production, inventory, recipes, and so on.

Foodservice programs, which may (or may not) interface with nutrient analysis and patient services programs, are those that manage purchasing and inventory data, produce food production forecasts, generate quantity recipes, compute costs, analyze use, calculate waste, and so on. These programs can also be used to measure productivity, do cost analysis, calculate meal equivalents, create purchase orders, and generate other similar types of data. It is common for these systems to be expandable and to have the ability to **integrate** with other program modules. For example, a foodservice may initially purchase an inventory system, then add a production control system, then a point-of-sale system to tie in cafeteria transactions, then the patient services system. However, the addition of too many modules may create problems and slow the system. This is especially true if the hardware does not support the number of applications used. Therefore, the temptation to overexpand an expandable system, adding modules just because they are available, should be avoided.

At this time, probably the only information processing application that technology cannot do well is the creation of a menu (that is, actual foods to be served, not a computer menu) for a foodservice operation. Many aspects of the menu-writing task are already supported by information technology. These include computer programs that track the nutrient content of menus, food costs, seasonal availability, point-of-sale data, recipes, and so on. Though it seems unlikely at the moment, given sufficient time and a detailed-enough database, even the difficult task of writing a foodservice menu may be carried out electronically.

In addition to those types of applications described, modules or freestanding programs are available for scheduling employees, screening patients for nutritional risk, calculating therapeutic diets, conducting nutritional assessments, computing kilocaloric requirements, identifying food/medication interactions, and so on. As was noted, many of these applications can be performed on handheld devices, information from which can be downloaded into desktop computers or computer networks as needed.

does it fit?

When specifying a new computer system, or an addition to an existing system, it is prudent to take a realistic look at the present *and future* needs of the facility. Because information processing systems are expensive to purchase, time-consuming to install, and likely to be used for a long time, the decision-making process needs to be a deliberative one. In addition, the final decision needs to be coordinated with IM.

It is best to start by conducting a needs assessment to figure out what the information handling requirements are. This should be done independent of knowing what any particular system has to offer, though it is helpful to know what kinds of data processing are available, generally. Next, a list of system requirements should be developed. At this point, some managers visit facilities where various information handling systems are in use. They speak with the managers and employees who work with the different systems to learn the pros and cons of each. It is at that point that it becomes necessary to determine if the coordination of old and new systems is desirable. The programs that are already in use at the facility should be evaluated to determine if any can be used or if an **upgrade** is available to meet current needs. Finally, the decision about what system is to be purchased can be made. There are situations in which it is necessary for several systems to be integrated and other circumstances where it is not desirable to integrate systems. Some examples follow.

If only the clinical dietitians need a food/medication interaction program, it might be best to use an existing program or to purchase a new program to perform that particular function at workstations or on netbooks or tablets that are used exclusively by clinical dietitians. It is not necessary to have a food/medication interaction database on the departmental system, because only a limited number of users have been identified.

Integrate. *To combine (one or more compatible systems or program modules).*

Upgrade. *To replace with a newer or better version of hardware or software.*

Likewise, a program that is capable of writing work schedules for employees would not have widespread use but could be installed on a single computer, rather than on the departmental system. It may not be essential to integrate either of these programs with other programs.

Nutrient analysis, on the other hand, is best installed as part of the larger package because it can be used to analyze individual patient menus, quantity recipes, cafeteria meals, nonselective meals, snacks, and foods consumed by patients on kilocalorie counts. It can be used by many individuals for a variety of applications related to both patient care and foodservice. This does not mean that an integrated nutrient analysis program will meet the needs of everyone in the department, however. Individual dietitians, like a metabolic research dietitian, may find that the nutrient analysis database is inadequate to meet the needs of the metabolic unit. This could necessitate the purchase of a more detailed program for that specific application.

ready-to-use packages

It is usually more cost-effective to purchase a ready-to-use computer package than it is to have a system custom designed for a single application. The ready-to-use programs often come with customer support for the end user and are not dependent on the one or two programmers who designed and, therefore, have intimate knowledge of the program. Larger, well-known vendors may be more reliable than small companies with only one or two products. In addition, these vendors may be willing to **customize** their software to meet the needs of a customer. For example, if a hospital foodservice determines that the patient service program must communicate with the existing patient information system, the vendor might develop the programs necessary to download information from one system to the other as a condition of the sale. This is beneficial to both the vendor and the customer, because the customer gets what is needed and the vendor has a product that can now be marketed as a value-added item to other customers who use the same patient ordering system. It is no longer necessary for dietetics professionals to develop customized information handling systems, because the variety of products on the market is adaptable to a wide range of needs.

Customize.
Develop or modify applications to fit the needs of a particular customer.

starting up from scratch

It is possible, with some computer programs, to install the system and begin using it immediately. Limited training may be required for individuals who are not familiar with computers, but many individuals can begin to use the program immediately, with no training whatsoever. The food/medication interaction program is an example of a stand-alone, self-contained program that can be accessed and used immediately upon installation. Foodservice systems, on the other hand, are seldom so easy to bring on-line. Usually a planned phase-in of a new system is necessary.

data entry. Though data entry is not required for all systems to operate well, a tremendous amount of data must be entered into most foodservice information handling systems before they are usable. For example, the database that exists in the program needs to be customized by adding recipes, menus, lists of ingredients and other goods kept in inventory, prices for those goods, and so on. This data entry may take weeks or even months to complete, depending on the resources that can be dedicated to it. It is one of the reasons that integrated systems are often implemented on a piece-by-piece basis. This allows part of the system to come on-line before the entire system is brought up. For example, an inventory program can be implemented if the items in inventory, the vendors, and the costs are entered into the computer. After this is completed, the recipes could be entered and coordinated with the ingredients available from inventory. Later, cafeteria point-of-sale data could be added in order to forecast production needs for the cafeteria. Other modules could be added even later.

Different data entry requirements exist for each part of the foodservice information system. Little hard data are located in the inventory database when it is purchased, because inventory is unique to each operation. Most of the extrinsic information regarding specifications, vendors, and prices is added on site. Alternatively, the nutrient analysis database comes with a generous number of foods and nutrients already included in data files. Nevertheless, in integrated systems, even the nutrient analysis program is not complete. It needs product-specific data for the foods provided by certain vendors, for the recipes used in the facility, and for any special items that are served. Any food that is produced and served in a foodservice but is not found in the nutrient analysis database must be entered or downloaded from the recipe file. If the food that is served differs from the "generic" version of that food (for example, if meat lasagna is in the database and the facility serves a low-fat, low-sodium vegetable lasagna), the database needs to be changed.

Because of the large amounts of data that need to be entered into a new foodservice computer system, the task is enormous. Once a program is adopted and operating, it is unlikely that the foodservice will be able to afford to buy a new system for quite a while, because the installation costs are so large. Upgrades of a vendor's programs are usually a viable alternative, because these will feature the ability to download information from one version of the program to the next. The relationship between a foodservice and its information system, like a marriage, is a long-term commitment.

implementation. Implementation of a computer system is a complex project that needs careful planning and thought. It is helpful to draw up an implementation plan on a Gantt chart to map out what tasks need to be done and to establish a timeline for the accomplishment of these tasks. In addition to data entry, which has been discussed, there are many other tasks related to bringing a system on-line.

One is the training of all staff who will be using the system. Training should be hands-on, in which staff actually run prototypes of the program on real terminals with simulated information. This helps staff to develop a feel for the keyboard and to visualize the screens that will be used. The training needs to be carried out in a systematic way over an adequate period of time. Employees must be allowed to practice until they are familiar and comfortable with the system. This is usually carried out as in-service training.

Another task is the development of policies and procedures and user manuals for the use of the system. The staff need to have these available ahead of time, too, so that they become adept at finding answers to common questions on their own. The manuals should be available at the time of the in-service training.

Office space may need to be redesigned to hold the equipment and make it accessible to all users. Wiring for some networked systems may disrupt the routine functioning of the operation for a while, so this should be done during nonpeak periods. Prior to start-up, an adequate volume of computer supplies must be available. Because there is no history of usage, this probably means that extra inventory will be purchased. Paper, labels, toner, and the like will be needed. There will also be some waste involved with these supplies until everyone is capable of using the new equipment effectively. New, ergonomically designed furniture and peripherals may need to be purchased and installed to allow employees to work comfortably and without injury.

troubleshooting common problems

The first problem that is likely to occur when the new system is implemented is that usual deadlines and timelines will not be met. This is due to unfamiliarity with the system and how it operates. Even if the system itself is faster and easier than the old way of doing things, the lack of routine and the need to think of each step that is being performed are likely to slow processes down. Adding extra staff for the first few days the system is in use can minimize this effect.

Likewise, there will probably be more than the usual number of errors during the start-up phase. The problems may result from inaccurate data entry, the system itself, operator errors, and so on. Consultants who are experts in the use of the system should be available for consultation during the start-up phase. They should be present on the premises, if at all possible. Sometimes they are available at a remote location from which they can access the system for diagnosis and treatment of the problems. These consultants should be able to talk workers through any problems with the operation of the system in a logical and easy-to-understand manner.

In addition, there should be individuals within the organization who understand the system well enough to be able to troubleshoot. This is especially true after the first few days of operation when the consultants are gone and the facility is left to its own resources. A common error that is made is that of training only one individual to be the in-house expert. This has two major effects. It provides no redundancy for times when that person is unavailable, which means that downtimes can be lengthy. It also makes that person indispensable, making it difficult to find a replacement should that person leave the position. This is one area where succession planning is essential and redundancy is prudent.

Some workers will find it especially stressful to try to adapt to an automated information system and may need to be transferred to different jobs. This will necessitate even more retraining, for them and for their replacements. It is helpful if this resistance can be detected during the training phase so that these employees can be offered other options. This will make the transition smoother and allow the employees to retain self-esteem.

Though it is unlikely that one can purchase, install, and implement a new information management system without some disruption to an organization, it is possible to manage the process. Personnel who are familiar with the system and consultants who have expertise in the implementation process can facilitate the changeover and minimize the problems that occur. The advantages of being able to manage information electronically justify the investment of time and money.

conclusion

In this chapter, information management was defined and information technology was described. There was an overview of information management issues, in general. Some of the discussion focused on the types of information processing systems that are used by dietetics professionals. Highlights of this chapter include the following concepts.

1. Information management is essential to how organizations operate. Information technology provides managers with more information, faster than ever before.
2. Intrinsic information is transformed by extrinsic information to generate output data.
3. Managers must find ways to utilize the information that they have without either becoming overburdened by too much data or settling for fewer data than are needed.
4. Information systems, both hardware and software, should be standardized, controlled, and integrated where appropriate.
5. Many types of information processing programs are available for dietetics professionals.
6. The selection and implementation of information processing systems may be complex and costly. Implementation should be well planned and scheduled so that the transition to the new system goes as smoothly as possible, with the least amount of disruption to workers and to production.

activities

activity 1

Hypothetically, you are in the market for a new computer. Consider the various computer applications that you are required to use for work and for school. You have a limited budget of $1,000 for both the hardware and the software. Apply the decision-making process that you studied in Chapter 4 to determine what hardware and software to purchase.

1. Describe what the computer is able to do in light of what your needs are.
2. List those items that you could not get that you wanted.
3. How will you compensate for these deficiencies?
4. List what extras you received that you did not need.
5. Do you anticipate using these extras? If yes, how will you use them?
6. What do you anticipate will be the usable life span of this computer?

activity 2

Make a Gantt chart for how you will make the transition from your present computer to the one you described in Activity 1. Include both the tasks to be done and a time frame for each task.

activity 3

Conduct an Internet search of three sites that provide information on judging the reliability of Internet sources. One of these sites should be the library of your own college or university. Compare and contrast the information gathered from each of these sources.

activity 4

Join a listserv that is related to an area of dietetics. You can locate such lists through the local dietetic association or on the ADA website at http://www.eatright.org. After two weeks, note what you have learned from subscribing to this service. Describe the value of this list to you, if any.

to study further

- Applegate, L. M., R. D. Austin and D. L. Soule. *Corporate Information Strategy and Management: Text and Cases*. 8th ed. Boston: McGraw-Hill, 2009.
- Ayres, E. J., J. L. Greer-Carney, P. E. Fatzinger McShane, et al. "Nutrition Informatics Competencies across All Levels of Practice: A National Delphi Study." *Journal of the Academy of Nutrition and Dietetics*. 112:2042–2052, 2012.
- Ayres, E. J. and L. B. Hoggle. "2011 Nutrition Informatics Member Survey." *Journal of the Academy of Nutrition and Dietetics*. 112:360–367, 2012.
- Ball, M. J., C. A. Weaver, and J. M. Kiel, eds. *Healthcare Information Management Systems: Cases, Strategies, and Solutions*. 3rd ed. New York: Springer-Verlag, 2010.
- Berg, M. *Health Information Management: Integrating Information Technology in Health Care Work*. New York: Routledge, 2004.
- Fitzsimmons, J. A., M. J. Fitzsimmons, and S. Bordoloi. *Service Management: Operations Strategy and Information Technology*. 8th ed. New York: McGraw-Hill, 2013.
- Gartee, R. *Electronic Health Records: Understanding and Using Computerized Medical Records*. 2nd ed. Upper Saddle River, NJ: Prentice Hall, 2012.
- Gartee, R. *Health Information Technology and Management*. Upper Saddle River, NJ: Pearson, 2011.
- Glandon, G. L., D. H. Samltz, D. J. Slovensky, et al. *Austin and Boxerman's Information Systems for Healthcare Management*. 7th ed. Chicago: Health Administration Press, 2008.
- Hamilton, B. *Electronic Health Records*. 3rd ed. New York: McGraw-Hill, 2013.
- Hoggle, L. B. "The Health Information Technology for Economic and Clinical Health (HITECH) Act and Nutrition Inclusion in Medicare/Medicaid Electronic Health Records: Leveraging Policy to Support Nutrition Care." *Journal of the Academy of Nutrition and Dietetics*. 112:1935–1940, 2012.
- Hoggle, L. B., M. A. Michael, S. M. Houston, and E. J. Ayres. "Nutrition Informatics." *Journal of the American Dietetic Association*. 106:134–139, 2006.
- Hristidis, V. *Information Discovery on Electronic Health Records*. Boca Raton, FL: Taylor & Francis, 2010.
- Pijpers, G. *Information Overload: A System for Better Managing Everyday Data*. Hoboken, NJ: J. Wiley & Sons, 2010.
- Turban, E., J. E. Aronson, and T. P. Liang. *Decision Support Systems and Intelligent Systems*. 7th ed. Upper Saddle River, NJ: Pearson/Prentice Hall, 2005.

scholarly journals

- *Cornell Hospitality Quarterly*
- *Health Informatics Journal*

- *Information and Management*
- *International Journal for Information Management*
- *Journal for Healthcare Quality*

other relevant periodicals

- *Healthcare Informatics*
- *Modern Healthcare*
- *Today's Dietitian*

relevant websites

- American Health Information Management Association http://www.ahima.org/
- American Medical Informatics Association http://www.amia.org/
- Healthcare and Information Management Systems Society http://www.himss.org/ASP/index.asp
- Health Information Technology http://www.healthit.gov/

other

- Academy of Nutrition and Dietetics Informatics Blog http://www.eatright.org/media/blog.aspx?blogid=6442451184

in practice

you, improved: understanding the promises and challenges
nutrition informatics poses for dietetics careers
Sara Aase

When Rush University Medical Center computerized and connected its patient care systems in 1995, the nutrition department made sure it was included. "The way we got our department networked was by selling people on the fact that we would be able to use our diet office management component," says Diane Sowa, MBA, RD, LDN, assistant director of clinical nutrition. That software product already stored and analyzed nutrient, intake, and recipe information. Hospital administrators realized that linking the diet office management system with real-time patient data, such as diet or discharge orders, would have a powerful effect. It would save time in data reentry, cut down on medical errors, help automate tray service by connecting with foodservice, and make patient care more effective. "For us, informatics is the ability to process data to help with problem solving in terms of nutrition care," Sowa says.

For the hospital's 676 patients, registered dietitians (RDs) enter diagnostic information using a fill-in-the-blank, clickable format. "We designed it by entering the most common problem, etiology, and signs and symptoms statements (PES) we typically see here," says Sowa. "And then the dietitian creates individualized PES statements." Automating the nutrition screen, which indicates nutrition risk based on information sheets RDs receive, streamlines daily workflow. RDs see the PES, plus body mass index (BMI) and other data entered by a nurse. These data trigger an automatic analysis of the gradient score indicating whether or not a patient needs to be seen immediately. "At-risk" status automatically generates a list of patients who need to be seen by the RD that day, along with their corresponding room numbers. The RD completes the nutrition assessment and initiates medical nutrition therapy (MNT) for malnourished patients and those on enteral and parenteral nutrition, as well as the same kind of analysis and alerts for patients requiring wound care and nutrition counseling. Based on a diet order entered electronically by a physician (which RDs may modify with approval), the flow sheet automatically computes daily calorie and protein needs from nutrition data. RDs can then auto-select a tube-feeding amount based on the patient's height and weight, which will then tell them the precise number of milliliters per hour the patient needs. Finally, the flow sheet information generates a nutrition assessment note, which the RD completes and signs.

Because of automation enabled by informatics, the time to complete nutrition assessments for patients at Rush Hospital has been cut in half. "Typically it would take 48 hours for all of that information to go full circle," Sowa says. "Now we can get it done within 24 hours." Improving efficiency has eliminated a lot of stress for RDs. "Our dietitians are seeing patients more quickly initially and are able to implement MNT sooner," Sowa says. "They can assess the success of the treatment plan more quickly and make changes as needed." It's also made patient care planning more consistent, accurate, and timely. Diet orders, for example, interface directly with the kitchen menu system, ensuring that the likelihood of a transcription error does not occur and increasing the speed at which the diet office receives the order. RDs also take handheld computers with them when they do patient rounds, entering patient care planning and documentation as they go. Because they've already completed the electronic "paperwork," when they're finished rounds, they're also finished with their work for the day.

Nutrition informatics is the "intersection of information, nutrition and technology."[1] Ideally, informatics makes it easier and faster for RDs to enter, retrieve, and use meaningful information, with the ultimate goal of improving patient care. "Informatics is the use of technology to make people better," says Pam Charney, PhD, RD, CNSD, a consultant and clinical coordinator at the School of Pharmacy, University of Washington, Seattle. Last summer Charney taught a 3-credit distance education course in nutrition informatics through the university. "It's about improving our use of knowledge."

With the push to establish electronic health records (EHRs) for every patient by 2014, all dietitians will be affected by informatics. "It doesn't matter if you're in a hospital environment, long-term care, business, community health, anything," says Curt Calder, MBA, RD, senior analyst and project manager of Clinical Information Systems at Intermountain Health Care in Provo, UT. "Informatics is going to touch you in one way or another." In 2001 Intermountain Health Care implemented an electronic records system serving 700 patients across 23 hospitals. Calder estimates it has probably saved full-time employees 10% of time once spent entering or reentering data. "We've plugged that time back into things that weren't getting done, such as discharge evaluations and instructions," he says. The informatics system went through another upgrade in 2006, with the goal of eliminating paper records completely within the next 2 years. Calder and others say RDs will see unprecedented opportunities to shape the field as demand for informatics skills grows. In this article, we'll take a look at how RDs are already using informatics, how the development of standards and educational tracks will influence the field, and the new opportunities that will evolve as nutrition informatics gains traction.

improving foodservice operations and clinical care

Foodservice managers have a long tenure with informatics, since the need to automate nutrient calculation for menus was an obvious one. Computrition, which sells nutrition informatics systems, for example, was born in 1980 in Chatsworth, CA. Today's systems automate recipe management and nutrition labeling and make it easier to manage purchasing, inventory, and production planning. "Those repetitive tasks like calculations for recipe production or recipe conversion can be done in the blink of an eye," says Dee Leggett, MBA, RD, president of DCL Consulting in Great Falls, VA. Over the course of her career, Leggett moved from clinical work and foodservice management to managing the foodservice systems and hospital-wide information systems for the Department of Defense, for whom she still contracts.

When combined with clinical services, a foodservice management system becomes a powerful tool—increasing patient safety and satisfaction while decreasing food waste and inventory costs. For example, at the National Institutes of Health (NIH), the kitchen roomservice call center automatically sees each patient's diet order, plus a list of allowed menu items. "They are not shuffling through paper menus and lists," says Lee Unangst, RD, dietitian informaticist at the NIH Clinical Center. If a doctor changes a diet order, the kitchen sees it immediately, as well as any special instructions for tray delivery, such as the need to add medications to be taken with food. New tray tracking features help prevent lost trays or service bottlenecks. "You can run monthly reports to see that your biggest delay is getting the tray out of the kitchen, or from the cart on the floor to the room," says Marty Yadrick, MS, MBA, RD, FADA, past ADA president and director of Nutrition Informatics for Computrition, which makes foodservice and nutrition care management systems. New wireless bedside features are popular, too. "RDs can enter preferences, make menu selections, or request diet overrides while bedside with their patients," Yadrick says. "That one-on-one patient contact over something as necessary and comforting as food is really important to patients."

The more interactive the clinical and foodservice systems, the greater the reduction in food waste and inventory, too. "People who use both sides of the software are amazed at the reduction in waste," Yadrick says. "You're preparing meals based on your patient census, not forecasted numbers," he says. "So you're not throwing out as much food, and you don't have tens of thousands of dollars in inventory just sitting around."

In 2003, the NIH Clinical Center upgraded its 25-year-old computer system with integrated foodservice and EHR systems. "Before that we used to have a lot of problems related to diet orders being missing," says Madeline Michael, MPH, RD, chief of Clinical Nutrition Services. "That's a big problem for patient safety." The NIH serves about 500 daily meals on its main campus in Bethesda, MD.

Like Rush University Medical Center, when NIH did its computer switch, it was also able to make data entry clickable, instead of requiring RDs to enter free text. One of the most ambitious aims for nutrition informatics right now is to standardize nutrition terms and codes, enabling the timeliness and accuracy of data retrieval—for research, billing, and greater efficiency and safety in patient care.[2] Being able to share information and understand the content of a term will make it easier to find meaningful patterns and target problems. "We have started to extract data to look at our workload volumes," Michael says. "We can see how many nutrition assessments, patient education, and research interventions we provided. Eventually we want to take a monthly look at the amount of workload per patient care unit and figure out our productivity per clinician and dietetic [technician] on that unit." Another benefit to informatics systems will be the ability to analyze patient data with an eye toward improving patient outcomes. "We'll start looking first at patients with BMIs over 40," says Sowa. "Our dietitians are absolutely overwhelmed by that diagnosis, so we want to look at those interventions first."

At the University of Michigan Pediatric Weight Management Center, physicians are using informatics in a pilot study to generate inspiring text messages to adolescent patients. For example, say the (fictional) name "Sherry Jones" scrolls across the computer screen, along with vital stats such as age, BMI, and details of her nutrition intervention plan for weight loss. A note in Sherry's file says she routinely skips breakfast, and that one of her weight-loss goals is to increase weekly intake of this meal. Based on this note, which includes Sherry's self-reported food preferences and wake-up time, the computer might generate an automatic text message to Sherry at 6:57 AM that reads: "How about yogurt and strawberries for breakfast today?"

Patients have loved the messages, says Susan Woolford, MD, MPH, the center's director. "We wondered what we could do to help them stay motivated between weekly visits, and because they all have phones, we thought that might be a great way to do it," she says. "They said the texts helped them keep the idea of making healthy choices top of mind."

coming career options

With the big push to create EHRs and adhere to meaningful use measures, RDs can anticipate that new and existing jobs will demand informatics skills. The Office of the National Coordinator of Health Information Technology (ONC) anticipates that an additional 51,000 professions need to be trained in order to assist with the EHR adoption program of the Health Information Technology for Economic and Clinical Health, or HITECH, Act.[2] Likewise, enthusiasm is growing for nutrition-focused informatics courses, and significant grant training opportunities are provided via HITECH funding. This fall, the first 10X10 offering (10,000 professionals trained in health informatics by 2010) for RDs by the American Medical Informatics Association (AMIA) wrapped up at the American Dietetic Association's (ADA's) 2010 Food & Nutrition Conference & Expo in Boston, MA. Made possible through ADA's collaboration with Oregon Health & Science University (OHSU), the 10X10 program offered RDs the chance to earn 51.5 CPE credits. "Already people are asking when it's being offered again," Yadrick says.

What kinds of career opportunities can you expect in informatics? How can you incorporate informatics into your area of expertise? Think about what kinds of skills you already use—and how technology could enhance them by solving problems. "The 2010 list might include managing health care data with electronic health records and personal health records," says Elaine Ayres, MS, RD, deputy chief of the Lab for Informatics Development at the NIH Clinical Center. "Or using social media and networking to reach out with context-specific messaging, or using large data repositories for data mining and research." Opportunities exist wherever you might help improve or design software or standards, or teach others about informatics concepts, technologies or best practices, design research protocols, or manage and understand the data informatics technology generates. For example, teachers; trainers; managers; dietetic technicians, registered; researchers; and consultants will use informatics. If you're technically inclined, there's plenty of room in information technology for software developers, Web or interface designers, or database experts with backgrounds as RDs. Mapping workflow and considering how technology may support more efficient processes will benefit RDs in all areas. At the CBORD Group, Inc (Ithaca, NY), for example, which produces food and nutrition service management software programs, all of the clinical trainers for the nutrition software suite are RDs, since they understand the RD's workflow. "A lot of us realized we like technology systems and teaching," says Margaret Dittloff, MS, RD, product manager of the Nutrition Service Suite. "We use those talents to implement systems, train people, do interface analysis or tech support, scripting or software engineering, or business analysis."

What about jobs 10 years out or more? "In 2020 dietitians might look to bionic garments that monitor body functions and anthropometrics," Ayres says. "Or to devices that can scan food to determine nutrient composition. Or to participating in virtual health care."

Depending on where you end up, your informatics job may be highly specific—writing software programs, for instance, or new electronic procedures for the Evidence Analysis Library, the Nutrition Care Process and Model, or quality management areas. "I think as electronic health records become more common, we'll see more and more specialized roles," says Unangst. On the other hand, as informatics and health evolve together, nutrition informatics will be an accepted part of a more broadly defined role—a required base of knowledge needed to do a job. Calder, for example, performs a grab bag of jobs that involve informatics as a senior analyst and project manager: designing protocols for tighter glucose control or smoking cessation, handling electronic records access and security issues, implementing systems, designing workflows, configuring systems, analyzing data, and troubleshooting software glitches. "Managers will have to understand informatics to be able to manage well," Unangst says. "As hospitals move to electronic records, you'll have to understand what's going on and make sure things are getting built in ways that benefit your staff."

challenges and opportunities

RDs say the biggest challenge for the field of nutrition informatics is education. Let's start with the unfortunate term *informatics*, which is off-putting. "A lot of dietitians who don't work in a clinical setting think, 'Oh, that doesn't affect me,'" says Nancy Collins, PhD, RD, LDN, who owns her own company in Florida and focuses on legal issues and wound care. Collins, a self-described "hoarder" of information, has eliminated the stacks of handouts that once overflowed in her office in favor of an online electronic database. "Everyone used to make fun of me for the state of my office because I held onto everything, but they would always call me looking for this or that handout. Now it's all online, accessible to anyone."

A lack of formal education tracks in nutrition informatics is another challenge—for students just entering dietetics, for established RDs who want to earn continuing education credits or advanced degrees, and for those aspiring to teach in the field of informatics themselves. Given the popularity of 10X10 and the urgency of EHR adoption, it's a void that soon should be filled. "There is and will be a huge need for clinicians who also have training and experience in clinical informatics," Charney says. "We're finding it's not enough to be a clinician who happens to like technology, or a computer person who happens to like the clinical side of things—we have to begin to develop advanced training for people on both sides of things."

A third challenge is the perception that nutrition isn't important to incorporate into electronic health systems, since RDs are not eligible providers for EHR adoption incentive programs.[3] But RDs already involved in informatics point out that seven of 10 of the top health risks (such as heart disease, cancer, stroke, diabetes, and kidney disease) involve nutrition, and that if RDs don't get involved in their institution's EHR committees, someone else without RD experience will build in nutrition-related functionality.

Flip that challenge, and it becomes unprecedented opportunity. Most hospitals, for example, are only at Stages 2 and 3 of a seven-stage pyramid that indicates full use of electronic medical records,[4] meaning that RDs can help build in the kind of functions they need as ancillary providers. "We understand what's hard for us and what we wish we could have," Dittloff says. Tight timelines for implementation are driving changes now. "Since the adoption of the HITECH Act there has been amazing acceleration to get to meaningful use for patient care," Calder says. "One of the greatest contributions dietitians can make is to add their advice to the design of their facility's electronic health record. You don't have to know a lot about informatics—you already bring the most critical knowledge about what you need to do your job."

making peace with computers

Fear of technology is valid, understandable, and should not be underestimated. Whose head isn't spinning these days trying to keep up with all of the newest social networks or iPhone apps? We know all too well that trying to learn technology or judge its usefulness to our lives can suck up as much time as it promises to save. On the other hand, because of its ubiquity, adjustment times are getting shorter. Calder and Michael, for example, say that it took staffs about a month to adjust to new systems and processes, and then they swore they'd never go back to the old ones.

And the more technology advances, the more it needs humans to drive it in order to actually deliver desired results. As informatics systems mature, they will require increasingly sophisticated ways of looking at and analyzing data for patterns—for example, matching best protocols to diagnoses, or learning whether follow-up interventions were successful. "We'd like to be able to identify protocols based on profiles, for example, around A1c levels," Michael says. One of the hoped-for outcomes of the HITECH Act is to enable analysis of nationally aggregated data for public health purposes. "For example, I could look at everyone in the Pacific Northwest with a particular nutrition diagnosis," Charney says. (Aggregate data would be stripped of identifying information.) "It could make it easier to track back foodborne illness outbreaks."

Like any technology, informatics systems are only as effective as the people building and managing them. The better you understand workplace roles and systems, the better you can articulate needs and how technology could meet them. "Lots of times people want a computer system, but they don't know what they want to fix," says Leggett. "Then they say the computer system wasn't any good." Many RDs will find themselves in a "translator" role between dietetics and information technology staff, a role Dittloff claims for herself. "My RD training helps me keep foremost in my mind that the goal is to try to provide whatever my colleagues need at the moment they need it to make the patient care experience better." The more conversant you are with the technology side of informatics, the more effective you'll be. "To walk the walk you have to be able to talk the talk," says Michael, who recalls her first exposure to informatics as akin to walking into a United Nations meeting and needing an interpreter headset. "Getting comfortable with the lingo is very important."

The more sophisticated nutrition informatics systems become, the more skilled with informatics RDs will need to be to manage them. "These systems generate and retain so much information that it can be hard to understand what you're looking at," Unangst says. Nutrition informatics is not an "install it and forget it" proposition—getting a system in place is just the beginning of ongoing requests for upgrades and new capabilities toward ongoing improvement. "They require continuous attention to understand how to improve what you're looking for or what you want to measure, and how to communicate that," Unangst says. In other words, more informatics could mean more job security. "It's the whole reason my job exists."

in practice references

1. Yadrick M. "Informatics 'Light.'" Nutrition Informatics Blog, American Dietetic Association Website. http://www.eatright.org/Media/Blog.aspx?id=4294968500&blogid=6442451184. Published September 15, 2010. Accessed October 5, 2010.

2. Hoggle L., Yadrick M., and Ayres E. "A Decade of Work Coming Together: Nutrition Care, Electronic Health Records, and the HITECH Act." J Am Diet Assoc. 2010; 110:1606–1614.

3. Hoggle L. "EHR Incentive Program—What Does This Have to Do with Dietitians?" Nutrition Informatics Blog, American Dietetic Association Website. http://www.eatright.org/Media/Blog.aspx?id=4294968297&blogid=6442451184. Published June 21, 2010. Accessed September 22, 2010.

4. Davis M. "The State of U.S. Hospitals Relative to Achieving Meaningful Use Measurements." Healthcare Information and Management Systems Society (HIMSS), HIMSS Analytics Website. 2009:1–18 www.himssanalytics.org/docs/HA_ARRA_100509.pdf. Accessed September 22, 2010.

5. This article was written by Sara Aase, an award-winning freelance writer in Minneapolis, MN.

PII: S0002-8223(10)01655-X

doi:10.1016/j.jada.2010.10.019

chapter references

1. Information Management. Dictionary.com. *The Free On-Line Dictionary of Computing.* Denis Howe. http://dictionary.reference.com/browse/Information Management. Accessed September 21, 2012.

2. Fouman, Michael. "Informatics." In *International Encyclopedia of Information and Library Science.* 2nd ed. J. Feather and P. Sturges, eds. Oxford, UK: Routledge, 2002.

3. Hoggle, Lindsey B. "What IS Nutrition Informatics?" Academy of Nutrition and Dietetics Nutrition Informatics Blog. http://www.eatright.org/Media/Blog.aspx?id=6442452276&blogid=6442451184&terms=Nutrition+Informatics. Published May 17, 2010. Accessed September 24, 2012.

4. Best, David P. "Business Process and Information Management." In *The Fourth Resource: Information and Its Management.* D. P. Best, ed. Brookfield, VT: Aslib/Gower, 1996.

5. Ibid.

6. Orna, Elizabeth. "Valuing Information: Problems and Opportunities." In *The Fourth Resource: Information and Its Management.* D. P. Best, ed. Brookfield, VT: Aslib/Gower, 1996.

7. Lacey, K. and E. Pritchett. "Nutrition Care Process and Model: ADA Adopts Road Map to Quality Care and Outcomes Management." *Journal of the American Dietetic Association.* 103:1061–1072, 2003.

8. Academy of Nutrition and Dietetics. *International Dietetics and Nutrition Terminology (IDNT) Reference Manual: Standardized Language for the Nutrition Care Process.* 4th ed. Chicago: 2013.

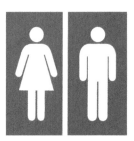

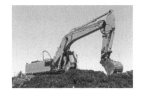

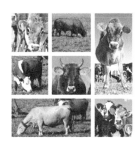

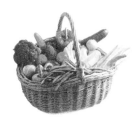

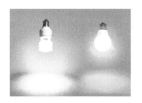

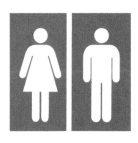

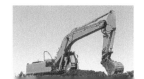

chapter seventeen

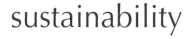

sustainability

learning objectives

1. Define *sustainability*.

2. Describe strategies used for energy conservation.

3. Determine why water conservation is an important aspect of sustainability.

4. Identify how recycling can be used for landfill diversion.

5. Discuss the use of composting for pre- and post-consumer food waste.

6. Define *foodshed*.

7. Differentiate among locally sourced, organic, and transgenic foods.

8. Discuss the rationale behind enforcing the humane treatment of animals used in food production.

9. State how efforts to promote social justice can impact farmworkers.

10. Discuss the certification of green restaurants, green businesses, and green buildings.

11. Identify educational strategies that have been implemented to foster sustainability related to food and nutrition.

overview

Sustainability is usually defined as meeting "the needs of the present without compromising the ability of future generations to meet their own needs."[1] As the population of the world continues to grow rapidly, it is incumbent upon all of us to find ways to lessen our impact on the environment so that those who come after us have adequate resources to live productive, comfortable lives.

This chapter will address many of the issues of sustainability that relate to food and nutrition. Certainly all of us are able to make changes in our own lives that will conserve resources. However, as dietetics professionals, we can also serve to educate those around us about the urgency of the problem. Those of us in clinical and community practice can encourage our clients to purchase seasonal foods that are available from environmentally friendly, local sources. Recycling can be done in offices and other businesses, and simple things like turning off lights and computer monitors help conserve energy. Even the use of reusable, rather than disposable, beverage containers is a behavior that can be modeled to clients and colleagues alike.

Dietetic professionals who work in foodservices have even greater opportunities to promote sustainability. Foodservice managers have the opportunity to manage the entirety of the operation, not just the production of food. Resource management includes managing both energy and water resources. Much of the waste generated by foodservices can be either recycled or composted. Food can be sourced from environmentally friendly farms that are fair and respectful to farm workers and treat livestock humanely. This chapter will explore the complexities involved as foodservices strive to become more sustainable. It will describe of some of the ways in which foodservices can and do meet this challenge.

In 2007, the Sustainable Food Systems Task Force of the American Dietetic Association (now the Academy of Nutrition and Dietetics) developed a Sustainable Food Systems Model (see Figure 17.1). It provides a graphic representation of the interactions among the production, transformation, distribution, access to, and consumption of food, and how these are impacted by resources and the external environment.

energy management

Many of us became aware of energy management when we first saw a U.S. Environmental Protection Agency (EPA) **fuel economy estimate** on a new car or the Department of Energy's (DOE) **energy guide label** on a major appliance that was purchased for home use. The information on these labels allowed us to make educated choices about purchases, not solely based on purchase price, but also based

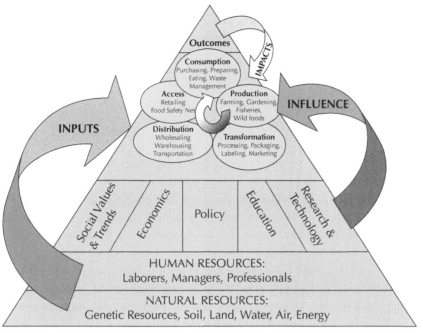

Healthy Land, Healthy People: Building a Better Understanding of Sustainable Food Systems for Food and Nutrition Professionals. Copyright © 2007 by Academy of Nutrition and Dietetics. Reprinted with permission.

Figure 17.1 Sustainable Food Systems Model.

on operating costs. Even though a fuel-efficient product may cost more to purchase, these often save money in the long run because of durability and energy conservation.

The EPA introduced a voluntary labeling program to identify and promote energy-efficient products in the U.S. in 1992. The designation is called **Energy Star**. Initially the designation was limited to computers and computer monitors. Now the agency has developed Energy Star designation for 60 different categories of products for home and office use.[2] Purchasing Energy Star office equipment such as computers, copiers, monitors, and lighting saves considerable energy and is a good place to begin working on sustainability efforts. But the savings is not just limited to which products we purchase. It also includes how we use that equipment. Turning monitors off during non-working hours saves additional energy, as do sensors that turn the lights off when a room is empty or dim them when there is adequate light coming in from the outside. Cycling equipment off when it is not in use saves energy for all types of equipment, not just those with the Energy Star label.

In terms of energy consumption, however, the biggest contributors are those systems that are involved in heat transfer, including furnaces, boilers, water heaters, cooking equipment, refrigeration, air conditioning units, freezers, and ice machines. These

Energy Star.
http://www. energystar.gov/

systems can be either gas or electric. Energy used for heat transfer is important for all types of facilities and businesses. Air temperature must be maintained at a comfortable level so that workers can be productive, and restroom facilities need to have hot water.

foodservice equipment

Though all businesses should be cognizant of energy conservation, foodservices are much more energy intensive than most other businesses. They rely on heating and cooling to prepare their products, to store them, and to maintain food safety. Typically a foodservice uses about five times as much energy per square foot as a retail or office facility.[3] See Table 17.1 to see how energy is consumed in a foodservice operation.

Energy Star designations are currently available for several types of gas and electric commercial foodservice appliances. These include fryers, ovens, steamers, hot food holding cabinets, refrigerators, ice machines, dishwashers, and griddles. As research is completed on other appliances, more types will be added to the list. In addition there are **lifecycle cost calculators** available for foodservice equipment and lighting to help someone purchasing new equipment make informed choices about the total cost of the appliance over time.

Lifecycle Cost Calculators. *Tools that are used to determine the total cost of purchasing, operating, and maintaining a piece of equipment for its expected lifetime.*

It should be noted that sometimes foodservice facilities in institutions do not pay their own overhead and have little incentive to purchase the piece of equipment with the lowest operating costs. It is shortsighted to do so, since the health of the parent organization is at stake in the long term as well as the foodservice department. Managers

Type of Equipment	Percent of Energy Consumed
Food preparation, including cooking equipment, hot beverage makers, toasters, hot holding equipment.	35%
HVAC, including heating, cooling, kitchen exhaust, and tempering makeup air.	28%
Sanitation, including dishwashing and heating water for pre-rinsing, dishwashing, and hand washing.	18%
Lighting.	13%
Refrigeration, including reach-in and walk-in refrigerators and freezers and ice machines.	6%

Table 17.1 Breakdown of Energy Use in a Full-Service Restaurant.[4]

management practice in dietetics

should include operating costs of equipment in every capital budget request, even if it does not have a direct impact on the department's bottom line. This way the organization has the information needed to make the best possible decision.

Just like computers and monitors, the foodservice appliances need to be maintained properly. The gaskets on both heating and cooling equipment need to be intact so as not to allow heat or cold to escape from the appliance while it is operating. Strip curtains in walk-in coolers need to hang straight down to floor level to be effective; they should not be tied back or cut off, as sometimes happens. Condensers for refrigerators and freezers should be free of built-up ice and dirt, and ice machines should not be located near cooking equipment.

Consideration needs to be given to how appliances are operated, too. During non-peak production hours, unused cooking equipment should be turned off, or at least turned down to an idle rate. For example, sometimes all ovens in a facility are turned on at the beginning of the workday and not turned off until the last cook leaves the premises at night. Depending on the type of facility and the menu being served, one oven may be all that is needed during the breakfast service. One may also be sufficient for the hours after the main evening meal has been served. In that case, it would be wise to turn only one oven on at the beginning of the day, use all ovens during the noon and evening meals, then leave only one oven on between the end of service and closing time. This not only reduces the energy used by the ovens, but it also helps decrease the need to cool the air in the kitchen, which also saves energy.

lighting

Lighting systems with occupancy sensors are relatively commonplace. Daylighting systems are available to harvest sunlight and adjust indoor lighting accordingly. It is appropriate to explore these energy-saving technologies when building or renovating a facility. However, even if this is not possible, energy-saving lighting technologies such as replacing incandescent bulbs with compact fluorescent (CFL) bulbs and light-emitting diode (LED) bulbs. Though these Energy Star–rated bulbs are more expensive to purchase, they last much longer than incandescent bulbs, actually saving both energy and money in the long term.

In fact, based on use of 3 hours per day, the average life of a 60-watt incandescent bulb is about 1,000 hours and that of a 13-watt CFL is between 6,000 and 15,000 hours.[5] The light output for each of these bulbs is similar. It is likely that CFLs will completely replace incandescent bulbs in North America in a few years. LED technology is developing rapidly and will probably come into widespread use within the next decade.

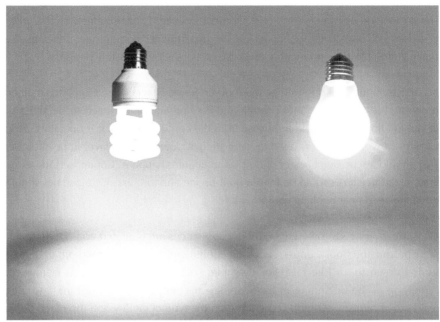

CFLs will replace incandescent bulbs in the near future.

water/waste water diversion

Just as we are learning ways to conserve energy, it is equally important to conserve other resources. Water is high on the list of vulnerable resources, since one of the effects of **global warming** appears to be the disruption in the usual rates of precipitation and periods of both drought and flooding in areas of the world not normally impacted by such weather.[6] In addition to these changes, the world population is growing and increasing amounts of fresh water will be needed for human consumption, for food production, and for sanitation.

Water is essential in all kinds of buildings including offices, healthcare facilities, retail organizations, hospitality services, and foodservices. It is also required for irrigation, both for food crops and for landscaping. It should be noted that when it comes to water, it is not just the cost of water that is of concern, but also the costs involved in heating or cooling the water, and the cost of disposing of and treating wastewater. Conservation of water saves dollars in many real ways.

sinks and restroom facilities

Once again, all businesses use water and most can improve water handling in the short term through the installation and use of low-flow valves placed on sinks and showers in patient or guest rooms, in office break rooms, restrooms, and in the kitchenettes found in hospital nursing units. Replacing fixtures is a more substantial investment and is often done in conjunction with major renovations and new construction. The use of low-flow toilets, sensor faucets, hot water recirculating systems, or tankless (instant) water heaters for restrooms are all strategies that decrease the use of water resources.

garbage disposals and pulpers

Foodservices are heavy users of water and are among the places where conservation efforts can have a major impact. **Garbage disposals** have been standard pieces of equipment in foodservice facilities since the middle of the last century. The amount of water that they use is dependent

Copyright © 2011 by Depositphotos/Peter Hansen.

Restroom facilities can be equipped with water conservation in mind.

on the size of the unit. However, suffice it to say that they use significant amounts of water to dilute and carry away ground-up solid waste. This is discharged directly into the sewer system and transported to water treatment plants. Some jurisdictions have banned the use of these units for all new construction due to excessive water consumption and the burden of treating large amounts of solid waste in water treatment facilities.[7] Others tax them so heavily that foodservice operators are reticent to install them. In operations where they are in use, efforts should be made to manage that use so that not everything that is able to be discarded through this system is put through the unit. For example, pre-consumer plant waste like melon rinds, carrot tops, and so forth can be composted rather than sent through a garbage disposer. Even post-consumer plate waste (which contains significant amounts of fat and protein) can be composted, though the high protein content of this type of waste means that it may attract scavengers and must be handled differently than waste that is composed of only plant parts.

Garbage Disposal. *A machine that uses large amounts of water as it grinds solid waste; discharges both into the sewer system.*

Another piece of equipment that is sometimes used to handle plate waste is a **pulper**. These machines act like disposals by grinding up waste, but they then separate solid from liquid waste and send only the liquids into the sewage system. The solid waste is compacted and transported to another site for digesting or composting. Early versions of pulpers were as water intensive as garbage disposals, but had the advantage of not sending solids to the water treatment plants. Newer versions recirculate the water, which cuts down both on water used and the amount of waste water that is transferred to the treatment plant. Any facility that is purchasing a new pulper should choose a model that recirculates water.

Pulper. *A machine that grinds solid waste, then extracts the solids so that only water is discharged into the sewer system.*

sustainability 545

sanitation equipment

Serviceware.
Dishes and flatware used for serving food.

Foodservice facilities have to have equipment to ensure that it they can adequately sanitize **serviceware**, pots and pans, and utensils. This equipment may be as simple as a three-compartment sink in small facilities, to a large, flight-type dishwasher in large institutions like university dining halls. In each case, hot water is a necessary part of the process. Both the water itself and the energy used to heat it need to be managed in much the same way as other resources.

Pre-Rinse Nozzle.
A device that is used in foodservice dishwashing areas that sprays water on dirty dishes to remove waste that is left on the plates before they are put into the warewasher.

Take for example the **pre-rinse nozzles** that have been used in dishrooms and potwashing areas in foodservices for decades. Early versions of these nozzles used about three gallons of water per minute. New versions do just as good a job of removing food waste from dishes with a flow rate of 1.6 gallons of water per minute or less. If such nozzles are used for only one hour a day, the water savings is 60 gallons of water per day. This does not include the cost of heating the water or the cost of wastewater treatment. It is estimated that the use of a water-efficient spray nozzle for three hours per day could save as much as $1,000 per year.[8] Typically these devices are available at substantial savings or no cost in order to encourage water conservation.

Warewashing is another area with heavy water usage and where efforts should be made to conserve water. In this case, however, the water usage is dependent on the machine that is being used. The principal way to conserve water with existing machines is to be certain that the machine is used only for full racks of dishes, or during peak periods. However, when machines are being replaced, it is appropriate to look at machines that are both energy and water efficient. Energy Star standards have been set for dishwashers; these standards address both energy and water consumption.[9] Some machines are designed to recycle water. For example, water that was used in the rinse cycle for one load of dishes may be used in the wash cycle for a subsequent load. Though there is definitely additional cost in heating water for use in high-temperature machines (needing 180°F water for the final rinse), that cost may be offset by the decreased need for chemical sanitizers. Energy-efficient booster heaters are ancillary to high-temperature dish machines.

Landfill. *A site that is designated as a dumping area for waste generated by a community.*

waste management

A topic of recent interest has been that of waste management. Too much waste is being created in North America and **landfills** are struggling to cope with all of the discarded materials. In an effort to decrease the amount of material going to land-fills, there has been exponential growth in **recycling**, which includes reducing the amount of waste overall, reusing whatever can be reused, recycling what cannot be reused, and purchasing recycled materials whenever possible. All of these concepts

Recycling.
The process of converting waste materials into new products.

management practice in dietetics

require that consumers be educated on why this is important and how to accomplish these goals.

landfill diversion

One of the major goals of recycling is to divert materials from landfills. In most businesses, there are ways to divert much of the waste that is generated by implementing recycling programs for that waste. Collecting and recycling paper, cardboard, glass, metal, and some plastics is commonplace to many offices, schools, and other businesses, including parks and entertainment venues. Batteries, electronic equipment, and toner cartridges can be recycled as well.

In foodservice, pre-consumer waste includes the packaging that the product comes in (cardboard, cans, bottles, bags, and so forth) as well as the discarded portion of the food being processed (like peels, cores, seeds, and hulls). Post-consumer foodservice waste is that which is left to be discarded after the customer has eaten. It includes food scraps, napkins, packaging, drink containers, and the like. Foodservices have differing strategies for dealing with waste that is compostable and waste that can be recycled in other ways.

First, reductions can be made by reducing the packaging that is used, both in the back of the house and in the dining area. Portion-controlled packets for condiments such as ketchup, mayonnaise, cream cheese, and coffee whitener can be replaced with larger self-service dispensers of these items. Individual servings of cereal can be replaced by putting bulk cereals in dispensers. Other ways to divert materials from the landfill include the use of reusable serviceware, as well as the recycling of metals, glass, and plastics. Many jurisdictions now require the separation of waste materials into three categories: compostable, recyclable, and other (that which goes to the landfill).

composting

Earlier a distinction was made between the composting of **pre-consumer waste** and that of **post-consumer waste**. When dealing with food waste, one major difference between the types of waste is the protein content of the waste material. Often pre-consumer waste is mostly plant materials from the back of the house, so **composting** can be done almost anywhere without problems. However, with the high protein content characteristic of post-consumer plate waste, the compost is likely to draw rodents and other scavengers, which are generally not welcome in urban areas. Thus, post-consumer food waste should be composted at more rural sites. Generally, commercial composting facilities are designed to handle this type of waste.

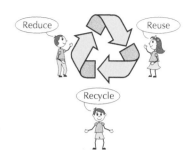

Recycling contributes to creating a sustainable environment.

Pre-consumer food waste. *Food waste generated during foodservice production; generally largely plant materials.*

Post-consumer food waste. *Food waste generated after consumers have consumed their meals; also known as plate waste.*

Composting. *The decomposition of organic material (like plants and food waste) into a material that can be used either to enhance soil or as a fertilizer.*

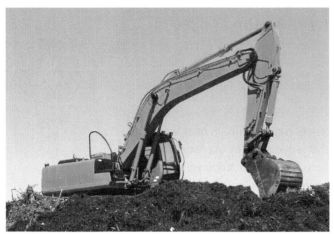

Copyright © 2012 by Depositphotos/Peter Zijlstra.

One of the newer ways to handle foodservice waste utilizes **food waste conversion technology**. This uses equipment that converts pre- and post-consumer food waste into an organic soil amendment in a matter of hours. The solid material from pulpers is delivered to a unit on site that composts those materials automatically. The unit is electrically operated and requires no additives or chemicals to complete the cycle. These units are available in sizes that work in medium- to large-scale foodservice facilities. The use of composting for food waste is one of the many ways that is being used to reduce the volume of material going to landfills.

Generally, post-consumer food waste is handled by commercial composting operations.

Food Waste Conversion Technology. *http://www. ecorect.com/*

Another way is to increase the use of products that are compostable. Disposable serviceware made from paper, sugarcane, bamboo, rice hulls, potato starch, or other organic materials can be composted along with the food waste. However, it should be noted that this is effective only if the compostable items are actually composted. Too often restaurants switch to compostable containers for their customers who then dispose of them by sending them to the landfill. Since the compostable products cost considerably more than traditional disposable serviceware, using it is wasteful unless customers are aware of how to divert these containers from the landfill to the composting process and make the effort to do this. With the use of recycling, composting, and similar strategies, it is possible to divert more than 80% of foodservice waste from landfills.

food

It is impossible to discuss sustainability without also talking about food, and that requires a bit of background information related to agriculture. This includes the production of both animal products (poultry, meat, and seafood, eggs, and dairy) and plant food crops. As the population continues to grow, there will be an increased need to transition to a more plant-based diet, both because of the cost involved in producing a diet centered on animal protein, and because of its impact on the environment. There is already a movement focused on using locally produced foodstuffs to reduce the impact of transporting large quantities of food from place to place, and it seems this is likely to continue for some time.

Foodshed. *The geographic region from which a community is fed.*

It is helpful to think in terms of a **foodshed**. This is the geographic area from which a community or a population center is fed. In the early twentieth century, foodsheds were local; that is, food was produced very close to where it was consumed. With advances in farming, food processing, transportation, and refrigeration over the course of the century, the foodshed expanded to include the entire country, and even the entire globe. Today, the trend is to return to a more localized foodshed, acquiring foods within a limited distance from the point of consumption as much as possible. Obviously, not all types of foods are produced in all geographic areas of North America, but it is definitely possible to use locally produced foods on a seasonal basis in most places.

organic

The Organic Foods Production Act was passed in 1990, which authorized the USDA to develop regulations relating to the production requirements and the labeling of **organic** foods. These regulations for plant crops, meat, poultry, dairy, eggs, and fish can be accessed at the USDA website. Though there is disagreement among experts about whether or not organically produced foods are more nutritious or healthier in other ways than conventionally produced foods, it is clear that organic production is better for the environment, since there are fewer synthetic fertilizers and pesticides used on the crops that can work their way into the groundwater. These can negatively impact waterways, fish, and other seafood. Organic animal products come from animals that are fed only organic feed and are given neither growth hormones nor antibiotics.

Organic. *Products, largely food, that have been certified by the USDA as meeting the standards set by the National Organics Program. See http:// www.usda.gov/wps/ portal/usda/ usdahome? navid= ORGANIC_ CERTIFICATION.*

It should also be noted that organic certification is a fairly costly undertaking. Large producers generally have more resources to obtain this certification than do small producers. Therefore, some small farmers who use organic farming practices cannot legally label their crops organic because they have not completed the certification process. It is not necessary to insist on "certified" organic if the local grower's farming practices are known to follow these standards.

Even if a foodservice operation wants to purchase locally produced organic foods, it can be a difficult goal to achieve. Sometimes the food is not available in the quantities required for a large foodservice operation. Sometimes the price point is too high, making the product unaffordable. Also, depending on the location of the foodservice, the definition of its foodshed may vary, either with the product being purchased or with the season of the year. As an example, it is unlikely that a foodservice in New England will be able to source local blueberries in January. Some facilities even have a tiered system for describing their foodshed, using a smaller radius from the facility for some products and a larger one for others. For instance, a foodservice in Florida may purchase citrus from within a 50-mile radius, but may have to expand that radius to 500 miles to purchase potatoes, and further than that to purchase coffee.

To meet the increasing demands for larger quantities of locally produced or organic foods, some small farmers are banding together to form cooperatives, which allows them to pool their products in a distribution center (regional food hubs). The distribution center then handles order processing and delivery of local products in sufficient quantities to meet the needs of large foodservices. Though this is not available in all locations yet, the trend seems to be gaining momentum.

biotechnology

Crops that have been developed using biotechnology are not allowed to be labeled organic. Nevertheless, these crops can and should be a part of a sustainable foods system. Drought-resistant crops that were developed using genetic engineering can reduce production losses when there is insufficient rain to support the growth of traditional crops. Herbicide-tolerant corn and soybeans allow for the application of weed-killing chemicals that reduce the number of times that a field needs to be plowed, saving on the use of petroleum-based fuel and minimizing soil erosion. Genetically modified plants can even be used for bioremediation; that is, to clean up soil and water that has been contaminated with toxins like heavy metals so that fields can become productive again.[10]

There has been much controversy surrounding the use of biotechnology in food production. However, it is unlikely that traditional farming methods will produce enough food to feed the world's population by the middle of this century. Crops need to be developed with the ability to adapt to variations in precipitation, temperature, soil salinity, and nitrogen content of the soil. They will also need to be resistant to insects and herbicide tolerant.[11] **Transgenic plants** will be essential if crop yields are to increase enough to meet the needs of the population.

Transgenic Plants.
Plants that have been created by transplanting a gene from a different species.

animal welfare

Another sustainability issue that must be addressed is the welfare of the animals used as food. Recently, there have been graphic depictions of the mistreatment of animals as they are making their way into the food supply. Such practices are inexcusable, both because of the suffering imposed on the animal and because of the food-safety issues that often accompany such practices. Of concern, too, is the overuse of antibiotics in concentrated animal feeding operations, which can lead to the development of antibiotic-resistant strains of bacteria.

Certified Humane Raised and Handled.
http://www.certi fiedhumane.org/

Several programs, such as "**Certified Humane Raised and Handled**," "**AGA Certified**," and others listed in the "In Practice" feature at the end of this chapter have been developed. Such programs set standards for the humane treatment of animals and monitor the compliance of producers. These voluntary certifications assure consumers that animals used as food sources of meat and poultry are treated as sentient creatures that are entitled to live in a natural, healthy, and low-stress environment.

AGA Certified.
http://www. americangrassfed. org/

management practice in dietetics

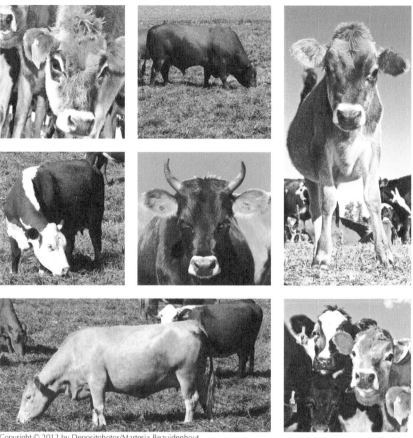

Humane treatment of cattle includes allowing them to engage in natural behaviors, like grazing.

cage-free eggs

Many of the eggs produced in North America are gathered from hens that spend their lives confined to cages. Lately, there has been an effort to treat laying hens more humanely by allowing them to move more freely in open areas of buildings that have bedding, perches, and nest boxes for laying eggs. More and more customers are demanding that restaurants and foodservices serve only cage-free eggs. Note though, that cage-free eggs are not the same as free-range eggs, which come from hens that have access to the outdoors.

sustainable seafood

Fish and other seafood are an important part of a healthful diet. Some of the seafood that is available in today's marketplace comes from fisheries, where various species are caught in the wild. Some fisheries are small and may focus on subsistence fishing or recreational fishing. Others are huge operations that harvest and process vast quantities of fish. Some species of seafood are plentiful, while other types are overfished and some are even endangered. Depending on the lifespan of a particular species, it may take decades for an overfished species to regenerate itself to its full potential.

Some freshwater fish (like catfish), marine fish (like sea bass), mollusks (like oysters), and crustaceans (like shrimp) thrive in nature and can be farmed. Seafood farming is also called **aquaculture**. It can be carried out in either fresh water or sea water. Though seafood farming is very different than land-based farming, it is common practice worldwide. In fact, 85% of the seafood that is consumed in the U.S. is imported, and 50% of that amount is farmed.[12] Aquaculture contributes to the supply of seafood available for human consumption and can also be used to help restore wild species that are being overfished.

Aquaculture. *The farming of fish.*

FishWatch. *http://www. fishwatch.gov/ index.htm*

Seafood Watch. *www.monterey bayaquarium.org/ cr/seafoodwatch. aspx*

Unfortunately, it is a very complex process to keep track of all of the information related to the sustainability of different types of seafood. Rating systems are available to assist foodservices in determining which species are available and whether or not a particular species is plentiful. The National Oceanic and Atmospheric Administration, a governmental agency, provides information through "**FishWatch**." "**Seafood Watch**," a subsidiary of the Monterey Bay Aquarium, identifies individual species of seafood and ranks each as one of the following: best choice; good alternative; or avoid. Other certifications are listed at the end of the chapter as part of the "In Practice" feature.

social justice

The workers who produce food should have safe work environments and are entitled to a competitive wage for their work. Farm workers should have access to safe and adequate working conditions, including water, shade, restroom facilities, and so forth. Beyond this, care should be taken to protect their health and safety, in part by limiting their exposure to pesticides, and in part by providing access to health care. Grievance procedures should be in place to protect farm workers from unfair labor practices.

Fair Trade Certification is available for some products that are grown in developing countries. This certification addresses issues that are similar to those listed above, but also protect the farmer's income with guidelines about fair pricing and price protection.

It should be noted that it will take time for most foodservices to make the transition toward using sustainably produced foods. Time and energy are required to determine which products meet the needs of an individual foodservice operation and what foods can be sourced in a particular geographic region. Prices must be negotiated in order to keep consumer prices affordable. Menus and recipes may need to be changed to accommodate new foods or different preparation methods. Marketing strategies must be adapted to the new normal. A good model might be to set a goal of purchasing 5% of sustainably produced foods during the first two years of the transition and increasing that percentage incrementally over time.

green foodservices

Over the past decade, there has been a great deal of movement in the industry toward sustainability. Pioneers in the movement were some small, individual restaurants that sourced fresh, seasonal, and local foods whenever possible. Notable among these is Chez Panisse, which opened its doors in California in 1971.[13] The first foodservice management company to embrace sustainability as part of its corporate culture was the Bon Appétit Management Company, which was founded in 1987.[14] Since those early days, many other restaurants, management companies, and self-operated onsite foodservices have joined the sustainability movement, and together, much progress is being made.

green restaurants

The **Green Restaurant Association** a non-profit agency that certifies restaurants as being green. It has developed standards related to energy, water, waste reduction, and sustainable food, much of which has been discussed in this chapter. In addition, there are standards for furnishings, building materials, and chemicals. A site inspection of the restaurant is completed and points are awarded based on how well the standards are being met. Restaurants can earn a two-, three-, or four-star rating from this agency.

Other organizations do offer such certifications, but operators should be wary of programs that issue certifications without a site inspection of the facility. Furthermore, the certification should not be tied to purchasing "green" products from the certifying agency. In general, non-profit accrediting agencies tend to be the most reputable.

An additional source for information about green restaurants is available from the National Restaurant Association through its **Conserve—Sustainability Education Program**. Also, **Green Seal** is a non-profit agency that evaluates products for environmental impact. It is an especially good source for information on cleaning products, paint, paper supplies, and the like. Finally, the U.S. Small Business Administration offers information on green certification and eco-labeling.

green businesses

Some foodservices prefer to be certified as a green business, rather than as a green restaurant. This is particularly true of onsite foodservices. Green business certification

Green Restaurant Association.
http://www. dinegreen.com/

Conserve— Sustainability Education Program.
http://conserve. restaurant.org/ index.cfm

Green Seal.
http://www. greenseal.org/

is a generally a function of the local (city or county) government. When seeking such certification from a non-governmental agency, it is probably best to avoid those certifications with a strong marketing focus. Purchasing a certificate of membership or a directory listing in return for a fee from a green organization does not make a business green. Scams are rampant, so buyer, beware.

green buildings

Leadership in Energy and Environmental Design.
http://www. newusgbc.org/

Leadership in Energy and Environmental Design (LEED) is a certification system developed by the U.S. Green Building Council (USGBC) in 2000. "LEED certification provides independent, third-party verification that a building, home or community was designed and built using strategies aimed at achieving high performance in key areas of human and environmental health: sustainable site development, water savings, energy efficiency, materials selection and indoor environmental quality."[15] The guidelines for obtaining LEED certification are continuing to evolve as new products and technologies enter the marketplace. Standards for existing structures differ from those set for new construction. This makes it possible to certify existing operations that have made significant strides in the area of sustainability. Levels of LEED certification are Certified, Silver, Gold, and Platinum, with Platinum Certification being the highest rating possible.

education

One significant way of encouraging people to develop sustainable lifestyles is to educate them to the advantages of making the necessary changes. Most of us are aware of recycling efforts and have used special receptacles for recycling paper, bottles, cans, and so forth. This is done both in work and in residential settings. It is relatively easy to do the right thing when the reasons for doing so are apparent and the environment (in this case the recycling receptacles) are visible and accessible.

However, change is not always this easy, especially when the results are invisible, or so far removed from the source that they seem irrelevant. Education is important, and can be achieved through the use of items as simple as table tents, or as sophisticated as professional media presentations.

Often the most effective education occurs when there is a measurable outcome. For example, some college dining halls collect and measure plate waste so that students can see how many pounds of food are discarded in a day. The result is usually so dramatic that students change their behavior, at least temporarily. Another strategy that has been used with success in some locations is "Trayless Tuesdays." In this scenario students continue to choose all the foods they care to eat, but that food has to be carried without a tray. Students take less food at a time and tend to consume it before going back to take more. Often they return for more only if they are still hungry after consuming the original portion. This strategy has decreased the amount of plate waste and has the added benefit of decreasing the number of items that need to be washed, saving water as well. It has been so successful in some schools that customers no longer use trays at all. "Trayless Tuesdays" has morphed into "Trayless Dining." The savings from both wasted food and decreased water and energy use can then be used to purchase more sustainably produced foods such as locally grown fruits and vegetables or cage-free eggs.

To-go containers for both beverages and for food products used to be (and sometimes still are) made of materials that had to be disposed of in landfills. Now many of these containers are compostable and can be disposed of along with plate waste; so can paper napkins. For some time, individuals have been using reusable beverage containers like coffee mugs, often with a discounted price for the beverage when the customers bring their own containers. As an extension of this concept, some onsite dining facilities are offering reusable to-go food containers to their customers. When returned, the foodservice provides the next purchase in a similar container at a discount. The original container is washed and sanitized for use in the future.

A number of different strategies have been utilized to encourage consumers to decrease the amount of red meat being consumed. This is often done in conjunction with encouraging the transition toward a more plant-based diet. "**Meatless Mondays**" is an approach that emphasizes both personal health and environmental health in its promotions. Because meat production is very energy (kilocalorie) and water intensive, another intervention that is being used in some onsite foodservices is the downsizing the portions of meat being served. Limiting the amount of meat served can lead to significant environmental savings.

Farmer's markets have grown in number and in influence in this century. More and more people purchase some of their foodstuffs in these settings each week. This is one of the centerpieces of the local food movement, since many of the products are grown in the region where they are sold. As noted earlier, it is incumbent on dietetic practitioners to educate their clients on the value of purchasing local products, but most foodservices cannot afford the time or the cost of purchasing this way. However, a growing trend among onsite foodservice is to bring the farmer's markets or **community supported agriculture** (CSA) systems to their sites, so that their customers have access to fresh local products for home use. Offering these services at worksites supports local agriculture as well as the customers, who do not have to drive to such farms or markets at other locations.

Community Supported Agriculture. *A system in which consumers purchase a membership in a CSA, in return for which they receive a box of freshly harvested farm products each week during the growing season.*

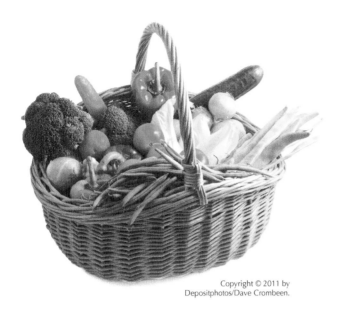

Copyright © 2011 by
Depositphotos/Dave Crombeen.

Typical CSA delivery.

Perhaps the most dramatic undertaking in sustainability education, though, is the **zero-waste event**. In these promotions, foodservices, often in conjunction with other organizations or groups, develop a series of educational programs for their customers while serving a meal of sustainable foods. All containers for food and beverages are either compostable or reusable. Demonstrations, workshops, or activities are included on such matters as gardening, composting, recycling, energy and water management, and so forth. These events serve to demonstrate what is being done in the area of sustainability as well as educating others about it. Though labor intensive, this type of event is very successful at getting the message out.

conclusion

In this chapter, sustainability was defined, and a variety of strategies were described that can contribute toward fostering an environment that will continue to support future generations. The major concepts addressed in this chapter include:

1. Management includes the conservation of energy and water resources, which impacts both the finances of the organization and the external environment.
2. Landfill diversion can be achieved using a variety of strategies, including recycling and composting of pre- and post-consumer food waste.
3. Organic foods, locally grown foods, and transgenic foods all are a part of a sustainable food system. These should be addressed together as a comprehensive system, rather than as competing entities.
4. Animal production should be tempered with humane practices to decrease stress on the animals and to mitigate food-safety issues.
5. Farm workers, both in developed and developing countries, are entitled to a living wage and a safe work environment.
6. Sustainable practices must be supported with ongoing education in order for consumers to know how and why to adopt such practices.

activities

activity 1

Plan a menu for your favorite meal and list all of the ingredients that you will need to prepare that meal. For whatever ingredients you already have on hand, review the packaging to determine the place where that product originated. For any ingredients that you do not have, go to a grocery store or farmer's market to determine where those products come from. You may need to do some research into the origin of some of the ingredients, since country of origin is not required for all foods. For example, coffee may or may not be labeled with information about whether it came from Colombia, Hawaii, or Uganda. When you have gathered all of this information, determine what the foodshed is for that meal. What changes can you make to this meal in order to decrease the size of the foodshed?

activity 2

Contact your local waste management company. In some cases, waste disposal may be handled by the local government's waste management agency. Most of the information needed for this activity may be available on their website.

Determine the following regarding waste management in your region:
    What percentage of waste goes to the community's landfill?
      Are any items banned from disposal in the landfill?
    What items, if any, are recycled?
      Does recycling require separation of waste, e.g., paper, metal, glass, or plastics?
      What items are not being recycled that could be?
Does the company or agency participate in composting?
      Does the material to be composted include only plant-based material?
      What happens to the compost, once it is finished?

activity 3

Do an Internet search looking for the term "Zero-Waste Event" and describe three strategies you found related consumer education for each of the following topics:

- Reduce
- Reuse
- Recycle

to study further

Materials to supplement this chapter can be found in the following sources.

American Dietetic Association. "Position of the American Dietetic Association: Food and Nutrition Professionals Can Implement Practices to Conserve Natural Resources and Support Ecological Sustainability." *Journal of the American Dietetic Association*. 107:1933–1043, 2007.

Henroid, D., J. Henderson, et al. "Creating Sustainability Strategic Plans for Healthcare Foodservice Operations." *Journal of the American Dietetic Association*. 109: A80, 2009.

Kunstler, J. H. *The Long Emergency: Surviving the Converging Catastrophes of the Twenty-First Century*. New York: Grove/Atlantic, Inc., 2005.

Lund, H. F. *The McGraw-Hill Recycling Handbook*. 2nd ed. New York: McGraw-Hill Professional, 2001.

National Research Council of the National Academies. *Toward Sustainable Agriculture Systems in the 21st Century*. Washington, DC: The National Academies Press, 2010.

Peregrin, T. "Sustainability in Foodservice Operations: An Update." *Journal of the American Dietetic Association*. 111:1286–1294, 2011.

Pollan, M. *The Omnivore's Dilemma: A Natural History of Four Meals*. New York: Penguin Press, 2006.

Pollan, M. *In Defense of Food: An Eater's Manifesto*. New York: Penguin Press, 2008.

scholarly journals

Journal of Agriculture, Food Systems and Community Development
Journal of Environmental Economics and Management
Journal of Sustainable Development

other relevant periodicals

Sustainable Farmer
Sustainable Living Magazine

relevant websites

Bon Appétit Management Company http://www.bamco.com/sustainable-food-service
University of California, Davis Dining Services http://dining.ucdavis.edu/sustainability.html

in practice

The University of California has developed a Sustainable Practices Policy which has been implemented throughout the ten campuses and five medical centers in the system. The Policy and Procedure related to Food Services appears below.

policy summary:

"The Sustainable Practices Policy ("Policy")[16] establishes goals in eight areas of sustainable practices: green building, clean energy, transportation, climate protection, sustainable operations, waste reduction and recycling, environmentally preferable purchasing, and sustainable foodservice."

policy text:

sustainable foodservices practices

1. Campus and Medical Center Foodservice Operations
    Campuses and Medical Centers shall develop sustainability goals and initiatives in each of the four categories of sustainable foodservice practices listed below.
    a. Food Procurement
       Each campus and Medical Center foodservice operation shall strive to procure 20% sustainable food products by the year 2020, while maintaining accessibility and affordability for all students and Medical Center foodservice patrons.
    b. Education
       Each campus and Medical Center shall provide patrons with access to educational materials that will help support their food choices.
    c. Engagement With External Stakeholders
       Campus and Medical Center departments, organizations, groups, and individuals shall engage in activities with their surrounding communities that support common goals regarding sustainable food systems.
    d. Sustainable Operations
       Campus and Medical Center foodservice operations shall strive to earn third-party "green business" certifications for sustainable dining operations.
2. Retail Foodservice Operations:
    a. Retail foodservice tenants located on campuses will strive to meet the policies in III.H.1.a-d. above. Given the constraints faced by nationally-branded franchises that must purchase food through corporate contracts, campus departments managing retail foodservice tenants will have the option of meeting III.H.1.a. (procuring 20% of all sustainable food products by the year 2020) by

aggregating the purchases of all retail entities under the jurisdiction of a single operational unit on campus.

b. Campuses will include Section H of this *Policy* in lease language as new leases and contracts are negotiated or existing leases are renewed. However, campuses will also work with tenants to advance sustainable foodservice practices as much as possible within the timeframe of current leases."

procedures

sustainable foodservices practices

1. Campus and Medical Center foodservice operations subject to this *Policy* shall include both self-operated and contract-operated foodservices.

2. In the context of this *Policy*, sustainable food is defined as food and beverage purchases that meet one or more of the criteria listed below, which are reviewed annually by the UC Sustainable Foodservices Working Group (under the UC Sustainability Steering Committee).

    i. Locally Grown[8]
    ii. Locally Raised, Handled, and Distributed
    iii. Fair Trade Certified
    iv. Domestic Fair Trade Certified
    v. Shade-Grown or Bird Friendly Coffee
    vi. Rainforest Alliance Certified
    vii. Food Alliance Certified
    viii. USDA Organic
    ix. AGA Grassfed
    x. Pasture Raised
    xi. Grass-finished/100% Grassfed
    xii. Certified Humane Raised & Handled
    xiii. Cage-free
    xiv. Protected Harvest Certified
    xv. Marine Stewardship Council
    xvi. Seafood Watch Guide "Best Choices" or "Good Alternatives"
    xvii. Farm/business is a cooperative or has profit sharing with all employees
    xviii. Farm/business social responsibility policy includes (1) union or prevailing wages, (2) transportation and/or housing support, and (3) health care benefits
    xix. Other practices or certified processes as determined by the campus and brought to the Sustainable Foodservices Working Group for review and possible addition in future Policy updates.

---

[8]Resulting from regional constraints, campus definitions of "Locally Grown" and "Locally Raised, Handled, and Distributed" may vary; however, Locally Grown and Locally Raised, Handled, and Distributed cannot be defined as over 500 miles.

management practice in dietetics

3. With the goal of achieving 20% sustainable food purchases, all Food Service Operations should track and report annually the percentage of total annual food budget spent on sustainable food.

4. If cost effective, each campus and Medical Center will certify one facility through a third-party green business certification program through one of the following: (1) city or county's "green business" program, (2) Green Seal's Restaurants and Food Services Operations certification program, or (3) the Green Restaurant Association certification program.

5. Campuses, Medical Centers, and retail foodservice operations will provide an annual progress report on these goals. Annual reports should include the individual campus and Medical Center's goals as well as the progress and timelines for the programs being implemented to reach those goals.

6. Campuses and Medical Centers are encouraged to form a campus-level food-services sustainability working group to facilitate the campus goal setting and implementation process.

7. The stakeholders who are involved with the implementation of the Sustainable Foodservice section of this *Policy* will participate in a systemwide working group to meet, network and to discuss their goals, best practices, and impediments to implementation.

8. Campuses and Medical Centers are encouraged to implement training programs for all foodservice staff on sustainable foodservice operations, as well as, where applicable, on sustainable food products being served to patrons, so that staff can effectively communicate with the patrons about the sustainable food options.

9. Campuses and Medical Centers are encouraged to participate in intercollegiate and national programs that raise awareness on dietary health, wellness and sustainability (e.g. the MyPyramid.gov Corporate Challenge and the Real Food Challenge).

10. Campuses and Medical Centers are encouraged to develop health and wellness standards for food service operators, including eliminating the use of trans-fat oils or products made with trans-fat.

11. Campuses and Medical Centers are encouraged to undertake additional initiatives that encourage healthy and sustainable food services operations. Examples include tray-less dining, beef-less or meat-less days, and preservative minimization programs."

references

1. Brundtland, Gro Harlem. *Our Common Future.* New York: Oxford University Press. 1987, p. 43.
2. "History of Energy Star." http://www.energystar.gov/index.cfm?c=about. ab_history. Accessed October 4, 2012.
3. Bell, Todd. "Introduction to Commercial Cooking Appliances and Equipment." Food Service Technology Center. Presentation on August 17, 2012.
4. Ibid.
5. "Why Choose Energy Star?" http://www.energystar.gov/index.cfm?c=cfls. pr_cfls_why. Accessed October 4, 2012.
6. Gore, Al. *An Inconvenient Truth: The Crisis of Global Warming.* New York: Rodale, Inc. 2007, p. 72.
7. Leibenluft, Jacob. "Should We Dispose of Disposals?" *Slate.* December 26, 2008. http://www.slate.com/articles/health_and_science/the_green_lantern/2008/09/should_we_dispose_of_disposals.html. Accessed October 15, 2012.
8. "Pre-Rinse Spray Valves." http://www.fishnick.com/equipment/sprayvalves/. Accessed October 9, 2012.
9. "Commercial Dishwashers for Businesses and Operators." http://www.energystar.gov/index.cfm?fuseaction=find_a_product.showProductGroup&pgw_code=COH. Accessed October 12, 2012.
10. Jamison-McClung, Denneal. "Biotechnology—Meeting Challenges in Human Health, Energy and Agriculture." UC Davis Biotechnology Program. Presentation on August 14, 2012.
11. Ibid.
12. Farmed Seafood. http://www.fishwatch.gov/farmed_seafood/index.htm. Accessed October 17, 2012.
13. About Chez Panisse. http://www.chezpanisse.com/about/chez-panisse/. Accessed October 17, 2012.
14. Bon Appétit Management Company. http://www.bamco.com/about-us/history-and-awards. Accessed October 18, 2012.
15. "What LEED Is." http://www.usgbc.org/DisplayPage.aspx?CMSPageID=1988&gclid=CIXQ3auG6LICFexFMgodMRkALQ. Accessed October 4, 2012.
16. Excerpts from: "Sustainable Practices Policy," http://www.ucop.edu/ucophome/coordrev/policy/sustainable-practices-policy.pdf. Copyright © 2011 by *The Regents of the University of California.* Reprinted with permission.

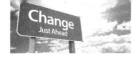

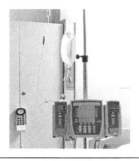

chapter eighteen

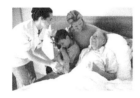

managing change

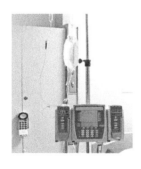

learning objectives

1. Discuss why change is considered to be inevitable.

2. Identify the factors that influence the rate of change in today's workplace.

3. Describe the reasons employees resist change.

4. List the types of change that typically occur in organizations.

5. Describe how change should be managed.

6. Differentiate between managing change and management, in general.

7. Discuss ways to minimize the stress associated with change.

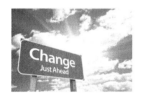

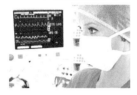

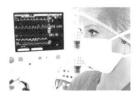

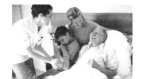

overview

It has been said that the two certainties in life are death and taxes. In today's world, there is another. Change is also inevitable. Change is being driven by a number of factors. Social, political, and economic forces have caused changes ranging from minimum-wage rulings to diversity in the workplace, from initiatives to eliminate workplace harassment to new programs for medical insurance, to name just a few. In addition, there are changes in science and technology that affect both what we do and how we do it. All these changes combine to make today's workplace a vibrant and exciting place to be.

The speed with which the changes are coming is unprecedented. Workers and managers are trying to cope with a workplace that is moving in "fast forward." It is difficult to always be in a change mode, not knowing what to expect and never being able to develop a reasonable routine. As soon as workers get comfortable with a new piece of equipment, a new set of rules, or a new way of doing their jobs, another change happens to upset the applecart. This constant stress eventually becomes too much to cope with and burnout may occur, both to managers and to employees.

This chapter attempts to make some sense out of the changes that are happening in the workplace. It begins with a discussion of the inevitability of change and the impact that the acceleration of change is having on organizations and workers. This introduction is followed by a description of the reasons people resist change and the types of change most likely to occur in the workplace. It will conclude with some methods used to manage change and how to minimize the stress of change through communication and other techniques.

Aside from the description of change and people's resistance to it, none of this material is new. It has been covered earlier in this text. The themes of leadership, trust, communication, and respect for employees are played out in the management of change, in much the same way as they have been in the management of staff, production, procurement, accountability programs, and other areas. These concepts are not new, but their application is.

the inevitability of change

Remember life before college? For many, things were pretty comfortable then. You knew what to expect and could rely on a certain degree of constancy in your life. You got up each morning in the same environment, ate familiar foods that were provided for you, went to school in the winter, and had free time in the summer. Perhaps you had a job on the side. Life was predictable and, therefore, easier. Do you want to go back to those simpler times? Did you enjoy life more when someone else took care of you?

Though some people will answer these questions with a resounding "Yes," most realize that it is not possible to go back. Even if they could, they would probably not be happy when they got there. Remember that those were the days when phones were only used for talking, computers were bulky desktop models, and connections to the Internet were painfully slow, if they were available at all. In the twentieth century alone, there were major changes like the automobile, television, racial integration, the demise of the Soviet Union, safe methods of birth control, the emergence of AIDS, air and space travel, human rights initiatives, and an awareness of humanity's impact on natural resources.

We look back at the past with nostalgia. We are comfortable with the status quo and find it natural to resist change. Nevertheless, once we accept change, it is impossible to return to the way it was in before. Sometimes we cannot even envision how it was. Can you, for example, imagine how your life would have been if you had never had access to television, an automobile, or the telephone?

Some changes, like those just mentioned, are imposed on us from the outside. Other changes are internal. We grow up. We learn things. We become independent. We take on responsibility. We gain experience. We grow older. During our middle years, we develop a fear of aging and wish that we could stop the clock. We can't, so we continue to transform ourselves. Change, both internal and external, is inevitable.

the acceleration of change

The major difference between change now and change as it occurred a century ago is the speed with which the external changes are happening. Science and technology build on what came before, so that the discoveries and inventions multiply exponentially. The current speed with which people, things, and information move from place to place was beyond imagination a century ago. The increase in information, along with the ready access to that information, means that change will take place even faster in the future.

These external changes are having an impact on the internal changes that people face. People are required to learn more, because there is more to learn. And what is learned in college is no longer enough to last a lifetime. One must keep on learning throughout adulthood. It is unlikely that anyone will ever be able to complete his or her education—the need for lifelong learning is essential. This is compounded by the fact that modern medicine has increased both the life expectancy and improved the quality of life for many individuals. This increased longevity, accompanied by the increased rate of change, means that individuals will need to accommodate more change than ever before. This acceleration of change will probably continue into the foreseeable future.

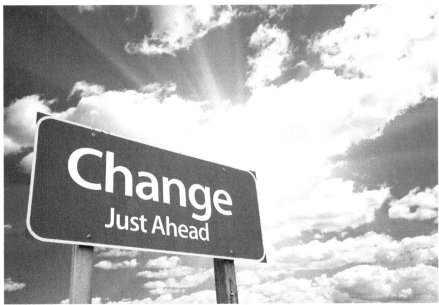

External changes are also having a major impact on businesses and organizations that are forced to change in response. Organizations must respond to global changes in the marketplace. In addition to changes in science and technology, the market is affected by social, political, and economic change. In turn, the changes within an organization will have an impact on individual workers.[1] It is this impact that is of concern to managers, because employees will need to be supported throughout the change process. If change is not managed, it will drive the organization into chaos.

In the environment of change, an organization needs to be flexible. Rules will be broken, guidelines will be altered, and traditional roles will be questioned. The status quo is not an acceptable goal. In the past, it was commonplace for a document (for example, a job description, a procedure, a recipe, or an operational plan) to be useful for several years. This is no longer true. Most of these documents must be reviewed and updated annually. Some need to be revised on an ongoing basis.

Unfortunately, flexibility on the part of the organization is disruptive to the workers in that organization. They are asked to do their jobs in different ways, or to do different jobs altogether. Sometimes their jobs are eliminated, and they find themselves unemployed. Their benefits are changing, so they are unsure of insurance coverage, paid time off policies, and so on. A change in management means that employees need to adjust to the new boss's way of getting things done. Then, too, the changes may happen in rapid succession, so that the workers barely adjust to one change before another happens. No wonder they sometimes feel like helpless victims. Under such circumstances, it is natural to resist change, either consciously or unconsciously.

management practice in dietetics

resistance to change

Some changes are welcome, like a move into a brand-new facility or the upgrading of a computer system. Other changes are less welcome, like layoffs or significant increases in workload. Whether the change is viewed as positive or negative will have an impact on how well people adjust to the change and how much resistance occurs. This perception is highly individual. One person can view an anticipated change as very positive while another will see the same change as extremely negative. Even the most positive change will generate some degree of resistance.

It has been said that a 20-50-30 rule applies to organizational change.[2] This means that, in general, about 20 percent of the people in an organization will embrace change and welcome it. Another 50 percent are ambivalent about the change. The remaining 30 percent are resistant to change and may even go so far as to sabotage or undermine the change process.

The percentages cited might not be accurate in all situations, but the fact remains that only a small proportion of staff will actually look forward to changes at the time they are introduced. Part of managing change, then, is to increase the percentage of individuals who view the change positively. Nearly 80 percent of an organization's staff will need to be convinced that the change is a good one and worth the stress involved in making the change. To meet this goal, management must first explore the reasons people resist change. These reasons are listed in Table 18.1.

Lack of understanding of the need for change

Lack of understanding of or a different sense of the context or environment

Belief that the proposed change violates the core values of the organization

Misunderstanding of the change and its implications

Belief that the change is not in the best interests of the organization

Lack of trust in those introducing the change

Lack of belief that the leadership is serious about making changes

Lack of belief that the leadership is capable of making the change happen

Perception that the change is unfairly selective

Adapted from: Bill Quirke, *Communicating Change*. McGraw Hill, 1995.

Table 18.1 Why People Resist Change[3]

lack of understanding of the need for change

Employees' jobs are very different from managers' jobs. Workers are not required to have or to utilize conceptual skills. For the most part, rank-and-file employees are task oriented. They are paid to tend to the trees, not to look at the forest. Because of this, they have a limited frame of reference for assessing the whole environment. True, they may notice that the number of customers in the cafeteria is lower than it used to be, or that the patient trayline now takes 20 minutes less than it used to take. However, these pieces of information will not be associated with a downturn in business, or a decrease in the number of hospitalized patients. They certainly are not equated with decreased revenues and a need to worry about money to make the next payroll. From the bottom up, it looks like large organizations have plenty of money, merely because of their size. The financial health of the organization has little relevance to the housekeeper who mops the office floor.

From the employee's perspective, the environment may look very stable, even if it is not. The same people come to work each day, do the same jobs that they have always done, and take home a paycheck as they have in the past. Frontline workers are not privy to information about budgets, costs, inventory, competitive forces, markets, productivity, and other things that have an impact on how the organization does business. Whatever information they do have may not be complete or correct, either in fact or through interpretation. Without the knowledge or understanding of the whole picture, it is difficult to see the need for change. The natural tendency is to think that everything is going on as usual and that there is no need to change.

lack of understanding of or a different sense of the context or environment

Often, managers and employees have a differing sense of what the environment is. For example, consider the dietitian who is working in a WIC clinic during an economic downturn. From that dietitian's perspective, the client needs are greater than they have been and the waiting lists for services are long. There is an obvious need to expand the program by hiring more staff to meet the needs of a larger target population. From the management's perspective, however, the economic downturn means lower levels of funding and a need to do more with less. Some programs may actually have to decrease the number of clients who are served because of budget cuts. Divergent perspectives of the same external environment make it difficult for an employee to feel any urgency to change, especially when the change is counter to what the employee thinks the change should be. In fact, from the employee's perspective, the manager may be playing the role of an alarmist. It is easy to see why the employee is likely to resist change under these circumstances.

*belief that the proposed change violates the core
values of the organization*

Employees have a sense of what the organization is all about. This is especially true if the organization has a written mission statement or a statement of purpose. Yet, even the most clearly written statement is subject to interpretation. For example, a school foodservice may provide required levels of nutrients in a meal that has standard portions of foods. The organization is meeting the governmental guidelines that mandate what should be served. However, the food server may believe that the job is to feed hungry children, not to provide a certain amount of nutrients. Feeding children may be viewed as inconsistent with limiting portion sizes. Thus, the employee may resist any change that enforces the use of standardized portions.

Another sensitive issue within the dietetics profession, especially for the managers of dietitians, relates to the charging for nutrition services. Many dietitians entered the profession for altruistic reasons. They often believe that everyone is entitled to food and nutrition services and that these services should be available to all, regardless of the individual's ability to pay. In hospitals, nutrition services used to be included under the umbrella of "room rate." This means that the fee that patients were charged for the room also included whatever food and nutrition services that were required. This tradition had its origin in an era when food was the only way to provide nutritional care to patients. In those days, most of the effort of dietitians was focused on getting food to the patients.

Times change, and technology has changed the ways in which some patients are fed. Though meals are still viewed as a fundamental part of the room rate, other nutrition services are not. For example, though some clients do eat what is traditionally known as "food," others have diagnoses that require them to be fed highly specialized formulas, either by tube or intravenously. The cost of some of these feedings, on a daily basis, can be more than 10 times the cost of food. Furthermore, to plan feeding regimens for clients with complex needs requires time-intensive consultation from a dietitian with highly specialized skills, which is also costly. It is obvious that such extensive nutrition services could not continue to be included as part of the room rate.

Clinical nutrition managers who wanted to continue providing these costly services to clients, soon learned that they could not afford to do so without increased revenues. Therefore, they set up fees for clinical nutrition services. However, in order to charge for these services, there must be a physician order. (Without an order, third-party payers are unlikely to pay for the service.) The dilemma is this—if the physician does not order the service, should it be rendered free of charge; is it the right of every patient to have these services?

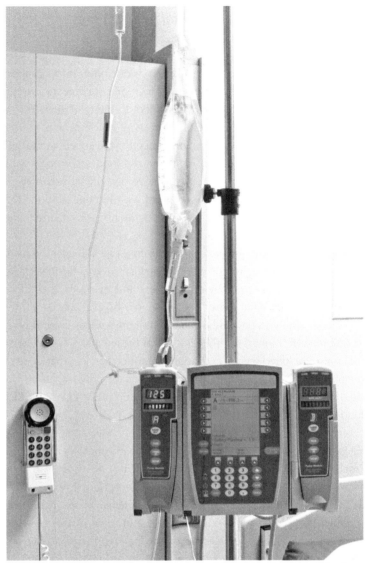

Feeding patients parenterally can be very expensive.

Considering the history of the profession, it is easy to see why clinical dietitians might choose to provide the service, even without a physician's order. It is, after all, what they were trained to do. However, this has the negative impact of devaluing the service. (Why would some clients pay when others get the same service for free?) The managers made a change to enable the services to continue to be available. Clinical dietitians, with a differing set of values, undermined their managers by providing the services without charge.

management practice in dietetics

Fortunately, clinical dietitians are changing their views on this issue. The importance being reimbursed for services is widely recognized as one of the strategies for the survival of the profession. There are not many professionals who continue to provide complex clinical services for free. Those who continue to do so are a luxury that health care organizations and the profession can no longer afford.

misunderstanding of the change and its implications

Food safety is a major concern in the foodservice industry. The Food and Drug Administration's Food Code, or variations of it, have been implemented throughout North America as the first line of prevention for food-borne illness. Implementation of these standards required foodservices to reevaluate their recipes, their menus, and their procedures (including receiving, storage, production, service, and reuse of foods). In many instances, this led to changes in how things were done in the kitchens of foodservice operations.

It is essential for managers to continue to update their knowledge of the food code, and to implement changes as the code is revised. Though foodservice workers are required to have a basic knowledge of food safety, they are often unaware of the reasons that underlie some of the procedures that they are asked to implement. For them, it may appear that management is just coming up with new ways to make the employees work harder. For example, a cook may want to bring out eight dozen eggs that will be needed for breakfast at 6 a.m., and put away any leftovers at 10 a.m. Now that cook is required to bring the eggs out a dozen at a time (so that eggs are not held between 41°F and 135°F for more than one hour). This means that the cook must make eight trips to the refrigerator instead of one.

If the cook is unaware of the food safety issues related to eggs, the change in procedure could be viewed as a burden, not an essential part of the job. When employees do not understand or do not agree with the rationale for a change, they will be reluctant to comply with new guidelines, rules, or procedures. Education is key to preventing this type of misunderstanding.

belief that the change is not in the best interests of the organization

Because employees and managers have different perspectives of the organization, it is possible that they will also have different beliefs about what is good for the organization. Consider the organization that recently furloughed 10 percent of the employees in a cost-containment move. There was a great deal of stress associated with those layoffs. Now, three months later, the management feels a need to unify the remaining staff and to give them a sense of pride and teamwork.

As an attempt to unify the staff, a decision is made to empower a committee of employees to select stylish new uniforms for the current workers. The management's objective is team-building, which from its perspective is good for the organization. The employees may view the new uniforms as a waste of money that could better be spent by bringing their former colleagues back to work, which is (in their opinion) what the organization really needs. To the managers, a one-time outlay of money is justified, but the workers may not differentiate between a one-time investment in uniforms versus the ongoing cost of labor. Once again, the workers are justified, from their perspective, in resisting the transition to the new attire.

lack of trust in those introducing the change

If employees trust their managers, it is easier for them to accept change than if there is a lack of trust. Without trust in management, employees do not believe what they are being told but look for the "real" agenda behind proposed changes. For example, consider a DTR who is asked to increase the number of patient screenings done each day. This DTR is told that this is necessary because another diet technician resigned and no replacement worker is available to carry out the screenings. If there is trust in the manager, the employee will probably be willing to try to comply with the request. However, if the DTR distrusts the manager, the request could be viewed as an effort by the manager to save money by not hiring a replacement. If this is the belief, the DTR is more likely to resist doing any extra work. Whether the DTR believes the manager or not is dependent on the degree of trust that exists.

lack of belief that the leadership is serious about making changes

The old adage "Actions speak louder than words" applies here. If a manager tells employees about a proposed change that subsequently does not happen, then the employees are not likely to believe that the manager will ever make the change. If this happens repeatedly, about many different things, the employee is likely to think that the manager is all talk and no action. This can happen in all areas of management. A history of this type of behavior makes implementing change difficult.

For example, a department director might tell employees that they will have their performance appraisals one month before their anniversary dates so that their pay raises will begin on time. However, the promise is never carried out because the managers become distracted by other projects in the department. Then the director indicates that all employees will be eligible to take a class on time management, but the class never materializes. Next the employees are told that there will be a company party during the holidays for them and their families, but the party doesn't happen. Faced with this pattern of behavior from the manager, an employee is likely to ignore any talk of change, because the manager is "all talk" and seldom follows through. It is easy to interpret the behavior as resistance to change, though it might be that the employee is just being realistic.

lack of belief that the leadership is capable of making the change happen

Sometimes the change that is proposed appears to be a difficult one, or one that has been tried before and failed. Under these circumstances, or in situations where managers are viewed as weak or indecisive, employees may feel that the management cannot accomplish what it set out to do. Difficult or complex changes must be carried out by managers who have the will, the authority, and the stamina to implement those changes.

Consider the patient services manager (PSM) in a health care facility who initiates a program to have all patient foods tasted by a panel composed of a chef/cook, a foodservices manager, and a clinical dietitian. Because this must occur before the start of tray assembly, it is imperative that all food be ready 10 minutes prior to the scheduled start time. This can be accomplished only with the cooperation of the participants in the taste panel. However, the PSM has no control over the cooks to get the product out early because cooks report to the production manager, nor does the PSM manage the clinical staff or the foodservices managers.

Because the PSM has no authority over the taste panel members, there are likely to be no negative consequences for participants who show up late, or not at all, for the taste panel. Shortly, they will consider their role on the panel as nonessential. The program will falter as attendance drops. Eventually the program will be phased out. (The program may never even get off the ground if similar programs have been unsuccessful during previous trials.) In this situation, the program failed because of lack of authority on the part of the manager in charge of the program. Employees seem to sense when this is about to happen and ignore the change because there appears to be little chance of its successful implementation.

perception that the change is unfairly selective

Sometimes a proposed change has a greater impact on one part of the workforce than it has on another. For example, computerization in a campus dining operation may eliminate the need for clerical staff but have no effect on the number of food production workers needed. Conversely, in the summers, some production workers may be asked to take time off because the students are gone for this time period, while the paperwork continues and the office staff is still needed. When layoffs occur, they seldom affect all areas proportionately. Usually some groups are harder hit than others are. Though the management reasons may be sound, it may be felt that only a certain group has been targeted. This causes employee dissatisfaction and leads to resistance to change.

kinds of organizational change

Now that the reasons for resistance to change have been considered, it is important to learn what types of changes occur in organizations. In general, there are three types of changes that organizations face. These are change in structure, change in the work processes (reengineering), or change in the culture of the organization. Any of these changes may be considered individually, but usually each has an impact on the others.

change in structure

Organizational structure refers to those characteristics of the organization that are reflected in the organizational chart. A change in structure can be a change in hierarchy, line/staff relationships, span of control, centralization, or departmentalization. Change in structure does not necessarily mean a change in the overall size of the organization, though that may occur as part of structural change. Change in structure could involve other modifications to an organization's structure, like personnel reassignments, the opening of an office or a clinic in an outlying location, or the addition of a new service (an eating disorders program or a high-risk pregnancy program). Other examples of change in structure include the change that separates clinical nutrition services from foodservices in a hospital, or one that consolidates housing, dining, and environmental services on a university campus.

In recent years, a common form of restructuring has involved making the organization smaller. This has been called *downsizing* or *rightsizing* and is frequently seen as a negative change. Rightsizing is often accompanied by the flattening of the organization, which includes eliminating levels of management, increasing each manager's span of control, and empowering employees to be more accountable for their own activities. Though downsizing might be a solution for some problems, it is not a panacea. Organizations need to be careful that downsizing does not become an end in itself. Prior to determining if cuts in staffing levels are necessary, there must be a clear understanding of the goals and mission of the organization and of the work that needs to be done. Downsizing should always be a part of the solution to a larger problem. It is the means to an end, not the ultimate goal.

The reduction in force that accompanies downsizing is always a cause for concern. If the layoffs are done strictly on the basis of seniority, the task is relatively easy but may leave the company with an aging and tired workforce: employees who are happy to have survived the layoffs, but who lack enthusiasm. If seniority is not used as a basis for the layoffs, the managers have more flexibility to choose which employees to retain. Managers need to exercise caution and be sure to use objective criteria in making their selections. These include the skills that the worker brings to the workplace, the productivity of the employee, and quality of work. It should not be based on the employee's age, gender, economic need, personality, or the fact that the worker is the boss's cousin. It is easy to play favorites and choose to retain workers who are well liked but do not have good skills. This is likely to be a significant error.

For example, a Clinical Nutrition Manager may need to reduce the staff of 10 people by 30 percent. It is possible to accomplish this by retaining all seven clinical dietitians and laying off the DTR and two diet clerks. However, this means that the dietitians would have to assume tasks like checking patient trays for accuracy, correcting menus, and screening patients. Though they can probably do these tasks, the dietitians may not be as good at them as the technicians and the clerks are. In addition, the tasks may not be professionally rewarding to them. Given the nature of the work to be done, it might be better to retain one clerk and one technician and lay off one clerk and two dietitians.

Some organizations restructure through growth. This means adding staff and, perhaps, layers of management. An example of this type of growth can be seen in entrepreneurial businesses that started in someone's "garage" and expanded into a multimillion-dollar software development company. These changes in structure, though positive for the organization as a whole, are as traumatizing to employees as downsizing. The production worker, who used to see the owner of the company every day, is now insulated from that executive by a manufacturing manager and a vice president of operations. The worker can no longer tell the owner when something is wrong. Long-term employees may feel alienated because their voices are not being heard and their opinions no longer seem to be important.

Acquisitions and mergers also lead to changes in structure that may or may not result in a change in the organization's size. Though there will undoubtedly be changes at the top of the organizational structure as a result of a merger, the employees at lower levels may not experience much impact from the change.

change in work process

Other changes that can occur in organizations are changes in work process, also known as reengineering. Reengineering may be driven by economic reasons but are more likely to be driven by changes in technology, equipment, or personnel. It is notable, too, that reengineering does not always result in decreased manpower or decreased costs. Reengineering may be done to improve quality or performance, which could actually result in increased demand for a product. This, in turn, could lead to the need for increased labor hours and a larger staff.

Classic examples of economically driven reengineering are the self-service delis and salad bars located in corporate dining facilities. In the past, foodservice employees assembled all sandwiches and salads in the kitchen. Individually plated items were then placed on the cafeteria lines and purchased by customers. The assembly of the products was costly from a labor standpoint. It also meant that the dishes were in use for long periods of time, during which the products were being assembled, stored, displayed, and consumed. The transition to self-service transferred much of the labor to the customer. Portion control is not a problem, because the customer paid for the product by weight. In addition, a more rapid turnover of dishes meant that inventory costs for these items were reduced. In this situation, the reduction in operating costs justified the initial expenditure for the equipment needed to install a self-service unit. The change in how sandwiches and salads were made was driven by the need to reduce costs.

A technologically driven change can be seen in institutional mail distribution systems. The emergence of networking technologies for desktop computers has decreased the need for paper to flow between departments in an organization. Documents can be transmitted electronically, stored, revised, and updated without ever being printed on paper; e-mail has largely replaced hard copies of memos and letters and even magazines and journals. If a printed copy is desired, it is sent electronically and printed where it is needed so that the hard copy does not need to be transported from one place to another. Postage is calculated and printed electronically. Bulk mailings are folded, stuffed into envelopes, and sealed using specialty equipment. These and other changes in mailroom technology have decreased the need for large numbers of workers in the mailrooms of corporations, hospitals, and universities. This is one simple example of how process change can be driven by technology.

In addition to desktop computers, other technological advances are driving changes in how nutritional professionals do their work. Debit cards are being used by food stamp recipients, children in school lunch programs, and college students in campus dining facilities. Bioelectrical impedance measures body composition and indirect calorimetry measures basal resting metabolic rate. Tube feedings and intravenous solutions are being delivered with precision using electronic pumps. Inventory is being controlled using barcode technology. Hospital patients with access to room service choose their food on a meal-by-meal basis over the phone or by using wireless devices, as illustrated on in-house video systems.

Change in standard equipment may also impact how jobs are done. A good sharp knife will improve the performance of a chef. Clamshell griddles, convection ovens, and combination steamers all allow food to be cooked faster than by conventional methods, which means that recipes and procedures must be changed. The installation of a new dishwasher will usually change how the dishroom crew gets their jobs done. Even the rearrangement of the equipment within a work area can facilitate the workflow.

Finally, the personnel involved in doing or supervising the job may cause work processes to be altered. A new person might have a better idea about how to do a task. For example, an RD or a DTR may streamline the screening process by using a check mark if lab values are normal, rather than writing down all of the actual values. A diet clerk may determine that it is more efficient to wear a telephone headset to keep both hands free for handling paperwork. Staff at a WIC clinic could schedule group appointments for follow-up visits rather than staggered appointments, so that the clients might attend nutrition education classes rather than have individual counseling sessions. A manager may decide to provide cooks with additional cutting boards so that they can be sent through the dishwasher between uses, rather than having to be sanitized by the cooks between tasks.

Process changes may be planned, but often they happen spontaneously. They may be earthshaking (like the installation of a new computer system) or innocuous. Sometimes they happen without fanfare. For example, an RD may feel that it is too cumbersome to calculate body mass index on all clients, so decides to use a smartphone app instead. This is a personal choice that alters a work process for one individual but has no impact on the rest of the workforce.

change in organizational culture

A change in culture is the most basic type of change that can happen in an organization. It is also the one that is most far-reaching. At the same time, a cultural change is one that is likely to be overlooked. Organizational culture is less tangible than either structure or process. Managers can plan and implement changes to the structure of an organization, and then sit back and measure how the changes are progressing. The same can be done with process changes. However, it is difficult to visualize modifying an organization's culture, so management is very uncomfortable in tackling this type of change.

Cultural changes can result from a change in leadership, in mission, in management style, or just through evolution. Many of these changes—such as an increase in empowerment for employees, a transition from a we/they adversarial relationship to "team spirit," or pulling together to achieve a common goal—are worthy cultural changes but are very difficult to evaluate. Managers want measurable outcomes, but cultural changes cannot always be measured in the short term. Culture is something that must be nurtured over time. In organizations that have strongly positive cultures, other types of changes are likely to succeed. Ironically, organizations with a strong positive culture may not require major change, because these organizations are constantly adapting to their environment, making small adjustments on an ongoing basis. It might be said that if a corporate culture is well managed, nurtured, and allowed to evolve, change will manage itself.

Changes in organizational culture are likely to occur most rapidly during mergers, acquisitions, and divestitures. When companies change ownership, there are some differences between the organizational cultures that will require adjustments in how individual employees behave. Mergers tend to be somewhat easier if the companies involved have similar cultures, so that the adjustments that individuals are required to make are minimal. Organizations with vastly different cultures have more difficulty during the transition from old to new. They need to devote adequate resources to merging the two cultures.

In health care, as in the rest of the business world, each institution has its own unique culture. Some facilities, like teaching medical centers, are considered "high tech." The care given is state of the art, from the technology and science perspectives. The focus on technology will contribute significantly to the culture of the workplace. At the other end of the spectrum are the "high-touch" facilities. Though they also offer quality medical care, the focus is on the *care*. (Many such facilities are affiliated with religious denominations.) It does not take much imagination to see how these different cultures and values would make a merger difficult.

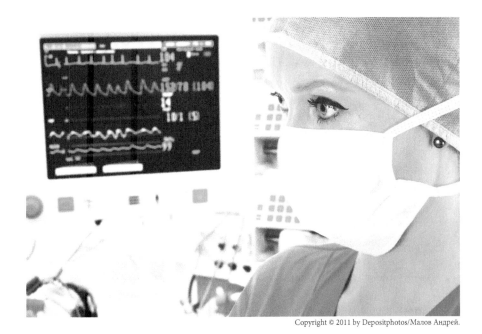

Some healthcare facilities are high tech …

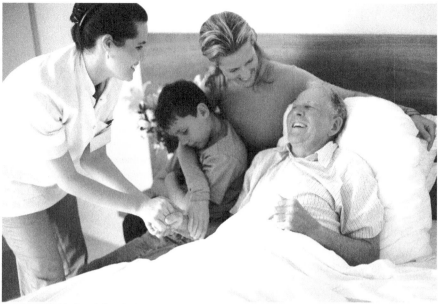

... others are high touch.

Despite the fact that organizational culture plays a central role in change management, it is often ignored during times of transition. Sometimes when the time for change arrives, it is too late to focus on culture. Under such circumstances, managers have to react in a timely manner and then revisit the cultural issues at a later date.

managing change

Managing change is a synthesis of much of what has been covered earlier in this text. It involves using the information that was discussed in the sections on leadership, communication, and decision making and applying it in situations that require major organizational change. Though managers routinely implement small changes, such as adjusting work schedules or reassigning tasks on a temporary basis, major changes are planned and implemented with greater deliberation, often with the help of a Gantt chart.

decision making

The process of managing change starts with problem identification. Recall that a problem is a discrepancy between what is and what should be. The problem that underlies the need for major change is seldom a simple one, like "there are too many employees." It is more likely to be that the company is losing money, that the customer is demanding something different, or that the cost of labor is too high. Management must be certain that it has identified the real problem and not merely a symptom. Problem identification may even involve anticipating a problem before it occurs. For example, a clinical nutrition manager may note that the facility is scheduled to transition to an electronic health record next year. The problem is one of training the clinical nutrition staff to use the new system before the system becomes operational.

Once the problem has been determined, the decision-making process is applied to establish what should be done to deal with the problem. Criteria must be established and weighted. Alternatives must be listed and analyzed. Then the decision is made, and the implementation is planned and set in motion. Finally, the results of the decision for change are evaluated.

Successful implementation of plans related to major changes, however, relies more heavily on communication and trust than does successful implementation for minor changes. If organizational leadership has used participatory management techniques, fostered open communication, shared information, earned and won the trust of personnel, and empowered employees to think for themselves, then implementing major change will be similar to implementing any other decision. The change will be handled routinely. However, if the organization is one in which communication is limited and information is hoarded, then there must be a new emphasis on communicating the impending changes with all levels of staff. Indeed, a change in the organizational culture may be necessary before a major change can succeed.

timing

One key factor that should be considered is timing. It is helpful to give personnel sufficient time to acclimate before implementing major changes. Employees need time to pass through five stages before adjustment to change will be complete. First they must become aware of the change, then understand it, support it, become actively involved, and finally committed to the change. These stages are listed in Table 17.2.

Personnel need time for discussion and to contribute their thoughts and ideas to the process of change. That means introducing the employees to the problem as soon as it is identified. If possible, staff should be allowed to participate in and contribute to discussions of the change at various levels. Though staff may not be called on to make a group decision related to major organizational change, they will feel a greater degree of ownership if their ideas are considered during the process. When employees are involved in setting and weighting criteria, in generating and analyzing alternatives, and in contributing to the implementation plan, many of the factors that cause staff to resist change are eliminated. In addition, management is gathering

Awareness
Understanding
Support
Involvement
Commitment

Adapted from: Bill Quirke, *Communicating Change*. McGraw Hill, 1995.

Table 18.2 Stages of Adjustment to Change[4]

management practice in dietetics

more information and developing more alternatives from which to choose. Managing change in this way creates a "win-win" scenario.

However, staff participation in change (like other forms of participative management) takes considerable time. Time is not always available when change is on the horizon. A crisis may dictate that an organization needs to cut costs dramatically and immediately in order to survive. In such cases, the time may have to be sacrificed to ensure the organization's existence. If changes are made quickly and without time for staff participation before the change, time after the event will be necessary for adjustment before the commitment stage is reached.

It should be noted that some managers identify a crisis when there is none. They want to move immediately to implement changes. This imperative to move quickly through the change process is often the result of the management's need to be doing something, rather than a real need for speed. Because time to adjust to change is necessary under any circumstances, the allocation of that time to a period either before or after the change is implemented should be a conscious decision. It is prudent to allow employees to get through as much of the adjustment period as possible prior to implementing major change, whenever this is feasible.

For example, if the change requires a reduction in the size of the workforce, allowing time for the adjustment period *before* the layoffs will provide adequate time for employees to adjust to the proposed change. Though this will cost some additional money, there is the benefit of giving managers more time to plan for a smooth transition from the old to the new structure. In this scenario, the adjustment period and the change itself are sequential steps; they do not occur at the same time. The employee is allowed to transition one step at a time.

If the adjustment period takes place *after* the reduction in force, there will be some monetary savings. However, productivity could decline dramatically during the adjustment period because the remaining workers will be dealing with both the change and the adjustment to the idea of the change, simultaneously. This compounds their stress levels; stress-related consequences could intensify. The time required to achieve commitment may increase when management uses this fast-track approach to change. In fact, commitment may never be achieved.

communication

In addition to identifying the problem correctly, generating trust, and using time deliberately, managers can employ some other techniques when implementing change. These have to do with how the change is communicated to the employees. Managers can "package" the message in the most positive light, minimizing problems and maximizing benefits. This is not to say that it is ever appropriate to lie to employees. Nonetheless, managers should be optimists rather than pessimists.

Those staff members who support the change can be recruited to help spread information about the new program to the remainder of the staff. These people may be given additional information about the change, and encouraged to share it with colleagues. This type of "cheerleading" can help to generate support for change. This technique may be used effectively to convince the employees who are ambivalent about the change to support it.

Finally, managers must be careful that the information that they pass along to their staff members is as correct and as clear as possible. Information should not be passed on prematurely, before decisions have been made. For instance, managers should not tell the staff that 20 percent of the workforce will be cut if the information they heard was that expenses have to be reduced by 20 percent. The information should be honest, presented in the best light possible, in the right amount, and without editorial comment. Managers must use good judgment in order to know the difference between fact and conjecture, and to pass on only the former. Employees should know what is relatively certain to happen but do not need to be informed of every possible alternative.

All of this information is useful in helping managers do their jobs during the change process. But the employee's perspective needs to be considered, as well. During times of change, either positive or negative, every employee and manager is under stress. There is a limit to each individual's ability to cope effectively with stress. The next section addresses this issue.

minimizing stress during change

Change, whether positive or negative, causes stress. Even the most positive change is accompanied by some degree of uncertainty. It is impossible to control for every contingency. When variables can be predicted, plans can be made to deal with those variables. However, during change, it is not likely that all of these factors will be known. The quirks, glitches, upsets, and surprises that accompany change increase resistance. Change upsets the status quo and takes away the comfort that comes with routines. In other words, any change causes some degree of stress.

Stress is also cumulative. If one is subjected to a major change in one's personal life, like marriage or divorce, changing jobs, purchasing a new home, and so on, one experiences significant stress. If several such changes occur in close proximity to one another, one's ability to cope is reduced. Changes in the work environment that take place when an individual's personal life is in upheaval are more stressful than changes at work when all is calm outside of the workplace. Because of differences in their personal lives, some people are better able to cope with workplace stress than are others. For the same reasons, an individual may handle workplace stress differently at different times. Unfortunately, organizations cannot time changes in the workplace so that they occur when workers are best able to cope with the additional stress. Still, there are some things that can be done to minimize the stress of change in the workplace.

trust

One major factor that determines how workers handle stress and change is the amount of trust that they have in the organization and its management. If there has been a history of broken promises and unfulfilled commitments, then the employee feels a greater degree of uncertainty than would be felt if there was a history of trust. If employees are told what to expect by someone they trust, they will be better prepared to handle stress.

communication

Communicating as much factual information as possible is also a benefit to employees. More information leads to a greater degree of certainty about what outcomes can be expected. Two-way communication is necessary so that staff can vent their frustrations and have their questions answered. As mentioned earlier, it is an added benefit to employees if they can contribute ideas that managers hear and acknowledge. This helps staff to feel that they have some role in the change process. They become active participants rather than bystanders.

transition time

There seems to be a threshold for the rate at which people can adjust to change. This must be considered if several changes need to be made. Multiple changes could be introduced at once, like a clinical nutrition service implementing a new patient information system at the same time as a different menu is introduced and a new formulary goes into effect. This frequently happens when a foodservice management company gets a contract with a health care foodservice operation. Sometimes the clinical nutrition manager is also new. Alternately, the changes could be made sequentially, first bringing in the new manager, then software, then implementing the menu, and finally introducing the formulary.

There are advantages and disadvantages to each method of introducing change. The larger, more complex group of simultaneous changes will generate intense stress for a relatively brief period of time. On the other hand, the sequential implementation of change will create less-intense stress over a longer period of time. The adjustment period for each change will be relatively short, but the total amount of time that it takes to complete all the changes will be considerable.

Managers can, therefore, choose to get through the stress as quickly as possible, or to transition more slowly. The latter choice may be better if it occurs in an environment with open communication and support. If the management is autocratic, it might be better to choose the more rapid transition time. Each manager must evaluate the options at the time of transition to determine how multiple changes are likely to be tolerated by staff.

employee assistance programs

Finally, when changes occur, large companies frequently offer Employee Assistance Programs (EAPs) to employees. Such programs can be geared toward those problems created by the change. If positions were eliminated and individuals lost their jobs, outplacement services are provided to assist employees in finding new jobs. If a change in structure requires that employees learn new jobs, retraining programs are established. At other times, stress management classes are appropriate. Normally, the Human Resources Department will administer these programs to help the employees get through organizational change successfully.

conclusion

This chapter has been drawn from the information that was presented in previous chapters and applied to the concept of managing change. The focus was on the types of changes that organizations face and the transitions that must occur to maneuver the organization through the transitions that are required of them. The concepts that were outlined in this chapter are listed below.

1. Change is inevitable and is taking place more rapidly than ever before.
2. People resist change for a variety of reasons, many of which have to do with miscommunication or misunderstanding.
3. Organizations undergo three basic types of changes—in structure, in work process, and in organizational culture.
4. Change is managed by establishing trust, using leadership effectively, making good decisions, and maintaining positive communication.
5. Employees should be given support and assistance to cope with the stress of change in the workplace.

activities

activity 1

List 10 major changes that have occurred in your life.

Rank these events in order of the amount of stress that they produced, from highest to lowest. Select one of the top three for analysis.

1. Describe how you handled the stress.
2. Is this the way that you usually deal with stress?
3. Do you deal differently with stress in your personal life than with stress at work or at school?
4. If yes, what is the difference?

activity 2

After students have completed the first individual activity, a class discussion should be held to:

1. Generate a list of the ways that individuals deal with stress.
2. Describe ways that groups deal with stress.
3. Determine how others—like teachers, families, and managers—help individuals and groups manage stress.

to study further

- Cameron, E. and M. Green. *Making Sense of Change Management: A Complete Guide to the Models, Tools & Techniques of Organizational Change.* 3rd ed. Philadelphia: Kogan Page, 2012.
- Cohen, D. S. *The Heart of Change Field Guide: Tools and Tactics for Leading Change in Your Organization.* Boston: Harvard Business School Press, 2005.
- *Harvard Business Review.* "Ten Must Reads on Change Management." Boston: Harvard Business Review Press, 2011.
- *Harvard Business Review.* "On Culture and Change." Boston: Harvard Business School Publishing, 2002.
- Harigopal, K. *Management of Organizational Change.* 2nd ed. Thousand Oaks, CA: Response Books, 2006.
- Hayes, J. *The Theory and Practice of Change Management.* 3rd ed. New York: Palgrave Macmillan, 2010.
- Jarratt, J. and J. B. Mahaffie. "Key Trends Affecting the Dietetics Profession and the American Dietetic Association." *Journal of the American Dietetic Association.* 102:1821–1839, 2002.
- Johnson, S. *Who Moved My Cheese?* New York: P.J. Putnam's Sons, 1998.
- Kotter, J. and H. Rathgeber. *Our Iceberg Is Melting: Changing and Succeeding Under Any Conditions.* New York: St. Martin's Press, 2005.
- Peregrin, T. "Guidelines for Successfully Managing Organizational Change." *Journal of the Academy of Nutrition and Dietetics.* 112:368–373, 2012.
- Porter, C. "A New Emphasis on Health Care Safety, Quality, and Cost Containment: How Will This Affect Dietetics Practice?" *Journal of the American Dietetic Association.* 104:1667–1670, 2004.
- Quinn, R. E. *Building the Bridge as You Walk on It: A Guide for Leading Change.* San Francisco: Jossey-Bass, 2004.
- Schein, E. H. *The Corporate Culture Survival Guide.* New and rev. ed. San Francisco: Jossey-Bass Publishers, 2009.
- Schein, E. H. *Organizational Culture and Leadership.* 4th ed. San Francisco: Jossey-Bass, 2010.
- Schein, Lawrence. *Post-Merger Integration: A Human Resources Perspective.* New York: The Conference Board, Inc., 2000.
- Schein, Lawrence. *Managing Culture in Mergers and Acquisitions.* New York: The Conference Board, Inc., 2001.
- Silverman, M. R. et al. "Current and Future Practice in Hospital Foodservice." *Journal of the American Dietetic Association.* 100:76–80, 2000.

scholarly journals

- *The Journal of Organizational Change Management*
- *Strategic Change*

management practice in dietetics

in practice

anticipating change

Though it is impossible to predict change with precision, some societal trends have begun that will have an impact on how dietetics professionals will need to practice during the twenty-first century. Three of these are presented here. The purpose of describing these trends is not to present a discussion of change management. No attempt will be made to propose solutions or strategies for your consideration. This is merely an attempt to provide "food for thought" so that you, as a dietetics professional, may be better prepared to address these and other changes that are destined to occur during your career.

how and where we eat

First, let's look at how we are eating. Households in North America were pretty self-sufficient a century ago. Much of what was used in the home was made or grown there. This included items of furniture, clothing, and, of course, food. Limited varieties of foods were available in the marketplace, and restaurants were a rarity, providing few options and choices for the consumer. Typically, at least one adult worked in the home full-time. Not only was most food prepared and consumed at home, but that food was consumed at family meals, scheduled into the routines of the day. Most families ate as a social unit at least twice (sometimes three times) a day, in the morning and in the evening. The foods consumed were prescribed by the cook, based on what was available, and few alternatives were offered. You either ate what was served, or you didn't eat.

Now families function differently. The definition of family is changing; much of the time, there is no adult at home during the day. Food is purchased in varying forms of readiness and either eaten cold or rethermed in the home. It is not being cooked there. (Homes are paralleling institutional foodservices in transitioning from cook-serve, to cook-chill modes of operation.) At the same time, a wide variety of products are available that allow family members to choose what to eat, and prepare single portions of that product whenever they want it. Schedules are dictated by outside events like team sports, classes, jobs, and the like, so family mealtimes may not be an option for some of us. The family meal, which used to be the norm, is disappearing. It is a holiday event rather than a twice-daily affair.

Increasingly, foods are taking on the form of "road food." We are getting good at "multitasking" so have learned to eat finger foods while driving to work and school. Breakfast sandwiches, energy bars, and snack foods are consumed on the go. Many folks actually store this type of food item in their vehicles, creating a replacement for the kitchen cupboard. Vehicles are designed with cup holders that used to hold either disposable cups or soda cans. Now, other products are designed to fit these holders; milk, soup, salads, yogurt, and meal replacement drinks are among those available, with more to come in the future. Furthermore, some accessories available for vehicles include refrigeration units and food warming units. And if we don't want to eat while driving, there are countless quick service restaurants ready to provide us with whatever we want, whenever we want it!

Who knows how the foods of the future will evolve, but if the current trend continues, the need to do any food preparation at home will fade away. In the future, the home kitchen may disappear entirely (going the way of the sewing room or the wood shop). If this happens, how will dietetics professionals be able to satisfy the needs of hospital-ized patients who are accustomed eating "on demand"? As to counseling patients on foods and food preparation techniques, is it realistic to expect clients to follow meal plans when they don't eat meals? Will we be ready and able to adapt to that change?

food intolerances and allergies

Nearly everyone knows that allergies to peanuts and shellfish can lead to anaphylaxis and death. Those who have food intolerances or allergies generally adapt by avoiding the offending food. Perhaps you know someone who must limit or eliminate milk because of a lactase deficiency. For severe allergies, some individuals must carry an EpiPen® so that they can inject life-saving epinephrine if exposed to the allergen.

There is a very real difference between a food allergy and a food intolerance. Moreover, not all of these allergies and intolerances are equally dangerous. Though some individuals become highly symptomatic in response to certain foods, others are merely uncomfortable for a short period of time. In developed countries where the Internet is widely available, some individuals may be too aware of potential food allergies and intolerances, almost to the point of hypochondria. When food sensitivi-ties are self-diagnosed, they may or may not be real at all.

For years, dietetics professionals have been working with patients with gluten-induced enteropathy, also called celiac disease or non-tropical sprue. The disease was difficult to treat with elimination diets since all sources of gluten, a protein found in many grains, needed to be eliminated. On this diet, patients must avoid wheat, rye, and barley in any form. Ready-prepared foods for this condition were limited, and items like bread and baked goods (which are typically wheat-based) had to be replaced with gluten-free products that were available only through mail order. Even foods that were OK to use one month may not be OK the next month if the manufacturing processes changed.

With the help of the Internet, many more people became aware of the condition. They began to experiment with the use of a gluten-free, or at least a reduced-gluten diet. Their interest sparked the food industry to develop more gluten-free products, which made their way into neighborhood grocery stores and restaurants. The marketing of these products further increased interest in gluten and, in due course, people began to diagnose themselves with gluten sensitivity.

It is impossible to determine how many of those who state that they are unable to consume gluten really have an intolerance of or a sensitivity to gluten. Some may actually have an allergy to wheat, which is different from gluten sensitivity. What is known, though, is that dietetic professionals had to adapt to this challenge by learning more about the underlying disorder and how to determine the extent to which the problem is real in a given individual. They also learned to be assertive about requesting a bona fide medical diagnosis before implementing such drastic dietary restrictions for their patients.

But the real problem is this … what is the next trend going to be? Will the Internet create a massive following for the raw food diet? Will super blue-green algae return to become the dietary supplement of the year? Will yogurt enemas come to be the recommended way in which to get probiotics? And will dietetics professionals be ready to face whatever that next movement will be?

high fructose corn syrup

There is a growing outcry against the widespread use of high fructose corn syrup (HFCS). It is used in the production of many different foods, the most prevalent of which are sweetened carbonated beverages. In some places, limits have been placed on the amount of the beverage that may be sold in a "to go" container. Other proposed interventions include a tax on these beverages or an outright ban on the use HFCS.

Proponents of these restrictions argue that HFCS is a major contributor to the over-weight and obesity epidemic that exists in North America. They believe that the rise in obesity has a direct relationship with the use of this sugar as an ingredient in food products.

Some take the opposing view, noting that consumption of HFCS beverages is and should be a personal choice. Since HFCS is chemically almost the same as sucrose (table sugar), it is unfair to single out the HFCS as being unhealthy. A further argument is that the negative effects are not caused by the HFCS per se, but the amount of total sugars that an individual consumes. Individuals should increase their energy expenditure if they do not want to gain weight.

It appears that there are several options for dealing with the controversy. First, a tax could be levied on HFCS-containing beverages, making it more expensive to purchase these products. It is even possible that the proceeds from this tax could be used for obesity prevention programs. Second, the amount of HFCS in a beverage could be decreased, to limit the number of total kilocalories being consumed. (This kind of "stealth nutrition" is already being used to decrease the sodium content of some canned foods.) Third, the use of HFCS in carbonated beverages could be banned entirely. (Historically, it has been demonstrated that when the public insists on the removal of an ingredient from a food product, manufacturers respond, as they did by lowering the trans fat content of many foods in the early part of this century.) The final option is to do nothing at all.

Which of these options appeals to you? Do you think that the government has the right or the duty to regulate what and how much individuals consume? What should dietetics students and dietetics professionals be doing NOW to address this issue?

These and other changes are inevitable. Will we view them as obstacles or as opportunities? With creativity and flexibility, we should be able to meet these and other challenges as they arise. But it requires the vision to think outside the box, and an attitude that allows us to be in that 20% of society who embraces change, rather than in the 30% who resists it.

references

1. Want, Jerome H. *Managing Radical Change: Beyond Survival in the New Business Age.* New York: John Wiley and Sons, 1995.
2. Laabs, Jennifer J. "Expert Advice on How to Move Forward with Change." *Personnel Journal* 75, July 1996:54–64.
3. Adapted from: Bill Quirke, *Communicating Change.* Copyright © 1995 by Bill Quirke. Reprinted with permission.
4. Ibid.

Index

Glossary

Accommodation. A situation in which members of a group feel that they have to accept the position of the dominant member of the group.

Accountability. The state of being responsible or liable for actions taken. Managers are accountable to suppliers, employees, customers, and other constituencies for what they do as well as for the work of their subordinates. Accountability includes a sense of duty to ensure that the proper services and goods are provided and individuals are treated fairly.

Accounting Period. The time period designated by an organization for purposes of financial reporting.

Accounts Payable. Money that is owed by a business to a creditor for the purchase of products, rent, mortgage payments, and other outstanding loans.

Accounts Receivable. Money that is owed to a business for products that have been delivered and invoiced.

Accreditation Council for Education in Nutrition and Dietetics. http://www.eatright.org/ACEND/

Accrued Liability. Expenses for which payment will be made in a future period, such as paid time off and income taxes.

Adequate. A criterion for management that considers if what was done was done in the correct amount.

Adjusted Occupied Beds. A measure generated through the use of a mathematical formula to adjust the actual number of occupied beds to reflect the work that is done in the hospital for patients who are not actually admitted for 24 hours or are not in residence at the time when the occupied bed census is taken. The formula is based on the hospital's usual activity patterns, volumes of outpatient visits, day surgeries, patient acuity, and so on.

Advertisement. A job recruitment method in which the organization has complete control over the content.

Affirmative Action. A federal law that requires giving hiring preference to previously disenfranchised workers.

AGA Certified. http://www.americangrassfed.org/

American Hospital Association. www.aha.org/

Americans with Disabilities Act Home Page. http://www.ada.gov/

Americans with Disabilities Act Home Page. http://www.ada.gov/

Americans with Disabilities Act. A federal law that enables people with different physical abilities to enter the mainstream with greater ease by mandating that organizations and businesses provide the appropriate accommodation (for example, accessible lavatories, parking, and so on) for all.

Analytic Decision Maker. A type of decision maker who enjoys solving problems, likes to seek alternatives and information, can tolerate ambiguity, and applies a rational, methodical approach to solve problems.

Analyze the Alternatives. The fifth step in the decision-making process; the process of comparing and examining the alternatives available by measuring them against the same standards, using only relevant criteria.

AND's Evidence Analysis Library. http://andevidencelibrary.com/

Anecdotal Information. Optional informal notes that are sometimes kept by a manager as a reminder of things that have occurred.

Annual Bonus. One type of pay for performance that is earned at the end of the year for outstanding performance during that year. It usually results from meeting a pre-established goal. This is a one-time bonus that does not change the base pay rate.

Appropriate. A criteria for management based on the ability to adapt to the specific environment.

Aquaculture. The farming of fish.

Arbitration. A hearing before someone empowered to resolve the dispute.

Archive. Stored information.

Armored Transport. Transport of money between retail facilities and commercial banks by licensed and bonded companies.

Artifacts. Tangible items and their placement, which are a part of nonverbal communication that can convey an unintended message.

As Purchased (AP). The amount of a product (food item) acquired before any production loss has occurred.

Assets. Items of value owned by a person or business (for example, checking and savings accounts, real estate, inventories, equipment, and so on).

Attrition. Loss of employees because the employees voluntarily choose to leave their jobs.

Autocratic Leadership. A leadership style illustrated by a leader who takes total control, assumes full authority, and takes full responsibility for the area managed.

Balance Sheet. A financial report that summarizes an organization's assets, liabilities, and owners' equity. It provides the user with a snapshot of the organization's financial status at a specific point in time.

Bank. The amount of money that the cash register drawer contains at the start of a shift.

Base Rate. The hourly rate of pay for workers who are paid by the hour.

Behavioral Decision Maker. A type of decision maker who uses intuition, feelings, and perceptions versus hard data, and who dislikes ambiguity.

Benchmarking. The practice of measuring an organization's performance and productivity against standards, either internal or external.

Bereavement Time. Paid time off when there is a death in the family.

Bid Purchasing. A type of purchasing that requires vendors to bid on the item or items an organization specifies in order to be eligible to get the business; used mostly for capital equipment and contracts. The business is generally awarded to the lowest bidder who meets the specifications.

Blind Receiving. The process of receiving material when the amount is not included on the shipping document, so the receiver must write in the amount that was delivered.

Body Language. A personal characteristic of nonverbal communication that includes the use and extent of facial expressions and gestures, and may have an impact on communication.

Bonded. To bind by an agreement to pay a certain amount of money upon failure to complete a job properly; insuring an organization against financial loss incurred by such.

Brainstorming. The informal process of tackling a given problem by contributing as many ideas as possible without analysis or criticism.

Budget Variance. Any deviation from the budget.

Budget. An estimate of the income and expenditures during a given period of time based on the mission, goals, and objectives of an organization. In other words, an organization's business plan expressed in financial terms.

Budgeted Balance Sheet. A statement of the assets and liabilities of an organization based on budget estimates.

Bureau of Labor Statistics. http://www.bls.gov/

Burnout. A physical consequence of stress in the workplace that can result from working long hours, being tired, dissatisfied, or angry with the work or work setting.

Buy Back. An option in which the employer pays the employee for accrued time off that was not used.

Cafeteria Package. A selection of benefits offered to employees from which they can pick and choose according to individual needs.

Calendar Year. A 12-month period that begins January 1 and ends December 31.

Capital Budget. Projects spending on items that are costly and durable such as land, buildings, and major pieces of equipment.

Capital Goods. Large equipment, considered fixed assets, that is durable and can be depreciated over a period of time.

Captive Clientele. Customers who must use a product or a service because they have no other options.

Career Employees. Workers who expect to continue working in a job as long as their work performance is adequate.

Career Ladder. A series of progressively more responsible positions that allows one to move from entry level to upper level management over time.

Cash Award. A pay-for-performance plan that awards cash to employees for being creative, innovative, helpful, or just a good citizen. It is usually a one-time award.

Cash Budget. An estimate of the anticipated cash flow (that is, cash on hand, accounts payable, accounts receivable, and the cost of credit) that can be used to project the availability of funds.

Cash Handling. The management of cash transactions (includes the receiving, storing, counting, recording, withdrawing, and depositing of cash).

Cash Receipts. The amount of money that is present in the cash register drawer at the end of the day minus the starting bank.

Cash Register Tapes. A record of cash transactions made and stored by the cash register that contains information about daily cash sales.

Cash Register. A machine that records and displays the details of a sales transaction (such as the quantity and price of items purchased), as well as acting as a storage unit for the cash involved in these transactions.

Casual Employee. A worker who is not guaranteed any set number of hours each week but who is scheduled for work as needed.

Cause. A documented, legitimate reason for terminating a nonprobationary employee.

Centralization. The concentration of decision making and power at the upper levels of an organization.

Certainty. A situation in which the outcome of a decision is known and expected.

Certified Humane Raised and Handled. http://www.certified-humane.org/

Chain of Command. The vertical relationships between members of an organization that are based on authority and power.

Channel. A communication pathway through which a message is transmitted.

Charisma. A characteristic in leaders that reflects their degree of personal magnetism and their ability to attract others and to be followed.

Chief Clinical Dietitian. A managerial title of a dietitian who manages the clinical nutrition area of a healthcare facility and also does direct patient care.

Civil Service Examinations. A highly structured group interview used for candidates for governmental positions.

Clinical Dietitians. Registered dietitians who work in a healthcare setting and provide nutritional care to patients; management skills are often required as part of the job.

Clinical Nutrition Manager. The manager who is responsible for the overall nutritional care of patients who are admitted to a healthcare facility. This person may not do direct patient care on a regular basis.

Coercive Power. A type of power managers have to punish, which can be seen in disciplining, suspending, or terminating employees for cause, or in laying off staff when needed.

Commercial Bank. A banking institution that handles the everyday financial transactions of businesses.

Commercial Foodservices. Foodservices that traditionally cater to customers who have choices in where to eat, and which are usually profit driven (for example, supermarkets, food courts, restaurants, and so on).

Communication. The interaction between two or more individuals that allows for information to move from one person to another, either on a person-to-person level or through the use of some type of media.

Community Dietitian or Community Nutritionist. An RD who works in community nutrition by giving direct care to a client or clients. WIC Home Page www.fns.usda. gov/wic/ National Dairy Council. www.nationaldairycouncil.org Nutrition Screening Initiative. http://www.hospitalmedicine.org/geriresource/toolbox/pdfs/determine.pdf

Community Supported Agriculture. A system in which consumers purchase a membership in a CSA, in return for which they receive a box of freshly harvested farm products each week during the growing season.

Compensation. The salary given for work performed.

Compensatory Time Off. A method used to give salaried employees who work long hours some extra time off to compensate them for unpaid overtime worked.

Composting. The decomposition of organic material (like plants and food waste) into a material that can be used either to enhance soil or as a fertilizer.

Computer Forecasting. Using computer-generated forecasts to determine production needs. Accuracy is dependent on reliable historical data.

Computer Menu. A list of the available commands and operations performed by a computer from which a user may select.

Conceptual Decision Maker. A type of decision maker characterized by being open to new ideas, looking at many alternatives, having a high tolerance for ambiguity, and relying on instinct versus logic and reason.

Conceptual Skills. Managerial skills related to working with abstract ideas and concepts.

Consensus Leadership. A leadership style that requires that decisions or plans be made by a group and is based on all members working together until agreement is reached.

Conserve—Sustainability Education Program. http://conserve. restaurant.org/index.cfm

Consolidated Balance Sheet. A report that consolidates all the data from the balance sheets of an organization from multiple years into one statement. It is used to document financial conditions over time for internal and external reporting purposes.

Consolidated Profit and Loss Statement. A report that merges all the data from the profit and loss statements of an organization from multiple years into one report. It can be used for identifying trends over time.

Consultant Fee. A designated amount of remuneration for a contract employee; the fee may be established for the project or as a monthly or hourly rate for the duration of the project.

Contingent Workers. Employees, such as temporary and contract employees, who know that their work positions are short-term or temporary.

Continuing Education. Educational activities that are conducted by an external organization and that take place outside of the workplace. Examples include trade shows, educational workshops or seminars, college or university courses, and so on.

Continuous Quality Improvement (CQI). The processes of identifying areas in a department that can be strengthened and working to make those areas better.

Contract Employee. A worker who is usually hired to complete a project and who is typically not part of the payroll.

Contract Management Companies. Organizations that provide foodservice to other organizations or institutions; contracts vary in the services provided.

Controlling. A management function that involves inspecting the work that is done, ensuring that standards are met, and monitoring that the work is done as planned.

Cook-Chill Foodservices. Foodservices where hot foods are pre-prepared then chilled and held at safe (cool) temperatures then are rethermalized just prior to service.

Cook-Serve Foodservices. Foodservices in which hot foods are cooked and held at safe (hot) temperatures until they are served.

Cost Center. Any unit within an organization that has expenses. Some cost centers, like foodservices and pharmacy, also generate revenues. Others, like payroll, human resources, and materials management, are not expected to generate a profit or to break even.

Cost Plus. A pricing method in which the purchaser pays the actual cost of the goods to the vendor, plus a markup (often a set percentage) to cover the vendor's handling costs and profit.

Cost-of-Living Adjustments (COLAs). Pay raises that are based on inflation rates and are used to keep an employee's purchasing power intact despite economic changes over time. These raises change the base pay rate permanently.

Creativity. A leadership trait that enables effective leaders to find solutions and new ways to get things done.

Cross-Training. Preparing employees to perform various jobs within a work setting.

Cultural Competence. The ability to provide linguistically and culturally appropriate services.

Culturally Diverse Organization. An organization that has a workforce representative of many different cultural groups.

Current Assets. Cash and all assets that are readily available and can be converted to cash within a short period of time (usually one year).

Current Liabilities. Short-term debt that is due to be paid in the near future.

Customize. Develop or modify applications to fit the needs of a particular customer.

Cycle Menu. A menu that varies from day to day, but repeats itself when the cycle is complete. The menu cycle may be a few days or several weeks in length.

Database. A set of related information that is organized and stored in a computer for access and is usually associated with software applications.

De Facto Decisions. Decisions that are made passively with no obvious objections expressed.

Decentralization. The ability for individuals at lower levels of an organization to make decisions appropriate to their own areas of responsibility.

Decisional Roles. A managerial role based on being an entrepreneur, disturbance handler, resource allocator, and negotiator; these roles allow a manager to take charge, make changes, handle conflicts, determine how resources are used, and arrange deals.

Decision-Making Process. The logical, stepwise approach that is used to make a choice between options, to solve a problem, or to resolve a dilemma.

Decode. Decipher the message that was received.

Delphi Technique. An approach to coming up with a group decision similar to the nominal group technique except that members do not meet but instead communicate and analyze ideas through written communication until consensus is reached.

Demands. Wants that are supported by resources, such as money, that allow the wants to be fulfilled.

Democratic Leadership. A leadership style based on "majority rules," in which decisions are made by the group rather than by the manager alone.

Departmental Policy and Procedure Manuals. Written or online documents, specific to a department, that guide the activities and work processes of that department.

Departmentalization. The specialization of groups in an organization, which may be based on product, function, clients, location, or work processes.

Depreciation. An accounting technique that spreads the expense of capital equipment or buildings over their life spans, because value decreases gradually with time. It is calculated by dividing the purchase price of an item by its expected lifetime.

Dietetic Technician, Registered (DTR). A technician who has completed registration eligibility requirements established by the Commission on Dietetic Registration, successfully passed the Registration Examination for Dietetic Technicians, and meets continuing education requirements.

Differential Wage Rates. Changes in the rate of pay, such as additional pay for working overtime, for performing exceptionally difficult work, for working in a different job, or the additional payment made to employees who do not receive benefits.

Direct Channel. A communication pathway in which the message sent is targeted to a specific group(s) or person(s).

Direct Labor Costs. Labor costs that are related to the actual performance of work (for example, base pay, overtime, pay in lieu of benefits, and so on). These are the projections that get written into the labor budget.

Direct Material Budget. The estimate of cost for raw materials to be used in the production of goods. This part of the operating budget is computed for departments that produce a tangible product.

Directive Decision Maker. A type of decision maker characterized by being efficient and logical, requiring little information to make a decision, looking at few alternatives, and exhibiting a low tolerance for ambiguity.

Disciplinary Action. The activity performed by a manager when implementing a step in progressive discipline in order to assist an employee to correct a behavioral or performance problem.

Disciplinary Process. A step-by-step method of dealing with performance problems in employees.

Distribution Channel. The route products follow from the manufacturer to the end user; may be direct and simple, or complex with the products changing ownership several times along the way.

Distribution. The method of delivering a product to the marketplace.

Diversity. In the workplace, this refers to ethnic, racial, gender, age, and other differences among workers.

Division of Labor. The practice of assigning each worker a few specialized tasks to perform, rather than a large number of more general tasks.

Documentation. A written record of the disciplinary actions taken.

DOE Energy Label Guide. http://energy.gov/energysaver/articles/tips-shopping-appliances

Downtime. The time during which a facility cannot function as usual, due to such disturbances as power outages and system failures.

Downward Mobility. When an employee reverts to a previous or lower position in an organization.

Dress for Success. The idea that an appropriate appearance and grooming style will create the desired effect during communication.

Drive. A major trait of effective leaders that describes their ambition, efforts, and risks they take in order to succeed.

Durable Goods. Products that can oftentimes be used and reused repeatedly and that have a life expectancy measured in years.

Economy of Scale. A concept that it is more efficient to complete a task once on a large scale versus repeating the same task on a smaller scale to reach the same output level.

Edible Portion (EP). The amount of food that can be consumed after accounting for preparation and/or cooking losses.6

Effective. A criteria for management focused on meeting defined goals and objectives.

Efficient. A criteria for management defined as doing things in the best way relative to resource utilization.

Electronic Health Record (EHR). Computer-based electronic data processing and storage of complete client/patient records that eliminates the need for hard copies of these documents.

Employee Assistance Programs. Plans that provide employees with support in dealing with personal crises that could negatively impact work performance.

Employee Discipline. A tool used by managers to improve poor performance and enforce appropriate behavior to ensure a productive and safe workplace.

Employee Grievances. A method for employees to use to resolve conflicts when they feel they have been treated unfairly by management.

Employee Handbook. A publication, either print or web-based, that can serve as a reference manual to employees after the orientation process is completed. It usually reiterates material covered during the orientation and addresses other frequently asked questions.

Employee Handbooks. Written or online documents produced by organizations to provide information to employees relating to the organization's mission, policies, rules, benefits, and so on.

Encode. Create a message and determine how it is to be sent.

Energy Star. http://www.energystar.gov/

Entry-Level. A beginning position in a profession (for example, an entry-level dietitian).

EPA Fuel Economy Estimate. http://www.fueleconomy.gov/

Equal Opportunity. A federal law that prohibits discrimination against certain groups, such as women or minorities, in the workforce.

Ergonomics. The physical aspects of work and movement; how movement relates to the performance of a task.

Essential Communications Documents. Types of written communication that are necessary (fundamental) to carrying out the business of an organization.

Establish Decision-Making Criteria. The second step in the decision-making process; determining which factors will have the most relevance in solving a given problem.

Evaluation. The eighth and last step of the decision-making process; receiving feedback about the decision that has been implemented—that is, was it effective, efficient, appropriate, and adequate?

Expense Budget. Component of the operating budget that deals with all anticipated costs, which can further be divided into a number of sub-budgets (for example, labor, material, overhead, and other expenses).

Expert Power. A type of power—also known as the power of knowledge, experience, and information—in which an individual can exert influence on others due to their knowledge in a certain field.

Expertise. An important leadership trait that reflects the training and knowledge a leader must have in his or her specific field.

External Benchmarking. The process of an organization comparing its performance and productivity with those of other comparable organizations to determine whether it is performing at, above, or below the industry standard.

External Customer. The end user of the product made by an organization.

Extrinsic Information. Information that is stored in a computer system for the purpose of processing intrinsic information. It includes the database and the program that contains necessary information for carrying out the actual processing.

Facilities Design. The layout of a workplace (including traffic patterns), which affects the flow of people, goods, and services within a designated space.

FDA Food Code. http://www.fda.gov/Food/FoodSafety/RetailFoodProtection/FoodCode/FoodCode2009/default.htm

FDA's Food Code. Food and Drug Administration guidelines that specify correct food-handling techniques.

Feedback. Outputs from a system that are recycled as inputs to prevent errors or to improve the system in the future.

Feedback. The responses generated during interpersonal communications are known as feedback.

Firewall. Software that protects a private network or organizational intranet from outside penetration.

Fiscal Year. A 12-month period for which an organization plans the use of its funds. It can begin on any date and end 365 days later (366 in leap years).

FishWatch. http://www.fishwatch.gov/index.htm

Fixed Assets. Nonliquid, tangible goods that have been capitalized and are being depreciated over time. Includes land, buildings, equipment, and any improvements like new carpeting, paint jobs, and the installation of security systems.

Fixed Budget. Budget plan for which funds are allocated for the entire fiscal year. It is also known as static budget and can be applied to either the zero-based budget or to the incremental budget.

Flexibility. A known leadership characteristic that enables leaders to react to new changes and adapt well, allowing them to make quick judgments and adjustments.

Food and Drug Administration. http://www.fda.gov/

Food Waste Conversion Technology. http://www.ecorect.com/

Foodservice Programs. An information processing system for foodservices used to manage purchasing and inventory data, produce food production forecasts, generate quantity recipes, compute costs, analyze use, calculate waste, and so on.

Foodshed. The geographic region from which a community is fed.

Forecasting. A tool used to predict the quantities of product needed.

Form. A description of the product, which may include weight, size, packaging, and so on.

Formal Leader. A type of leader who is usually a manager and is recognized as one with a position and title that reflect the individual's status.

Four P's of Marketing. Product, place, promotion, and price; sometimes called the marketing mix.

Frequency of Delivery. The number of times deliveries are made by a vendor to a purchasing organization, which could be daily, weekly, or monthly.

Frontline Managers. Managers who oversee employees responsible for production; need a high level of technical skills, good human relations skills, and some conceptual skills.

Fruits and Veggies—More Matters. www.fruitsandveggiesmorematters.org

Full-Time Employee. An individual who is designated to work a certain number of hours a week who is considered "full time" by the employer (typically 40 hours/week).

Full-Time Equivalent (FTE). A standard term used to describe the number of full-time positions worked by all employees, including full-time, part-time, short-hour, and casual. One FTE is usually equal to 40 hours per week or 2,080 hours per year.

Gantt Chart. A two-dimensional diagram of a master schedule on which activities are listed on the left side of the figure and times are represented across the top. It depicts the movement of work through time.

Garbage Disposal. A machine that uses large amounts of water as it grinds solid waste; discharges both into the sewer system.

Global Warming. Increase in the temperature of the earth's oceans and atmosphere over time, generally thought to be due to human activity.

Goods. Tangible products. Ownership is transferred when goods are sold.

Green Restaurant Association. http://www.dinegreen.com/

Green Seal. http://www.greenseal.org/

Groceries. Food products that are shelf-stable at room temperature.

Grooming. The personal appearance, style, and attire of an individual, which has an impact on communication.

Group Interview. An interview in which more than one person interviews the candidate.

Groupthink. A characteristic of groups that evolves when the cohesiveness of the group becomes more important than the problem that needs to be solved; in this situation, members feel loyal to each other and may not want to jeopardize this unity by expressing opposing opinions.

HACCP (Hazard Analysis and Critical Control Point). Process that promotes food-safety protocols and outlines steps in the preparation of a food item starting from its point of delivery all the way to consumption.

Health Canada. http://www.hc-sc.gc.ca/index-eng.php

Healthcare Insurance Portability and Accountability Act. http://www.hhs.gov/ocr/privacy/

Hearing. A physical sense that is involuntary and passive and often done automatically without paying attention.

Hierarchy. A description of the vertical relationships in an organization, which dictates the reporting relationship among workers and the various levels of management.

High-Density Shelving. A type of storage unit that moves on tracks built into the storeroom. It saves space and promotes efficiency.

HIPAA. http://www.hhs.gov/ocr/privacy/hipaa/understanding/index.html.

Hiring Decision. The selection of the best candidate for the position.

Hiring Incentives. Rewards or bonuses that are given to job candidates to entice them to accept a position.

Hourly Worker. An employee who is paid a set rate for each hour worked, which is at least the minimum wage set by the government.

http://www.servsafe.com/home

Human Resource Policy and Procedure Manuals. Written or online documents used as a management tool to direct the actions of management relative to employee relations.

Human Resources Department. The department within an organization that is responsible for personnel matters, setting policy and procedures related to employees, and training managers in how to deal with human relations issues.

Human Resources. The people who work in an organization.

Human Skills. A managerial skill set composed of personal attributes, knowledge, and learned behavior that enables managers to work effectively and communicate with others.

Identify the Alternatives. The fourth step in the decision-making process; the act of determining the different options available to solve the problem at hand.

Implement the Decision. The seventh step in the decision-making process; the act of carrying out the decision that has been made; often involves communicating exactly what is to happen based on the decision.

Incremental Budget. A type of operating budget that is based on the previous year's budget and a predetermined increment. This increment may depend on a number of factors such as inflation rate, labor contracts, profitability, operating losses, restructuring, reengineering, and so on.

Incumbent. The person who currently holds the position.

Indirect Channel. A communication pathway in which the receiver is not specified.

Indirect Labor Costs. Labor costs over which managers have little control. These include benefits like insurance, taxes, and paid time off, which are not always included in the labor budget.

Indirect Material Budget. The estimate of the cost of materials that are used, but not associated with production.

Informal Leader. A type of leader who exhibits many characteristics of the formal leader but is not recognized as a leader by an organization and holds no title or authority.

Informatics. The science of information, which "studies the representation, processing, and communication in natural and artificial systems."

Information Management (IM). An area of management that includes "the planning, budgeting, control and exploiting of the information resources of an organisation."

Information Overload. Having too much data, which may impede management processes and interfere with decision making.

Information Shortages. The condition that exists when data are deficient or when not enough information is available to get a job completed.

Informational Roles. A managerial role in which the manager monitors and disseminates information or acts as a spokesperson for the organization.

Ingredient Room. A designated area of a food production facility in which the items needed to prepare a certain recipe are measured and assembled; some pre-preparation may also be done here.

Input Errors. Errors that occur while entering data (intrinsic information) into a system that often account for the failure of information systems to produce the desired results.

Inputs. Resources brought into a system; for example, money, people, technology, and materials.

Inseparability. A characteristic of services in which a product cannot be separated from its provider.

In-Services. Educational activities that are designed to update and introduce employees to new issues or topics pertinent to their jobs and organization, or to review and refresh employees on material that is already known. They usually occur at the workplace and during work hours.

Institutional Memory. The historical precedent of an organization that can be used in the decision-making process.

Intangible. Something that cannot be held, touched, or seen—like services.

Integrate. To combine (one or more compatible systems or program modules).

Integrity. An essential leadership characteristic that is seen in a leader's reliability, fairness, and credibility to others.

Intelligence. A major leadership characteristic that includes the ability to acquire and retain knowledge, and to respond quickly and successfully to a given situation.

Interface. Connection that allows communication and interaction between two software systems.

Internal Benchmarking. The process of comparing an organization's current data on productivity with its own past records to determine how its current performance compares with past performance.

Internal Congruity. Consistency within the organization, related to managers, employees, processes, communications, philosophy, culture, and so on. It is the thread that unifies the whole.

Internal Customers. Those individuals within an organization who provide direct service to the external customers.

International Food Information Council Foundation. http://www.foodinsight.org/

Interpersonal Roles. A managerial role in which a manager acts as a figurehead, a leader, or a liaison.

Interpret. Assign meaning to the message based on personal experiences.

Interview Schedule. A list of all of the questions that will be asked of each candidate in an employment interview; the agenda for the interview.

Intranet. An organization's internal communications system, available for sharing information within the organization, but not accessible to the public.

Intrinsic Information. Information that is processed; it includes the data that are entered into the system (input) as well as the data that are produced by the system (output).

Inventory. The material and goods kept on hand.

Invoice Receiving. The receiving of goods in which the amount of material sent is included on the shipping document and the receiver verifies that the amount listed is correct.

Invoice. The bill that is issued for a product that has been delivered. It may accompany the delivery or be issued separately.

Item Name. The name of the product that is purchased; may be generic or brand specific.

Job Analysis. A detailed description of the daily duties to be carried out in a specific job, often including time frames for each job activity.

Job Description. A listing of the general duties related to a job or job classification.

Job Enlargement. The practice of increasing the tasks done within a specific job; increasing the number and types of skills workers use in their jobs.

Job Enrichment. The practice of adding variety and, simultaneously, increasing the knowledge required to do a job. Job enrichment activities should be designed to respond to each employee's unique characteristics.

Job Hot Lines. A telephone service that lists employment opportunities.

Job Mobility. The ability of an employee to change jobs. Moves can be downward, upward, or lateral within an organization, or can be a move to another organization.

Job Reengineering. The process of restructuring jobs to fit the needs of employees and to respond to the continuously changing environment, technology, and needs of society.

Job Rotation. The practice of having workers do different jobs at different times to improve job satisfaction and minimize the potential for repetitive stress injury.

Job Specification. A list of requirements for a specific job, which can be evaluated objectively and that apply to all candidates for that job.

Job-Sharing. The concept of having two employees share one full-time job.

Joint Commission on Accreditation of Healthcare Organizations. http://www.jointcommission.org/

Just-in-Time. A type of delivery that is designed to reduce inventory by having goods arrive as needed for immediate use.

Labor Budget. A prediction of the labor costs needed to get work done; does not always include the cost of benefits. It can be written as part of the expense budget or as a separate part of the operating budget.

Labor Schedule. A management tool used to designate the hours and days each employee is to work.

Landfill. A site that is designated as a dumping area for waste generated by a community.

Lateral Move. When an employee takes a new position at the same organizational level as the former position. This is sometimes done so the employee can learn new skills.

Leaders. Individuals who are considered good managers, work well with staff, and demonstrate respect, concern, and empathy for employees.

Leadership in Energy and Environmental Design. http://www.newusgbc.org/

Leading. A management function that deals with the direction, motivation, and coordination of staff and their activities.

Legal Document. A written record that is required to serve as verifiable evidence that something has occurred.

Legitimate Power. A type of power that usually differentiates the formal from the informal leader and is related to the position held by the individual who exerts the power.

Liabilities. Debts or other financial obligations of a business (for example, payroll, rent, invoices owed for goods and services recently purchased, loan or interest payments, and so on).

Lifecycle Cost Calculators. Tools that are used to determine the total cost of purchasing, operating, and maintaining a piece of equipment for its expected lifetime.

Line Managers. Managers whose reporting relationships, both upward and downward, are vertical.

Lines of Authority. The vertical relationships within an organization; chain of command.

Liquid Assets. Items, like inventory, that can easily be converted to cash. See current assets.

Listening. An active process that requires effort or attention from the listener; used to decode messages.

Listserve. An electronic mailing list that is used as a means of communication among a group of colleagues wishing to interact with one another in areas of mutual interest.

Local Area Network (LAN). A type of data communications network in which a group of computers are interconnected in a small geographic area such as adjacent buildings.

Log-on. To start a session with a system by giving a user name and password as a means of user identification and authentication.

Longevity of Documents. The length of time a specific type of written document must be kept.

Long-Term Debt. Any debt that becomes payable after a year. Includes such items as mortgages, long-term leases, and warranties on goods sold.

Long-Term Plans. The projected outcomes or strategic plans of an organization based on its mission or philosophy; usually covering a period of from three to five years. These are sometimes called outcome goals.

Make the Decision. The sixth step in the decision-making process; involves choosing which alternative(s) will best solve the problem based on the analysis that has been done.

Management. Planning, organizing, leading, and controlling the use of resources to achieve objectives.

Managers. Individuals found within organizations who can effectively manage (plan, organize, and control) finances, production, and purchasing, but may not be considered effective leaders.

Managers. People who oversee and direct the work of others.

Manual Tally. The physical counting of orders received to determine production needs.

Market Positioning. Presenting a product to the target market, emphasizing the characteristics of the product that are most important to those consumers; equating the product with its benefits.

Market Research. The gathering of information about consumers' wants, needs, and demands to identify target markets and develop the marketing mix for those markets.

Market Segmentation. The identification and measurement of those characteristics that are present in a population subgroup that is likely to purchase a specific product.

Marketing Mix. A combination of product, price, promotion, and place as they contribute to the marketing of a product.

Marketing Perspective. A view of the marketplace that considers production, sales, products, and promotion in light of the consumers' needs, wants, and demands.

Marketing. A management tool that focuses on identifying the needs, wants, and demands of customers and developing products to meet those needs.

Marketplace. The milieu in which goods are exchanged; can be viewed from the perspective of production, product, selling, marketing, or social marketing.

Mass Marketing. The marketing of a product to the population at large without discriminating among population subgroups.

Master Budget. Consists of an operating budget, a capital budget, a cash budget, and a budgeted balance sheet.

Master Schedule. A time-based written outline, usually for complex or non-routine jobs, that plans the movement of work across time and is used to follow progress and keep work on time.

Material Management. The process of controlling the acquisition and distribution of material within an organization.

Meal Equivalents. A measure of foodservice productivity defined as the amount of all food sales divided by the average cost of a meal (entrée, starch, side dish, and dessert) within the facility.

Meals. A group of foods that are usually eaten together; typically, a meal includes an entrée, a starch, a side dish, and a dessert (it may also include an appetizer and/or a salad).

The number of meals prepared is often used to quantify the productivity of cooks.

Mediation. Negotiation between two parties, using a neutral intermediary to assist in settling a dispute.

Mentor. A person whom one with less experience may consult for advice and guidance.

Merit Increase. Pay raises that are based on employee performance. These raises change the base pay rate permanently.

Message. The information that is communicated by the sender to the receiver.

Micromanagement. The act of providing intensive supervision to subordinates by constantly checking and verifying their progress.

Middle Managers. Managers whose level is above that of frontline managers, but who are subordinate to top-level managers; need technical and conceptual skills in equal amounts and good human relations skills.

Middlemen. Individuals or groups who work in the distribution channel, moving the product from the producer or manufacturer to the consumer.

Miscellaneous. Any additional information the purchaser includes for the vendor's information to ensure receiving the correct product under the right conditions.

Mission Statement. The statement of philosophy or purpose that drives an organization.

Mobile Food Vendors. Food trucks or carts that move from place to place. Originally these were used where restaurants were not located; they have recently expanded their market to other locations.

Motivation. A common trait in leaders essential to their realization of a vision or goal and part of their need to be a leader.

Multicultural Organization. An organization that values, encourages, and affirms diverse cultural modes, in which each point of view is valid and different cultures contribute to decision making.

Multiple Vendor Purchasing. Procurement of goods from several vendors; may be motivated by the desire to improve selection or the need to get the lowest price.

Multi-Skilling. The process whereby workers learn to perform new tasks and to develop techniques that, in turn, enlarge their jobs.

MyPlate. http://www.choosemyplate.gov/

National Dairy Council. http://www.nationaldairycouncil.org

National School Lunch Program. http://www.fns.usda.gov/cnd/ Lunch/ School Meals. http://www.fns.usda.gov/cnd/

Needs. Things required for a state of well-being, such as physical (food, safety, and shelter) and mental (belonging, affection, and self-expression) well-being.

Networking. An optional and informal type of communication that can be either oral or written. It includes information exchange among colleagues and peers in related fields of interest.

Newsletters. A type of optional communications document that relates useful information about or to employees.

Noise. Interference factors that can affect a message and distort it (for example, physical environment, external factors like illness, bad timing, and so on).

Nominal Group Technique. A methodical, rational approach to making a group decision in which each member contributes ideas, and alternatives are ranked to deduce a sensible, fair decision.

Nondurable Goods. Products that get used up quickly and that have a life expectancy usually measured in days or months.

Non-Programmed Decisions. Decisions that are used to resolve unstructured problems; these decisions require much research and thought.

Nutrient Analysis Program. A program that consists of a database listing of food items and nutrients. It can be used to determine the nutrient composition of foods, recipes, or diets of individuals and groups.

Nutrition Informatics. "The effective retrieval, organization, storage and optimum use of information, data, and knowledge for food and nutrition related problem solving and decision making. Informatics is supported by the use of information standards, information processes and information technology."

Occupational Safety and Health Administration. http://www.osha.gov/

Occupational Safety and Health Administration—Ergonomics Page. http://www.osha.gov/SLTC/ergonomics/ index.html

Occupied Beds. A measure hospitals use to quantify the work that they do; the number of patients who occupy a bed in the facility on a specific day for a 24-hour period. These data are often obtained by determining the number of patients who are physically present at a specific hour during the night (for example, 2 a.m.).

Odd Lot. An amount of a product that is different from how a product is typically packaged. Orders in odd lots require the vendor to open packages to deliver the specified amount.

On-Call. A position that requires the employee to be available to come to work on short notice during unscheduled hours, if needed.

Online Survey Tool. An Internet tool that allows for the administration of online surveys. Examples include SurveyMonkey, SurveyGizmo, Kwiksurveys, and others.

Onsite Foodservices. Foodservices that typically serve people who have little choice in where they eat and that are usually not profit driven (for example, healthcare facilities, schools, prisons, and so on). These are also called noncommercial foodservices.

Open Storeroom. A storage system in which any employee can obtain goods from the storeroom at any time.

Operating Budget. Budget that takes into account the revenue, expense, direct labor, direct material, and overhead budgets as well as other operating expenses. It is used in projecting the income of an organization and in allocating funds within an organization.

Operating Statement. A document prepared by the accounting department of an organization at the end of an accounting period that compares actual fiscal performance to the budget (also called a performance report).

Optional Communications Document. Any type of written document that is not considered essential to the functioning of an organization.

Organic. Products, largely food, that have been certified by the USDA as meeting the standards set by the National Organics Program. See http://www.usda.gov/wps/portal/usda/usdahome?navid= ORGANIC_CERTIFICATION.

Organization Chart. A graphic representation of an organization's structure.

Organization. A systematic arrangement of people to accomplish a specific purpose.

Organizational Culture. The "personality" of an organization.

Organizing. A management function that deals with establishing an orderly, systematic method of dealing with issues.

Orientation Checklist. A document that lists all of the items that are to be accomplished or introduced during a new employee orientation.

Orientation Packet. An information packet handed out during an orientation that may include such items as information on benefits, a map of the facility, a list of commonly used telephone numbers and Internet addresses, a copy of the organization chart, and so on.

Orientation. The process of introducing a new employee to an organization, job, and work unit.

Other Operating Expenses. Subdivision of the operating budget that encompasses all other anticipated costs of operation. Items usually included are telephone bills, copying charges, printing, office supplies, books, travel, journals, postage, fees and licenses, and so on. Organizations that do not use sub-budgets would also include the costs of labor, overhead, and material under this heading.

Outcome Measurement. A type of productivity measure that determines whether or not the product did what it was supposed to do.

Outcomes. The term used for outputs in clinical or community nutrition.

Outputs. The results that occur when inputs are transformed in a system.

Overhead. The general expenses associated with the operation of a facility that include rent, taxes, utilities, repairs, and maintenance.

Owner's Equity. The term used to describe the ownership equity of a business with only one owner.

Ownership Equity. An owner's net investment in a business after providing for full payment of all creditors; the difference between assets and liabilities. When assets are in excess of liabilities by a considerable amount, equity is said to be high. When assets and liabilities are not significantly different, equity is said to be low.

Packaging. How the message is conveyed.

Packing Slip. A shipping document used to verify the receipt of a product, which is later compared to the invoice.

Padding. The practice of ordering and producing more product than is actually needed in order to avoid shortages.

Paid Time Off (PTO). The time an employee can be absent from work with pay.

Paper Review. An initial screening of the applications to eliminate candidates who do not meet the job specifications.

Par Level. The minimum amount of a specific item that is to be kept on hand at all times. Sometimes the term par stock is also used.

Participative Leadership. A commonly used leadership style in which the leader gathers information and seeks the opinions of colleagues and/or subordinates before taking action.

Part-Time Employee. An individual who works a certain number of hours a week that is less than what is considered "full time" by the employer (usually less than 40 hours/week).

Pass-Through Refrigerators. A small cold storage unit with doors on opposite sides so that foods can be put in on one side and taken out on the other. Frequently these are built into walls, so that one side is in a kitchen and the other side is in a cafeteria.

Patient Information Systems. The management information system that is used for the processing of some patient information (patient records, orders, laboratory tests, and billing and financial information) in health care facilities.

Patient Services Manager. A managerial position responsible for managing the foodservice for patients and coordinating the patient foodservice with the clinical nutrition staff.

Patient Services Program. An information processing system used by dietetics professionals to process information related to patient meals and meal service.

Pay for Performance. Incentive-pay programs that may be used alone or in combination with other compensation plans to reward employees based on performance. These are one-time incentives that do not change the base pay rate.

Payroll Liability. Any salaries and wages that are owed to employees on the day that the balance sheet is prepared.

Percentage Forecasting. Determining how much of a specific item is needed as a percentage of the total number of items needed.

Performance Appraisal. A tool used by managers to evaluate personnel and to help employees identify their strengths as well as areas that need improvement.

Performance Specifications. Written descriptions of how a piece of equipment is required to act, including factors that relate to speed, safety, production capacity, accuracy, and so on.

Perishable Goods. Products with a very short lifespan due to a high potential for deterioration or spoilage.

Perishables. Food purchases characterized by a limited shelf life and usually requiring cold storage such as refrigeration or freezing.

Perpetual Inventory. An ongoing inventory control system that tracks the amount of material on hand by taking an initial physical inventory and adding goods that have been purchased and subtracting goods that have been distributed or used in production.

Petty Cash. Money that is kept on hand for making emergency purchases or for minor expenditures that cannot be made through regular vendors in a timely manner.

Physical Characteristics. The physical appearance and shape of an individual, which may subtly affect communication.

Physical Inventory. The process of counting each item that is in storage at a specific time to determine what product is on hand.

Place. The location where the product is available to the consumer.

Planning. A management function that involves developing mission statements, setting goals, and outlining the steps needed to meet those goals.

Point of Sale. An inventory system in which the cash register is linked to inventory control, automatically subtracting an item as it is used or sold.

Point-of-Sale (POS) Systems. Cash register computer systems that are capable of tracking individual items sold and deducting those items from inventory.

Policy and Procedure (P&P). A written standard used within an organization to describe what is to be done and how to do it. Usually policies and procedures are written for tasks that are done repeatedly and by more than one individual.

Policy Statement. The component of a P&P that states what is to be done.

Politically Correct. A designation for terminology that is non-offensive or neutral to replace words or phrases in common usage that may be disparaging, offensive, or insensitive.

Portion Control. A form of production control to regulate serving size.

Post-consumer food waste. Food waste generated after consumers have consumed their meals; also known as plate waste.

Power. The source of a leader's influence over subordinates. It may originate from the leader, from the subordinate, from the position, or from the leader's ability to dispense rewards or punishment.

Pre-consumer food waste. Food waste generated during foodservice production; generally largely plant materials.

Prepaid Expenses. Expenses that are paid for in advance, such as insurance.

Pre-Rinse Nozzle. A device that is used in foodservice dishwashing areas that sprays water on dirty dishes to remove waste that is left on the plates before they are put into the warewasher.

Press Ganey. http://www.pressganey.com/index.aspx

Price. The cost of a product to consumers; the only component in the marketing mix that concerns itself with revenue and profit.

Pricing Unit. The unit on which the price of the item is based.

Primary Data. Information gathered for the sole purpose of the party who requires the information.

Prime Vendor. The supplier that provides most of the material purchased by an organization.

Pro Bono. Professional services provided free of charge.

Probationary Employee. A newly hired employee who has not yet demonstrated that he can successfully perform the job for which he was hired. The employee is given a set period of time, often 60 or 90 days, to learn the job.

Problem Avoider. A decision-making style in which the person does not recognize a problem or chooses to avoid it; one who may make the choice not to make a decision.

Problem Identification. The first step in the decision-making process; the act of finding a problem and acknowledging that it exists.

Problem Seeker. A decision-making style in which the person is proactive and deals with potential problems before they become obvious.

Problem Solver. A decision-making style in which the person recognizes existing problems and deals with them in a timely manner.

Problem. A difference between what is and what should be.

Procedure. The step-by-step description of a P&P that states the actions to take, the order in which they should occur, and the timelines to be followed.

Process Design. The methods and procedures used to facilitate the movement of people, work, and materials through space and time.

Procurement. Purchasing, or otherwise obtaining, material for use in an organization.

Product Perspective. A view of the marketplace that focuses on the product, its value, desirable features, or performance.

Production Control. The process of monitoring production during and after it has occurred to determine if plans are being met and to make adjustments as required.

Production Meetings. Planned or scheduled times when employees and managers gather to discuss production issues. Often used for information dissemination and for problem solving.

Production Perspective. A view of the marketplace based on the idea of growing, manufacturing, or creating a product for the marketplace.

Production Schedule. A document that specifies what is produced, how much, at what time, and by whom.

Production. The process of converting inputs into products such as goods, services, or ideas.

Productivity. Measurement of the relationship between outputs or products and inputs such as time, money, labor, and raw material. Productivity may be measured quantitatively, qualitatively, or in terms of outcomes.

Professionals. Individuals who have extensive formal education in a field and have acquired the knowledge and skills to make independent judgments and to function in that field with minimum supervision.

Profit and Loss Statement (P&L). A document generated by the accounting department of an organization that lists all the actual data accumulated for the accounting period, including controllable as well as uncontrollable revenues and expenses. It also shows a business's net profits or losses.

Profit Center. Any department within an organization with an income that exceeds operating costs.

Program. The set of instructions that a computer follows when processing information. A program utilizes information from a database to transform input into output.

Programmable Decisions. Decisions that, though not yet programmed, are of the routine type that can be programmed.

Programmed Decisions. Decisions that are made routinely, often relying on precedent, where information can be transferred from one similar situation to the next; usually used to solve structured problems.

Progressive Discipline. A disciplinary process characterized by the use of more drastic penalties for each repeated instance of poor performance.

Project Teams. A type of self-managed team whose duties do not include day-to-day operational issues but, instead, a specific issue for which they are free to set deadlines and processes.

Promotion. The methods used to attract consumers to a product to convince them to purchase it.

Proprietary Information. Knowledge about an organization that must be restricted to certain individuals within the organization or to members of that organization only.

Proxemics. A component of nonverbal communication that defines the spatial relationship between the sender and the receiver of a message.

Public Health Nutritionist. A dietitian/manager in community nutrition who has an advanced degree in public health nutrition, and whose managerial roles include overseeing community nutrition agencies or programs.

Pulper. A machine that grinds solid waste, then extracts the solids so that only water is discharged into the sewer system.

Purchasing Authority. A measure of a manager's control over the procurement of material; the amount a manager is allowed to spend without obtaining permission from his or her supervisor.

Purchasing Cooperative. A group of buyers who join together for the purpose of negotiating better purchasing contracts with vendors.

Qualitative Measurement. A type of productivity measure that is concerned with the accuracy and quality of what is produced.

Quality Assurance (QA). The process of identifying and solving problems within a department or area of an organization.

Quality Control (QC). A method to determine if the products being made meet minimum standards of acceptability.

Quality. A description of the minimum acceptable characteristics of an item, which can be represented using brand names, government grades, or detailed descriptions.

Quantitative Measure. A type of productivity measure that focuses on the quantity of product produced.

Quantity. The amount of a product to be purchased, often stated in multiples that relate to how the product is typically packaged (that is, each, case, box, dozen, gallon, pound, and so on).

Quick Service Restaurants. Foodservice organizations that provide fast meals, which may be eaten on the premise or carried out. (These are also called fast-food restaurants.)

Reach-In Refrigerator. A small cold storage unit in which all contents can be reached through a door located on the front of the unit.

Reactive. A characteristic of a problem solver who acts on problems after they have become obvious.

Real Time. An accounting of what is happening as it happens.

Receiver. The person who gets the message from the sender.

Receiving. The process of accounting for material that is delivered to an organization.

Recruiting Firms. Agencies that specialize in matching qualified candidates to available jobs.

Recruitment. The process of finding qualified applicants for open positions in an organization.

Recycling. The process of converting waste materials into new products.

Reductions in Force (RIFs). A decrease in the workforce, also called layoffs. Employees may be either transferred or terminated.

Referent Power. A type of power that comes from the relationship between a leader and his or her followers and is not related to the leader's position but to the ability to create and share a vision.

Registered Dietitians (RD). A dietitian who has completed the registration eligibility requirements established by the Commission on Dietetic Registration, successfully passed the Registration Examination for Dietitians, and meets continuing education requirements.

Reorder Point. The inventory level that is set for an item that triggers the placement of an order for more of that item so that the stock on hand does not fall below the par level.

Repetitive Stress Injury. Physical harm resulting from the strain of repeatedly doing the same task in the same way.

Replacements. Products that are purchased to replace items that have been lost, broken, stolen, or worn out with use.

Retail. A type of supplier, usually not covered by a purchasing agreement, which offers materials to the general public at higher prices than those charged by wholesale vendors. Sometimes used by organizations for last-minute or emergency purchases.

Retailers. An organization or individual who sells products directly to the end user of the product.

Revenue Budget. The projection of the income of an organization or a department based on the sale of products. It is a part of the operating budget.

Revenue Center. Any department within an organization that generates an income.

Reward Power. A type of power that is based on the ability to reward employees in terms of material goods (for example, pay raise or privileged parking) or praise (for example, public acknowledgment).

Risk Management. That type of management concerned with minimizing the liability of an organization in areas such as work-related illness, job-induced injury or stress, and products whose performance fails to meet set standards.

Risk. The unknown or uncertain factors or outcomes involved in making a decision.

Safe. A place or container used to secure valuables from theft.

Salaried Worker. An employee who has a set (usually annual) salary and who is expected to work until the job is completed.

Scope. An optional component of the policy section of a P&P that lists the individuals or groups impacted by the policy.

Seafood Watch. www.montereybayaquarium.org/cr/seafood-watch.aspx

Search Committees. A group of personnel who form a team to screen and interview candidates for some upper-management, administrative, and academic positions.

Search Engines. An Internet tool that allows you to do keyword searches for information. Examples include Google, Yahoo!, Lycos, Ask, Metacrawler, and others.

Secondary Data. Information that has already been compiled by another source.

Self-Confidence. A major leadership trait that involves having enough confidence and security in one's self to make decisions, take risks, and admit to making mistakes.

Self-Managed Teams. Work groups that function without a designated manager and involve the team members in decision making and in working together to manage themselves.

Self-Operated Foodservices. A foodservice in which the organization that receives the service owns and operates the foodservice.

Selling Perspective. A view of the marketplace based on getting customers to purchase the product.

Semi-Structured Interview. A type of interview that takes on a conversational tone but is somewhat organized by an outline of topics to be covered and an idea of how questions will be asked.

Sender. The person who creates and transmits a message to another person or people.

Service Perishability. A characteristic of services that implies that a service cannot be stored and used later; the service must be utilized upon delivery.

Serviceware. Dishes and flatware used for serving food.

ServSafe.

Setting. The physical environment in which communication takes place.

Shelf Life. The amount of time groceries can be used until they expire; indicated by a "use by" date.

Short-Hour Employee. An individual who works a predetermined number of hours a week that is less than half time (typically less than 20 hours a week).

Short-Term Plans. The interim plans of an organization geared toward fulfilling long-term goals; usually projected in days, weeks, or months. These are sometimes called process goals.

Sick Time. Paid time off to be used for illness or injury.

Single Rate. Pay raises that are universal and given to all employees either on an anniversary date or on an annual basis. It rewards employees equally, as long as their work falls within the standard range. This pay increase results in a permanent adjustment in the base pay rate.

Single-Use Menu. A menu that is designed to be used only once.

Skilled Worker. An individual who has special training or skills to perform a specific job (for example, cooks, secretaries, exterminators).

Small Equipment. Reusable equipment that costs more than supplies and has a longer life expectancy.

Social Marketing Perspective. A view of the marketplace that balances the needs, wants, and demands of consumers with those of the organization and those of society.

Social Security Administration. http://socialsecurity.gov/

Social Security. http://www.ssa.gov/

Span of Control. A measure of the influence a manager has on an organization; usually measured by the number of people who report to the manager.

Specialization. The process of acquiring in-depth knowledge and skills in a narrow area of a profession.

Specifications. Written descriptions of the material to be purchased, including item name, form, quantity, quality, and pricing unit.

Spreadsheet. A tool that allows input of numerical data into rows and columns for computation and analysis.

Staff Managers. Managers who oversee supportive departments or groups; they report laterally, not vertically.

Staffing. The determination of the type and number of employees that are needed to carry out the work of an organization.

Standardization. To make common or compatible.

Standardized Recipe. A production control that gives a known quantity of known quality ingredients to establish amounts needed to continuously reproduce the same high-quality product.

Statement of Purpose. Part of a P&P that explains rationale for a policy and may include how the policy relates to an organization's philosophy.

Static Menu. A menu that is used from day to day; it usually has a wide range of items from which the customer can choose.

Stock Rotation. The method used to move stock so that goods do not expire and older goods are used before newer ones.

Stockholders' Equity. The term used to describe the ownership equity of a corporation for which there is more than one owner.

Storage Area. A designated space used to hold and secure raw material until it is needed for production.

Strategic Plans. Global plans that set the direction for the organization within the context of its internal and external environments.

Structured Interview. An interview that follows a predetermined agenda.

Structured Problems. A discrepancy between what is and what should be that is both routine and predictable.

Subjective Forecasting. A forecasting method that uses information, experience, and intuition to determine the amount of product needed.

Succession Planning. A staffing strategy that anticipates what jobs will open due to retirements and promotions, and prepares other individuals to be eligible to move into these positions.

Supervisors. Individuals with authority to oversee and direct the work of subordinates as well as having responsibility for their own work.

Supplementary Channel. A secondary pathway used to transmit a message in another way to reinforce the message.

Supplies. Products characterized by having no finite shelf life.

Suspension. The third step in the employee disciplinary process, in which the employee is given time off, usually without pay, to demonstrate the seriousness of the problem.

Sustainability. Meeting "the needs of the present without compromising the ability of future generations to meet their own needs."

System Constraints. Limitations that are innate in a system, in light of the particular application in which the system is being used. Examples include speed, size of data-base, user-friendliness, reliability, format of output reports, and so on.

Tangible. Something that can be seen, touched, and felt.

Target Marketing. The marketing of a product to a unique subgroup within the population rather than to the population at large.

Task Analysis. The process of observing, in detail, each aspect of a job to determine if increases in efficiency or safety can be achieved.

Technical Skills. Managerial skills related to the production work of the organization.

Technical Specifications. Written descriptions for capital goods or other products that specify functions that can be determined by an objective test or measurement; includes such factors as type of material, dimensions, and weights.

Telecommuting. To access the intranet of an organization from a remote computer.

Temporary Workers. Employees who are hired for a finite period of time, as for a project, to cover a leave of absence, or when there is a transient need for more employees.

Termination. The final action in the employee disciplinary process, which leads to the end of employment and results after repeated failure of the employee to correct the problem.

The "Virtual" Nutrition Center. http://www.martindalecenter.com/Nutrition.html

Tickler File. A method of reminding oneself of "loose ends" that need follow-up. Often used for tracking procurement discrepancies such as back orders, cancellations, and shortages to ensure smooth production and proper payment, and to document vendor performance.

Timing of the Deliveries. The time of day deliveries should arrive; should correspond with production needs and the receiving personnel's schedule to ensure a smooth delivery and proper storage of goods.

Timing. A strategy for when communication will take place in relation to the present situation and the kind of message relayed.

Top-Level Managers. Managers who direct the activities of large segments of an organization rather than the actual production; need a high level of conceptual skills, good human relations skills, and some technical skills.

Total Quality Management (TQM). The application of quality management processes throughout the organization. This includes working on problems and strengthening areas that cross departmental lines.

Touching Behavior. A characteristic of nonverbal communication that describes the extent and ways an individual extends physical contact to others and the kind of message that contact transmits.

Transformation. The production or work of an organization that changes inputs into outputs.

Transformational Leadership. A leadership style that transforms employees who merely carry out their duties to employees who feel comfortable in contributing their input to the management process.

Transforming Leadership. A leadership style that prepares the subordinate to take over management functions and, in some cases, to become the successor to the manager.

Transgenic Plants. Plants that have been created by transplanting a gene from a different species.

Transmit. Send a message to one or more people (for example, in person, in print, or by using technologies like faxes, modems, phones, and so on).

Trayline. An assembly line for patient trays in some healthcare foodservices.

U.S. Department of Agriculture. http://www.usda.gov/wps/portal/usda/usdahome

U.S. Dept. of Labor. http://www.dol.gov/

U.S. Equal Employment Opportunity Commission. http://www.eeoc.gov/

Uncertainty. A situation in which the outcomes of a decision cannot be predicted with any degree of accuracy.

Unearned Revenue. Liability incurred from the advanced payments for products that have not yet been delivered.

Unskilled Workers. Employees who bring no marketable skills to the job and are trained in the workplace to perform the required tasks (for example, receptionists, cashiers, foodservice workers).

Unstructured Interview. An interview that resembles an informal conversation.

Unstructured Problems. A discrepancy between what is and what should be that is new, unusual, and often unpredictable.

Upgrade. To replace with a newer or better version of hardware or software.

Upward Mobility. When an employee is promoted to a higher position in an organization.

Use-by Date. The expiration date on a product, which indicates the last date the product should be used.

User Manuals. Online publications made available to employees in an organization for the purpose of communicating to them such information about how to operate and use equipment, programs, and information systems.

Vacation Time. Paid time off from work designated for leisure activities or rest.

Variability. A characteristic of services that indicates that services are not uniform, due to factors such as the provider of the service, the consumer, and the circumstances under which the service takes place.

Variable Budget. Budget plan for which expenses will vary in response to actual production, volume, or revenues. It is also referred to as flexible budget and can be used in conjunction with either the zero-based budget or the incremental budget.

Variable Pay. A compensation plan in which an employee receives a base salary or hourly wage and then an added bonus based on performance.

Variance Analysis. A statement prepared by managers to account for any deviation from the budget.

Verbal Warning. The first step in employee discipline, which includes identification of the problem and information sharing between the manager and the employee.

Walk-In Refrigerators. A type of cold storage that is large enough for people to enter.

Wants. Socially accepted ways to meet needs.

Warehouse Club Buying. An informal type of purchasing that is characterized by self-service; buying is usually cost-effective for small operations.

Websites. An Internet-based medium that uses electronic, written communication to convey information to many people.

Weight the Decision-Making Criteria. The third step in the decision-making process; assigning each established criterion a ranking in terms of importance to the decision that is to be made.

Wholesaler. An organization or person who buys products from the grower or producer and sells them to the retailer who, in turn, sells the products to the end user.

Without Cause. The case in which a probationary employee may be dismissed for whatever reason the manager feels is appropriate.

Word of Mouth. An informal method of information exchange that relies on verbal communication between individuals.

Work Simplification. The process of changing how a job is performed to decrease the energy expenditure and increase the output of a worker.

Worker. A person who does the work of the organization or produces the product.

Workflow. The way in which people and products move through a workplace.

Written Communication. A type of communication that uses written words to convey the message, either in hard copy or electronic format.

Written Warning. The second, more formal step in employee discipline, which includes stating the problem and noting repetition over time. Information sharing between the manager and the employee is also part of this step.

Yield. The amount of a product available for consumption from a specified quantity of ingredients after adjusting for losses that occur during production and service.

Zero-Based Budget. A type of operating budget that is based on estimated need for the coming year, without relying on last year's budget as a starting point. It requires managers to write budgets from scratch and to justify every dollar of proposed spending.

CPSIA information can be obtained at www.ICGtesting.com
Printed in the USA
LVOW02s0416160514

386053LV00001B/2/P